INTRAVENOUS IMMUNOGLOBULINS IN CLINICAL PRACTICE

COMPLIMENTS OF

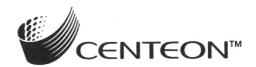
CENTEON™

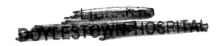

INTRAVENOUS IMMUNOGLOBULINS IN CLINICAL PRACTICE

EDITED BY

MARTIN L. LEE
School of Public Health
University of California
Los Angeles, California

VIBEKE STRAND
Stanford University
San Francisco, California

MARCEL DEKKER, INC.   NEW YORK · BASEL · HONG KONG

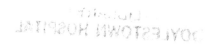

Library of Congress Cataloging-in-Publication Data

Intravenous immunoglobulins in clinical practice / edited by Martin L. Lee, Vibeke Strand.
    p. cm.
   Includes index.
   ISBN 0-8247-9881-3 (hardcover : alk. paper)
   1. Immunoglobulins—Therapeutic use. 2. Intravenous therapy. I. Lee, Martin L. II Strand,
Vibeke.
   [DNLM: 1. Immunoglobulins, Intravenous—therapeutic use. QW 601 I616 1997]
RM282.I44I586 1997
615'.37—dc21
DNLM/DLC
for Library of Congress
                                        97-25515
                                           CIP

The publisher offers discounts on this book when ordered in bulk quantities. For more information, write to Special Sales/Professional Marketing at the address below.

This book is printed on acid-free paper.

MARCEL DEKKER, INC.
270 Madison Avenue, New York, New York 10016
http://www.dekker.com

Current printing (last digit):
10 9 8 7 6 5 4 3 2

PRINTED IN THE UNITED STATES OF AMERICA

Preface

In the 1940s Cohn and colleagues developed a relatively straightforward chemical process for fractionating human blood into many of its significant component proteins, thus enabling the production of the first immunoglobulin concentrates (although suitable for intramuscular use only). In the following decade, Bruton and others recognized the genetic basis of various types of primary immunodeficiency syndromes and further characterized them. These two discoveries allowed for the regular treatment of patients using replacement infusions of human immunoglobulins and the concomitant improvement in quality of life and, ultimately, survival. Subsequently, specific immunoglobulin preparations were produced for treatment of or prophylaxis against specific pathogens such as hepatitis B, polio, tetanus, and pertussis. All of these so-called hyperimmune globulins were administered by the intramuscular route.

It became quite clear that this means of administration was not adequate for both the provider and the patient. Injections were quite painful; doses were limited in size and frequency; muscle proteases degraded much of the infused immune globulins; and the remaining protein reached the circulation only after significant delay. Attempts to inject material directly into the vasculature proved to be dangerous, and occasionally catastrophic, apparently as a result of the IgG aggregates that formed as part of the fractionation process. Subsequent developments employing first partial enzyme digestion (using proteases such as pepsin and papain) and then improvements in the fractionation process allowed for the ultimate production of true intravenous immunoglobulin (IVIG) concentrates.

Since the late 1970s when these concentrates became widely available, their use has grown exponentially. The serendipitous discovery by Imbach, Barandun, and colleagues in 1980 that IVIG could reverse the autoimmune thrombocytopenia in a young patient with severe chronic ITP and secondary hypogammaglobulinemia opened another avenue of applications: the treatment of autoimmune diseases.

Our goal in compiling this volume was to summarize critically the large array of clinical literature available on the use of IVIG preparations. Indeed, a review of MEDLINE citations since 1980 showed more than 1800 entries. Much of the work over the past several years has involved controlled clinical trials, putting research in this area on a firm, scientific footing. This is the focus of our book.

In recent years, studies have shown that IVIG may be useful in treating various primary and secondary immunodeficiencies. With regard to the latter, successful trials have been conducted in AIDS patients, premature neonates, individuals with multiple myeloma and chronic lymphocytic leukemia, bone marrow and liver transplantees, patients after high-risk (for infection) abdominal surgeries, and thermal burn victims.

A vast literature has also developed on the prophylaxis and treatment of numerous autoimmune diseases. Although the mechanisms of action of IVIG are incompletely understood, the range of successful applications is remarkable. Nonetheless, the number of large-scale controlled studies in this area remains small. This is changing, particularly with the recent publication by van der Meché and colleagues of a successful trial of IVIG in the treatment of acute Guillain-Barré syndrome.

In this book, many of the leading authorities on clinical applications of IVIG in their respective fields of medical research discuss work done to date. We sincerely believe that the reviews contained herein are comprehensive, but recognize the explosive growth of this literature. This volume will serve as a good overview for both clinician and researcher wishing to survey current information available on the clinical use of IVIG.

We are grateful to so many people for their invaluable assistance and support with this project. We want to offer our sincere gratitude to the contributors to this book. Their efforts clearly demonstrated a commitment to furthering knowledge about this important therapeutic agent.

We also wish to express our appreciation to Ms. Shirley Sutjiadi for providing invaluable administrative assistance in organizing this volume, and Dr. Ed Gomperts and Dr. Gordon Bray for providing many of the resources needed to complete our effort.

And, of course, we owe our families a large debt of gratitude. M. L. would like to thank his wife, Marilyn, and his two sons, Eliot and Danny, for their love and support. V. S. appreciates all the encouragement and understanding her husband, Jack, provided.

Martin L. Lee
Vibeke Strand

Contents

Preface   *iii*
Contributors   *ix*

I. Overview

  1. Pharmacokinetics of Intravenous Immunoglobulin Preparations   1
    Andreas Morell

  2. Pharmacoeconomics of Intravenous Immunoglobulin   19
    Martin L. Lee and Vibeke Strand

  3. Proposed Mechanisms for the Efficacy of Intravenous
    Immunoglobulin Treatment   23
    Vibeke Strand

  4. Production and Properties of Intravenous Immunogloblins   37
    John A. Hooper

  5. Nonviral Side Effects of Intravenous Immunoglobulins   57
    Mario Dicato, C. Duhem, and F. Ries

  6. Viral Safety of IVIG   67
    Peng Lee Yap

  7. Alternative Methods for the Administration of Intravenous
    Immunoglobulins   107
    Martin L. Lee

II. Infectious Disease Applications

  8. IVIG in Bone Marrow Transplantation   113
    Maurice J. Wolin and Robert Peter Gale

  9. Use of Intravenous Immunoglobulins for the Prevention and
    Treatment of Viral Infections in Solid Organ Transplantation   119
    Jeffrey A. DesJardin and David R. Snydman

10. Intravenous Immunoglobulin Use in the Newborn Infant:
    Treatment and Prevention of Infection   135
    Rajam S. Ramamurthy

11. Use of Intravenous Immunoglobulins in High-Risk Surgical
    Procedures and in Posttrauma Patients   151
    Giorgio Zanetti and Michel-Pierre Glauser

12. Intravenous Gammaglobulin Regimen for HIV-Infected Children:
    Infection Prophylaxis and Immunomodulation   159
    Arye Rubinstein

13. Use of Intravenous Immune Globulin in Adults with HIV Disease   167
    David J. Rechtman

14. Treatment of Primary Immunodeficiency Diseases with
    Gammaglobulin   175
    Richard I. Schiff

15. Intravenous Immunoglobulin Treatment for IgG Subclass
    Deficiency   193
    Thomas F. Smith

16. Prevention of Infections in B-Cell Lymphoproliferative Diseases 203
    Helen Griffiths and Helen Chapel

17. Etiology and Prevention of Infection Following Thermal Injury   225
    Khan Z. Shirani, George M. Vaughan, Albert T. McManus,
    Arthur D. Mason, Jr., and Basil A. Pruitt, Jr.

18. Prevention and Treatment of Viral Infection   243
    Martha M. Eibl and Hermann M. Wolf

19. Intravenous Immunoglobulin Therapy of Neonates with Nonpolio
    Enteroviral Infections   257
    Harry L. Keyserling

20. Treatment of Chronic Fatigue Syndrome   267
    Andrew R. Lloyd and Denis Wakefield

III. Autoimmune Disease Applications: Pediatric

21. Intravenous Gammaglobulin Therapy for Autoimmune
    Thrombocytopenic Purpura, Neutropenia, and Hemolytic Anemia   275
    James B. Bussel

22. Use of IVIG in Kawasaki Syndrome 293
Marian E. Melish

23. Juvenile Rheumatoid Arthritis 309
Thomas A. Griffin and Edward H. Giannini

24. Intravenously Administered Gammaglobulin for the Prevention
or Modulation of Insulin-Dependent Diabetes Mellitus 317
John M Dwyer and Stephen Colagiuri

IV. Autoimmune Disease Applications: Adult

25. Advances in the Treatment of Alloimmune-Mediated Platelet
Disorders with Intravenous Immunoglobulin 327
Thomas S. Kickler

26. Guillain-Barré Syndrome 337
Frans G. A. van der Meché and Pieter A. van Doorn

27. Chronic Inflammatory Demyelinating Polyneuropathy 349
Pieter A. van Doorn and Frans G. A. van der Meché

28. Intravenous Immunoglobulin in the Management of Myasthenia
Gravis 363
David Grob

29. Multiple Sclerosis 381
Anat Achiron

30. Polymyositis/Dermatomyositis 399
Lori B. Tucker and Earl D. Silverman

31. Use of Intravenous Immunoglobulin in Therapy of Rheumatoid
Arthritis 409
David E. Yocum

32. Treatment of Systemic Lupus Erythematosus with Pooled Human
Intravenous Immunoglobulin 415
Stanley C. Jordan

33. Intravenous Immunoglobulin Therapy of Systemic Necrotizing
Vasculitis 425
Leonard H. Calabrese

34. Lambert-Eaton Myasthenic Syndrome 431
John Newsom-Davis

35. Intravenous Gammaglobulin in the Treatment of Recurrent
     Pregnancy Loss   439
     Ann L. Parke

36. Intravenous Immunoglobulin and Other Autoimmune Diseases   447
     Martin L. Lee

37. Intravenous Immunoglobulin Therapy in Idiopathic Inflammatory
     Bowel Diseases   451
     Douglas S. Levine

V. Hyperimmunoglobulins

38. Development of Hyperimmune Immunoglobulins   467
     William J. Landsperger and Roger Lundblad

     Index   *503*

Contributors

Anat Achiron, MD., Ph.D. Director, Multiple Sclerosis Center, Sheba Medical Center, Tel-Hashomer, Israel

James B. Bussel, M.D. Associate Professor, Department of Pediatrics, Division of Hematology/Oncology, The New York Hospital–Cornell Medical Center, New York, New York

Leonard H. Calabrese, D.O. Vice Chairman and Head of Clinical Immunology, Department of Rheumatic and Immunologic Disease, Cleveland Clinic Foundation, Cleveland, Ohio

Helen Chapel, M.D., M.R.C.P., F.R.C.Path. Consultant Immunologist and Senior Clinical Lecturer, Department of Immunology, Oxford Radcliffe Hospital, Oxford, England

Stephen Colagiuri, M.D. The University of New South Wales, Sydney, Australia

Mario Dicato, M.D. Central Hospital of Luxembourg, Luxembourg, Belgium

Jeffrey A. DesJardin, M.D. Department of Geographic Medicine and Infectious Diseases, New England Medical Center and Tufts University School of Medicine, Boston, Massachusetts

C. Duhem, M.D. Central Hospital of Luxembourg, Luxembourg, Belgium

John M Dwyer, M.D., B.S., F.R.A.C.P., Ph.D. Professor, Department of Medicine, The University of New South Wales, Sydney, Australia

Martha M. Eibl, M.D. Professor, Institute of Immunology, University of Vienna, Vienna, Austria

Robert Peter Gale, M.D., Ph.D., F.A.C.P. Corporate Director, Blood Cell and Bone Marrow Transplantation, Salick Health Care, Inc., Los Angeles, California

Edward H. Giannini, M.Sc. Dr. P.H. Professor, William S. Rowe Division of Rheumatology, Department of Pediatrics, Children's Hospital Medical Center, University of Cincinnati College of Medicine, Cincinnati, Ohio

Michel-Pierre Glauser, M.D. Professor, Division of Infectious Diseases, Department of Medicine, University Hospital, Lausanne, Switzerland

Thomas A. Griffin, M.D., Ph.D. William S. Rowe Division of Rheumatology, Children's Hospital Medical Center, University of Cincinnati College of Medicine, Cincinnati, Ohio

Helen Griffiths, M.D., F.R.C.Path. Associate Specialist, Department of Immunology, Oxford Radcliffe Hospital, Oxford, England

David Grob, M.D. Director Emeritus, Department of Medicine, Maimonides Medical Center, and Professor, State University of New York Health Science Center, Brooklyn, New York

John A. Hooper, Ph.D. President, BioCatalyst Consultants, Liberty, Missouri

Stanley C. Jordan, M.D. Director, Transplant Immunology, Department of Pediatrics, Cedars-Sinai Medical Center, Los Angeles, California

Harry L. Keyserling, M.D. Associate Professor, Department of Pediatrics, Emory University School of Medicine, Atlanta, Georgia

Thomas S. Kickler, M.D. Professor of Pathology, Medicine, and Oncology, Johns Hopkins University School of Medicine, Baltimore, Maryland

William J. Landsperger, Ph.D. Senior Research Scientist, Department of Science and Technology, Hyland Division Research and Development, Baxter Healthcare Corporation, Duarte, California

Martin L. Lee, Ph.D., C.Stat. Lecturer, School of Public Health, University of California, Los Angeles, California.

Douglas S. Levine, M.D. Associate Professor, Department of Medicine, University of Washington, Seattle, Washington

Andrew R. Lloyd, M.B.B.S, M.D., F.R.A.C.P. Associate Professor, Department of Infectious Diseases, Prince Henry Hospital, Sydney, Australia.

Roger Lundblad, Ph.D. Department of Science and Technology, Hyland Division Research and Development, Baxter Healthcare Corporation, Duarte, California

Arthur D. Mason, Jr., M.D. U.S. Army Institute of Surgical Research, Fort Sam Houston, Texas

Albert T. McManus, Ph.D. Acting Chief, Laboratory Division, U.S. Army Institute of Surgical Research, Fort Sam Houston, Texas

Marian E. Melish, M.D. University of Hawaii and Kapiolani Medical Center for Women and Children, Honolulu, Hawaii

Andreas Morell, M.D. Chief Medical Officer, ZLB Central Laboratory, Blood Transfusion Service, Swiss Red Cross, Bern, Switzerland

John Newsom-Davis, M.A., M.D., F.R.C.P., F.R.A. Professor, Department of Clinical Neurology, University of Oxford, Oxford, England

Ann L. Parke, M.D. Professor, Department of Medicine, University of Connecticut Health Center, Farmington, Connecticut

Basil A. Pruitt, Jr., M.D., F.A.C.S. Clinical Professor, Department of Surgery, University of Texas Health Science Center, San Antonio, Texas

Rajam S. Ramamurthy, M.D. Professor, Department of Pediatrics, Division of Neonatology, University of Texas Health Science Center, San Antonio, Texas

David J. Rechtman, M.D. President, PharmaMedical Consultants International, Missoula, Montana

F. Ries, M.D. Central Hospital of Luxembourg, Luxembourg, Belgium

Arye Rubinstein, M.D. Professor of Pediatrics, Mibrobiology, and Immunology, Department of Pediatrics, Albert Einstein College of Medicine, Bronx, New York

Richard I. Schiff, M.D., Ph.D. Director, Clinical Immunology, Miami Children's Hospital, Miami, Florida

Khan Z. Shirani, M.D., Col mc. Chief, Clinical Division, U.S. Army Institute of Surgical Research, Fort Sam Houston, Texas

Earl D. Silverman, M.D., F.R.C.P. (C) Associate Professor of Pediatrics and Immunology, Department of Pediatric Rheumatology, The Hospital for Sick Children, University of Toronto, Toronto, Ontario, Canada

Thomas F. Smith, M.D. Professor, Department of Pediatrics, Washington University School of Medicine, St. Louis Children's Hospital, St. Louis, Missouri

David R. Snydman, M.D. Director, Clinical Microbiology, New England Medical Center, and Professor of Medicine and Pathology, Tufts University School of Medicine, Boston, Massachusetts.

Vibeke Strand, M.D. Clinical Associate Professor of Medicine, Division of Immunology, Stanford University, San Francisco, California

Lori B. Tucker, M.D.   Assistant Professor of Pediatrics, Division of Pediatric Rheumatology, New England Medical Center, Boston, Massachusetts

Frans G.A. van der Meché, M.D., Ph.D.   Professor, Department of Neurology, University Hospital Rotterdam, Rotterdam, The Netherlands

Pieter A. van Doorn, M.D., Ph.D.   Department of Neurology, University Hospital Rotterdam, Rotterdam, The Netherlands

George M. Vaughan, M.D., Col mc.   Chief, Internal Medicine Branch, U.S. Army Institute of Surgical Research, Fort Sam Houston, Texas

Denis Wakefield, M.D.   Department of Immunology, Prince Henry Hospital, Sydney, Australia

Hermann M. Wolf, M.D.   Institute of Immunology, University of Vienna, Vienna, Austria

Maurice J. Wolin, M.D.   Medical Director, Chiron Therapeutics, Emeryville, California

Peng Lee Yap, B.Sc., M.B.Ch.B., Ph.D., F.R.C.Path., F.R.C.P.E.   Consultant in Blood Transfusion and Immunology, Edinburgh & S.E. Scotland Blood Transfusion Service, Edinburgh, Scotland

David E. Yocum, M.D.   Director, Arizona Arthritis Center, Arizona Health Sciences Center, University of Arizona, Tucson, Arizona

Giorgio Zanetti, M.D.   Division of Infectious Diseases, Department of Internal Medicine, University Hospital, Lausanne, Switzerland

1

Pharmacokinetics of Intravenous Immunoglobulin Preparations

Andreas Morell
ZLB Central Laboratory, Blood Transfusion Service, Swiss Red Cross, Bern, Switzerland

INTRODUCTION

Much of our current understanding of the pharmacokinetics of IgG has emerged from research in the late 1960s which was mainly devoted to the assessment of normal metabolic properties of IgG in humans (1). These early studies were done with IgG isolated from human plasma, which was radiolabeled with iodine isotopes, and given intravenously as tracer doses. Later, pharmacokinetic studies were performed with commercial IVIG preparations in order to characterize their intact or modified IgG molecules. Basically, three approaches can be used to generate pharmacokinetic data of IVIG preparations:

1.   In the 1970s, some studies were done with radiolabeled IgG of IVIG preparations. Today, this approach is no longer feasible, mainly for ethical considerations.

2.   Pharmacokinetics of most IVIG preparations were obtained by analysis of the plasma disappearance curves after infusion in patients with congenital humoral immunodeficiencies.

3.   A more sophisticated approach consisted in the analysis of the plasma disappearance of specific IgG antibodies present in the infused IVIG but not produced by the subjects participating in the study. In normal individuals, pharmacokinetics obtained by this method may be closest to a hypothetical "true" in vivo behavior of IVIG.

The purpose of this article is to review available information on the pharmacokinetics of commercial IVIG preparations in immunologically normal subjects and in patients.

ANALYSIS OF PHARMACOKINETIC DATA

Tracer studies with radioiodinated plasma proteins indicated that their catabolism followed multicompartmental first-order kinetics (1). According to Nosslin, the protein is distributed in an intravascular pool and in one or more extravascular pools (2). After equilibration between intravascular and extravascular body compartments, the labeled protein is eliminated from the plasma at a constant rate, as illustrated in Figure 1 by a

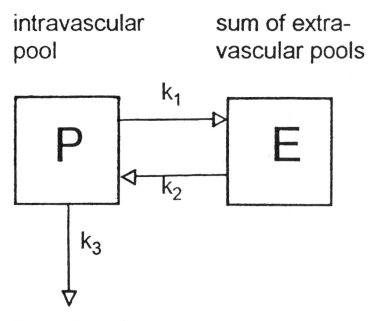

Figure 1 Two-compartment model consisting of an intravascular plasma pool (P) and an extravascular pool (E) representing the sum of all extravascular pools. The exchange flow between pools have rate constants K_1 and K_2. The catabolic rate constant is designated as K_3 (see Refs. 1,2).

hypothetical two-compartment model consisting of a plasma pool and a sum of several extravascular pools.

Most methods for data analysis were derived from the plasma radioactivity curve and were based on the general assumptions that synthesis and catabolism took place in a compartment in close contact with the intravascular space, that the study subjects were in steady state concerning IgG metabolism, and that metabolism of the labeled protein was identical with that of the native unlabeled protein (1). Figure 2a shows a semilogarithmic plot of the time-dependent decline of ^{125}I-labeled IgG representing the disappearance of the tracer from the plasma in a normal subject. Graphical or mathematical methods allow estimations of the distribution in intra- and extravascular pools, of the fraction that is catabolized daily (fractional catabolic rate, FCR) and of the half-life ($T_{1/2}$). If plasma IgG concentrations and the plasma volume are known, total circulating and total body IgG pools as well as the rate of daily IgG synthesis can be determined. Table 1 summarizes the normal values for IgG and IgG subclass metabolism in humans which were obtained in tracer studies under steady-state conditions (3,4).

Pharmacokinetic models for the analysis of IVIG preparations follow the same rules. Figure 2b shows an idealized IgG plasma disappearance curve in an agammaglobulinemic patient after IVIG infusion, where logarithms of plasma IgG concentrations are plotted against the post infusion time. Identical graphs are obtained if values on the ordinate are expressed as units of antibodies, as fractions of the infused IVIG, or as percentage of the peak IgG or antibody concentrations. From these experimental curves, pharmacokinetic parameters are calculated using mathematical models or by graphical analysis of the curves (5,6).

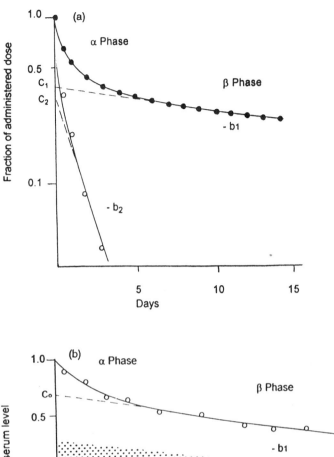

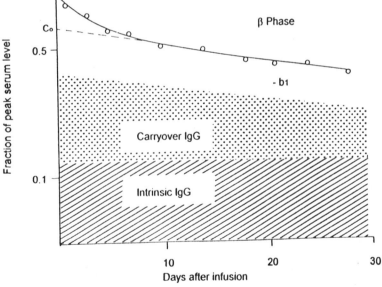

Figure 2 Idealized semilogarithmic plots of plasma disappearance curves. (a) Time-dependent decline of ^{125}I-labeled IgG in a normal person (tracer study). The solid circles represent measured values expressed as fraction of the injected dose. The α phase is further subdivided by "curve peeling," as indicated by open circles. The β phase is characterized by the slope $-b_1$. Slopes, extrapolations, and intercepts are explained in the text (see Ref. 1). (b) Time-dependent disappearance of infused IgG in a patient with congenital humoral immunodeficiency after IVIG infusion. Open circles represent IgG plasma concentrations expressed as a fraction of peak levels. Extrapolation of the final slope $-b_1$ to the ordinate and intercept C_0 are explained in the text. Both the α and β phases may be influenced by intrinsic IgG synthesis of the patient and by extrinsic carryover IgG from previous IVIG infusions (see Refs. 5,24).

Table 1 Pharmacokinetics of Normal IgG in Normal Individuals (mean values ± 1 SD)

	Total IgG	IgG1	IgG2	IgG3	IgG4
Half-life (days)	23 ± 4	21 ± 5	20 ± 2	7 ± 1	21 ± 3
Fraction (%) of intravascular pool catabolized daily (FCR)	7 ± 2	8 ± 2	7 ± 0.3	17 ± 1	7 ± 1
Distribution (% intravascular)	45 ± 5				
Pool sizes (g/kg)					
intravascular pool	0.49 ± 0.12				
total body pool	1.09 ± 0.26				
Synthetic rate (mg/kg/day)	34 ± 11				

Sources: IgG data were derived from Waldmann and Terry (3); IgG subclass data from Ref. 4.

In both parts of Figure 2, the initial phase (α phase) of the curves is characterized by a rapid decline of the infused material in the plasma. This decrease of the tracer or of the administered IVIG is rather complex and corresponds to the combined influences of distribution in the body and catabolism. After approximately 5–7 days this phase is followed by the final phase (β phase), which is a straight line in the semilogarithmic plot with a slope designated $-b_1$. Extrapolation of this line to the ordinate determines an intercept C_1 (Fig. 2a). By subtracting the extrapolated line from the original curve ("curve peeling"), the α phase can be characterized by a new curve with a slope $-b_2$ and an intercept C_2. As a result, the original plasma curve is described by the sum of two exponentials:

$$C = C_1 \cdot e^{-b_1 t} + C_2 \cdot e^{-b_2 t}$$

where C is the concentration of IVIG in the plasma, C_1 and C_2 are the intercepts, and $-b_1$ and $-b_2$ are the slopes of the two phases. Sometimes, the α phase can be further resolved by "curve peeling," and a third exponential is obtained. However, in many studies the experimental data do not allow a resolution of the plasma curve, and pharmacokinetic calculations are based on the β phase:

$$C = C_0 \cdot e^{-kt}$$

where the intercept C_0 represents the IVIG concentration in the plasma if the distribution had been instantaneous, and k is the slope of the β phase, designated as elimination constant (Fig. 2b). The half-life ($T_{1/2}$), defined as the time required for half of the IVIG to be catabolized, is proportional to the elimination constant k.

$$T_{1/2} = \frac{\ln 2}{k} = \frac{0.693}{k}$$

It should be noted that the elimination constant obtained by this method gives the catabolic rate as a fraction of the whole body, whereas if the α phase is included in the calculations, the resulting elimination constant describes the fractional catabolic rate as the fraction of the intravascular pool that is catabolized daily (1).

In general, kinetics of the initial α phase are important, if IVIG is considered for treatment of acute infections, since IgG and antibody levels reached in the first few hours or days after infusion may be critical. However, data on this phase are scarce. On the other hand, kinetics of the terminal β phase used for $T_{1/2}$ calculations are decisive when a prolonged replacement therapy is envisaged, as in patients with agammaglobulinemia. In fact, the $T_{1/2}$ was determined for all IVIG preparations. Other pharmacokinetic parameters known for some IVIGs are the volume of distribution in the body and the total clearance—i.e., the volume of plasma cleared of IVIG per unit of time. Clearance data are considered helpful since they characterize the catabolic rate of IVIG and are independent of metabolic mechanisms and compartmental distribution (5). However, since different mathematical models were used for these calculations, a comparison of the values published for IVIG preparations is somewhat problematic.

PHARMACOKINETICS OF IVIG PREPARATIONS IN NORMAL SUBJECTS

Pharmacokinetics of some IVIG preparations performed in healthy subjects were published in the literature whereas information on others was provided by manufacturers in package inserts or promotional printed matter. In most studies, the catabolism of specific IgG antibodies rather than that of total IVIG was analyzed. This approach allowed an observation period of up to several weeks until antibody levels had decreased to preinfusion values. Table 2 summarizes available data (7–10). The $T_{1/2}$ values of some antibody specificities in IVIG were comparable to the $T_{1/2}$ of normal IgG. Possible reasons for the relatively short $T_{1/2}$ of anti-CMV are discussed below. According to tracer studies and product information material, the distribution of IVIG preparations in the body was in the same range as that observed with normal IgG, with an intravascular portion of 41–57% (7; product information provided by manufacturers).

For two preparations apparent distribution volumes of 0.09 and 0.13 L/kg were calculated (9,10). The total clearance of anti-HBs in IVIG was calculated to be 0.14 ml per min or approximately 2.9 ml/kg/day (9). In general, pharmacokinetic parameters of these IVIG preparations appear to be close to values obtained by IgG tracer studies in normal subjects (1).

However, pharmacokinetics of enzymatically modified IVIG preparations were clearly different. These preparations consisted either of $F(ab')_2$ fragments after pepsin

Table 2 Half-Lives of IVIG and IgG Antibodies in Normal Individuals (range of reported values)

IVIG and antibodies	$T_{1/2}$ (days)	References
Total IVIG	14–24	Product information provided by manufacturers (7)
Antibodies to:		
hepatitis B surface antigen (HBsAg)	16–26	Product information provided by manufacturers (8–10)
cytomegalovirus (CMV)	9–12	Product information provided by manufacturers
tetanus toxoid	12–34	Product information provided by manufacturers (8)
S. pneumoniae type 1	14–35	Product information provided by manufacturers

digestion (11), or of a mixture of Fab and Fc fragments and intact IgG molecules after plasmin treatment of IgG (12,13). The half-life of the $F(ab')_2$ preparation was found to be 2 days, and the total clearance was 3.5 ml/min, or 72 ml/kg/day. The volume of distribution after equilibration of this preparation suggested that approximately 60% of the $F(ab')_2$ fragments were present in the extravascular space. In the plasmin-treated preparation the Fab fragments were cleared at a fast rate, whereas the Fc fragments had a $T_{1/2}$ between 6 and 9.5 days. The plasmin-resistant portion, approximately one-third of the preparation, consisted of intact IgG molecules with a half-life of 22 days and a distribution in the body comparable to that of normal IgG (50% intravascular). These studies indicate that molecular sites on the Fc portion are important for the control of IgG catabolism (14).

PHARMACOKINETICS OF IVIG IN PATIENTS WITH CONGENITAL HUMORAL IMMUNODEFICIENCIES

Patients with congenital agamma- or hypogammaglobulinemia represent a prime indication for replacement therapy with IVIG preparations. Due to the lack of intrinsic immunoglobulin production these patients have low IgG and antibody serum levels and are thus ideal subjects for pharmacokinetic studies. As a corollary, all available IVIG preparations have been investigated in such patients. Results were either published or provided by the manufacturers in promotional printed material.

Typical studies included eight or more patients with X-linked agammaglobulinemia or common variable immunodeficiency syndrome who were already on replacement therapy with IVIG preparations. If the previously administered IVIG differed from the study preparation, a "washout" period had to be permitted before the onset of the trial. The study dose was in most instances 0.4 g/kg/month. This dosage corresponding to somewhat less than the normal intravascular IgG pool (Table 1) increased the IgG serum concentration from the trough level measured before to a peak level of more than twice the preinfusion value approximately 15 min after infusion. Serum samples were collected usually at 2- to 3-day intervals until 4 weeks after infusion and evaluated for IgG and antibody concentrations. Some of the data obtained with three IVIG preparations are given in Table 3 (15–21). Peak levels obtained with this dosage exceeded preinfusion serum IgG levels by approximately 7–10 g/L. Figure 2b demonstrates the decrease of the IgG concentration in an immunodeficient patient after IVIG infusion. It was observed that in this situation the α phase of the curve was relatively flat when compared with IgG tracer decay curves. From extrapolation of the final slope to the ordinate (intercept C_o in Fig. 2b), it appears that approximately 70% of the IVIG was available in the intravascular space which differed from the 40–60% observed in normal individuals.

Table 3 shows that at day 7, when the infused material had equilibrated between intra- and extravascular spaces, the serum IgG levels were still increased, whereas at day 28, they were close to preinfusion values. Thus, under these conditions there was no apparent accumulation of IgG in the body. Analysis of the final β phase of experimental curves yielded half-life values which were prolonged when compared with previously discussed data. This can be explained by the important relationship between IgG serum concentration and the catabolic rate: radioactive tracer studies have shown that in agammaglobulinemic patients the $T_{1/2}$ of IgG was greatly prolonged, whereas in myeloma or other patients with high IgG levels, it was shortened (1,3,4).

Table 3 In Vivo Behavior of IVIG Preparations After Infusion of 0.4 g/kg Body Weight in Patients with Congenital Humoral Immunodeficiency

	IVIG preparation		
	Gammagard	Sandoglobulin	Gamimune-N
IgG plasma concentrations (g/L):			
preinfusion	3.90	5.41	6.37
15 min after infusion (peak)	13.72	12.32	14.89
day 7	6.93	8.62	10.80[a]
day 28	3.79	5.78	6.60[a]
Half-life (days)	26	32	35

[a]Extrapolated from Figure 1 in Ref. 15. Data are taken from Refs. 15–21.

Half-lives of most other IVIG preparations determined in immunodeficient patients varied also between 26 and 35 days according to product information provided by manufacturers and the literature (5,22,23). Of two IVIG preparations, half-lives of IgG subclasses were determined: the $T_{1/2}$ of IgG1, IgG2, and IgG4 were approximately 30 days as observed for total IgG, whereas the $T_{1/2}$ of IgG3 was approximately 20 days (18–21). Schiff and colleagues (5,16,23) calculated the total clearance of IVIG and IgG antibodies in immunodeficient patients. Values for different preparations were between 1.6 and 2.4 ml/kg/day.

Pharmacokinetics of antibodies directed against bacterial and viral antigens in immunodeficient patients showed a variable pattern (Table 4). Half-lives of antibodies against *Streptococcus pneumoniae* capsular polysaccharides, the core lipopolysaccha-

Table 4 Half-Life of IgG Antibodies in Patients with Congenital Humoral Immunodeficiencies After IVIG Infusions (mean values or ranges)

Antibody specificity	$T_{1/2}$ (days)	IVIG preparation
Bacterial polysaccharides		
S. pneumoniae, types 1, 6A, 7, 3	26–32	Gammagard, Gamimune-N, Sandoglobulin
Core lipopolysaccharide, *S. minnesota,* Re 595 mutant	30	Gammagard
S. pyogenes, group A	36	Sandoglobulin
H. influenzae, type B	23	Sandoglobulin
Tetanus toxoid	21–27	Gammagard, Gamimune-N, Iveegam, Intraglobin
Viral antigens		
Hepatitis B surface antigen	32	Sandoglobulin
Cytomegalovirus	32	Sandoglobulin

Sources: Data are taken from product information provided by manufacturers and from Refs. 5,16,18,19,21–23.

ride of gram-negative bacteria, and streptococcal group A carbohydrate were between 26 and 36 days (5,16,18,19,21–23). Antibodies against *Haemophilus influenzae* type b polysaccharide had a somewhat shorter survival of 23 days. Interestingly, the $T_{1/2}$ of IgG2 antibodies against *H. influenzae* was 33 days, whereas IgG1 antibodies of this specificity had a much shorter half-life—10 days (Fig. 3). This could mean that consumption of the IgG1 antibody isotype was selectively increased in these chronically infected patients. The $T_{1/2}$ values of antibodies against tetanus toxoid were between 21 and 27 days; those of antibodies against viral antigens were 32 days.

There are certain problems inherent in these investigations that need to be addressed. First of all, results may be influenced by a carryover effect of extrinsic IgG from previous IVIG infusions (Fig. 2b). This material is catabolized at the same rate as the study IVIG but its presence in the body changes the α phase of the infused IVIG (5,24). In addition, almost all patients with humoral immunodeficiency have some residual intrinsic IgG synthesis which affects serum IgG concentrations during the study period and alters the final slope of the IgG decay curve. It may in fact be partially responsible for the observed prolongation of the $T_{1/2}$ in these patients (5).

How do pharmacokinetics translate into dosage recommendations for patients? As already stated, 4 weeks after an IVIG infusion of 0.4 g/kg body weight, postinfusion IgG levels have returned to preinfusion values, indicating that 100% of the infused dose was catabolized. As a consequence, smaller doses and/or longer intervals between infusions will decrease, whereas higher doses and shorter intervals will raise trough IgG levels. After a series of high-dose infusions, a new equilibrium will be reached according to the observation that IgG catabolism is concentration-dependent, as demonstrated in

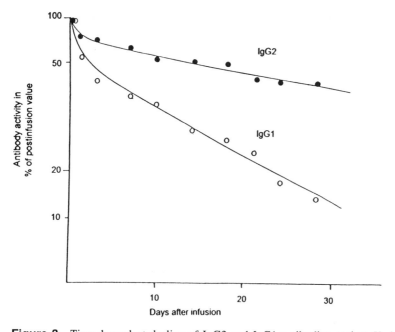

Figure 3 Time-dependent decline of IgG2 and IgG1 antibodies against *H. influenzae* type b polysaccharide in a patient with congenital humoral immunodeficiency following IVIG infusion of 0.4 g/kg body weight. Note rapid disappearance of IgG1 antibodies (A. Morell, unpublished results).

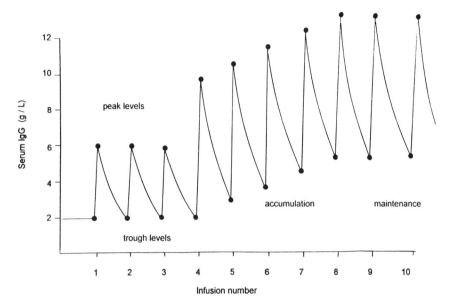

Figure 4 Serum IgG levels in a patient with congenital humoral immunodeficiency before (trough levels) and immediately after (peak levels) IVIG infusions. The figure demonstrates the influence of low- and high-dosage regimens: the accumulation phase induced by higher dosage (infusion 4) is followed by a new equilibrium or maintenance phase after infusion 8 (see Refs. 24–26).

Figure 4 (24–26). As there exists no fixed IgG serum concentration ensuring absence of acute infections in immunodeficient patients, IVIG dosage has to be individualized (26,27). Administration of 0.4 g/kg every 3–4 weeks is usually sufficient to keep trough IgG levels above 5 g/L, which is often considered a critical threshold. However, some patients may require higher doses (27).

PHARMACOKINETICS OF IVIG IN NEONATES AND INFANTS

Due to an active transplacental transport mechanism operating in the last 2 months of gestation, term-born neonates have slightly higher IgG serum levels than their mothers (28). During the first weeks of life, maternal IgG is known to be catabolized by the babies with an apparent $T_{1/2}$ of 30 days, and IgG serum concentrations decline to a nadir reached at approximately 3 months of age (29). Premature neonates have low serum IgG levels depending on their gestational age at birth. This is considered a risk factor for severe infections, i.e., neonatal sepsis, and represents the rationale for IVIG prophylaxis and treatment (30). Several clinical trials have provided information on the in vivo behavior of single or repeated infusions of IVIG. A summary of some relevant studies is provided in Table 5 (31–40).

In a prophylactic trial, Chirico and co-workers treated high-risk preterm neonates with weekly IVIG doses of 0.5 g/kg body weight (31). The resulting increase in serum IgG levels was most pronounced in babies weighing less than 1500 g. Levels of

Table 5 Pharmacokinetics of IVIG in Low-Birth-Weight Neonates (values expressed as means ± SD, or as ranges)

Reference	Dosage	$T_{1/2}$ (days)	Volume of distribution (L/kg)	Clearance (ml/kg/day)
Chirico et al. (31)	0.5 g/kg every week	23	ND[a]	ND
Weisman et al. (33)	0.5 g/kg single dose	31 ± 5	0.07 ± 0.02	4.2 ± 1.0
Weisman et al. (34)	0.25–1 g/kg single dose	24 ± 7	0.04 ± 0.01	3.0 ± 0.8
Weisman et al. (35)	0.5 g/kg single dose	29 ± 20	ND	ND
Noya et al. (36)	0.5–0.75 g/kg single dose	23 ± 6	ND	ND
Noya et al. (37)	0.5–1.0 g/kg single dose	20–29	0.13–0.26	3.7–5.6
Kyllonen et al. (38)	0.5–1.3 g/kg every 2 weeks	16–32	0.11 ± 0.01	2.0–2.8
Kinney et al. (39)	0.75 g/kg every 2 weeks	16–21	0.08 ± 0.01	ND
Groothuis et al. (40)	0.5–0.75 g/kg every month	21–28	ND	ND

[a]ND, not determined.

total IgG and of antibodies to group B streptococci, *E. coli*, and CMV were still above background after 4–6 days. Assuming a biexponential plasma elimination, the $T_{1/2}$ of the IVIG was estimated to be at least 23 days (32). However, the interval of 1 week between infusions did not allow precise calculations.

Three detailed studies of IVIG pharmacokinetics were undertaken by Weisman et al. In a first trial, these authors treated a group of neonates with a single IVIG dose of 0.5 g/kg and noticed an approximately twofold rise in serum IgG and an even more pronounced increase of antibodies against group B streptococci. Determinations of IgG and antibody levels at various times after infusion yielded an IVIG decay curve with a rapidly declining α phase and a slow terminal β phase, which was used to calculate a $T_{1/2}$ of 31 ± 5 days. The apparent distribution volume and the total clearance were considered to be close to values observed in adults (33). When these authors studied another IVIG in neonates, they noticed that a low dose of 0.25 g/kg induced only a transient rise whereas doses of 0.5 and 1 g/kg significantly increased IgG and group B streptococcal antibody levels for more than 14 days. From the terminal slope of the decay curve a $T_{1/2}$ of 24 days was calculated (34). In a recent large trial Weisman et al. treated premature neonates with a single dose of 0.5 g IVIG/kg body weight which increased IgG serum levels from 5.5 g/L to 12.5 g/L. The half-life calculated from data obtained 1, 2, and 8 weeks after infusion was 29 ± 20 days (35).

Similar results were reported by Noya and co-workers, who administered single doses of 0.5 and 0.75 g/kg to two groups of very low-birth-weight neonates (36). Serum IgG increased more than threefold in the high-dose and more than doubled in the low-dose group of infants. The subsequent decrease showed an initial rapid distribution phase followed by a much longer elimination phase from which a $T_{1/2}$ value of 23 ± 6 days was calculated in both groups of infants. After approximately 21 to 28 days, IgG serum levels had returned to preinfusion values but were still above 3 g/L. In another study with a different IVIG preparation, Noya et al. confirmed and extended these results (37).

Other investigators determined the dosage of IVIG and the dosing intervals required to maintain serum IgG levels above a target concentration of 7 g/L, which is close to the lower limit of IgG in cord blood of term-born infants (38). It was hypothesized that sustaining this target level could reduce the incidence of infections. For this purpose, low-birth-weight neonates received IVIG infusions of 0.5 g/kg. If IgG levels in day 2 or 6 postinfusion serum samples were below the target, the IVIG dose was increased to 0.7 g/kg or higher: to maintain the target level, infants with a birth weight of less than 1 kg required 0.9 g/kg and those with more than 1 kg needed 0.7 g/kg every 2 weeks. In babies with a birth weight of less than 1 kg, the average $T_{1/2}$ of 16 ± 6 days after the first dose increased significantly to 27 ± 4 days after subsequent IVIG infusions. In babies with a higher birth weight, the $T_{1/2}$ was 28 days after the first dose and 32 days after the last. The volume of distribution was 0.11 ± 0.011 L/kg, and mean clearance values ranged from 2.0 to 2.8 ml/kg/day.

This target level concept, the adjustment of the IVIG dosage to achieve and maintain an "optimal" IgG serum concentration of 7 g/L, was taken up in a large prophylactic trial in very low-birth-weight neonates (41). By using an IVIG regimen of 0.9 g/kg in infants below and of 0.7 g/kg in newborns above birth weights of 1000 g, the target was met or even exceeded: mean IgG trough levels increased from 3.8 to 7.7 g/L in the first group and were maintained between 6 and 7 g/L in the second group of infants.

In their trial on the efficacy and pharmacokinetics of IVIG, Kinney and co-workers treated high-risk neonates with IVIG doses of 0.75 g/kg immediately after admission to the hospital and then every 14 days for up to 3 months (39). This schedule maintained serum IgG levels above 5 g/L in babies weighing less than 1 kg and above 7 g/L in those weighing more than 1.5 kg. Pharmacokinetics could be analyzed from serum samples collected during the first 3 days after IVIG infusions and at days 7 and 14. As shown in Table 5 the $T_{1/2}$ of 16–21 days was somewhat shorter than that observed in other studies.

Finally, Groothuis et al. studied pharmacokinetics of antibodies against respiratory syncytial virus (RSV) in infants at risk for RSV infections (40). The patients were given monthly infusions of a special lot of an IVIG preparation selected for high content of RSV-specific antibodies. Three groups of children received either 0.5, 0.6, or 0.75 g IVIG/kg body weight per infusion; serum could be obtained prior to, and at days 1, 2, and 14 after, each infusion. The $T_{1/2}$ value was 28 days in children with the highest IVIG dose but shorter in the other two groups. As expected, the increase of antibodies was most pronounced with the highest dose where the successive IVIG doses at monthly intervals induced a slight but not statistically significant increase of the preinfusion antibody titers. The authors concluded a monthly dose of 0.75 g/kg to be sufficient to achieve and maintain a desired anti-RSV titer.

There are a number of problems that may limit the validity of pharmacokinetic studies in newborns. First of all, newborns are not in steady-state conditions, even when IVIG is replaced at regular doses and intervals. Term-born neonates produce detectable amounts of IgG in early months of life, which could result in a slight overestimation of the half-life of infused IgG (34). On the other hand, the rapid growth of new-borns causes expansion of body compartments during the observation time, which results in a dilution of the infused IVIG and in a shortening of the $T_{1/2}$. In general, the metabolic rate and the turnover of plasma proteins like IgG is correlated with the body size, as shown in different animal species (1). Thus, one would anticipate shorter $T_{1/2}$ values in infants than in adults, particularly in newborns with hypermetabolism due to fever and infection who were included in some studies. However, this is obviously not the case: data in Table 5 suggest that pharmacokinetics of IVIG in newborns appear to be similar to those in adults.

PHARMACOKINETICS OF IVIG IN PATIENTS WITH SECONDARY IMMUNODEFICIENCIES

Management of various secondary immunodeficiencies includes passive immunotherapy with IVIG. One of the most prominent conditions is immunodeficiency in allogeneic bone marrow transplant (BMT) recipients. A number of studies were devoted to the assessment of pharmacokinetics of IVIG and IgG antibodies in BMT patients. Results of $T_{1/2}$ determinations were conflicting since various investigators observed surprisingly short values whereas others reported survival times comparable with those found in patients with congenital humoral immunodeficiency or in normal subjects. Some of these studies are briefly summarized here and results are presented in Table 6 (42–49).

Rand and co-workers treated 27 patients with a high-dose IVIG regimen of 0.5 g/kg weekly beginning 1 week before until 98 days following BMT (42). The $T_{1/2}$ of CMV antibodies infused as a component of the IVIG was 3.4 days after the first dose and increased to 6.1 days after the fifth. Total IVIG half-life was estimated to be 5–10 days. There was a clear-cut accumulation of IVIG which increased from a mean of 8.2 $\pm$ 2.2 g/L to 14.7 $\pm$ 2.1 g/L and a concomitant more than sixfold increase of anti-CMV titers during the study. These values were observed in CMV-seronegative patients who had received only screened CMV-negative blood products and of whom serum samples were taken 1, 4, and 7 days after IVIG infusions. In a subsequent study, using another IVIG preparation at dose regimens of 0.25 and 0.5 g/kg body weight infused every 2 weeks, Rand et al. noticed significant increases of total IgG and of anti-CMV titers after the high IVIG dosage. Determinations in serum samples taken at days 1 to 7 yielded a mean $T_{1/2}$ of 6.2 days. The volume of distribution was 0.135 $\pm$ 0.014 L/kg, and the total body clearance varied between 0.46 and 0.61 mL/h/kg. There was little accumulation of IVIG in these patients even with the higher regimen. Similar results were reported by Bosi et al. (44), who after a single IVIG administration of 0.5 g/kg found a $T_{1/2}$ for CMV antibodies of 5.6 days (range 3.5–12.5 days). Even shorter $T_{1/2}$ values, 30–70 h, were observed by Hagenbeek (45).

Reasons that could possibly explain this rapid elimination are the short observation time after IVIG infusions and the application of one-compartment models in these studies. As a consequence, the data may primarily reflect the α phase of distribution in the body (Fig. 2). Moreover, determinations of anti-CMV activity in serum samples are crucial: some studies were based on neutralization titer assays whereas in others quantitative methods of analysis were applied. Evidently, quantitative determinations, e.g., enzyme immunoassays, allowing the assessment of low serum levels, are preferable. Possibly, other factors such as hypercatabolism due to fever, total body irradia-

Table 6 Half-Life of IVIG and IgG Antibodies to CMV in Patients with Secondary Immunodeficiencies

Reference	Preparation	Dosage	$T_{1/2}$ (days)	Comments
1. Patients after bone marrow transplantation				
Rand et al. (42)	IVIG	0.5 g/kg every week	6.1 ± 5.1	1 week observation time
Rand et al. (43)	IVIG	0.25–0.5 g/kg every 2 weeks	6.2	1 week observation time; one-compartment model
Gratwohl et al. (46)	IVIG	0.5 g/kg every week	30	29 days observation time after last infusion
Metselaar et al. (48)	CMV-IVIG[a]	1.0 ml/kg at 1–3 week intervals	14	increase of $T_{1/2}$ from 5 to 14 days at longer observation time
Reusser et al. (47)	CMV-IVIG	0.1 g/kg every 20 days	20 ± 8	20 days observation time. Further increase of $T_{1/2}$ to 25 days after second infusion
Drobyski et al. (49)	CMV-mAb[b]	0.05–0.5 mg/kg every 3 weeks	17 ± 3	38 days observation time; two-compartment model
2. Patients with chronic lymphocytic leukemia				
Huser et al. (8)	IVIG	0.14–0.36 g/kg every month	32	28 days observation time; steady state after third infusion, trough levels above 6 g/L at higher dosage
Chapel et al. (51)	IVIG	0.4 g/kg every 3 weeks	39 ± 10	21 days observation time; steady state after five infusions, trough levels above 6 g/L

[a]CMV hyperimmune globulin preparation.
[b]CMV monoclonal antibody preparation.

tion, and ablative chemotherapy in some patients also contributed to the short half-life observed in these studies.

Gratwohl et al. treated five patients with weekly IVIG doses of 0.5 g/kg starting 3 days before until 88 days after BMT (46). Under this regimen, total IgG trough levels increased from 8.8 ± 1.8 g/L before to 27.1 ± 1.9 g/L at the end of the infusion series, and anti-CMV levels rose from <1 to 3.7 units/mL. After the infusions were stopped, the accumulated IgG dropped to half of the peak level within 29 days. A similar elimination was observed for anti-CMV and other IgG antibodies, suggesting a $T_{1/2}$ of approximately 30 days.

Several studies with anti-CMV hyperimmune IgG preparation are in line with this observation. Reusser et al. infused BMT patients with a prophylactic dose of 0.1 g/kg every 20 days (47). They reported a half-life of 20 ± 13 days after the first infusion and a half-life of 25 ± 13 days after a subsequent infusion of this hyperimmune globulin in CMV-seronegative patients. These pharmacokinetics were assessed in serum specimens spanning 20 days after infusion. Using the same anti-CMV hyperimmune globulin, Metselaar and co-workers found $T_{1/2}$ values of 13–17 days for anti-CMV antibodies in CMV-seronegative cardiac transplant recipients (48). Finally, a pharmacokinetic study with monoclonal human IgG1 anti-CMV antibodies in BMT patients yielded a $T_{1/2}$ of 14–20 days (49). The authors applied a two-compartment model and based their calculations on serum values obtained between day 1 and day 38 after infusion. Thus, some of the reported data suggest that $T_{1/2}$ values in transplant patients may depend at least in part on the applied pharmacokinetic models and on the length of postinfusion observation time.

IVIG replacement therapy was furthermore shown to be beneficial to patients with low-grade B-cell tumors such as chronic lymphocytic leukemia (CLL) or low-grade non-Hodgkin's lymphoma (NHL). These patients often have severely decreased levels of serum immunoglobulin and of specific antibodies (27,50). Pharmacokinetic data would thus help to determine optimal IVIG dosage and time intervals between infusions. Huser et al. (8) observed that in some CLL patients the $T_{1/2}$ of IVIG was prolonged (Table 6). In their thorough study, Chapel et al. investigated the kinetics of IVIG in patients who were treated with IVIG infusions of 0.4 g/kg every 3 weeks for 1 year (51). Their low original IgG serum levels increased by >8 g/L after the first infusion. After the fifth infusion individual IgG serum trough levels stayed between 6 and 9 g/L in the patients, indicating that IVIG replacement was equal to catabolism. The $T_{1/2}$ was assessed on serum samples collected until day 21 after the last infusion. The range of the $T_{1/2}$ in these patients was between 25 and 57 days with a mean value of 39 ± 10 days, which is close to the findings in patients with primary humoral immunodeficiency.

Sklenar et al. studied kinetics of 12 different pneumococcal antibodies in three groups of CLL patients who received IVIG infusions of either 0.1 g/kg, 0.4 g/kg, or 0.8 g/kg every 3 weeks for 4 months (52). These regimens caused a dose-dependent increase of all antibodies above a protective level of 200 ng/mL of antibody N. After the fourth infusion trough levels of all antibody specificities remained constant, suggesting steady-state conditions. After the last infusion the authors followed the antibody and total IgG elimination rates. The time that elapsed until antibody levels had decreased to 50% of peak levels was between 8.5 ± 6.9 weeks for the smallest and 7.1 ± 1.3 weeks for the largest dose regimen. Similar elimination rates of 6–7 weeks were found for total IgG, which is considerably longer than the $T_{1/2}$ reported by Chapel and Lee

(51). The authors concluded that a dose of 0.4 g/kg every 3 weeks was optimal for replacement of antipneumococcal antibodies in CLL patients.

SUMMARY AND CONCLUSIONS

Pharmacokinetics of most IVIG preparations reflect metabolic properties of normal IgG. After IVIG infusion in normal individuals and patients, serial determinations of total IgG and of IgG antibodies result in biphasic plasma or serum disappearance curves with an initial, α phase representing early catabolism and distribution between body compartments, and a final, β phase representing catabolism. Pharmacokinetic parameters were derived from these curves usually by applying suitable two-compartment mathematical models. The biological half-life or $T_{1/2}$ was the only parameter consistently determined for all IVIG preparations. In immunologically normal persons, the $T_{1/2}$ values of IVIG preparations were between 14 and 24 days, and those of various IgG antibodies between 12 and 35 days. Some of these variations were probably due to individual differences in the IgG catabolism. However, the wide range of $T_{1/2}$ values may at least in part also reflect molecular disparities of IVIG preparations and methodological differences between the studies.

In patients with congenital humoral immunodeficiencies, the $T_{1/2}$ of the infused total IgG was in general prolonged. The same phenomenon was observed for the IgG subclasses and IgG antibodies in IVIG, suggesting a relationship between IgG serum concentration and catabolism, as was described for normal IgG. Pharmacokinetics of IVIG in neonates at high risk for infection were found to be comparable with those in normal adult individuals: several groups of investigators reported $T_{1/2}$ values between 16 and >30 days. A number of studies were devoted to the assessment of IVIG pharmacokinetics in bone marrow transplant patients. Reported results for $T_{1/2}$ values of total IgG and IgG antibodies were conflicting: some investigators found short half-lives for total IgG and CMV antibodies, whereas in other studies $T_{1/2}$ values were in the normal range. Finally, in patients with chronic lymphocytic leukemia and related disorders, the $T_{1/2}$ of the infused preparations appeared to be prolonged, as in patients with congenital humoral immunodeficiencies. Pharmacokinetics of IVIG preparations in patients may be subject to even more pronounced individual variations than in normal persons. Furthermore, steady-state conditions that have to be assumed for most two-compartment models are in fact rarely approximated. One-compartment models with short observation times applied by some investigators may characterize mainly the initial α phase but may seriously underestimate the $T_{1/2}$. One also has to consider that some patients were in a state of hypercatabolism due to fever, malignancy, and radiation or chemotherapy. In spite of all these limitations, the evaluation of pharmacokinetic properties of IVIG preparations has provided information useful for the planning of prophylactic and therapeutic regimens and dosing intervals in patients.

REFERENCES

1. Waldmann TA, Strober W. Metabolism of immunoglobulins. Progr Allergy 1969; 13:1–110.
2. Nosslin B. Analysis of disappearance time-curves after single injections of labelled proteins.

In: Protein Turnover. Ciba Foundation Symposium 9 (new series). Amsterdam, New York: Associated Scientific Publishers, 1973:113–130.

3. Waldmann TA, Terry WD. Familial hypercatabolic hypoproteinemia. A disorder of endogenous catabolism of albumin and immunoglobulin. J Clin Invest 1990; 86:2093–2098.

4. Morell A, Terry WD, Waldmann TA. Metabolic properties of IgG subclasses in man. J Clin Invest 1970; 49:673–680.

5. Schiff RI. Intravenous immunoglobulins for treatment of antibody deficiencies. In: Good RA, Lindenlaub E, eds. The Nature, Cellular, and Biochemical Basis and Management of Immunodeficiencies. Symposia Medica Hoechst 21. Stuttgart: Schattauer FK Verlag, 1987:523–541.

6. Notari R. Biopharmaceutics and Clinical Pharmacokinetics. New York: Marcel Dekker, 1987.

7. Morell A, Schürch B, Ryser D, et al. In vivo behaviour of gamma globulin preparations. Vox Sang 1980; 38:272–283.

8. Huser HJ, Schwander D, Wegmann A, et al. Verträglichkeit und Verweildauer eines intravenösen Immunglobulinpräparates bei immunologisch gesunden Personen und Verträglichkeit bei Patienten mit Hypogammaglobulinämie infolge chronischer lymphatischer Leukämie. Schweiz Med Wschr 1986; 116:151–156.

9. Glöckner WM. Kinetik von Immunglobulin G nach intravenöser oder intramuskulärer Applikation. In: Kornhuber B, ed. Patient, Infektion, Immunglobulin. Heidelberg: Springer Verlag, 1984:33–38.

10. Eriksson O. Determination of half life in healthy volunteers of anti HBs in Gammonativ. Technical Report No 81 98 093, 1981. Stockholm: Kabi Vitrum AB, Research Department.

11. Theobald K, Högy B. Pharmacokinetics of single and multiple infusion of 5S intravenous immunoglobulin. Vox Sang 1995; 68:5–8.

12. Barandun S, Castel V, Makula MF, et al. Clinical tolerance and catabolism of plasmin-treated γ-globulin for intravenous application. Vox Sang 1975; 28:157–175.

13. Janeway CA, Merler E, Rosen FS, et al. Intravenous gamma-globulin. Metabolism of gamma-globulin fragments in normal and agammaglobulinemic persons. N Engl J Med 1968; 278:919–923.

14. Winkelhake JL. Immunoglobulin structure and effector functions. Immunochemistry 1978; 15:695–714.

15. Pirofsky B. Safety and toxicity of a new serum immunoglobulin G intravenous preparation, IGIV pH 4.25. Rev Infect Dis 1986; 8(suppl 4):457–463.

16. Schiff RI. Half-life and clearance of pH 6.8 and pH 4.25 immunoglobulin G intravenous preparations in patients with primary disorders of humoral immunity. Rev Infect Dis 1986; 8(suppl 4):449–456.

17. Pirofsky B. Clinical use of a new pH 4.25 intravenous immunoglobulin preparation (Gamimune-N). J Infect 1987; 15(suppl 1):29–37.

18. Mankarious S, Lee M, Fischer S, et al. The half-lives of IgG subclasses and specific antibodies in patients with primary immunodeficiency who are receiving intravenously admininstered immunoglobulin. J Lab Clin Med 1988; 112:634–640.

19. Lee ML, Mankarious S, Ochs H, et al. The pharmacokinetics of total IgG, IgG subclasses, and type specific antibodies in immunodeficient patients. Immunol Invest 1991; 20:193–198.

20. Ochs HD, Morell A, Skvaril F, et al. Survival of IgG subclasses following administration of intravenous gammaglobulin in patients with primary immunodeficiency diseases. In: Morell A, Nydegger UE, eds. Clinical use of intravenous immunoglobulins. New York: Academic Press, 1986:77–85.

21. Fischer SH, Ochs HD, Wedgwood RJ, et al. Survival of antigen-specific antibody following administration of intravenous immunoglobulin in patients with primary immunodeficiency diseases. Monogr Allergy 1988; 23:225–235.

22. Eibl M. Intravenous immunoglobulins: Clinical and experimental studies. In: Alving BM, Finlayson JS, eds. Immunoglobulins: Characteristics and Uses of Intravenous Preparations.

Bethesda: U.S. Dept. Health Human Serv.; Publ. Health Service, FDA, DHHS Publication No. (FDA)-80-9005, 1979:23–30.

23. Schiff RI, Rudd C. Alterations in the half-life and clearance of IgG during therapy with intravenous γ-globulin in 16 patients with severe primary humoral immunodeficiency. J Clin Immunol 1986; 6:256–264.

24. Ochs HD, Fischer SH, Wedgwood RJ, et al. Comparison of high-dose and low-dose intravenous immunoglobulin therapy in patients with primary immunodeficiency diseases. Am J Med 1984; 76(3A):78–82.

25. Roifman CM, Levison H, Gelfand EW. High-dose versus low-dose intravenous immunoglobulin in hypogammaglobulinemia and chronic lung disease. Lancet 1987; 2:1075–1077.

26. Leen CLS, Yap PL, McClelland DBL. Increase of serum immunoglobulin level into the normal range in primary hypogammaglobulinemia by dosage individualization of intravenous immunoglobulin. Vox Sang 1986; 51:278–286.

27. NIH Consensus Development Conference 1990. Intravenous immunoglobulin, prevention and treatment of disease. JAMA 1990; 264:3189–3193.

28. Brambell FWR. The transmission of immunity from mother to young and the catabolism of immunoglobulins. Lancet 1966; 2:1087–1093.

29. Weiner AS. The half-life of passively acquired antibody globulin molecules in infants. J Exp Med 1951; 94:213–221.

30. Wilson CB. Immunologic basis for increased susceptibility of the neonate to infection. J Pediatr 1986; 108:1–12.

31. Chirico G, Rondini G, Plebani A, et al. Intravenous gammaglobulin therapy for prophylaxis of infection in high risk neonates. J Pediatr 1987; 110:437–442.

32. Nolan BM, Kauffman R. Pharmacokinetics and effectiveness of intravenous immunoglobulins in neonates. J Pediatr 1988; 112:325–326.

33. Weisman LE, Fischer GW, Hemming VG, et al. Pharmacokinetics of intravenous immunoglobulin (Sandoglobulin) in neonates. Pediatr Infect Dis 1986; 5(suppl 3):185–188.

34. Weisman LE, Fischer GW, Marinelli P, et al. Pharmacokinetics of intravenous immunoglobulin in neonates. Vox Sang 1989; 57:243–248.

35. Weisman LE, Stoll BJ, Kueser TJ, et al. Intravenous immune globulin prophylaxis of late-onset sepsis in premature neonates. J Pediatr 1994; 125:922–930.

36. Noya FJD, Rench MA, Garcia-Prats JA, et al. Disposition of an immunoglobulin intravenous preparation in very low birth weight neonates. J Pediatr 1988; 112:278–283.

37. Noya FJD, Rench MA, Courtney JT, et al. Pharmacokinetics of intravenous immunoglobulin in very low birth weight neonates. Pediatr Infect Dis J 1989; 8:759–763.

38. Kyllonen KS, Clapp DW, Kliegman RM, et al. Dosage of intravenously administered immune globulin and dosing intervals required to maintain target levels of immunoglobulin G in low birth weight infants. J Pediatr 1989; 115:1013–1016.

39. Kinney J, Mundorf L, Gleason C, et al. Efficacy and pharmacokinetics of intravenous immune globulin administered to high-risk neonates. Am J Dis Child 1991; 145:1233–1238.

40. Groothuis JR, Levin MJ, Rodriguez W, et al. Use of intravenous gamma globulin to passively immunize high-risk children against respiratory syncytial virus: safety and pharmacokinetics. Antimicrob Agents Chemother 1991; 35:1469–1473.

41. Fanaroff AA, Sheldon BC, Korones B, et al. A controlled trial of intravenous immune globulin to reduce nosocomial infections in very-low-birth-weight infants. N Engl J Med 1994; 330:1107–1113.

42. Rand KH, Houk H, Ganju A, et al. Pharmacokinetics of cytomegalovirus specific IgG antibody following intravenous immunoglobulin in bone marrow transplant recipients. Bone Marrow Transplant 1989; 4:679–683.

43. Rand KH, Gibbs K, Derendorf H, et al. Pharmacokinetics of intravenous immunoglobulin (Gammagard) in bone marrow transplant patients. J Clin Pharmacol 1991; 31:1151–1154.

44. Bosi A, de Majo E, Guidi S, et al. Kinetics of anti-CMV antibodies after administration of

intravenous immunoglobulins to bone marrow transplant recipients. Haematologica 1990; 75:109–112.

45. Hagenbeek A, Brummelhuis HGJ, Donkers A, et al. Rapid clearance of cytomegalovirus-specific IgG after repeated intravenous infusions of human immunoglobulin into allogeneic bone marrow transplant recipients. J Infect Dis 1987; 155:897–902.

46. Gratwohl A, Doran JE, Bachmann P, et al. Serum concentrations of immunoglobulins and of antibody isotypes in bone marrow transplant recipients treated with high doses of polyspecific immunoglobulin or with cytomegalovirus hyperimmune globulin. Bone Marrow Transplant 1991; 8:275–282.

47. Reusser P, Osterwalder B, Gratama JW, et al. Kinetics of cytomegalovirus IgG following infusion of a hyperimmune globulin preparation in allogeneic marrow transplant recipients. Bone Marrow Transplant 1989; 4:267–272.

48. Metselaar HJ, Velzing J, Rothbarth PH, et al. A pharmacokinetic study of anti-cytomegalovirus hyperimmunoglobulins in cytomegalovirus seronegative cardiac transplant recipients. Transplant Proc 1987; 19:4063–4065.

49. Drobyski WR, Gottlieb M, Carrigan D, et al. Phase I study of safety and pharmacokinetics of a human anticytomegalovirus monoclonal antibody in allogeneic bone marrow transplant recipients. Transplantation 1991; 51:1190–1196.

50. Cooperative group for the study of immunoglobulin in chronic lymphocytic leukemia. Intravenous immunoglobulin for the prevention of infection in chronic lymphocytic leukemia. N Engl J Med 1988; 319:902–907.

51. Chapel HM, Lee M. Immunoglobulin replacement in patients with chronic lymphocytic leukemia (CLL): kinetics of immunoglobulin metabolism. J Clin Immunol 1992; 12:17–20.

52. Sklenar I, Schiffman G, Jonsson V, et al. Effect of various doses of intravenous polyclonal IgG on in vivo levels of 12 pneumococcal antibodies in patients with chronic lymphocytic leukaemia and multiple myeloma. Oncology 1993; 50:466–477.

2

Pharmacoeconomics of Intravenous Immunoglobulin

Martin L. Lee
*School of Public Health, University of California,
Los Angeles, California*

Vibeke Strand
Stanford University, Stanford, California

INTRODUCTION

The notion of using classic economic arguments to assess the potential benefit of a new therapeutic intervention has become quite widespread over the past few years. One might argue, in fact, that the economic justification for the use of a new therapy has become as important as the need for demonstrating its effectiveness.

With regard to the use of intravenous immunoglobulin (IVIG) administration, it is generally perceived that use of such an expensive treatment should be rationed. Yet, there has been little formal economic evaluation of IVIG therapy.

This chapter will briefly review the economic data that have been generated in the treatment of Kawasaki disease, chronic lymphocytic leukemia (CLL), home infusion (for primary immunodeficiency syndromes), and in other miscellaneous settings.

KAWASAKI DISEASE

Klassen and colleagues evaluated the economics of IVIG for the treatment of the acute phase of Kawasaki disease (1). In this assessment, three possible courses of action were considered (based on prior literature; see the relevant chapter in this text on Kawasaki disease): aspirin alone at 100 mg/kg/day for 14 days followed by 3–5 mg/kg/day for a variable period; IVIG at 400 mg/kg for 4 consecutive days (designated as the low-dose option); or IVIG at 2 g/kg for 1 day (designated as the high-dose option). Aspirin was also included in each of the IVIG treatment options.

Costs considered included those for treatment, hospitalization time, clinic visits, laboratory testing, and physician services.

The primary serious outcome of Kawasaki disease, coronary artery abnormalities, was used to assess the relative efficaciousness of the three treatment modalities. A sensitivity analysis was included to allow for varying rates of occurrence of coronary artery aneurysms, duration of hospitalization, and treatment (particularly IVIG) cost.

Results indicated that the cost of care for 100 patients with Kawasaki disease would be reduced by $323,400 (approximately $32,000 per patient) if the high-dose IVIG option was utilized instead of aspirin alone, due to the 14 cases of coronary artery abnormalities prevented. High-dose IVIG was superior to the low-dose option by about $118,000 (or approximately $12,000 per patient) because of the average reduction of two cases of aneurysm. However, the authors pointed out that the high-dose regimen could be more expensive than the low-dose (by $8500/100 patients) if patients in both groups were hospitalized for 5 days. They viewed this not to be a likely circumstance, given the reduced morbidity in the IVIG treatment groups.

As a result of this analysis, high-dose IVIG was endorsed as the treatment of choice for Kawasaki syndrome because of its therapeutic effectiveness and its resultant economic benefit.

CHRONIC LYMPHOCYTIC LEUKEMIA (CLL)

A randomized, double-blind, placebo-controlled trial successfully demonstrated that IVIG administered on a regular, prophylactic basis significantly reduces the incidence of serious bacterial infections in patients with CLL who are at risk for these infections (2). (This study is discussed in detail in the chapter on IVIG and B-cell lymphoproliferative diseases.) After these results were published, Weeks and colleagues performed an economic evaluation of IVIG treatment in this context using a decision-analytic model (3).

Their model was based on the comparison of two approaches to infection prophylaxis: regular IVIG infusions (at 400 mg/kg every 3 weeks), or no prophylaxis. Considered in this analysis were the direct costs of the treatment, its complications, and treating the outcome (infections). A utility evaluation (based on querying 10 oncologists) was included in the model in order to place a value on the following clinical states: CLL without infection; CLL with a trivial infection; CLL with a moderate infection; CLL with a major infection; and an intravenous immune globulin infusion.

Based on their analyses, a gain in 1 quality-adjusted life year (QALY)—i.e., a year of life after adjusting for the utility or value assessments associated with this year—by the use of IVIG prophylaxis would cost approximately $6 million. This is an astoundingly large figure when placed in the context of, say, hospital hemodialysis, which is estimated to cost about $54,000/QALY (4). The authors admitted, however, that the cost would be substantially lower if various other costs, including treatment effectiveness (particularly with regards to reducing mortality in this patient population), and other assumptions were all to move in the beneficial direction. They did not necessarily view this as a likely scenario.

Subsequently, Lee and Courter (5) critiqued the Weeks analysis (3). The original clinical trial was designed to demonstrate a reduction in serious infections, which was viewed as a surrogate measure for mortality; therefore, the patients were not followed for a sufficient amount of time to assess this latter outcome. Indeed, patients were selected for participation in the trial on the basis of their predicted ability to survive the year on study. In addition, subsequent evaluations of this treatment modality have indicated that a subset of patients more likely to benefit from treatment could be identified, and reduction in the amount of IVIG administration was still effective. As a result, the requirements of Weeks et al. for a reduced cost of care were being met.

Another substantial criticism of the Weeks study, namely, the use of physicians rather than patients to evaluate utilities, was specifically addressed in a separate study (6). Indeed, Gill and Feinstein (7) have persuasively argued that such assessments must specifically be conducted with patients, with physician opinions viewed as secondary.

As a result, Lee et al. (6) conducted a study in 12 patients with either CLL (n = 9) or multiple myeloma (n = 3), another B-cell disease also treated with IVIG. In this small evaluation, patients who had previously received or were receiving IVIG were queried regarding their feelings about the treatment and its consequences. From the responses and with a modest assumption concerning the mortality benefit from IVIG usage, the cost of gaining one QALY could be reduced to approximately $95,000, a much more defensible figure.

The controversy in this area reveals that the use of IVIG in this therapeutic area is not universally agreed upon. Further research and evaluation are needed to better define its role in the treatment armamentarium.

HOME INFUSION THERAPY

Formal economic evaluations of IVIG in the home care setting have not been conducted, but some data are available to assess its cost and benefit. The costs of various available IVIG products vary widely (8); it is critical to carefully evaluate the different preparations.

Daly and colleagues administered quality-of-life questionnaires to 37 home care individuals versus 29 patients treated in a traditional clinic setting (9) and showed that home-based therapy is preferred to clinic-based. The individuals surveyed had various primary antibody deficiencies. Rodriguez et al. have also reported similar findings in an evaluation of 38 patients or relatives of patients (10).

Recently, Gardulf et al., based on their experience in Sweden, have argued that the use of subcutaneous rather than intravenous infusions administered at home could reduce the cost per patient per year by $10,000 (11). As a result of this finding, it is presumed that IVIG may be cheaper to administer in the home care setting on a cost-utility basis.

OTHER APPLICATIONS

Francioni and colleagues in an open trial of 12 patients with systemic lupus erythematosus (SLE) refractory to conventional treatments noted an improvement in the quality of life of these individuals (12). Because of the high cost of IVIG, they recommended its use particularly for those not responding to other therapies and those with infectious complications.

In patients with idiopathic thrombocytopenia purpura (ITP), Massolo et al. have noted that IVIG reduces the need for hospitalization (particularly in children), the requirements for platelet transfusions, and the use of steroids (13). As a result, they noted that the "social cost" of treating ITP is not higher in children when IVIG is used.

CONCLUSION

The limited number of studies and evaluations of the economic cost of IVIG appear to indicate that it may not be as high as the popular perception. Clearly, more research is needed in this regard.

REFERENCES

1. Klassen TP, Rowe PC, Gafino A. Economic evaluation of intravenous immune globulin therapy for Kawasaki Syndrome. J Pediatr 1993; 122:538–542.
2. Cooperative Group of the Study of Immunoglobulin in Chronic Lymphocytic Leukemia. Intravenous immunoglobulin for the prevention of infection in chronic lymphocytic leukemia. N Engl J Med 1988; 319:902–907.
3. Weeks JC, Tierney MR, Weinstein MC. Cost effectiveness of prophylactic intravenous immune globulin in chronic lymphocytic leukemia. N Engl J Med 1991; 325:81–86.
4. Feeny D, Labelle R, Torrance GW. Integrating economic evaluations and quality of life assessments. In: Spilker B, ed. Quality of Life Assessments in Clinical Trials. New York: Raven Press, 1990:71–83.
5. Lee ML, Courter SG. Quality of life assessment versus clinical outcome measures: an example. Drug Inform J 1994; 28:39–43.
6. Lee ML, Chapel H, Brennan V, Gamm H, Dicato M, Courter SG. Quality-of-life assessments and clinical outcome measures in patients with B-cell lymphoproliferative disease receiving intravenous immunoglobulin. In: Strand V, Simon L, Johnson K, eds. Early Decisions in DMARD Development IV: Biologic Agents in Autoimmune Diseases. Atlanta: Arthritis Foundation, 1996:183–189.
7. Gill TM, Feinstein AR. A critical appraisal of the quality of quality-of-life measurements. JAMA 1994; 272:619–626.
8. Bielory L, Long GC. Home infusion therapy: comparison of costs for intravenous immunoglobulin. NJ Med 1993; 90:512–515.
9. Daly PB, Evans JH, Kobayashi RH, et al. Home-based immunoglobulin infusion therapy: quality of life and patient health perception. Ann Allergy 1991; 67:504–510.
10. Rodriguez M, Procupet A, Heras J. Cost-effectiveness of home administration versus hospital administration of intravenous immunoglobulin. Med Clin 1991; 96:47–51.
11. Gardulf A, Anderson V, Bjorkander J, et al. Subcutaneous immunoglobulin replacement in patients with primary antibody deficiencies: Safety and costs. Lancet 1995; 345:365–69.
12. Francioni C, Fioravanti A, Gelli R, Megale F, Marcolongo R. Long-term treatment with i.v. immunoglobulin in the therapy of systemic lupus erythematosus. Rec Prog Med 1993; 84:679–686.
13. Massolo F, Flori C, Cellini M, Baraldi C, Iori G. Use of high-dose intravenous immunoglobulins in pediatric hematology. Pediatr Med Chirurg 1994; 16:37–41.

3

Proposed Mechanisms for the Efficacy of Intravenous Immunoglobulin Treatment

Vibeke Strand
Stanford University, San Francisco, California

INTRODUCTION

This chapter reviews the mechanisms postulated to account for the benefits of intravenous immunoglobulin (IVIG) infusions in treating autoimmune diseases and as infection prophylaxis in cases of acquired immune deficiencies. There are a limited number of FDA-labeled clinical indications for the use of IVIG in the U.S.: as replacement therapy in primary immunodeficiency diseases; as treatment of idiopathic thrombocytopenia purpura (ITP); and as prophylaxis for bacterial infections in B-cell chronic lymphocytic leukemia (CLL), for pediatric HIV infection, and for local and systemic infections, interstitial pneumonia, and acute graft vs. host disease (GvHD) after bone marrow transplantation. However, based on the positive clinical experience in the treatment of ITP and Kawasaki disease (KD), IVIG administration has been investigated in a variety of autoimmune diseases and acquired immune deficiencies. (Table 1). Prospective randomized controlled trials are lacking in most of these clinical indications, and the underlying pathophysiological disease processes are not well understood. The mechanisms of action hypothesized to account for the benefits of IVIG administration are largely derived from in vitro data and published reports of small uncontrolled clinical trials and thus may not be applicable to all clinical situations. Nonetheless, our understanding has advanced considerably in the past several years.

The Y-shaped immunoglobulin G molecule is comprised of the amino terminal end with two antigen combining sites: the variable, or $F(ab')_2$, region; and the constant, or crystallizable, Fc region. Each immunoglobulin molecule is specific to its antigen; this specificity resides within the variable $F(ab')_2$ or hypercomplementarity region. Within the constant Fc region of the molecule, common to all IgG molecules of that individual, reside multiple biological functions, including binding to complement and to cell surface Fc receptors (FcR) on reticuloendothelial (RE) cells. Complement activation results in opsonization, phagocytosis, lysis (complement-dependent cytotoxicity), and stimulation of polymorphonuclear cell (PMN) function, including agglutination, chemotaxis, and oxidative metabolism. FcR binding allows macrophages to phagocytize antigen-antibody (Ag-Ab) complexes, and causes mast cell and basophil activation and degranulation.

Table 1 Autoimmune Diseases in Which IVIG Treatment
Has Been Investigated

Dermatological
   Bullous pemphigoid
Organ-specific
   Insulin–dependent diabetes
   Autoimmune thyroiditis/Graves' ophthalmopathy
Inflammatory bowel disease
   Crohn disease
   Ulcerative colitis
Hematological
   Idiopathic thrombocytopenia purpura
   HIV–associated thrombocytopenia
   Autoimmune neutropenia
   Autoimmune hemolytic anemia
   Acquired factor VIII inhibitor
Neurological
   Myasthenia gravis/Lambert–Eaton syndrome
   Guillain-Barré syndrome
   Chronic inflammatory demyelinating polyneuropathy
   Multiple sclerosis
   Intractable childhood seizures
   Amyotrophic lateral sclerosis
Vasculitides
   Kawasaki disease
   ANCA+ vasculitis
Multiple organ system
   Systemic lupus erythematosus
   Antiphospholipid antibody syndrome
   Dermatomyositis/Polymyositis
   Rheumatoid arthritis
   Juvenile rheumatoid arthritis
   Graft vs. host disease
Recurrent fetal loss $\pm$ antiphospholipid antibody syndrome
Chronic fatigue syndrome

Many of the immunomodulatory effects attributed to IVIG administration may occur because of complementary interactions between autoantibody $F(ab')_2$ variable (V) regions (idiotypes) and V regions present in the administered IgG (anti-idiotypes) preparation. The term "connectivity" refers to the ability of these idiotype-anti-idiotype reactions to control humoral and cellular immune responses. It is now recognized that autoantibodies to a broad variety of self antigens are present in the sera of healthy individuals, as well as those with autoimmune disease (1). It is estimated that 1 g of IVIG contains approximately 4×10^{18} molecules, capable of recognizing >10 million antigenic determinants (2). Concentrated IVIG preparations are pooled from 10,000–15,000 donors and can be expected to contain a vast assortment of autoantibody idiotypes (ids) and anti-idiotypes (anti-ids). Products pooled from multiparous women and older donors with broader expression of public idiotopes are therefore thought to be more effective (3). IgG dimers, formed because of id-anti-id complementarity, are plentiful in IVIG preparations and may function in several ways: to prevent autoantibody binding to antigen; when bound to FcR on phagocytic cells, to act as superopsonins facilitating RE system clearance; when bound to FcR on B cells, to inhibit autoantibody production; and when recognized by T cells, to downregulate cell activation and proliferation.

Other processes may account for the acute and short-term effects observed after IVIG treatment. In addition to a broad spectrum of autoantibodies based on donor number and population, pooled IVIG preparations contain antibodies to specific infectious antigens and superantigens. The infusion of large amounts of antibody may change antigen-antibody ratios, thereby altering immune complex tissue deposition and solubilization. Fluctuations in serum levels change the catabolic rate of IgG, transiently altering levels of endogenous and exogenous immunoglobulin. Table 2 lists the short-term effects attributed to IVIG administration.

Work by Dietrich, Kaveri, Kazatchkine, and others supports the hypothesis that id-anti-id regulatory mechanisms predominantly account for the beneficial effects of IVIG administration. IVIG infusions may passively transfer autoantibody anti-idiotypes and actively alter endogenous regulation of autoantibody expression through id anti-id interactions. Prolonged benefit may also be attributed to Fc-dependent changes in B-cell and autoantibody production. Interactions with other cell surface antigens and alterations

Table 2 Short-Term Effects of IVIG Administration

Fc-dependent interactions
    Inhibition of complement-mediated damage
    Blockade of FcR binding on RE cells
        Decreased FcR clearance of Ab-coated cells
        Fc-dependent feedback inhibition of auto-Ab synthesis
        FcR expression rapidly regenerated; effect short-lived
    Alteration of NK cell function
$F(ab')_2$ or V region–dependent interactions
    Contain Abs reactive with idiotypic region of autoAbs → formation of
    id-anti-id dimers
        Neutralization of auto-Ab: prevent binding to its antigen
        Downregulation of auto-Ab production: id-anti-id dimers bind to B cell FcR
        Stimulation of anti-id Ab production
    Neutralization/removal of superantigens
Fc and $F(ab')_2$-dependent mechanisms
    Change structure or solubilize deposited immune complexes (ICs)
        Decrease circulating ICs
        Decrease C1q and anti C3 binding of ICs
        Alter ratio of Ag + Ab ↔ AgAb (circ) ↔ AgAb (tissue)
    Immunoregulatory
        Modulates cytokine and cytokine antagonist production
        Reversal of endothelial cell activation, adhesion molecule expression
        Decreased lymphocyte proliferation
        Increased NK cell function and number
Increased catabolism of IgG

Table 3 Long-Term Effects of IVIG Administration

Passive neutralization of auto-Abs
Downregulation of B-cell function and suppression of auto-Ab synthesis
Induction of disease specific anti-id Ab response
Id-anti-id–mediated selection of T-cell repertoire
Interaction with other cell surface antigens
    Via Ab to the beta chain of T-cell receptor
    Via Ab to CD4, CD5
    Via soluble MHC class I and II Ag; soluble CD4, CD8
Alterations in cytokine and cytokine antagonist production
Decreased endothelial cell activation and adhesion molecule expression

---

in cytokine secretion may additionally account for modulation of T- and B-cell activation and function. Table 3 lists the mechanisms believed responsible for the long-term or immunomodulatory effects of IVIG treatment.

Fc-DEPENDENT INTERACTIONS

IVIG binds the activated C3b and C4b components of complement, inhibits their binding to target cells, and solubilizes circulating immune complexes (4). Basta et al. have demonstrated that IVIG administration protects guinea pigs from death in the complement-mediated Forssman shock model, and postulate that this mechanism is particularly important in the reversal of thrombocytopenia, hemolytic anemia, and leukopenia (5,6). C3 and C4 bind to the Fc fragment of IgG, forming heterodimers, which act as "superopsonins," sponging up activated complement; yet they are resistant to complement degradation (7). Consistent with this hypothesis, marked increases in the number of IgG molecules bound to red blood cells (RBCs) have been observed in patients with autoimmune hemolytic anemia after treatment with IVIG, concomitantly with decreased C3 binding and prolongation of RBC survival in the circulation.

Decreased FcR binding on RE cells is frequently cited as a predominant mechanism accounting for the immediate benefit of IVIG treatment in ITP and in cytopenias secondary to SLE (8–11). This response may be mediated by competitive binding to FcR, which blocks binding of Ab-coated cells, as well as downregulation of FcR expression by small immune complexes present in IVIG preparations. Several clinical observations support this hypothesis: following treatment with IVIG in patients with ITP infused autologous RBCs coated with anti-RhD antibodies survived longer (12); in patients with refractory ITP, administration of anti-Fcγ receptor antibodies was beneficial (13). In vitro incubation with IVIG resulted in decreased phagocytosis of anti-Rh-D-coated RBCs by adherent peripheral blood mononuclear cells (PBMCs) (14). Although this mechanism may account for the rapid onset of effect after IVIG treatment, it does not explain long-term benefit. Cell surface FcRs are regenerated over time; exogenous IgG is estimated to remain in the circulation for 4–6 weeks.

Another Fc-mediated mechanism explaining the effect of IVIG infusions may be alteration of NK cell function. Following treatment of ITP and autoimmune neutropenia, peripheral circulating numbers of NK cells increased (15). Finberg reported similar findings in patients with KD and refractory seizure disorders, suggesting that IVIG inhibits margination of NK cells by downmodulating endothelial cell activation and adhesion molecule expression (16,17). Saulsbury (among others) has pointed out that the rapidity of improvement observed in patients with KD argues for other mechanisms, suggesting that microbial superantigens mediate these disease manifestations (18).

F(ab')$_2$ OR V-REGION-DEPENDENT INTERACTIONS

Passive infusion of anti-idiotypes in IVIG preparations may neutralize the effects of circulating autoantibody and downregulate its production when id-anti-id dimers bind to FcR on B cells. It may also stimulate the formation of regulatory IgG (and IgM) anti-id antibodies.

Passive neutralization of antiphospholipid (APL) antibodies may result from id-anti-id interactions. IVIG preparations can neutralize lupus anticoagulant activity in vitro (19,20). In the experimental APL syndrome, induced by transfer of anticardiolipin antibodies to naive mice, IVIG treatment resulted in significantly less fetal resorptions than in untreated cohorts (21).

In vitro F(ab')$_2$ fragments present in IVIG preparations neutralized and/or inhibited antigen binding to antibodies to factor VIII, group IIb/IIIa surface antigen on platelets, double-stranded deoxyribonucleic acid (dsDNA), thyroglobulin, intrinsic factor, myeloperoxidase, and anti-neutrophil cytoplasmic antigen (ANCA) (22–26). These disease-associated idiotypes are frequently dominant and cross-reactive, and recognize molecules that have been evolutionarily conserved (27,28). Affinity columns of sepharose bound IVIG F(ab')$_2$ fragments often selectively bind these autoantibodies in higher amounts than are measured in patients' sera (29,30). Several authors have reported the presence of anti-id antibodies in sera of patients in remission (31), suggesting that IVIG administration may restore a more normal pattern of serum autoantibody levels (32,33).

Clinical observations following IVIG treatment in myasthenia gravis, SLE, ANCA-positive vasculitides, Guillain-Barré syndrome, and anti–factor VIII autoimmune disease suggest that responders develop anti-idiotype antibodies specific to the implicated autoantibody (34,35). Silvestris and colleagues assayed 11 IVIG preparations and found high reactivity to anti-DNA-IgG-ids, predictive of nephritis, in two (36). Evans and Abdou showed that pooled IVIG preparations contained anti-id antibodies against anti-DNA antibodies which specifically inhibited binding of SLE sera to DNA but did not affect binding of antitetanus toxoid antibodies to tetanus toxoid (37). The anti-id antibody was eluted from anti-DNA affinity columns following depletion of anti-DNA, anti-Fc, and anti-F(ab')$_2$ portions of normal IgG. In vitro incubation of this anti-id antibody with PBMCs from SLE patients specifically downregulated spontaneous secretion of anti-DNA antibodies and had no effect on polyclonal IgG secretion (38).

Pooled IVIG preparations also contain anti-id antibodies to ANCA (35); inhibition of ANCA binding in vitro by IVIG F(ab')$_2$ fragments correlates with reported decreases in ANCA titers in patients with vasculitis following IVIG treatment (39,40). Transient increases in ANCA binding frequently occur during and immediately after IVIG infusions, followed by sustained decreases 10–40 days later, attributed to id anti-id regulation.

Similarly, specific downregulation of autoantibody production may account for the beneficial effects of IVIG treatment in patients with platelet and RBC alloimmunization. IVIG administration to 19 patients refractory to HLA-matched platelet

Table 4 Use of IVIG as Infection Prophylaxis

Hematological malignancies
   Chronic lymphocytic leukemia
   Multiple myeloma
   Low-grade B-cell lymphoma
Immune deficiency following chemotherapy, irradiation
Prophylaxis of CMV infection
   Bone marrow transplantation
   Solid organ transplantation
   HIV infection
Prophylaxis in HIV-positive adults and children
Prophylaxis in renal insufficiency
Prophylaxis in hepatic failure
Prophylaxis in burns

transfusions resulted in prolonged platelet recoveries in 13, all of whom had decreased levels of platelet-associated immunoglobulin (41). IVIG has also been effective in allowing organ transplantation in patients highly sensitized to MHC class I antigens (42). Based in part on studies in the severe combined immunodeficiency disease (SCID hu) immune deficient mouse, induced IgM as well as IgG anti-id antibodies may regulate autoantibody production. Consistent with this hypothesis, increased levels of anti-id IgM antibodies have been reported following IVIG treatment of alloimmunization, SLE, and vasculitis (42,43).

The salutory effects of IVIG therapy in primary and acquired immune deficiencies has in part been attributed to specific neutralization of common infectious antigens (Table 4). Evidence to support a similar role in autoimmune disease treatment has been lacking, despite a commonly held belief that KD is of infectious etiology. Recently, Takei at al. published in vitro data indicating the presence of high-titer antibodies to staphylococcal superantigens in commercial preparations of IVIG, capable of inhibiting T-cell responses (44).

MECHANISMS ATTRIBUTABLE TO Fc-
AND F(ab')₂-DEPENDENT INTERACTIONS

In vitro data from early use of IVIG preparations suggested that it solubilized tissue-bound or circulating immune complexes. Recently, less importance has been attributed to this mechanism, although clinical observations support its occurrence. Tomino demonstrated that incubation of renal biopsy specimens with human sera or IVIG solubilized intraglomerular deposits of IgG immune complexes, attributing clinical benefit in SLE to this effect (45). Subsequently, IVIG administration improved creatinine clearance and decreased proteinuria in a series of nine SLE patients with renal disease refractory to steroids and cytoxan; in vitro incubation with IVIG resulted in dissociation of glomerular deposits (46). Following IVIG therapy, Akashi and Jordan, respectively, reported dramatic improvement in two patients with SLE and one with Stevens-Johnson syndrome (47,48). However, in a series of six SLE patients with cytopenias or renal and/or cutaneous manifestations, in vivo evidence of decreased C1q binding of immune complexes failed to correlate with clinical improvement after treatment with IVIG (49). Schifferli reported transient but asymptomatic increases in serum creatinine in eight patients with SLE following IVIG administration; only two had impairment of renal function prior to treatment (50). Others have also observed exacerbation of lupus nephritis despite initial dramatic improvement (51,52). Although data are anecdotal, worsened renal disease in patients with SLE may occur due to enhanced immune complex formation; IVIG infusions must therefore be utilized with caution.

Leung et al. reported increased numbers of circulating activated T cells and spontaneous IgG and IgM secretion in patients with KD, which decreased after treatment in the first controlled trial of IVIG (53). During the acute phase of the disease, IL-1, TNF-α, IFN-γ, and IL-6 levels were elevated, which was associated with activation of vascular endothelial cells and upregulation of E selectin expression (54,55). Furukawa et al. reported that elevations of soluble (or circulating) ICAM-1 correlated with the presence of coronary artery disease in KD (56); flow cytometry indicated that activated T cells were temporarily removed from the peripheral circulation (57). Together, these data indicate that IVIG administration reduces inflammatory cytokine secretion, endothelial cell activation, and adhesion molecule expression, thereby preventing further vascular damage.

Modulation of cytokine secretion may be a primary or secondary effect. Several investigators have reported downmodulation of monocyte secretion of the proinflammatory cytokines—IL-6, IL-1, TNF-α, and IL-2—after in vitro incubation of PBMCS or stimulated macrophages with IVIG (58–60), which may explain its early beneficial effects in KD. Based on its salutory effects in multiple sclerosis (MS) and in animal models of autoimmunity, Achiron et al. hypothesized that IVIG exerts its therapeutic effect by inhibiting the consequences of T-cell activation, such as TNF-α production (61). Bendtzen et al. first reported the presence of naturally occurring autoantibodies to IL-1 in sera from normal individuals (62), another possible means for IVIG regulation of cytokine secretion. Recent publications have reported rapid increases in plasma levels of IL-1 receptor antagonist and soluble TNF-α receptors as well as IL-6, IL-8, IFN-γ, and/or TNF-α following IVIG infusion in patients with primary hypogammaglobulinemia or secondary epilepsy (63,64), suggesting agonistic as well as antagonistic effects on cytokine secretion.

The variable region-dependent immunomodulatory effects of IVIG do not appear to be restricted to B-cell activation and function. IVIG preparations contain antibodies to the first complementarity-determining region (cdr-1) of the T-cell receptor (TcR) Vb chain (65). Antibodies to these epitopes have been detected in patients with SLE and RA, as well as normal individuals, expression increased with age suggesting a naturally occurring mechanism that may regulate TcR expression and function (66). In a T-cell–dependent animal model of autoimmune uveitis, treatment with IVIG decreased specific autoantibody mediated T-cell proliferative responses and cytokine secretion (67). Soluble MHC classes I and II (including CD4) are present in IVIG preparations (68); these molecules may directly downmodulate specific T–B-cell interactions (69). In addition, IVIG preparations contain antibodies to the CD5 cell surface antigen (Ag), which may function to regulate B-cell production of auto-Abs (70).

Recent work suggests that IVIG infusions directly affect cell activation and proliferation. Van Schaik and others have demonstrated dose-dependent inhibition of antigen (MLR: mixed lymphocyte reactions) and mitogen (PHA and recombinant IL-2) stimulated proliferation of PBMCs and EBV-transformed cell lines following incubation with supraphysiologic concentrations of IVIG equivalent to current high-dose IV regimens (250–500 mg/kg body weight) (71–73). In PBMC cultures, in vitro exposure to IVIG reduced total immunoglobulin secretion, presumably by direct and indirect effects on B cells and antigen-presenting cells (74).

INCREASED CATABOLISM OF IgG

In patients with normal immunoglobulin levels, the fractional rate of IgG catabolism increases in direct proportion to its concentration in plasma. Following administration of high (400–500 mg/kg) doses of IVIG, plasma levels of IgG are estimated to reach ≥200% of normal. At these levels, the fractional catabolic rate may increases to 180%, and the half-life decrease from 21 to 12 days (75). Increased catabolism may explain some of the immediate effects of therapeutic IVIG infusions and why they been reported as effective as intensive plasmapheresis (with cyclophosphamide) in Guillain-Barré syndrome (76). Alterations in IgG catabolism and FcR expression and function presumably act synergistically with specific id-anti-id modulation of T- and B-cell responses.

DERMATOMYOSITIS EXAMPLE

In the Dalakas study of patients with dermatomyositis, repetitive muscle biopsies were performed in patients who demonstrated improvement in muscle strength. Although treatment was blinded, only the patients who received IVIG improved (77). Posttreatment biopsies revealed abundant deposits of IgG around muscle fibers and capillaries, suggesting that the Fc portion of administered IgG bound directly to FcR on vessel walls. CD8-positive T-cell inflammatory infiltrates resolved; MHC I expression, prominent on the periphery of muscle fascicles pretreatment, was barely detectable, as was ICAM-I on endothelial cells. Deposits of complement membrane attack complexes on capillaries and necrotic muscle fibers were absent after treatment. Regenerating muscle fibers, prominent before treatment, became sparse, and the mean number of capillaries increased. Following treatment with IVIG, in vitro uptake of C3 by sensitized RBCs was decreased in patients who responded (78). Together, these observations provide evidence that IVIG administration downregulates T-cell activation, cytokine secretion, vascular endothelial cell activation, and adhesion molecule expression, and prevents complement-mediated damage.

LONG-TERM IMMUNOMODULATORY EFFECTS

Prolonged effects have been reported following IVIG treatment, after serum levels of IgG and catabolism of exogenous immunoglobulin would have normalized, implying direct modulation of T and/or B cell function. In addition to Fc and id-anti-id–mediated mechanisms, interactions with other cell surface antigens presumably alter cytokine secretion, endothelial cell activation, and lymphocyte function. Multiple effects, both $F(ab')_2$ and Fc-dependent, described previously, may interact both acutely and over time. As clinical responses are variable across diseases, and in patients with similar disease manifestations, it is difficult to predict the benefit of IVIG administration in a given clinical situation. Further work in the context of randomized controlled clinical trials will be necessary to better define the efficacy and mechanism of IVIG treatment in autoimmune diseases. Nonetheless, data strongly suggest that high-dose administration can actively modulate immune responses as well as passively neutralize autoantibody-induced effects.

PROPHYLACTIC USE OF IVIG IN ACQUIRED IMMUNE DEFICIENCIES

Following use as replacement therapy in patients with primary antibody deficiencies, high-dose IVIG administration has prevented infection in individuals with acquired immune deficiencies in the setting of hematological malignancies, solid tumors following intensive chemotherapy and/or irradiation, chronic renal or hepatic insufficiency, burns, HIV infection, and transplantation (Table 4).

Cytomegalovirus (CMV) infections can be a serious complication following bone marrow and organ transplantation, and in AIDS. Because subclinical infection is so pervasive in the general population, clinical disease may rapidly occur in the setting of immunosuppression due to reactivation of latent infection or transplantation of CMV-positive tissue into a seronegative host. Although primary efforts are concentrated on preventing transmission of CMV to seronegative recipients, hyperimmune Ig and IVIG are routinely utilized as prophylactic treatment. Clinical effects have not correlated with titers of CMV antibodies, and preference for CMV hyperimmune globulin vs. IVIG preparations remains controversial. Transplant recipients who are seropositive for CMV have a greater incidence of infection; prophylactic treatment with IVIG has decreased the occurrence of interstitial pneumonitis (79). In CMV seronegative recipients, IVIG administration has reduced the incidence not only of CMV infections, but also of acute GvHD. In a randomized controlled multicenter trial, regular administration of IVIG to patients with chronic lymphocytic leukemia (CLL) decreased the incidence of moderate infections (80). Currently, it is recommended to administer IVIG to patients with low-grade B-cell malignancies (CLL, lymphoma, multiple myeloma) if they have low levels of antibodies to pneumococcal capsular polysaccharides or serum IgG or have survived a severe infection (81,82).

Although adult patients with HIV infection frequently have hyperglobulinemia, defects in T-cell function and antibody synthesis are well documented. Children with AIDS have poor primary antibody responses and suffer from infections similar to children born with primary hypogammaglobulinemia. Despite results of several small uncontrolled series indicating successful prophylaxis against viral and bacterial (but not opportunistic) infections in children and adults, an NIH-sponsored trial in children with AIDS failed to show benefit (83). Because zidovudine was not routinely administered, its findings remain controversial. Use of IVIG is still advocated in children with AIDS; further trials will be necessary to define whether IVIG has a therapeutic role in HIV infection in both children and adults.

Although IVIG treatment offers prophylaxis against infection because of passive administration of antibodies to common organisms, additional effects are believed to mediate benefit (84) (Table 5). In early or persistent low-grade infection IVIG may neutralize infectious antigens and superantigens; prevent viral and bacterial antigen binding to complement and/or target cells; increase opsonization; and remove circulating immune complexes in antigen excess. Many of the id-anti-id mechanisms leading to

Table 5 Effects of IVIG Administration in Infections

Binding and neutralization of infectious Ag, toxins
Restore normal levels of Ab to common organisms
Blockade of binding of viruses and bacteria to target cells
Neutralizing Abs vs. superantigens
Increased opsonization
PMN function requires normal levels of IgG
C3 + Fd of IgG = complex that acts as superopsonin
Increased NK and bone marrow macrophage function
Removal of circulating ICs in Ag excess which are immunosuppressive
Reduction in inflammatory cytokine levels

downregulation of cytokine secretion, endothelial cell activation and lymphocyte function, which are hypothesized to improve autoimmune disease, may also prevent infection or lessen its consequences.

CONCLUSIONS

IVIG administration may be effective in the treatment of a variety of autoimmune diseases and as prophylaxis against viral and bacterial infections in certain settings of acquired immune deficiency. Data to explain its benefit are largely derived from uncontrolled studies in small numbers of patients and in vitro data which may poorly predict in vivo effects. High doses of IVIG are hypothesized to modulate T- and B-cell function indirectly through Fc and $F(ab')_2$-dependent mechanisms and directly by alterations in cell surface antigen expression, inflammatory cytokine secretion, endothelial cell activation, adhesion molecule expression, and lymphocyte activation and function. Although well tolerated, IVIG therapy is expensive. Further work in the context of randomized controlled clinical trials will be necessary to better define its therapeutic role in treating autoimmune diseases and infection in acquired immune deficiencies.

REFERENCES

1. Hurez V, Kaveri SV, Kazatchkine NLD. Expression and control of IgG autoreactivity in normal human serum. Eur J Immunol 1993; 23:783–789.
2. Imbach P. Immune thrombocytopenic purpura and intravenous immunoglobulin. Cancer 1991; 68:1422–1425.
3. Dietrich G, Algiman M, Sultan Y, Nydegger UE, Kazatchkine M. Origin of anti-idiotypic activity against anti factor VIII autoantibodies in pools of normal human immunoglobulin G (IVIG). Blood 1992; 79:2946–2951.
4. Lin R, Racis S. In vivo reduction of circulating C1q binding immune complexes by intravenous gammaglobulin administration. Int Arch Allergy Appl Immunol 1986; 79:286–290.
5. Basta M, Kirshborn P, Frank MM, Fries LF. Mechanism of therapeutic effects of high dose intravenous immunoglobulin: alteration of acute, complement-dependent immune damage in a guinea pig model. J Clin Invest 1989; 84:1974–1981.
6. Basta M, Fries LP, Frank MM. High doses of intravenous Ig inhibit in vitro uptake of C4 fragments onto sensitized erythrocytes. Blood 1991; 77:376–380.

7. Frank M, Basta M, Fries L. The effects of intravenous immune globulin on complement-dependent immune damage of cells and tissues. Clin Immunol Immunopathol 1992; 62:S82–S86.
8. Ballow M. Mechanisms of action of intravenous imune serum globulin therapy. Pediatr Infect Dis J 1994; 13:806–811.
9. Gelfand E. Treatment of autoimmune diseases with intravenous immune globulin. Sem Heamtol 1992; 29:127–33.
10. Dwyer J. Manipulating the immune system with immune globulin. N Engl J Med 1992; 326:107–116.
11. Rosen F. Putative mechanisms of the effect of intravenous gamma-globulin. Clin Immunol Immunopathol 1993; 67:S41–S43.
12. Fehr J, Hofmann V, Kappeler V. Transient reversal of thrombocytopenia in ITP by high dose intravenous gamma globulin. N Engl J Med 1982; 306:1254–1258.
13. Clarkson S, Bussel J, Kimberly R, Valinsky J, Nachman R, Unkeless J. Treatment of refractory ITP with anti Fc gamma receptor antibody. N Engl J Med 1986; 314:1236–1239.
14. Sheth K, Al-Sedairy S, Lee J. Effectiveness of intravenous immune globulin preparations in prevention of phagocytosis of anti-Rh-D-coated erythrocytes by mononuclear phagocytes. Vox Sang 1993; 65:190–193.
15. Engelhard D, Waner JL, Kapoor N, Good RA. Effect of intravenous immune globulin on NK cell activity: possible association with autoimmune neutropenia and idiopathic thrombocytopenia. J Pediatr 1986; 108:77–81.
16. Finberg R, Newburger J, Mikati M, Heller A, Burns J. Effect of high doses of intravenously administered immune globulin on natural killer cell activity in peripheral blood. J Pediatr 1992; 120:376–380.
17. Saulsbury F. The effect of intravenous immune globulin on lymphocyte populations in children with Kawasaki syndrome. Clin Exp Rheumatol 1992; 10:617–620.
18. Rich R. Intravenous IgG: supertherapy for superantigens? [editorial; comment]. J Clin Invest 1993; 91:378.
19. Said P, Martinuzzo M, Carreras L. Neutralization of lupus anticoagulant activity by human immunolglobulin in vitro. Nouv Rev Fr Hematol 1992; 34:37–42.
20. Matsuda J, Gohchi K, Kawasugi K, Tsukamoto M, Saitoh N, Kinoshita T. In vitro lupus anticoagulant neutralizing activity of intravenous immunoglobulin (letter). Thromb Res 1993; 70:190–10.
21. Bakimer R, Guilburd B, Zurgil N, Shoenfeld Y. The effect of intravenous gamma-globulin on the induction of experimental antiphospholipid syndrome. Clin Immunol Immunopathol 1993; 69:97–102.
22. Kaveri S, Dietrich G, Hurez V, Kazatchkine M. Intravenous immune globulin in the treatment of autoimmune diseases. Clin Exp Immunol 1991; 86:192–198.
23. Kaveri S, Dietrich G, Kazatchkine M. Can intravenous immunoglobulin treatment regulate autoimmune responses? Semin Hematol 1992;29(3 suppl 2):64–71.
24. Kaveri S, Mouthon L, Kazatchkine M. Immunomodulating effects of intravenous immunoglobulin in autoimmune and inflammatory diseases. J Neuro Neurosurg Psych 1994; 57(suppl):6–8.
25. Kaveri S, Want H, Rowen D, Kazatchkine M, Kohler H. Monoclonal anti-idiotypic antibodies against human anti-thyroglobulin autoantibodies recognize idiotopes shared by disease associated and natural anti-thyroglobulin autoantibodies. Clin Immunol Immunopathol 1993; 69:333–340.
26. Pall AA, Varagunam V, Adu D, Smith N et al: Anti idiotypic activity against anti myeloperoxidase antibodies in pooled human immunoglobulin. Clin Exp Immunol 1994; 59:257–262.
27. Dietrich G, Kazatchkine M. Normal immunoglobulin G (IgG) for therapeutic use (intravenous Ig) contain antiidiotypic specificities against an immunodominant, disease-associated, cross-reactive idiotype of human anti-thyroglobulin autoantibodies. Clin Invest 1990; 85:620–626.

28. Kaveri S, Want H, Rowen D, Kazatchkine M, Kohler H. Monoclonal anti-idiotypic anti-bodies against human anti-thyroglobulin autoantibodies recognize idiotopes shared by disease associated and natural anti-thyroglobulin autoantibodies. Clin Immunol Immunopathol 1993; 69:333–340.

29. Dietrich G, Kaveri S, Kazatchkine M. A V region connected autoreactive subfraction of normal human immunoglobulin G. Eur J Immunol 1992; 22:1701–1706.

30. Ronda N, Haury M, Nobrega A, Coutinho A, Kazatchkine M. Selectivity of recognition of variable (V) regions of autoantibodies by intravenous immunoglobulin. Clin Immunol Immunopathol 1994; 70:124–128.

31. Sultan T, Kazatchkine MD, Malsonneuve P, Nydegger UE. Anti-idiotypic suppression of autoantibodies to factor VIII (antihemophilic factor) by high-dose intravenous gammaglobulin. Lancet 1984; 2:765–768.

32. Hurez V, Kaveri SV, Kazatchkine MD. Normal polyspecific immunoglobulin G (IVIG) in the treatment of autoimmune disease. J Autoimmun 1993; 6:675–681.

33. Rossi F, Kazatchkine MD. Antiidiotypes against autoantibodies in pooled human polyspecific IG. J Immunol 1989; 143: 4104–4109.

34. Kaveri S, Dietrich G, Kazatchkine M. Can intravenous immunoglobulin treatment regulate autoimmune responses? Semin Hematol 1992; 29(3 suppl 2):64–71.

35. Rossi F, Jayne D, Lockwood C, Kazatchkine M. Anti-idiotypes against anti-neutrophil cytoplasmic antigen autoantibodies in normal human polyspecific IgG for therapeutic use and in the remission sera of patients with systemic vasculitis. Clin Exp Immunol 1991; 83:298–303.

36. Silvestris F, Cafforio P, Dammacco F. Pathogenic anti-DNA idiotype-reactive IgG in IVIG preparations. Clin Exp Immunol 1994; 97:19–25.

37. Evans M. Detection and purification of antiidiotypic antibody against anti-DNA in intravenous immune globulin. J Clin Immunol 1991; 11:291–295.

38. Evans M, Abdou N. In vitro modulation of anti-DNA secreting peripheral blood mononuclear cells of lupus patients by anti-idiotypic antibody of pooled human intravenous immune globulin. Lupus 1993; 2:371–375.

39. Jayne D, Esnault V, Lockwood C. ANCA anti-idiotype antibodies and the treatment of systemic vasculitis with intravenous immunoglobulin. J Autoimmun 1993; 6:207–219.

40. Jayne D, Lockwood C. Pooled intravenous immunoglobulin in the management of systemic vasculitis. Adv Exp Med Biol 1993; 336:469–72.

41. Ziegler A, Shadduck R, Rosenfeld CS. High dose IVIG improves response to single donor platelets in patients refractory to platelet transfusion. Blood 1987; 70:1433–1439.

42. Tyan D, Li V, Czer L, Trento A, Jordan SC. Differential inhibition of anti-HLA lymphocytotoxic antibody activity by pooled human gamma globulin. Transplantation 1994; 57:553–562.

43. Jordan SC, Toyoda M. Treatment of autoimmune diseases and systemic vasculitis with pooled human intravenous immune globulin. Clin Exp Immunol 1994; 97(suppl):31–38.

44. Takei S, Arora YK, Walker SM: Intravenous immunoglobulin contains specific antidies inhibitory to activation of T cells by staphylococcal toxin superantigens. J Clin Invest 1993; 91:602–607.

45. Tomino Y, Sakai H, Takaya M, et al. Solubilization of intraglomerular deposits of IgG immune complexes by human sera or gamma globulin in patients with lupus nephritis. Clin Exp Immunol 1984; 58:42–48.

46. Lin C-V, Hsu H-C, Chiang H. Improvement of histological and immunological change in steroid and immunosuppressive drug resistant lupus nephritis by high dose intravenous gamma globulin. Nephron 1989; 53:303–310.

47. Akashi K, Nagasawa K, Mayumi T, Yokota E, Ochi N, Kusaba T. Successful treatment of refractory SE with intravenous immunoglobulins. J Rheumatol 1990; 17:375–379.

48. Jordan SC. Remarkable benefit in a patient with Stevens Johnson syndrome. Unpublished report.

49. Lin R, Racis S. In vivo reduction of circulating C1q binding immune complexes by intravenous gammaglobulin administration. Int Arch Allergy Appl Immunol 1986; 79:286–290.
50. Schifferli J, Leski M, Favre H, Imbach P, Nydegger U, Davies K. High dose intravenous IgG treatment and renal function. Lancet 1991; 337:457–458.
51. Barron K, Sher M. Intravenous immunoglobulin therapy: magic or black magic. J Rheumatol 1992; 19:94–97.
52. Winder A, Molad Y, Ostfeld I, Kenet G, Pinkhas J, Sidi Y. Treatment of systemic lupus erythematosus by prolonged administration of high dose intravenous immunoglobulin: report of 2 cases. J Rheumatol 1993; 20:495–498.
53. Leung D, Burns J, Newburger J, Geha R. Reversal of lymphocyte activation in vivo in the Kawasaki syndrome by intravenous gammaglobulin. J Clin Invest 1987; 79:468–472.
54. Leung D, Kurt-Jones E, Newburger J, Cotran R, Burns J, Pober J. Endothelial. cell activation and high interleukin-1 secretion in the pathogenesis of acute Kawasaki disease Lancet 1989; 1298–1302.
55. Leung D. The immunoregulatory effects of intravenous immune globulin in Kawasaki disease and other autoimmune diseases. In: Ballow M, ed. IVIG Therapy Today. 1992: 93–104.
56. Furukawa S, Khozoh I, Matsubara T, et al. Increased levels of circulating ICAM-1 in Kawasaki disease. Arth Rheum 1992; 35:672–677.
57. Furukawa S, Matsubara T, Tsuji K, Okumura K, Yabuta K. Transient depletion of T cells with bright CD11a/CD18 expression from peripheral circulation during acute Kawasaki disease. Scand J Rheumatol 1993; 31:377–380.
58. Andersson IP, Andersson UG, Human intravenous immunoglobulin modulates monokine production in vitro. Immunology 1990; 71:372–376.
59. Shimozato T, Iwata M, Kawada H, Tamura N. Human immunoglobulin preparations for intravenous use induces elevation of cellular cyclic adenosine 3'5' monophosphate levels, resulting in suppression of TNFα and IL-1 production. Immunology 1991; 72:497–501.
60. Toyoda M, Zhang Z-M, Petrosian A, Galera O, Wang S-J, Jordan SC. Modulation of immunoglobulin production and cytookine MRNA expression in peripheral blood mononuclear cells by IVIG, J Clin Immunol 1994; 14:178–189.
61. Achiron A, Margalit R, Hershkoviz R, et al. Intravenous immunoglobulin treatment of experimental T cell-mediated autoimmune disease. Upregulation of T cell proliferation and downregulation of TNFα secretion. J Clin Invest 1994; 93:600–605.
62. Svenson M, Hansen MB, Bendtzen K. Distribution and characterization of autoantibodies to IL-1a in normal human sera. Scand J Immunol 1990; 32:695–701.
63. Aukrust P, Froland P, Liabakk N-B et al. Release of cytokines, soluble cytokine receptors, and interleukin-1 receptor antagonist after IVIG administration in vivo. Blood 1994; 84:2136–2143.
64. Ling Z, Yeoh E, Webb B, Farrell K, Doucette J, Matheson D. Intravenous immunoglobulin induces interferon-gamma and interleukin-6 in vivo. J Clin Immunol 1993; 13:302–309.
65. Marchalonis JJ, Kaymaz H, Schluter SF, Yocum DE. Human autoantibodies to a synthetic putative T cell receptor B chain regulatory idiotype: expression in autoimmunity and aging. Exp Clin Immunogenet 1993; 10:1–15.
66. Marchalonis JJ, Schluter SF, Wang E, et al. Synthetic autoantigens of immunoglobulins and T cell receptors: their recognition in aging, infection and autoimmunity. PSEBM 1994; 207:129–147.
67. Saoudi A, Hurez V, deKozak Y, et al. Human immunoglobulin preparations for intravenous use prevent experimental autoimmune uveoretinitis. Int Immunol 1993; 5:1559–1567.
68. Santoso S. Quantitation of soluble HLA class I antigen in human albumin and immunoglobulin preparations for IV use by solid phase immunoassay. Vox Sang 1992; 62:29–33.
69. Blasczyk R, Westhoff U, Grosse-Wilde H. Soluble CD4, CD8, and HLA molecules in commercial immunoglobulin preparations. Lancet 1993; 341:789–790.
70. Vassilev T, Gelin C, Kaveri S, Zilber M, Boumsell L, Kazatchkine M. Antibodies to the

CD5 molecule in normal human immunoglobulins for therapeutic use. Clin Exp Immunol 1993; 92:369–372.

71. vanSchaik I, Lundkvist I, Vermeulen M, Brand A. Polyvalent immunoglobulin for intravenous use interferes with cell proliferation in vitro. J Clin Immunol 1992; 12:325–334.

72. Klaesson S, Ringden O, Markling L, Remberger M, Lundkvist I. Immune modulatory effects of immunoglobulins on cell-mediated immune responses in vitro. Scand J Immunol 1993; 38:477–484.

73. Sbrana S, Ruocco L, Vnacore R, Azzara A, Ambrogi F. In vitro effects of an immunoglobulin preparation for intravenous use on T-cell activation. Allerg Immunol (Paris) 1993; 25:35–37.

74. Kondo N, Ozawa T, Musihake K, et al. Suppression of immunoglobulin production of lymphocytes by intravenous immunoglobulin. J Clin Immunol 1991; 11:152–158.

75. Masson PL. Elimination of infectious antigens and increases of IgG catabolism as possible modes of action of IVIG. J Autoimmun 1993; 6:683–689.

76. vanderMeche FGA, Schmitz PIM, Group tDG-BS. A randomized controlled trial comparing intravenous immune globulin and plasma exchange in Guillain Barre syndrome. N Engl J Med 1992; 326:1123–1129.

77. Dalakas M, Illa I, Dambrosia J, et al. A controlled trial of high dose intravenous immune globulin infusions as treatment for dermatomyositis. N Engl J Med 1993; 329:1993–2000.

78. Basta M, Dalakas MC. High dose Intravenous immunoglobulin exerts its beneficial effect in patients with dermatomyositis by blocking endomysial deposition of activated complement fragments. J Clin Invest 1994; 94:1729–1735.

79. Sullivan KM, Kopecky KJ, Jocom J, et al. Immunomodulatory and antimicrobial efficacy of IVIG in bone marrow transplantation. N Engl J Med 1990; 323:705–712.

80. Cooperative Group for the Study of Immunoglobulin in CLL. Intravenous immunoglobulin for the presentation of infection in CLL, a randomized controlled clinical trial. N Engl J Med 1988; 319:902–907.

81. Griffiths H, Lea J, Bunch C, Lee M, Chapel H. Predictors of infection in chronic lymphocytic leukemia. Clin Exp Immunol 1992; 89:374.

82. Chapel HM, Lee M, Hargreaves R, et al. Randomized trial of IVIG as prophylaxis against infection in plateau phase multiple myeloma. Lancet 1994; 343:1059–1063.

83. National Institute of Child Heath and Human Development IVIG Study Group. IVIG for the prevention of bacterial infections in children with sympotmatic HIV infection. N Engl J Med 1991; 325:73–80.

84. Hammarstrom L, Gardulf A, Hammarstrom V, et al. Systemic and topical immunoglobulin treatment in immunocompromised patients. Immunol Rev 1994; 139:43–70.

4

Production and Properties of Intravenous Immunoglobulins

John A. Hooper
BioCatalyst Consultants, Liberty, Missouri

INTRODUCTION

In the past 15 years, the number of clinical applications of intravenous immunoglobulin (IVIG) has grown far beyond expectations. Originally intended to supply antibodies to patients with primary immunodeficiency disorders who are antibody-deficient, IVIGs have been found to benefit many other types of patients. This is because IVIG contains thousands of different antibodies, each of which may have the potential to produce a clinical effect.

Because the concentration of any single antibody in a "normal" IVIG preparation is relatively low, high doses are required for clinical efficacy. The combination of high doses and expanding clinical applications has made the cost of IVIG therapy a health care issue.

The purpose of this review is to describe how commercial IVIGs are produced and to discuss differences in products that might have a clinical impact. This review will describe procedures that eliminate viruses during IVIG manufacture and will summarize the virus reduction data available for commercial IVIG preparations.

COLD ETHANOL FRACTIONATION

The process used to fractionate large volumes of human plasma was developed in the early 1940s by E. J. Cohn and his co-workers in the Department of Physical Chemistry at Harvard Medical School (1). Although originally intended to produce albumin solutions for use as a blood substitute during World War II, the Cohn fractionation procedure has proven to be useful in the large-scale separation of classes of therapeutic plasma proteins (2,3).

The cold ethanol fractionation process as developed by Cohn is generally used to produce three protein fractions: an IgG concentrate, an intermediate in the production of coagulation factors VII and IX, and human serum albumin. Albumin is the only fraction that does not require additional purification prior to use in humans. The proteins in the other fractions must be isolated by additional purification procedures or must be subjected to other special processes.

INTRAMUSCULAR IMMUNOGLOBULINS

IgG produced by cold ethanol fractionation is suitable for intramuscular or subcutaneous injections and is an intermediate in IVIG production. Most manufacturers use essentially the same method (1,2). However, a modified cold ethanol fractionation process developed by Kistler and Nitschmann is used by several European fractionators (4).

When the process is controlled carefully, Cohn fractionation produces an IgG fraction with a purity greater than 97% (w/w) (5). Since it was designed to obtain high yields, the Kistler-Nitschmann process produces an IgG fraction that contains higher levels of impurities (4).

Contaminants of these IgG fractions include IgA, IgM, albumin, prekallikrein activator, prekallikrein, activated coagulation factors (especially XIa), complement proteins, plasmin, and plasminogen. Despite their relatively low levels, many of these contaminants can produce adverse reactions during intravenous infusion (5). Moreover, plasmin and plasminogen are responsible for the production of IgG fragments that correlate with reductions in antibody activities during production and storage of immunoglobulin preparations (6,7).

Historically, the IgG produced by cold ethanol fractionation was freeze-dried to remove the ethanol and to produce a stable intermediate fraction. However, freeze-drying IgG in the presence of ethanol promotes the formation of IgG aggregates at the expense of IgG monomer (5). The relationship between IgG aggregates and side reactions from IV infusions of immunoglobulins has been the topic of many discussions (3,5,8).

Intramuscular immunoglobulin (IMIG) is usually formulated at a protein concentration of 165 mg/ml and contains 0.3 M glycine, 0.9 % (w/v) sodium chloride, and 0.1 g/L merthiolate. IMIG solutions are adjusted to pH 6.8 ± 0.4 and are stored as solutions at 5 °C. With time, IMIG preparations tend to develop precipitates and/or relatively large particles. This physical instability is caused by the natural tendency of purified IgG in solution at neutral pH to form aggregates.

INTRAVENOUS IMMUNOGLOBULINS

Virtually all commercial IVIGs are produced from large pools of human plasma by first using a cold ethanol fractionation process. However, the IgG concentrate obtained by plasma fractionation must be subjected to additional processing to produce material for IV injection. The processes used after cold ethanol fractionation differ from product to product and have a substantial impact on the differences observed between IVIG products.

In 1962, spontaneous complement activation (anticomplement activity) by IgG aggregates was proposed as the principal cause of adverse side reactions when IMIG was injected intravenously (8). The terms "anticomplement activity" and "aggregates" came to be used interchangeably, and hemolytic tests for anticomplement activity became routine tests of IVIG safety.

The desire to eliminate anticomplement activity had a significant impact on the development of commercial IVIG preparations (3,5). Many IVIG manufacturing procedures reduced anticomplement activity by enzymatic digestion or chemical modification. Early enzymatic processes utilized pepsin, a nonspecific protease which hydrolyzes proteins at many different sites and produces $(Fab')_2$ as the principal IgG fragment (9,10).

To preserve more of the IgG in its intact biologically active form, some IVIG manufacturers began to limit enzymatic digestions by reducing the amount of pepsin added to the IgG solution (8). Others used the more specific enzyme plasmin which hydrolyzes IgG at fewer sites and produces Fab and Fc fragments (11).

Later, several plasma fractionation companies developed IVIG products in which anticomplement activities were suppressed by chemical modification. The goal of chemical modification was to reduce anticomplement activity without producing any IgG fragments. By reacting with amino acids in the Fc region of the IgG molecule, modified IVIG products were obtained which were structurally intact and were low in anticomplement activity (12–14).

Proteolytic digestion and chemical modification of IgG to suppress spontaneous complement activation had several unintended consequences. Complement activation by antigen-antibody complexes plays an important role in the killing of encapsulated bacteria by leukocytes (15). It is also likely that antibodies with chemically and physically altered Fc regions are rapidly removed from the circulation by the reticuloendothelial system. Thus, antibodies in enzyme-digested and chemically modified IVIGs have been shown to have reduced bacterial opsonizing activities (16–21) and shortened circulating half-lives (22–25).

Table 1 lists 39 commercial IVIG preparations that are sold in the United States, Europe, or Japan. Eighteen products are produced by treating the IgG obtained by cold ethanol precipitation with proteolytic enzymes or with chemicals that bind irreversibly to the IgG molecule. The other products are produced by a wide variety of processes, many of which provide additional purity.

Thirteen of the IVIG products listed in Table 1 are produced using additional purification procedures. Ion exchange adsorption with diethylaminoethyl (DEAE) chromatography media is used by several manufacturers to purify the IgG obtained by cold alcohol fractionation. One manufacturer utilizes a carboxymethyl (CM) ion exchange adsorption process. Another purification step involves fractional precipitation with polyethylene glycol.

Seven IVIGs are made by alcohol fractionation and diafiltration to remove alcohol. One IVIG is produced directly from plasma by DEAE column chromatography without prior fractionation with alcohol.

Of the IVIGs listed in Table 1, 14 are formulated as solutions and 25 are freeze-dried. Historically, IVIGs were freeze-dried to obtain an IgG preparation that would be stable for 2–3 years. Purified IgG solutions formulated at neutral pH are physically unstable and after a period of time (hours to days) will precipitate and form visible particles.

In 1986, McCue and co-workers reported on the development of a stable IVIG solution (26). This product represented a major advance in IVIG product formulation. There were two key elements in the development of this product: (1) adjustment of the pH to 4.25 to obtain a clear, physically stable IgG solution; and (2) the realization that patients might tolerate IgG solutions formulated at a pH significantly lower than the customary range of 6.4–7.2.

Thirty-one of the IVIGs listed in Table 1 are produced from plasma obtained from "unselected" donors. The term "unselected" is used to designate plasma donations obtained at random. Normal, or standard, IVIG produced from such plasma contains

Table 1 Commercial IVIG Preparations

Type of IgG process	Trade name(s)	Manufacturer	Country	Plasma	State
Pepsin digestion	Gamma F	Japan Red Cross	Japan	U	D
	Globulin V	Centeon (Armour)	Japan	U	D
	Glovenin	Nichiyaku	Japan	U	D
	Immunoglobulin IV	Kaketsuken	Japan	U	D
Pepsin digestion, heat plasmin digestion	Gamma-Venin P	Centeon (Hoechst)	Japan	U	D
	Merieux-VG	Merieux	Japan	U	D
	Venoglobulin	Green Cross Corp.	Japan	U	D
Pepsin treatment, pH 4	Sandoglobulin, Sanglopor	Swiss Red Cross	Switzerland	U	D
	pH 4 Polyvalentes	Biotransfusion	France	U	D
	Immunoglobulin IV	Blood Transfusion Service	Scotland	U	D
	Immunoglobulin IV	Netherlands Red Cross	Netherlands	U	D
Sulfonation	Venimmun	Centeon (Hoechst)	Germany	U	D
	Venilon	Kaketsuken	Japan	U	L
β-Propiolactonation	Intraglobin	Biotest	Germany	U	L
	Cytotect	Biotest	Germany	S	L
	Varitect	Biotest	Germany	S	L
	Pentaglobin	Biotest	Germany	U	L
	Hepatect	Biotest	Germany	S	L
Trypsin, PEG, DEAE	Endobulin, Iveegam	Immuno AG	Austria	U	D
DEAE, S/D	Gammonativ N	Pharmacia-Upjohn (Kabi)	Sweden	U	D
	Immunoglobulin IV	BPL	England	U	D

Method	Product	Manufacturer	Country		
DEAE, S/D, diafiltration	Gammagard S/D	Baxter	US	U	D
	Polygam S/D	Baxter (for ARC)	US	U	D
PEG, DEAE, heat	Alphaglobin, Flebogamma	Green Cross Corp.	Spain	U	L
	Venoglobulin IH	Green Cross Corp.	Japan	U	L
PEG, DEAE, S/D	Venoglobulin S	Green Cross Corp. (Alpha)	US	U	L
PEG, DEAE	Venoglobulin I	Green Cross Corp.	Japan, US	U	D
	Glovenin I	Nihon Seiyaku	Japan	U	D
PEG, HES	Globulin N	Centeon (Armour)	Japan	U	D
CM ion exchange	Globuman	Swiss Serum and Vaccine Inst.	Switzerland	U	D
PEG, caprylate, DEAE, heat	Nordimmun	Novo Nordisk	Denmark	U	D
Diafiltration, heat	Gammar P IV	Centeon (Armour)	US	U	D
Diafiltration, pH 4.25	Gamimune N, Polyglobin N	Bayer	US	U	L
	Psomaglobin	Bayer	Germany	S	L
	Cytoglobin	Bayer	Germany	S	L
Diafiltration, pH 4, S/D	Octagam	Octapharma	Austria	U	L
Diafiltration, S/D	CytoGam	Mass. Public Health Labs	US	S	D
Diafiltration, S/D	RespiGam	Mass. Public Health Labs	US	S	L
DEAE column, S/D	WinRho SD	RH Pharmaceuticals	Canada	S	D

U = unselected; S = selected; D = dried; L = liquid.

a wide variety of antibodies that represents the cumulative exposure of the donors to the environment. Except for antibodies stimulated by childhood or adult immunizations, the concentration of each antibody in normal IVIG is relatively low—i.e., on the order of nanograms to a few micrograms per milliliter.

Nine products listed in Table 1 are produced from "selected" donors or donations in which plasma is segregated on the basis of antibody content. These products are known as specific immunoglobulins (SIGs) and contain elevated levels of clinically relevant antibodies. SIGs, also known as hyperimmunes, are intended to provide greater clinical efficacy using relatively small doses of immunoglobulin. All of the SIGs in Table 1 are produced by testing donors or donations for high levels of naturally occurring antibodies. SIGs produced by vaccinating donors are currently being developed.

VIRUS REMOVAL DURING IVIG MANUFACTURE

Table 2 summarizes data on the removal of viruses during IVIG manufacturing processes. Cold ethanol fractionation has long been considered a process that inactivates and removes viruses during the manufacture of plasma proteins, especially immunoglobulins. In the 1970s, investigators demonstrated that hepatitis B virus (HBV) distributed to fractions I (fibrinogen), III (IgM), IV (coagulation proteins), and V (albumin) but not to fraction II (IgG) during Cohn fractionation (27,28). Some HBV inactivation was also demonstrated (28). In another study, a small amount of hepatitis B surface antigen was detected in fraction II (29).

In 1985, Piskiewicz and co-workers showed that HIV-1 is rapidly inactivated by cold 20% (v/v) ethanol (30). In 1986, Wells et al. demonstrated that Cohn fractionation of plasma to fraction II reduced the amount of infectious HIV-1 by more than 10^{15} in vitro infectious units per milliliter (31). A somewhat smaller reduction of HIV-1 was observed by Mitra and co-workers (32). However, these investigators also noted that HIV-1 levels were reduced $> 10^4$-fold in purified IgG solutions after 3 days at either pH 6.8 or pH 4.25 at a temperature of 27°C. The same results were obtained after an 8-h incubation at 45 °C (32).

In other studies, Henin and co-workers showed that HIV-1 was removed by the Kistler-Nitschmann fractionation procedure (33). The authors also confirmed the observation of Piskiewicz et al. (30) that HIV is inactivated by 20% (v/v) ethanol.

Recent experiments (34) using the polymerase chain reaction (PCR) to measure hepatitis C virus (HCV) ribonucleic acid demonstrated that cold ethanol fractionation removes much HCV RNA by partitioning. Although most HCV RNA was found in cryoprecipitate, fraction I, and fraction III, some PCR reactive material was detected in fraction II (34). In a subsequent study, complete elimination of HCV antibodies from plasma pools was shown to increase the proportion of HCV RNA that distributed to fraction II (35). Removal of HCV antibodies by the multiantigen screening test also correlated with the appearance of HCV RNA in the final product of an IVIG preparation (36).

Virus elimination processes fall into two main categories—partitioning and inactivating. Virus removal by partitioning may occur when virus particles are precipitated along with proteins into discard fractions or when they are adsorbed during clarification filtration procedures that use a finely divided solid as a filter aid. Virus inactivation may occur during heating, freeze-drying, pH adjustment to high or low values, incubation with organic solvents, treatment with detergents, chemical modification,

Table 2 Virus Elimination Data for IVIG Manufacturing Procedures

Virus	Model for	Process	Log reduction	Reference
HIV-1		Cohn-Oncley fractionation	> 5.9	Piszkiewitz (56)
HIV-1		Cohn-Oncley fractionation	> 15	Wells (31)
HIV-1		Cohn-Oncley fractionation	> 5	Mitra (32)
HIV-1		Cohn-Oncley fractionation	11	Uemura (57)
HIV-1		Cohn-Oncley fractionation	> 24.5	Baxter (53)
HIV-1		Cohn-Oncley fractionation	> 5.5	Octapharma (58)
HIV-1		Cohn-Oncley fractionation	> 16.1	Eriksson (59)
HIV-1		Kistler-Nitschmann fractionation	> 10	Hénin (33)
HIV-1		PEG precipitation/bentonite filtration	2	Uemura (57)
HIV-1		β-propiolactone	> 4.5	Prince (45)
HIV-1		Heat, 1 h, 60 °C	> 4.6	Uemura (57)
HIV-1		Heat, 0.5 h, 60 °C	> 5.7	Centeon (54)
HIV-1		Pepsin, pH 4, 16 h, 37 °C	> 6	Kempf (52)
HIV-1		pH 4, 16 h, 37 °C	> 6	Kempf (52)
HIV-1		pH 4, 24 h	> 5.5	Octapharma (58)
HIV-1		pH 4.25, 21 days, 20 °C	> 5.7	Bayer (60)
HIV-1		pH 6.8, 72 h, 27 °C	> 4.0	Mitra (32)
HIV-1		pH 6.8, 8 h, 45 °C	> 4.0	Mitra (32)
HIV-1		DEAE Sephadex adsorption	1.0	Piszkiewicz (56)
HIV-1		DEAE Sephadex adsorption	7.4	Massot (61)
HIV-1		Solvent-detergent	> 8.4	Baxter (53)
HIV-1		Solvent-detergent	> 5.0	Eriksson (59)
HIV-1		Solvent-detergent	> 10	Uemura (57)
HIV-1		Solvent-detergent	> 5.3	Octapharma (58)
HIV-1		Solvent-detergent	> 5.7	Baxter (53)
HIV-2		Solvent-detergent	> 4.8	Uemura (57)
HIV-2		Cohn-Oncley fractionation	> 5.4	Trepo (28)

(continued)

Table 2 Continued

Virus	Model for	Process	Log reduction	Reference
HBV		Cohn-Oncley fractionation	>5.6	Schroeder (27)
HBV		DEAE Sephadex chromatography	>4	Zolton (62)
HBV		QAE Sephadex chromatography	>5	Zolton (62)
NANB		β-propiolactone, UV light	>4.0	Prince (63)
NANB		β-propiolactone, 5 h, 23 °C	>3.5	Stephan (46)
HCV		Cohn-Oncley fractionation (a)	>4.7	Yei (34)
HCV		Cohn-Oncley fractionation (b)	>3.5	Tankersley (35)
HCV		4% (w/v) PEG precipitation	>4.0	Uemura (57)
HCV		pH 4.25, 21 days, 21 °C	>3.0	Louie (51)
HCV		Solvent-detergent	>3.0	Uemura (57)
HCV		Heat, 1 h, 60 °C	2.0	Uemura (57)
Sindbis	HCV	Cohn-Oncley	>9.6	Baxter (53)
Sindbis	HCV	Cohn Oncley	>6.4	Octapharma (58)
Sindbis	HCV	4% (w/v) PEG precipitation	>1.9	Uemura (57)
Sindbis	HCV	Solvent-detergent	>5.9	Uemura (57)
Sindbis	HCV	Solvent-detergent	>5.1	Baxter (53)
Sindbis	HCV	Solvent-detergent	>7.8	Octapharma (58)
Sindbis	HCV	Solvent-detergent	>5.2	Eriksson (59)
Sindbis	HCV	Heat, 1 h, 60 °C	>5.1	Uemura (57)
Sindbis	HCV	Heat, 2 h, 60 °C	>7.7	Centeon (54)
Sindbis	HCV	pH 4, 24 h	>8.9	Octapharma (58)
BVDV	HCV	Cohn-Oncley fractionation	3.4	Bayer (60)
BVDV	HCV	pH 4.25, 21 days, 20 °C	>3.2	Bayer (60)
BVDV	HCV	8% (w/v) PEG precipitation	2.3	Massot (61)
BVDV	HCV	DEAE Sephadex adsorption	0.8	Massot (61)
BVDV	HCV	Heat, 4 h, 60 °C	>6.5	Massot (61)
BVDV	HCV	Pepsin, pH 4, 10 h, 37 °C	>5.2	Sandoz (55)
BVDV	HCV	pH 4, 10 h, 37 °C	>5.0	Sandoz (55)
Semliki Forest virus	HCV	Pepsin, pH 4, 16 h, 37 °C	>6.8	Kempf (52)

Semliki Forest virus	HCV	pH 4, 16 h, 37 °C	>6.8	Kempf (52)
Pseudorabies	Enveloped DNA virus	Cohn-Oncley fractionation	>5.1	Bayer (60)
Pseudorabies	Enveloped DNA virus	Cohn-Oncley fractionation	>7.3	Octapharma (58)
Pseudorabies	Enveloped DNA virus	pH 4.25, 21 days, 20 °C	>3.4	Bayer (60)
Pseudorabies	Enveloped DNA virus	pH 4, 24 h	>5.9	Octapharma (58)
Pseudorabies	Enveloped DNA virus	Solvent-detergent	>4.3	Baxter (53)
Pseudorabies	Enveloped DNA virus	Solvent-detergent	>8.4	Octapharma (58)
Pseudorabies	Enveloped DNA virus	8% (w/v) PEG precipitation	3.3	Massot (61)
Pseudorabies	Enveloped DNA virus	DEAE Sephadex	>5.7	Massot (61)
Pseudorabies	Enveloped DNA virus	Heat, 6 h, 60 °C	>4.3	Centeon (54)
Pseudorabies	Enveloped DNA virus	Heat, 12 h, 60 °C	>5.6	Massot (61)
Pseudorabies	Enveloped DNA virus	Pepsin, pH 4, 10 h, 37 °C	>5.5	Sandoz (55)
Pseudorabies	Enveloped DNA virus	pH 4, 10 h, 37 °C	>5.3	Sandoz (55)
VSV	Enveloped RNA virus	4% (w/v) PEG precipitation	>3.9	Uemura (57)
VSV	Enveloped RNA virus	Solvent-detergent	>6.0	Baxter (53)
VSV	Enveloped RNA virus	Solvent-detergent	>5.5	Uemura (57)
VSV	Enveloped RNA virus	Solvent-detergent	>5.3	Octapharma (58)
VSV	Enveloped RNA virus	Solvent-detergent	>4.0	Eriksson (59)
VSV	Enveloped RNA virus	Heat, 1 h, 60 °C	>5.4	Uemura (57)
VSV	Enveloped RNA virus	Heat, 0.5 h, 60 °C	>7.0	Centeon (54)
Simian virus 40	Nonenveloped, DNA	Pepsin, pH 4, 16 h, 37 °C	>5.7	Kempf (52)
Simian virus 40	Nonenveloped, DNA	Cohn-Oncley fractionation	>5.0	Bayer (60)
Simian virus 40	Nonenveloped, DNA	8% (w/v) PEG precipitation	2.6	Massot (61)
Simian virus 40	Nonenveloped, DNA	DEAE Sephadex	1.9	Massot (61)
Simian virus 40	Nonenveloped, DNA	Heat, 60 °C, 12 h	>3.2	Massot (61)
Encephalomyocarditis	Nonenveloped, RNA	pH 4.25, 21 days, 20 °C	0.2	Bayer (60)
Encephalomyocarditis	Nonenveloped, RNA	Cohn-Oncley fractionation	>7.5	Baxter (53)
Bovine parvovirus	Parvovirus B-19	Heat, 60 °C, 10 h	>4.7	Centeon (54)
Bovine parvovirus	Parvovirus B-19	Pepsin, pH 4, 10 h, 37 °C	>4.7	Sandoz (55)
Bovine parvovirus	Parvovirus B-19	pH 4, 10 h, 37 °C	>4.1	Sandoz (55)

enzymatic digestion, oxidation reactions, or exposure to ionizing radiation. Antibodies that bind to viruses and prevent them from being infective (virus neutralization) may also be considered as inactivating (37–39).

Heating albumin solutions for 10 h at 60 °C was the first virus inactivation procedure applied to a plasma protein solution (1). Although no obvious physicochemical changes have been noted in heat-treated albumin solutions, proteins with measurable biological activity are usually inactivated by heat (40). However, dried factor VIII concentrates were subjected to heat treatments because of the high probability that they were contaminated with viruses.

Virus inactivation results obtained by heating dried coagulation proteins were mixed. Although HIV-1 was inactivated by heating for 10 h at 60 °C, non-A, non-B hepatitis was not inactivated (41). Other manufacturers who used temperatures up to 80 °C for 72 h obtained a greater degree of virus inactivation (42). In general, virus inactivation by heating dried coagulation proteins was incomplete and variable since the amount of virus inactivation depended on the residual moisture content of the product (43). Moreover, the heated proteins became relatively insoluble and demonstrated significant losses in biological activity.

One of the first processes validated as a virus inactivation step for immunoglobulins was developed in 1975 by Stephan (12). Originally intended to reduce anticomplement activity, this process involves chemical modification of an intermediate IgG fraction with β-propiolactone. Subsequent studies demonstrated that β-propiolactone inactivated HBV (44), HIV-1 (45), and NANB hepatitis (46).

In 1988, Funakoshi and his colleagues (47) reported that when IgG solutions that contained 33% (v/v) sorbitol were heated for 10 h at 60 °C, eight study viruses, including HIV and Sindbis (a surrogate for NANB hepatitis), were inactivated.

Also in 1988, Horowitz reported that the solvent/detergent process, originally developed to inactivate viruses in factor VIII concentrates (48), was an effective virucidal process for IgG solutions (49). Subsequently, solvent/detergent virus inactivation has shown to be a very reliable virus inactivation procedure for a wide variety of natural and recombinant proteins including immunoglobulins (50). Importantly, the biological activities of these proteins are not altered by conditions that inactivate viruses (48–50).

In other studies, inactivation of hepatitis C and bovine viral diarrhea virus (BVDV) has been reported in a liquid IVIG preparation formulated at pH 4.25 and incubated for 21 days at 21 °C (51). The kinetics of the inactivation showed that BVDV (a surrogate for HCV) was slowly inactivated over the 21-day study period. In contrast to their earlier experience with HIV-1 (32), the authors observed that BVDV inactivation was pH-dependent with reductions of 10-fold at pH 6, 100-fold at pH 4.5, and 10,000-fold at pH 4.0 in samples incubated for 21 days at 21 °C (51).

Pepsin digestion at pH 4 and 37 °C has also been shown to inactivate several enveloped viruses (52). Experiments with vesicular stomatitis virus demonstrated that both low pH 4 and pepsin contributed to inactivation of this virus (52).

Few data are available on the elimination of nonenveloped viruses during IVIG manufacture. Encephalomyocarditis (EMC) virus has been shown to be removed during cold ethanol fractionation (53) and has been inactivated by heating for 10 h at 60 °C (54). Bovine parvovirus has been inactivated when incubated with or without pepsin at pH 4 for 10 h at 37 °C (55).

COMPOSITION OF IVIG

Table 3 shows data on the composition of 14 different IVIG preparations. In this study, samples were purchased on the open market; were reconstituted according to the manufacturers' instructions (if necessary); were sterile filtered; were dispensed into sterile, encoded containers; were refrigerated or frozen; and were sent to several different laboratories for testing. The samples were tested in parallel, and the code was not broken until the tests had been completed and the data were summarized.

Consistent with previous studies (5), IgG size distribution measured by high-performance liquid chromatography varied by product. For most samples, monomeric IgG ranged from 85–99% of the total IgG in the sample. Gamma F, which is produced with pepsin digestion, contained relatively high levels of IgG fragments and low (77%) monomer. IgG dimer levels in the IVIG samples varied from <1–13%, and high-molecular-weight material (IgG polymer) was usually <1%. Four products contained IgG fragments: two that are prepared by enzyme treatment, and two that are formulated as liquids.

Purity, which is defined as the absence of non-IgG proteins, varied substantially among the products (Table 3). The IgA content of an IVIG provides the only firm clinical correlation with a product characteristic measured in vitro. Gammagard S/D, which contains the lowest IgA level, is the only product that has been safety administered for several years to primary immunodeficient patients with antibodies to IgA and proven sensitivity to IgA (64). Consequently, this is the only IVIG with no known contraindications.

ANTIBODY ACTIVITIES OF IVIG

Since the active ingredients of immunoglobulins are antibodies, qualitative and quantitative studies of IVIG antibody activities are essential. A significant amount of variation in the levels of opsonic antibodies to several neonatal bacterial pathogens in IVIG preparations was recently been reported by Weisman and his co-workers (65).

The Weisman study was conducted because clinical reports on the use of IVIG to prevent bacterial infections in low-birth-weight neonates had been inconsistent (66,67). The authors were greatly impressed with the high degree of variation observed in the quantity of each opsonic bacterial antibody studied in the different lots of IVIG regardless of manufacturer (65). The data also showed significant product to product variation for most of the antibodies studied (65).

In this study, Weisman et al. reported that the titers of opsonic antibody to *Staphylococcus epidermidis, Escherichia coli,* and *Haemophylus influenzae* were consistently low in all samples tested (65). In other studies from the same laboratory, Fischer and co-workers (68) reported on opsonic antibody levels to *S. epidermidis* in three commercial IVIG products. No IVIG preparation had consistent opsonic antibody levels. Some lots contained relatively high levels of opsonic antibody to *S. epidermidis* while other lots contained little or no activity. IVIG lots containing relatively "high" levels of opsonic antibody were protective against lethal *S. epidermidis* infections in a suckling rat model (68).

Table 3 Composition of IVIG Preparations

Product	Protein (mg/ml)	IgA (µg/ml)	IgM (µg/ml)	Albumin (mg/ml)	IgG mono (%)	IgG dimer (%)	IgG poly (%)	IgG frag (%)
Cytoglobin	54 ± 1	110 ± 60	10 ± 6	<0.8	98	2	<1	<1
Cytotect	98 ± 2	100 ± 0	39 ± 1	0.8 ± 0	85	13	2	
CytoGam	49	374	19	9.7	97	3	<1	
Gamimune N	51 ± 2	148 ± 55	76 ± 15	nd	99	<1		<1
Gamma F	55	31	nd	nd	77	2		21
Gammagard S/D	51 ± 1	1.0 ± 0.1	nd	2.2 ± 0.1	95	4	<1	
Gammar IV	56 ± 2	36 ± 4	nd	25 ± 2	88	10	2	
Glovenin I	50 ± 1	139 ± 77	nd	nd	92	8		
IG Polyvalentes	48 ± 0	48 ± 6	5 ± 6	<0.8	92	7	1	1
Sandoglobulin	46 ± 4	1066 ± 41	51 ± 10	1.2 ± 0.4	92	7	<1	
Venilon	54	–	26	0.9	89	11	<1	
Venoglobulin I	57 ± 2	303 ± 313	1.2 ± 0.1	9.3 ± 0	90	10	<1	
Venoglobulin IH	50	14	nd	nd	89	11		
Venoglobulin S	47 ± 0	10 ± 2	nd	nd	90	10	<1	

The data are expressed as mean ± standard deviation when more than one lot was tested.
nd = Not detected.

Table 4 Bacterial Antibodies in IVIG Preparations

Product	S. minn R595 EIA titer[a]	P. aerug Type 1 EIA titer[a]	E. coli 0.11:B4 LPS EIA titer[a]	E. coli J5 LPS EIA titer[a]	E. coli J5 Lipid A EIA titer[a]	S. pneumo 14 Opsonic titer[b]	GBS III Opsonic titer[b]	H. Influ b Opsonic titer[b]
Cytoglobin	295	102	22	102	729	—	—	—
Cytotect	43	108	5	27	79	—	—	—
CytoGam	238	54	5	34	263	—	—	—
Gaminune N	258 ± 39	57 ± 10	13 ± 8	30 ± 5	315 ± 32	12.6	3.5	4.0
Gamma F	<5	<5	<5	<5	<5	20.0	10.0	5.0
Gammagard S/D	277 ± 94	132 ± 36	12 ± 11	46 ± 11	273 ± 43	10.0	12.6	2.5
Gammar IV	83 ± 16	90 ± 18	18 ± 9	29 ± 10	122 ± 27	12.6	17.8	5
Glovenin I	47	208	16	62	167	20.0	3.5	2.5
IG Polyvalentes	186 ± 148	34 ± 8	8 ± 5	31 ± 6	1002 ± 577	15.9	12.6	5.0
Sandoglobulin	56 ± 12	89 ± 22	21 ± 5	34 ± 15	113 ± 4	12.6	14.1	6.3
Venilon	37	49	11	60	167	5.0	14.0	2.5
Venoglobulin I	93 ± 8	142 ± 26	21 ± 10	83 ± 6	245 ± 97	12.6	14.1	10.0
Venoglobulin IH	147	79	7	57	179	10.0	10.0	2.5
Venoglobulin S	205	36	7	33	253	10.0	10.0	5.0

[a]The data are expressed as arithmetic means ± standard deviation when more than one lot was tested.
[b]The data are expressed as geometric mean titers.

Table 5 Virus Antibodies in IVIG Preparations

Product	HAV (titer)	HBV (mIU/ml)	CMV (PEI U/ml)	EBV-VCA (EIA titer)	VZV (EIA titer)	Rubella (IU/ml)
Cytoglobin	200 ± 0	1610 ± 919	154 ± 13	7680 ± 3620	1920 ± 0	26 ± 0
Cytotect	333 ± 115	770 ± 581	50 ± 2	512 ± 0	960 ± 0	41 ± 0
CytoGam	200	850	111	5120	1920	26
Gamimune N	200 ± 0	697 ± 185	32 ± 23	4266 ± 1478	1920 ± 0	26 ± 0
Gamma F	100	700	<6.4	2560	120	13
Gammagard S/D	267 ± 115	627 ± 23	35 ± 0	5120 ± 0	1600 ± 550	24 ± 3
Gammar IV	167 ± 58	527 ± 25	27 ± 1	5120 ± 0	960 ± 0	24 ± 3
Glovenin I	150 ± 70	445 ± 5	23 ± 4	2560 ± 0	330 ± 212	10 ± 0
IG Polyvalentes	400 ± 0	1120 ± 225	20 ± 9	3413 ± 1478	1280 ± 554	26 ± 0
Sandoglobulin	100 ± 0	307 ± 120	16 ± 3	2560 ± 0	2240 ± 1460	24 ± 3
Venilon	100	150	29	1280	960	10
Venoglobulin I	333 ± 115	230 ± 36	18 ± 3	5120 ± 0	1920 ± 1663	22 ± 3
Venoglobulin IH	400	410	31	5120	960	26
Venoglobulin S	200 ± 0	660 ± 127	30 ± 2	3840 ± 1810	1920 ± 0	23 ± 4

The data are expressed as mean ± standard deviation when more than one lot was tested.

S. epidermidis was the most frequent cause of infections in two clinical trials of two different IVIGs in low-birth-weight neonates (66,67). The second most frequent cause of infections was *Staphylococcus aureus* (66,67). It is possible that variation in the content of *S. epidermidis* antibody in the products used in these trials may have contributed to the differences in clinical outcomes—i.e., successful prevention of late-onset bacterial infections by Baker and associates (66), and the failure to prevent late-onset bacterial infections by Fanaroff and co-workers (67).

Tables 4–6 summarize antibody data obtained in the blinded study described previously. It is interesting to note the relatively low levels of several bacterial antibodies in the products produced by pepsin digestion and by chemical modification (Table 4). This pattern has been observed in previous studies conducted in several laboratories (5,16–21). A similar pattern of product to product differences are observed in some antiviral titers (Table 5) and in virus-neutralizing activities (Table 6).

Overall, the antibody data in Tables 4–6 confirm the observations of Weisman et al. (65) and Fischer et al. (68) that antibody levels in different lots and in different products are inconsistent. Unfortunately, the contribution of assay to assay variation of the various antibody test procedures has not been determined. Thus, quantitative comparisons based on small studies, and small numbers of samples, are risky. It should be mentioned that only single lots of some of the products listed in Tables 4–6 were available for this study. Therefore, the data for these products may not be representative and should be interpreted cautiously.

FUTURE DIRECTIONS

Currently, a great deal of attention is being focused on immunomodulatory applications of IVIG, especially in the treatment of autoimmune disorders. Much of the informa-

Table 6 Virus-Neutralizing Titers in IVIG Preparations

Product	RSV type A[a]	RSV type B[a]	Parainfluenza 3[a]	CMV[b]
Cytoglobin	nt	nt	nt	>2700
Cytotect	nt	nt	nt	650 ± 433
CytoGam	nt	nt	nt	>2700
Gamimune N	314	35	131	1620 ± 990
Gamma F	693	103	184	<300
Gammagard S/D	271	34	253	2340 ± 805
Gammar IV	230	38	191	900 ± 0
Glovenin I	162	19	33	900 ± 3
IG Polyvalentes	212	21	182	<300
Sandoglobulin	209	27	122	300 ± 0
Venilon	139	26	76	300
Venoglobulin I	169	15	56	2340 ± 800
Venoglobulin IH	304	35	140	2700
Venoglobulin S	258	20	125	900
RSVIG Control	2108	149	121	nt

[a]The data are expressed as geometric mean titers.
[b]The data are arithmetic means ± standard deviation.
nt = Not tested.

tion on immunomodulation with IVIGs is anecdotal, and controlled clinical trials are needed to clarify issues of clinical efficacy and to identify the antibodies responsible for the clinical effects.

It is likely that future immunoglobulin products with enhanced clinical efficacy will be developed to prevent, and perhaps to treat, microbial infections. Currently, there are efforts to develop specific immunoglobulins by immunizing donors with experimental vaccines in order to obtain plasma that contains high levels of clinically relevant antibodies. Other initiatives involve development of monoclonal antibodies that can be produced in sufficient quantities to be used in current and future patient populations.

Studies on viral safety will continue to address other methods of virus removal. One of the most attractive possibilities for virus removal is the use of a final filtration procedure to remove all types of viruses without altering the antibody biological activities of the immunoglobulin. It is possible that such procedures will be needed to prevent transmission of viruses not yet discovered.

REFERENCES

1. Cohn EJ, Strong LE, Hughes WL Jr, et al. Preparation and properties of serum and plasma proteins III: a system for the separation into fractions of the protein and lipoprotein components of biological tissues and fluids. J Am Chem Soc 1946; 68:459–475.
2. Oncley JL, Melin M, Richert DA, Cameron JW, Gross PM Jr. The separation of the antibodies, isoagglutinins, prothrombin, plasminogen and beta-lipoprotein into subfractions of human plasma. J Am Chem Soc 1949; 71:541–550.
3. Aronson DL, Finlayson JS. Historical and future therapeutic plasma derivatives (Epilogue). Semin Thrombos Hemostas 1980; VI:1231–1239.
4. Kistler P, Nitschmann Hs. Large scale production of human plasma fractions: eight years experience with the alcohol fractionation procedure of Nitschmann, Kistler and Lergier. Vox Sang 1962; 7:414–424.
5. Hooper JA, Alpern M, Mankarious S. Immunoglobulin manufacturing procedures. In: Krijnen HW, Strengers PFW, van Aken WG, eds. Immunoglobulins. Amsterdam: Central Laboratory of the Netherlands Red Cross Blood Transfusion Service, 1988:361–380.
6. Painter RH, Minta JO. Stability of immune serum globulin during storage: effects of modifications in the fractionation scheme. Vox Sang 1969; 17:434–444.
7. Tankersley DL, Alving BM, Yi M, Blou MG, Mason BL, Finlayson JS. Predictive tests for fragmentation of immune globulins. In: Alving BM, Finlayson JS, eds. Immunoglobulins. Characteristics and Uses of Intravenous Preparations. Washington: US Government Printing Office, 1980:173–177.
8. Barandun S, Kistler P, Jeunet F, Isliker H. Intravenous administration of human gamma globulin. Vox Sang 1962; 7:157–174.
9. Smyth DG. Techniques in enzymic hydrolysis. In Hirs CHW, ed. Methods in Enzymology XI: Enzyme Structure. New York: Academic Press, 1967: 214–236.
10. Schultze HG, Schwick HG. Über neue Möglichkeiten intravenöser Gammaglobulin-Applikation. Dt Med Wschr 1962; 87:1643–1650.
11. Sgouris JT. The preparation of plasmin-treated immune serum globulin for intravenous application. Vox Sang 1967; 13:71–84.
12. Stephan W. Undegraded human immunoglobulin for intravenous use. Vox Sang 1975; 28:422–437.
13. Masuho Y, Tomibe K, Matsuzawa K, Ohtsu A. Development of an intravenous gamma-globulin with Fc activities. I. Preparation and characteristics of S-sulfonated human gamma-globulin. Vox Sang 1977; 32:175–181.

14. Schroeder DD, Tankersley DL, Lundblad JL. A new preparation of modified immune serum globulin (human) suitable for intravenous administration. I. Standardization of the reduction and alkylation reaction. Vox Sang 1981; 40:373–382.

15. Yang KD, Bathras JM, Shigeoka AO, James J, Pincus SH, Hill H. Mechanisms of bacterial opsonization by immune globulin intravenous: correlation of complement consumption with opsonic activity and protective efficacy. J Infect Dis 1989; 159:701–707.

16. Pollack M. Antibody activity against *Psuedomonas aeruginosa* in immune globulins prepared for intravenous use in humans. J Infect Dis 1983; 147:1090–1098.

17. Kim KS, Wass CA, Kang JH, Anthony B. Functional activities of various preparations of human intravenous immunoglobulin against type III group B streptococcus. J Infect Dis 1986; 153:1092–1097.

18. Bender S, Hetherington S. *Haemophilus influenzae* type b opsonins of intravenous immunoglobulins. J Clin Immunol 1987; 7:475–480.

19. Steele RW, Steele RW. Functional capacity of immunoglobulin G preparations and the F(ab')$_2$ split product. J Clin Microbiol 1989; 27:640–664.

20. van Furth R, Braat AGP, Leijh PCJ, Gardi A. Opsonic and physicochemical characteristics of intravenous immunoglobulin preparations. Vox Sang 1987; 53:70–75.

21. Alpern M, Garciacelay Z, Hooper J. Opsonophagocytic activity of intravenous immunoglobulins. Lancet 1987; ii:97.

22. Janeway CA, Merler E, Rosen FS, et al. Intravenous gamma globulin. Metabolism of gamma globulin fragments in normal and agammaglobulinemic persons. N Engl J Med 1968; 278:919–923.

23. Winston DJ, Ho WG, Rasmussen LE, et al. Use of intravenous immune globulin in patients receiving bone marrow transplants. J Clin Immunol 1982; 2(April suppl):42S–47S.

24. Hagenbeek A, Brummelhuis GJ, Donkers A, et al. Rapid clearance of cytomegalovirus-specific IgG after repeated intravenous infusions of human immunoglobulin into allogeneic bone marrow transplant recipients. J Infect Dis 1987; 155:897–902.

25. Rand KH, Gibbs K, Derendorf H, Graham-Pole J. Pharmacokinetics of intravenous immunoglobulin (Gammagard) in bone marrow transplant patients. J Clin Pharmacol 1991; 31:1151–1154.

26. McCue JP, Hein RH, Tenold R. Three generations of immunoglobulin G preparations for clinical use. Rev Infect Dis 1986; 8(suppl):S374–S381.

27. Schroeder DD, Mozen MM. Australia antigen: distribution during Cohn fractionation of human plasma. Science 1970; 168:1462–1464.

28. Trepo C, Hantz O, Jacquier MF, Nemoz G, Cappel R, Trepo D. Different fates of hepatitis B virus markers during plasma fractionation. Vox Sang 1978; 35:143–148.

29. Berg R, Bjorling H, Bertnsen K, Espmark A. Recovery of Australia antigen from human plasma products separated by a modified Cohn fractionation. Vox Sang 1972; 22:1–13.

30. Piszkiewicz D, Kingdon H, Apfelzweig R, et al. Inactivation of HTLV-III/LAV during plasma fractionation. Lancet 1985; ii:1188–1189.

31. Wells MA, Wittek AE, Epstein JS, et al. Inactivation and partition of human T-cell lymphotrophic virus, type III, during ethanol fractionation of plasma. Transfusion 1986; 26:210–213.

32. Mitra G, Wong MF, Mozen MM, McDougal JS, Levy JA. Elimination of infectious retroviruses during preparation of immunoglobulins. Transfusion 1986; 26:394–397.

33. Hénin Y, Maréchal V, Barré-Sihnoussi F, Chermann JC, Morgenthaler JJ. Inactivation and partition of human immunodeficiency virus during Kistler and Nitschmann fractionation of human blood plasma. Vox Sang 1988; 54:48–83.

34. Yei S, Yu MW, Tankersley DL. Partitioning of hepatitis C virus during Cohn-Oncley fractionation of plasma. Transfusion 1992; 32:824–828.

35. Tankersley DL. Requirements on donor selection and how to achieve viral inactivation in the production process. In: Intravenous Immunoglobulins and Safety Against Blood Borne Infections. Gothenburg, Oct 20, 1994.

36. Yu MW, Mason BL, Guo ZP, et al. Hepatitis C transmission associated with intravenous immunoglobulin. Lancet 1995; 345:1173–1174.

37. Tabor E, Gerety RJ. Transmission of hepatitis B by immune serum globulin. Lancet 1979; ii:1293.

38. Tabor E, Aronson DL, Gerety RJ. Removal of hepatitis B virus infectivity from factor IX complex by hepatitis B immune globulin. Lancet 1980; ii:68–70.

39. Finlayson JS, Tankersley DL. Anti-HCV screening and plasma fractionation: the case against. Lancet 1990; 335:1274–1275.

40. Dixon M, Webb EC. Heat inactivation of enzymes. In: Enzymes. New York: Academic Press, 1964:145–150.

41. Piszkiewicz D, Thomas W, Lieu MY, et al. Virus inactivation by heat treatment of lyophilized coagulation factor concentrates. Curr Stud Hematol Blood Transfus 1989; 56:44–54.

42. Colvin BT, Rizza CR, Hill FGH, et al. Effect of dry-heating of coagulation factor concentrates at +80 °C for 72 hours on transmission of non-A non-B hepatitis. Lancet 1988; ii:814–816.

43. Suomeia H. Inactivation of viruses in blood and plasma products. Transfus Med Rev 1993; VII:42–57.

44. Prince AM, Stephan W, Brotman B. β-Propiolactone/ultraviolet irradiation: a review of its effectiveness for inactivation of viruses in blood derivatives. Rev Infect Dis 1983; 5:92–107.

45. Prince AM, Horowitz B, Dichtelmüller H, Stephan W, Gallo RC. Quantitative assays for evaluation of HTLV-III inactivation procedures: Tri(N-butyl)phosphate: sodium cholate and β-propiolactone. Cancer Res 1985; 45:4592s–4594s.

46. Stephan W, Dichtelmüller H, Prince AM, Brotman B, Huima T. Inactivation of the Hutchinson strain of hepatitis non-A, non-B virus in intravenous immunoglobulin by β-propiolactone. J Med Virol 1988; 26:227–232.

47. Funakoshi S, Uemura Y, Yamamoto N. Virus inactivation and elimination by liquid heat treatment and PEG fractionation in the manufacture of immune globulin intravenous. In: Krijnen HW, Strengers PFW, van Aken WG, eds. Immunoglobulins. Amsterdam: Central Laboratory of the Netherlands Red Cross Blood Transfusion Service, 1988:313–325.

48. Horowitz B, Wiebe ME, Lippin A, Stryker MH. Inactivation of viruses in labile blood derivatives. I. Disruption of lipid-enveloped viruses by tri(n-butyl)phosphate detergent combinations. Transfusion 1985; 25:516–522.

49. Horowitz B. Preparation of virus sterilized immune globulin solutions by treatment with organic solvent/detergent mixtures. In: Krijnen HW, PFW Strengers, van Aken WG, eds. Immunoglobulins. Amsterdam: Central Laboratory of the Netherlands Red Cross Blood Transfusion Service, 1988:285–295.

50. Horowitz B, Prince AM, Horowitz MS, Watklevicz C. Viral safety of solvent-detergent treated blood products. Dev Biol Stand 1993; 81:147–161.

51. Louie RE, Galloway CJ, Dumas ML, Wong MF, Mitra G. Inactivation of hepatitis C virus in low pH intravenous immunoglobulin. Biologicals 1994; 22:13–19.

52. Kempf C, Jentsch P, Poirier B, et al. Virus inactivation during production of intrtavenous immunoglobulin. Transfusion 1991; 31:423–427.

53. Gammagard®S/D package insert. Data on file, Baxter Healthcare Corporation, Hyland Division, Glendale, California, 1994.

54. Gammar®-P IV promotional brochure. Data on file, Armour Pharmaceutical Company, Kankakee, Illinois, 1995.

55. Sandoglobulin® promotional brochure (UK). Data on file, Sandoz Pharma Ltd., Basel, Switzerland, 1993.

56. Piszkiewicz D, Andrews J, Holst S, et al. Safety of immunoglobulin preparations containing antibody to LAV/HTLV-III. In: Vossen J, Griscelli C, eds. Progress in Immunodeficiency Research and Therapy II. Amsterdam: Elsevier, 1986:197–200.

57. Uemura Y, Yang UHJ, Heldebrant CM, Takechi K, Yokoyama K. Inactivation and elimination of viruses during preparation of human intravenous immunoglobulin. Vox Sang 1994; 67:246–254.
58. Octagam® promotional brochure. Data on file, Octapharma Pharmazeuitka, Vienna, Austria, 1995.
59. Eriksson B, Westman L, Jernberg M. Virus validation of plasma-derived products produced by Pharmacia, with particular reference to immunoglobulins. Blood Coag Fibrinolysis 1994; 5(suppl 3):S37–S44.
60. Gamimune® N promotional brochure. Data on file, Miles, Pharmaceutical Division, Biological Products Business Unit, West Haven, Connecticut, 1994.
61. Massot M, Ristol P, López MT, et al. Validatiion of the inactivation and removal of viruses during the manufacturing process of liquid pasteurized human intravenous immunoglobulin. In: Caragol I, Español T, Fontan G, Matamoros N, eds. Progress in Immune Deficiency. Barcelona: Springer-Verlag Ibérica, 1995:275–276.
62. Zolton RP, Padvelskis JV. Evaluation of an ion-exchange procedure for removal of hepatitis type B contamination from human gamma globulin products. Vox Sang 1984; 47:114–121.
63. Prince AM, Stephan W, Dichtelmüller, Brotman B, Huima T. Inactivation of the Hutchinson strain of non-A, non-B hepatitis virus by combined use of β-propiolactone and ultraviolet irradiation. J Med Virol 1985; 16:119–125.
64. Cunningham-Rundles C, Zhou Z, Mankarious S, Courter S. Long-term use of IgA-depleted intravenous immunoglobulin in immunodeficient subjects with anti-IgA antibodies. J Clin Immunol 1993; 13:272–278.
65. Weisman LE, Cruess DF, Fischer GW. Opsonic activity of commercially available standard intravenous immunoglobulin preparations. Pediatr Infect Dis 1994; 13:1122–1125.
66. Baker CJ, Melish MM, Hall RT, et al. Intravenous immune globulin for the prevention of nosocomial infection in low-birth-weight neonates. N Engl J Med 1992; 327:213–219.
67. Fanaroff AA, Korones SB, Wright LL, et al. A controlled trial of intravenous immune globulin to reduce nosocomial infections in very-low-birth-weight infants. N Engl J Med 1994; 330:1107–1113.
68. Fischer GW, Cieslak TJ, Wilson SR, Weisman LE, Hemming VG. Opsonic antibodies to *Staphylococcus epidermidis*: in vitro and in vivo studies using human intravenous immune globulin. J Infect Dis 1994; 169:324–329.

5

Nonviral Side Effects of Intravenous Immunoglobulins

Mario Dicato, C. Duhem, and F. Ries
Central Hospital of Luxembourg, Luxembourg, Belgium

INTRODUCTION

Intravenous immune globulins (IVIGs) are safe biological products currently used in a broad spectrum of diseases. In the past, replacement therapy for primary immunodeficiency syndromes was provided through intramuscular injections. In the early 1980s, highly purified monomeric suspensions of IgG for intravenous use became available, and 15 years later nearly 20 commercial preparations of IVIG are at the disposal of the clinician. Indications for IVIG use extended to acquired immune defects and diseases for which an underlying immunological dysregulation is suspected.

The large field of application of IVIG has been recently reviewed, as were their immunomodulatory and anti-inflammatory mechanisms of action (1,2). This growing usage has increased the need for high-quality IVIG, and indeed the large experience acquired with these products, even in high dosage, confirms that side effects are rare and often mild.

This chapter reviews the adverse reactions after IVIG therapy reported to date in the literature. In some of these, the causal role of the immunoglobulins is just suspected from a circumstantial relation in their occurrence, and the presumed mechanisms are largely speculative, particularly in rare autoimmune disease, where the spontaneous evolution of the disease is sometimes unforeseeable and for which symptoms of the primary disease can be mistaken as side effects of IVIG.

SIDE EFFECTS OF IVIG

The side effects of IVIG can be separated into undesirable effects of their active components, the IgGs, and adverse reactions due to the "impurity" of the commercial preparation, other immunoglobulins, soluble substances, or viruses. However, some of the mechanisms of these side effects are still hypothetical and probably complex. Their enumeration will thus be made according to their major manifestations, irrespective of their putative cause. The problem of viral contamination of the batches is reviewed in another chapter of this book.

Generalized Reactions

Generalized reactions occur in 1–15% of cases (generally less than 5%) during and/or shortly after the administration of IVIG. Most begin 15–30 min after the onset of the infusion; they are often mild and self-limited and include pyrogenic reactions, minor systemic symptoms such as myalgia, fever, chills, headache, low back pain, nausea or vomiting, vasomotor and cardiovascular manifestations marked by changes in blood pressure, and tachycardia, shortness of breath, and chest tightness (3–6).

These reactions are generally attributed to aggregated immunoglobulin molecules, generating activation of the complement system. The kinetics of formation of such aggregates can be influenced by the rate of infusion of the IVIG, explaining the clear relation between this parameter and the occurrence of a generalized reaction. These complications can also be due to antigen–antibody reactions, to potential contaminants, or sometimes to the stabilizer used during the manufacturing process.

It has been recently demonstrated that a significant and rapid increase in plasma levels of some cytokines like IL-6, IL-8, and tumor necrosis factor alpha (TNF-α) was seen 1 h after IVIG infusion. This can partly mediate some adverse reactions of IVIG while other effects on cytokines and cytokine receptor network (induction of soluble TNF receptors and IL-1 receptor release) may be important for the therapeutic efficacy of IVIG in several immune-mediated disorders (7).

There are rare reported cases of general symptoms with delayed onset, beginning a few days after IVIG infusion, suggesting a type III allergic reaction (8).

Hypersensitivity and Anaphylactic Reactions

Severe and even fatal anaphylactoid reactions have been observed during IVIG treatment. These dramatic reactions, though reported as extremely rare, should be kept in mind by anyone using IVIG treatment, even very occasionally. Their real incidence is difficult to appreciate, but they occur preferentially in patients with IgA deficiency (9,10). In these patients anaphylactic shock is correlated with the presence in the serum of anti-IgA antibodies. These antibodies are of the IgG and the IgE isotypes. The presence of IgE anti-IgA, detected by ELISA in some patients, explains the scenario of these severe reactions in their chronology, their violence, and their requirement of very low IgA amount in IVIG batches to develop (10). Among hypogammaglobulinemic patients, although showing a poor antibody synthesis to common antigens, those with combined subclass deficiency (IgG2 and IgA deficiencies, for example) are more exposed to develop this complication. Patients with autoimmune diseases present an increased prevalence of selective IgA deficiency when compared to normal blood donors (1/50 in systemic lupus or juvenile rheumatoid arthritis, 1/200 in myasthenia gravis, and 1/700 in a normal caucasian population). Furthermore, anti-IgA antibodies seem to be more frequent in those IgA-deficient subjects with autoimmune diseases (11). Seriously ill patients with a compromised cardiac function are at increased risk of vasomotor cardiac complications, manifested by an increased blood pressure and/or cardiac failure. The kallikrein activity of some IVIG preparations has been incriminated as contributing to these adverse vasomotor reactions. Moreover, the volume of fluid delivered with IVIG (700 ml with standard preparations) is intolerable in a subset of fluid-restricted patients with congestive heart failure, especially at a high infusion rate.

Neurological Complications

As noted previously, headache is commonly observed in patients receiving IVIG, but this is efficiently palliated by analgesic and/or antihistaminic drugs.

Acute aseptic meningitis has been reported as a cause of recurrent IVIG-associated headache, occurring in a context of fever, meningism, nausea, and vomiting, beginning a few hours to a few days after IVIG infusions. To date, 14 documented cases have been described in the literature. In most cases, this clinical picture recurred after any subsequent retreatment with IVIG. The mechanisms underlying this complication remain poorly understood although sporadic observations of a significant blood eosinophilia suggest an immunoallergic basis in some of them (3,12,15). Several cases of aseptic meningitis have been associated with the use of drugs such as isoniazid and sulfamethiazole or in patients with systemic lupus erythematosus receiving anti-inflammatory drugs.

Still more intriguing, a case of recurrent migraine has been described after IVIG therapy, suggested by the typical symptoms at presentation and the efficient prevention by propanolol before subsequent IVIG infusions. The association of IVIG and migraine is hypothetical but is strongly suspected on the basis of the chronological relation between the events in a 45-year-old man devoid of personal or family history of migraine, although any plausible physiopathology is difficult to formulate (16).

Stroke as a side effect of IVIG treatment will be discussed later.

Renal Complications

Acute renal failure related to IVIG infusions has been reported in 21 cases. When it occurred, the best evidence for a cause-and-effect relationship was the close temporal association between IVIG treatment and the onset of clinical and biological symptoms of renal failure, as well as the patient's return to pretreatment creatinine levels after stopping the drug, with the exception of a young woman who had to be hemodialized and subsequently transplanted (17,25).

A renal biopsy was performed in five of these 21 patients, and some pathological features in three of these cases suggested a high solute load-induced damage of the proximal tubule, similar to that associated with the use of dextran or mannitol. Indeed, in these patients, osmotic nephrosis is probably the most frequent mechanism leading to a reversible impairment of renal function. This can be due to immunoglobulins themselves (macroaggregates) or to certain components of some IVIG batches like sucrose (added as stabilizing agent). This latter has been reported with the use of high-dose IVIG preparation containing up to 1.67 g of sucrose per gram protein.

Less frequently, a glomerular injury can be the cause of renal failure as shown in the case of a 39-year-old woman with mixed cryoglobulinemia associated with lymphoma (20). Prophylactic infusions of IVIG were undertaken in this patient because of severe hypogammaglobulinemia and recurrent infections, but she developed acute, severe, mixed cryoglobulinemic nephropathy with evidence of antigen-antibody complex deposition after a single infusion of IVIG. In another case, a proliferative glomerulopathy was observed, and antibody-antigen deposits activating the complement system were assumed.

In some cases, a functional mechanism is evoked for renal dysfunction, explained by a disturbance of glomerular perfusion, especially after high doses of IVIG infused at a high rate (modification of oncotic pressure generating a lowering of the glomerular filtration rate). In one case, this complication needed a plasmapheresis to restore a normal renal function (25). In most of the reported cases, a preinfusion impairment of renal function was observed, and IVIG treatment only contributed to the degradation of creatinine levels in patients with mild chronic renal insufficiency. This underlines the importance of measuring renal function in patients for whom IVIG treatment is planned, at least before the first infusion.

Hematological Complications

Neutropenia has been reported to complicate some treatments with IVIG, the main mechanism being unknown. One case of neonatal immune neutropenia following the administration of intravenous globulins has been described. In this infant, treated for alloimmune thrombocytopenia, antineutrophil-specific antibodies were detected in the child's serum but not in the maternal serum (26). In this pediatric case, the neutropenia (less than $500/mm^3$) was supposed to result from the administration of IVIG batches in which antineutrophil antibodies were detected, but this is probably far from being a frequent mechanism in patients presenting such a complication which is otherwise mild and transitory most of the time.

Ten cases of acute Coombs-positive hemolytic anemia developing during or shortly after IVIG infusions have been published (27,29), two of them being particularly severe—in a 30-year-old man and in a 9-month-old infant, treated respectively for immune thrombocytopenic purpura (ITP) and Kawasaki disease. In both cases, hemolysis mediated by antibodies to blood group antigens (anti-A and anti-D) could be demonstrated. When high doses of IVIG are infused, especially at high rates, their isoagglutinin content can be sufficient to explain a Coombs-positive hemolytic anemia. Decreased haptogloblin levels and mild reticulocytosis can be observed in normal volunteers receiving IVIG but without any change in hemoglobin levels, suggesting that clinically insignificant (because well-compensated) hemolysis may occur during IVIG treatment.

Thrombotic Complications

Four cases of fatal stroke in elderly patients (62–83 years old), all receiving IVIG for ITP, have been reported (30,31). The authors postulated that IVIG infusions could be responsible for an enhancement of adenosine triphosphate release from platelets, favoring their aggregation and, subsequently, thrombotic events, as suggested by in vitro aggregometry studies. However, these data were not confirmed by others. In some cases with ITP the rise in platelet count after IVIG treatment (that can be dramatic) might play a role in generating a vaso-occlusive event.

More recently, the effect of high-dose IVIG on blood rheology both in vitro and in vivo has been described (32). These data show that the increased viscosity after IVIG infusions can significantly impair blood flow and could generate myocardial infarction or stroke in predisposed patients, especially the elderly. However, in spite of all these elegant studies and hypotheses, few severe thrombotic episodes have been encountered with IVIG therapy. Moreover, in the mentioned case reports, the etiological link between the treatment and cardiovascular events occurring with increased frequency in an old and severely ill population is not that obvious.

Contamination of IVIG Batches

This short section refers to immunologically active proteins detected in some IVIG preparations that could be clinically relevant. Viral contamination is discussed elsewhere.

The levels of soluble HLA class II molecules (sHLA-DR, DQ, and DP) in IVIG preparations appear to exceed those measured in the plasma of healthy individuals, suggesting a concentration process during manufacturing; based on the total dosage of IVIG per infusion, these contaminating sHLA class II molecules may become immunogenic. In contrast, HLA class I molecules (A, B, C) are undetectable (33).

Significant levels of soluble CD4 and CD8 molecules have been detected in some commercial preparations of IVIG. Seventeen of these were tested by ELISA for the presence of proteins and cytokines such as interferon-gamma (IFN-γ), TNF, IL-1, IL-2, and IL-4. Out of these substances, only IFN-γ was present at measurable concentrations. The clinical relevance of these observations remains unclear (34,35).

One case of uveitis has been reported in a 9-year-old hypogammaglobulinemic patient, which was attributed to a localized vasculitis. Anticytoplasmic antibody (ANCA) activity was detected in IVIG batches and was proposed as the cause of the vasculitis. However, the causative role for ANCA in vasculitis in this child remains unproven (the young patient might have an underlying localized uveitis). Attempts to reproduce this disease in animals by the same mechanism have failed. Moreover, a transient peak in serum ANCA activity has been noted after IVIG infusion, attributed to displacement of ANCA from tissue sites (36,37).

Miscellaneous Side Effects

Some side effects of IVIG are mentioned in the literature as sporadic case reports. Generally, the assessment of a real relationship is sustained only by the temporal association between the observation and the IVIG infusion in the absence of any other obvious etiological agent, but most of the time no clear physiopathogenic explanation can be given.

Alopecia

Three cases of alopecia developing after IVIG treatment have been reported. The three women (19, 42, and 61 years old) were treated for ITP and complained of diffuse alopecia up to 4 weeks after infusions. Their hair regrew within the 4 weeks following the withdrawal of IVIG. Two additional cases have been mentioned by IVIG manufacturers. An immunological basis for alcopecia is possible, despite the negativity of immunofluorescence studies performed on the scalp biopsies of two of these patients.

Hypothermia

We made the curious observation of a transitory hypothermia (to 35 °C) in a 59-year-old CLL patient beginning a few hours after every IVIG infusion from the second one. The pathogenesis of this peculiarity remains speculative and may be due to perturbation in bradykinin pathway.

Interference with Vaccination

It should be noted that, while passive immunotherapy, particularly against some viruses (CMV, HIV, . . .), is one of the objectives of IVIG administration, interference with the active antibody response to live viral vaccines (such as rubella and measles) is certainly an undesirable side effect. Antibody response to measle vaccine is inhibited for up to 5 months after standard doses of IVIG and reponses to rubella vaccine only for 2 months (39). Moreover, this must be adjusted on the basis of the dose of immune globulins. Thus, an interval of at least 3–4 months should be respected between the last administration of IVIG (especially at high dose) and live viral vaccines in young patients.

MANAGEMENT AND PREVENTION OF IVIG SIDE EFFECTS

The management of the side effects of IVIG is symptomatic, and in view of their mildness, they rarely require any aggressive treatment with the exception of very uncommon anaphylactic reactions or cardiovascular complications. Depending on the particular manifestations, drugs palliating the symptoms are analgesics, antipyretic drugs, or antihistaminic drugs. For those occurring during IVIG infusion, a transitory stop or a lowering of the flow rate decreases or abolishes the symptoms most of the time. To optimize the prevention of side effects of IVIG and make them yet safer drugs, special measures should be taken at three levels: the manufacturer, ensuring an optimal purification of its product; the clinician, respecting some rules of administration; and the patient, to be screened for risk factors predisposing to complications.

Purification of IVIG

One batch of IVIG results from the processing of the plasma of 3,000–15,000 donors making a 100% guarantee of purity almost impossible concerning viral and protein contaminants. However, if additional steps in production can now improve the inactivation of lipid-enveloped viruses, other, still unknown viruses can always present future problems per screening being generalized where feasible (for further discussion see Chapter 6). The presence of potentially active and deleterious antibodies (like ANCA) always remains a possibility in individual IVIG batches. However, in regard to the acquired clinical experience, this does not seem to be really significant.

Screening of the Patient

Most of the severe reactions to IVIG have been observed in patients with anti-IgA antibodies. This eventuality should thus ideally be assessed by systematic screening before any instauration and particularly reinstauration of treatment in IgA-deficient patients, especially those with hypogammaglobulinemia or autoimmune diseases. However, a complete and reliable detection of those specific antibodies is hard to achieve. If IgG anti-IgA can be titrated by passive hemagglutination, the determination of IgE anti-IgA (supposed to be responsible of some of the most severe reactions) requires a sensitive ELISA test that cannot be performed in the routine. On the other hand, when IVIG treatment is indicated in a known IgA-deficient patient, low IgA-containing IVIG preparations should be preferred; the concentration of IgA in IVIG batches can vary by a factor of 1 to 100 in the different specialties.

Drug Administration

Rate of infusion

In the clinical practice, the rate of IVIG infusion is generally low at the beginning and then increases every 15–30 min, based on patient's tolerance, but the administration of a "standard dose" (400 mg/kg) may take up to 8 h in some patients; in most cases, symptoms such as fever and chills can be alleviated by lowering the infusion rate or briefly stopping it. A phase I rate escalation study was conducted in patients undergoing bone marrow transplantation and receiving IVIG prophylactically (500 mg/kg/week) to determine the minimal period of infusion of concentrated IVIG (10%) that was acceptably tolerated. After a first 6-h infusion, 40 patients were randomized to receive the same IVIG amount over a period of 2, 3, 4, or 5 h. The conclusion of this study was that at this dose IVIG could be infused over a 3-h period with a good tolerance (40).

However, in spite of these data and a large clinical experience confirming them, small, nonrandomized studies clearly show that IVIG can be administered safely with few adverse reactions at high infusion rates. Recently, in a series of 27 patients it was known that infusion rates can be raised up to 860 mg/kg/min without generating any prohibitive occurrence of adverse events, most of them being mild to moderate.

These data about safety of high IVIG infusion rates (> 500 mg/kg/h) could seem inconsistent with the common recommendations of manufacturers and the daily experience of clinicians. Nevertheless, these apparently conflicting data could be explained by a hypothesis of optimal formation of immune circulating complexes (ICC): in parallel to the in vitro antibody-antigen complex formation curve, the ICC probably responsible for most immediate reactions to IVIG could optimally form in vivo, intravenously, between two extreme flow rates, high (> 500 mg/kg/h) "in excess of antibody" (=IVIG) and low (< 150 mg/kg/h) in excess of intravenous "antigens."

These data about rapid infusions of IVIG should be verified in a large randomized study before being applied in the routine, but if they are confirmed, this could spare significant hospital stay, which can be particularly important for outpatient treatment. A safe way of proceeding is to give the first administration at a standard rate and then speed up the rate after having checked the patient for creatinine levels and M component.

Premedication

For patients presenting with repeated reactions unresponsive to reduction of the infusion rate of IVIG, premedication with hydrocortisone (100 mg IV) or an antihistaminic drug can be considered and is generally efficacious.

CONCLUSIONS

In spite of their multiple mechanisms of action, some of which are still poorly understood, IVIGs are safe products. Although severe adverse experiences have been reported, they are largely anecdotal and causative; the role of IVIG in their pathogenesis is often equivocal. The benefits of IVIG have been described for a growing number of diseases where immunoregulatory disorders are suspected and for which satisfactory alternative treatment is lacking.

REFERENCES

1. Dwyer JM. Manipulating the immune system with immune globulin. N Engl J Med 1992; 326:107–116.
2. NIH Consensus Conference. Intravenous immune globulin: prevention and treatment of disease. JAMA 1990; 264:3189–3193.
3. Schiavotto C, Rugerri M, Rodeghie F. Adverse reactions after high-dose intravenous immunoglobulins: incidence in 83 patients treated for idiopathic thrombopenic purpura (ITP) and review of the literature. Haematologica 1993; 78(6, suppl 2):35–40.
4. Misbah SA, Chapel HM. Adverse effects of intravenous immunoglobulins. Drug Saf 1993; 9(4):254–262.
5. Duhem C, Ries F, Dicato M. Side-effects of intravenous immune globulins. Clin Exp Immunol 1994; 97(suppl 1):79–83.
6. Camp-Sorrell D, Wujcik D. Intravenous immunoglobulin administration: an evaluation of vital sign monitoring. Oncol Nurs Forum 1994; 21(3):531–535.
7. Aukrust P, Froland SS, Liabakk NB, et al. Release of cytokines, soluble cytokine receptors and interleukin-1-receptor antagonist after intravenous immune immunoglobulin administration in vivo. Blood 1994; 84(7):2136–2143.
8. Hachimi-Idrissi S, De Scheffer J, De Waele M, Dab I, Otten J. Type III allergic reaction after infusion of immunoglobulins. Lancet 1990; 336:55.
9. McCluskey DR, Boyd NA. Anaphylaxis with intravenous gammaglobulin. Lancet 1990; 336:874.
10. Burks AW, Sampson HA, Buckley RH. Anaphylactic reactions after gammaglobulin administration in patients with hypogammaglobulinemia. Detection of IgE antibodies to IgA. N Engl J Med 1986; 314:560–563.
11. Liblau R, Morel E, Bach JF. Autoimmune diseases, IgA deficiency and intravenous immunoglobulin treatment. Am J Med 1992; 93:114–115.
12. Casteels-Van Dale M, Wijn Daele L, Hunninck K, Gillis P. Intravenous immune globulin and acute aseptic meningitis. N Engl J Med 1990; 323:614–615.
13. Kato E, Shindo S, Eto Y, et al. Administration of immune globulin associated with aseptic meningitis. JAMA 1988; 22:3269–3270.
14. Watson J, Gibson J, Joshua DE, Kronenberg H. Aseptic meningitis associated with high-dose intravenous immunoglobulin therapy. J Neurol Neurosurg Psychiatr 1991; 54:275–276.
15. Vera-Ramirez M, Charlet M, Parry GJ. Recurrent aseptic meningitis complicating intravenous immunoglobulin therapy for chronic inflammatory demyelinating polyardiculoneuropathy. Neurology 1992; 43:1636–1637.
16. Constantinescu CS, Chang AP, McClusckey LF. Recurrent migraine and intravenous immune globulin therapy. N Engl J Med 1993; 329:583–584.
17. Rault R, Piraino B, Johnston JR, Okal A. Pulmonary and renal toxicity of intravenous immunoglobulin. Clin Nephrol 1991; 36:83–86.
18. Kobosko J, Nicol P. Renal toxicity of intravenous immunoglobulin. Clin Nephrol 1992; 37:216–217.
19. Tab E, Hajinazarian M, Bay W, Neff J. Mendell JR. Acute renal failure resulting from intravenous immunoglobulin therapy. Arch Neurol 1993; 50:137–139.
20. Barton JC, Herera GA, Galla JH, Bertoli LF, Work J, Koopman WJ. Acute cryoglobulinemic failure after intravenous infusion of gammaglobulin. Am J Med 1987; 82:624–629.
21. Schifferli J, Leski M, Favre H, Imbach P, Nydegger U, Davies K. High-dose intravenous IgG treatment and renal function. Lancet 1991; 337:457–458.
22. Ashsan N, Palmer BF, Wheeler D, Greenlee RG, Toto RD. Intravenous immunoglobulin-induced osmotic nephrosis. Arch Intern Med 1994; 154(7):1985–1987.
23. Ruggeri M, Castaman G., De Nardi G, Rodeghi F. Acute renal failure after high-dose

intravenous immune globulin in a patient with idiopathic thrombocytopenic purpura. Haematologica 1993; 78(5):338–339.

24. Ellie E, Combe C, Ferrer Y. High-dose immune globulins and acute renal failure. N Engl J Med 1992; 327(14):1032–1033.

25. Poullin P, Moulin B, Ollier J, Benaicha M, Olmer M, Gabriel B. Complications renales des immunoglobulines intraveineuses; rôle des facteurs hémodynamiques rénaux. Presse Med 1995; 24(9):441–444.

26. Lassiter HA, Bibb KW, Bertolone SJ, Patel CC, Stroncek DF. Neonatal immune neutropenia following the administration of intravenous immune globulin. Am J Pediatr Hematol Oncol 1993; 15(1):120–123.

27. Brox AG, Cournoyer D, Sternbach M, Spurll G. Hemolytic anemia following intravenous gammaglobulin administration. Am J Med 1992; 93:114–115.

28. Comtenzo RL, Malachowski ME, Messner HC, Fulton DR, Berkman EM. Immune hemolysis disseminated intravascular coagulation and serum sickness after large dose of immune globulin given intravenously for Kawasaki disease. J Pediatr 1992; 120:926–928.

29. Salama A, Mueller-Eckhardt C, Kieffel V. Effect of intravenous immunoglobulin in immune thrombocytopenia. Lancet 1983; ii:193–195.

30. Woodruff RK, Griff AP, Firkin FL, Smith IL. Fatal thrombic events during treatment of autoimmune thrombocytopenia with intravenous immunoglobulins in elderly patients. Lancet 1986; ii:217–218.

31. Frame WD, Crawford RJ. Thrombotic events after intravenous immunoglobulin. Lancet 1986; ii:468.

32. Reinhart WH, Bechtold PE. Effect of high-dose intravenous immunoglobulin therapy on blood rheology. Lancet 1992; 339:662–664.

33. Grosse-Wilde H, Balsczyk R, Westhoff V. Soluble HLA class I and class II concentrations in commercial immunglobulin preparations. Tissue Antigens 1992; 39:74–77.

34. Blaczyk R, Westhoff V, Grosse-Wilde H. Soluble CD4-CD8 and HLA molecules in commercial immunoglobulin preparations. Lancet 1993; 341:789–790.

35. Lam L, Whitsett CF, McNichol JM, Hodge TW. Immunologically active proteins in intravenous immunoglobulins. Lancet 1993; 342:678.

36. Ayliffe W, Haeney M, Roberts SC, Lavin M. Uveitis after antineutrophil cytoplasmic antibody contamination of immunoglobulin replacement therapy. Lancet 1992; 339:558–559.

37. Donatini G, Goetz J, Hauptmann G. Uveitis and antineutrophil cytoplasmic antibody in immunoglobulin. Lancet 1992; 339:1175–1176.

38. Chan-Lam D, Fitzsimons EJ, Douglas WS. Alopecia after immunoglobulin infusions. Lancet 1987; i:1436.

39. Siber GR, Werner BG, Halsey NA, et al. Interference of immune globulin with muscles and rubella immunization. J Pediatr 1993; 122(2):204–211.

40. Iapoliti C, Williams LA, Huber S. Toxicity of rapidly infused concentrated intravenous immunoglobulin. Clin Pharm 1992; 11:1022–1026.

6

Viral Safety of IVIG

Peng Lee Yap

*Edinburgh & S. E. Scotland Blood Transfusion Service,
Edinburgh, Scotland*

INTRODUCTION

Human immunoglobulin G preparations suitable for intravenous administration (IVIG) are widely used for the prophylaxis of infection in patients with primary and secondary immunodeficiency and for the treatment of a wide variety of diseases thought to be immunologically mediated (see elsewhere in this volume). Until the 1980s, IVIG preparations were thought not to transmit viral infections, unlike plasma-derived coagulation factor concentrates, which were known to transmit a variety of viral infections, prior to the introduction of viral inactivation steps, such as heat or solvent-detergent treatment (Table 1). However, in the past two decades there have been reports of the transmission of hepatitis by a variety of IVIG preparations (1–22) leading to serious concern about the safety of IVIG preparations with respect to the transmission of virus infections.

In these reports (Table 2), the virus (or viruses) causing the hepatitis could not be identified as most of the patients who were initially studied suffered from either X-linked agammaglobulinemia (XLA) or common variable immunodeficiency (CVI) and therefore were unable to mount an antibody response, although hepatitis B transmission could be excluded, as some of the patients were hepatitis B surface antigen (HBsAg)-negative. Hepatitis A was excluded on epidemiological grounds, and the form of hepatitis associated with IVIG therapy was therefore initially described as non-A, non-B hepatitis (NANBH). However, following the discovery of the hepatitis C virus (HCV) (23), it was shown to be implicated in NANBH associated with IVIG preparations (24). This was not completely unexpected since HCV had previously been demonstrated to be the cause of NANBH associated with blood transfusion (25) and with coagulation factor concentrate therapy (26). Furthermore, the interval between exposure to the implicated IVIG batches and the detection of raised alanine aminotransferase (ALT) levels and the histological appearance of liver biopsies in patients with IVIG-associated NANBH was similar to that of NANBH associated with coagulation factor concentrate therapy (2,3).

This review will consider the different reported episodes of virus transmission associated with IVIG, the various viruses that have been transmitted or could be transmitted by immunoglobulin preparations, and the factors that may be involved in HCV

Table 1 Viruses Transmitted by Human Plasma Derivatives

Virus	Diameter (nm)	Nucleic acid	Strandedness	Transmitted of coagulation factors	Transmitted of immunoglobulin preparations	Comment
Hepatitis A[a]	27	RNA[b]		Yes	No	Antibodies in IVIG probably protective.
Hepatitis B	42	DNA	Partially Double	Yes	Yes	Old reports; no reports since HBsAg screening introduced.
Hepatitis C	30–60	RNA	Single	Yes	Yes	Many reports for IVIG—see Table 2.
Hepatitis delta	36	RNA	Single	Yes	No	HBsAg screening is probably a safety factor.
HIV-1	100	RNA	Single	Yes	No	One unsubstantiated report of retrovirus transmission.
Parvovirus B19[a]	24	DNA	Single	Yes	No	Antibodies in IVIG probably protective.

[a]No lipid envelope.
[b]This RNA is symmetrical.

Table 2 Episodes of HCV Transmission by Intravenous Immunoglobulin Where Preparation Involved Was Identified

Preparation	Publication year (Ref.)	Year of occurrence	Patients	Production method (finishing step)	Batches involved	Final formulation	Comment
IV IgG (BPL)	1984 (1,2)	1983	12/12	Gel filtration	1	Freeze-dried	Experimental preparation
IV IgG (Baxter Pilot Plant)	1985 (3,4)	1984	7/16	Ion exchange[a]	2	Freeze-dried	Pilot plant preparation
Gammonativ (Kabi)	1986 (5)	1985	4/?	Ion exchange[a]	NS[b]	Freeze-dried	Licensed (Sweden)
Gammonativ (Kabi)	1988 (7)	1985	16/77	Ion exchange[a]	Many	Freeze-dried	Licensed (Sweden)
IV IgG (SNBTS)	1989 (8)	1988	4/34	pH4 + pepsin	1	Freeze-dried	Licensed (U.K.)
Anti-D (East Germany)	1991 (12)	1979	2533	Ion exchange[c]	Many	Freeze-dried—	
IV IgG (FRC BTS)	1993 (9)	1985	4/8	Ion exchange[c]	NS	Freeze-dried	Experimental preparation
Anti-D (Ireland)	1994 (13)	1977	1037	Ion exchange[c]	Many	Freeze-dried	Licensed (Ireland)
Gammagard (Baxter)	1994 (14,15,19–22)	1993	>100	Ion exchange[c]	Many	Freeze-dried	Licensed (U.S.)
Venoglobulin (Alpha)	1995 (18)	1994	1[d]	PEG precipitation and ion exchange	NS	Freeze-dried	Licensed (U.S.)

Source: Reprinted from Yap, 1996, by permission of the Editor, Clinical and Experimental Immunology.
[a]Ion exchange chromatography was carried out using DEAE-Sephadex.
[b]NS—not stated.
[c]Starting material was plasma; no cold ethanol fractionation step was used prior to ion exchange chromatography.
[d]Single case report.

transmission by IVIG preparations including various aspects of the immunoglobulin manufacturing procedure (Table 3). It will also consider procedures that might improve the safety of IVIG preparations, and consider factors essential for the safety of IVIG preparations.

HISTORICAL BACKGROUND

The risk of viral contamination is a feature common to all biologicals (of which IVIG preparations are one) whose production involves the use of material of animal or human origin. Viral contamination of a biological may arise from the source material (such as human blood) or from various substances or solutions introduced during the production process. In the past, a number of biologicals administered to humans have been contaminated with viruses, and in several instances the contaminating virus was identified only many years after the product had been introduced into routine clinical use, since such transmission episodes occurred prior to adequate knowledge concerning the nature of the infectious agents. Many of the resulting infections in recipients have had serious or fatal consequences, and the primary cause of these viral transmissions by biologicals has been contamination of the starting or source materials. Examples include yellow fever vaccine that was contaminated by avian leukosis virus by virtue of its production in infected hens eggs, while SV40 was a contaminant of poliovirus and adenovirus vaccines prepared in the 1950s on primary cultures of kidney cells obtained from rhesus monkeys that harbored a clinically inapparent infection with SV40. Human growth hormone and gonadotropins extracted from the pituitaries of cadavers have also been implicated in the transmission of the etiological agent responsible for Creutzfeldt-Jakob disease.

Viral contamination of a biological can also arise from the use of infected material during production or as an excipient, and as far back as the late 1930s and early 1940s it was observed that some individuals vaccinated with yellow fever vaccine developed jaundice and hepatitis. This vaccine had been contaminated with HBV present in human serum which had been added as a stabilizer. Hepatitis was also associated with other vaccines that also contained homologous blood (27,28), and by the end of

Table 3 Factors Relevant to the Risk of Transmission of Viral Infections by Intravenous Immunoglobulin

---

Effective use of donor exclusion criteria
Donor screening for viral infections (HIV-1, HIV-2, HBV, HCV)
Size of plasma pool and number of donors in pool
Testing of plasma pools for evidence of viral infection (HIV-1, HIV-2, HBV, HCV)
Use of cold ethanol fractionation
Virucidal finishing steps after cold ethanol fractionation
Presence of neutralizing antibodies throughout the IVIG manufacturing process
GMP including particularly segregation and containment of process after the viral
    inactivation step
Final formulation of preparation and conditions for storage prior to administration
Testing of final IVIG batches for evidence of viral contamination

---

the 1940s and early 1950s it was clear that the hepatitis suffered by vaccine recipients was due in part to the use of human blood as part of the vaccine (29).

Surprisingly, immunoglobulin preparations prepared by cold ethanol fractionation in the 1940s did not transmit hepatitis; this was demonstrated by one early study, which showed that an intramuscular immunoglobulin preparation could be prepared from icteric plasma, which did not transmit hepatitis when injected into volunteers. However, this plasma, when injected into other volunteers, transmitted hepatitis (30). Subsequently, it was shown that other products from the same plasma such as fibrinogen and coagulation factor VIII and IX concentrates also transmitted hepatitis, leading to the belief that cold ethanol fractionation was the unique factor responsible for the viral safety of immunoglobulin preparations.

The issue of the viral safety of blood products, including immunoglobulin preparations, was considered in detail in a review in 1957 by Pennell, who prophetically suggested that "no fraction prepared from pooled plasma by any technique (could) be presumed to be free from the virus of homologous serum hepatitis unless shown to be so by volunteer studies or by application of an effective sterilising technique" (31). In this review, it was pointed out the early studies had indicated that only immunoglobulin preparations derived from methods 6 and 9 in the cold ethanol fractionation procedure developed by Cohn and his colleagues (32) or the Nitschmann modification (33) were free of virus contamination without specific sterilization. Problems with hepatitis transmission by immunoglobulin preparations using the zinc method (method 12) (34) and the Kekwick ether procedure (35) were highlighted, demonstrating that immunoglobulin preparations were still able to transmit viral infections despite the presumed presence of specific antibody against the contaminating virus. It was therefore suggested that the freedom from viral transmission was not solely due to the presence of antibody in the immunoglobulin preparation against the particular virus, and Pennell concluded that there appeared to be "no ready (specific) explanation for the freedom of cold ethanol gammaglobulin" from hepatitis transmission. The importance of cold ethanol fractionation was subsequently further emphasized by the recent reports that immunoglobulin products prepared by non cold ethanol fractionation (9,12,13) methods were associated with HCV transmission (see below).

In addition to the above reports of hepatitis transmission by vaccines and some blood products, the importance of using plasma free of viral contamination for the production of immunoglobulins was further highlighted by the sporadic reports of HBV transmission by intramuscular immunoglobulin preparations (36–40). In addition, there was also a report that an antihistamine preparation containing immunoglobulin was also reported to have been implicated in numerous cases of HBV infection in Italy (41). At this time, the presence of hepatitis B surface antigen (HBsAg) in immunoglobulin preparations was also reported in many different immunoglobulin preparations (41–44). These reports were attributed either to the use of contaminated plasma prior to fractionation or to suboptimal fractionation methods or to contamination during the fractionation procedure, but after the routine introduction of HBsAg screening of blood donors, there were subsequently no reports of HBV transmission by immunoglobulin preparations, thus demonstrating the importance of the removal of the relevant virus in the initial plasma pool used for the manufacture of this blood product.

By the 1960s attempts were being made to administer IgG intravenously for the treatment of patients with XLA or CVI (see elsewhere in this volume), and a number of different IVIG preparations that were free of immediate adverse reactions were developed prior to 1983. At that time, it was generally accepted that both intramuscular and intravenous immunoglobulin preparations did not transmit viral infections unlike coagulation factor concentrates which did transmit a number of different hepatitis viruses (Table 1), even though both types of blood products had been derived from the same plasma pools that resulted in safe immunoglobulin preparations. There were therefore no specific studies performed to evaluate the viral safety of IVIG preparations until the first report in 1983 (see below).

TRANSMISSION OF NON-A, NON-B HEPATITIS
BY EXPERIMENTAL IVIG PREPARATIONS

In 1983, the first report of NANBH occurring in immunodeficient patients receiving an experimental IVIG preparation were published (1), and further details were subsequently reported (2). This was unexpected, as NANBH associated with any of the IVIG preparations available at the time had not been previously reported. In this episode, the donors had been screened for HBsAg, and standard cold ethanol fractionation technology had been used. The manufacturer involved (then called the Blood Products Laboratory, now called the Bioproducts Laboratory, BPL) had produced intramuscular immunoglobulin preparations derived from cold ethanol fractionation for over 20 years without any reports of viral transmission (R. S. Lane, personal communication).

In the experimental process, Cohn fraction II from a plasma pool derived from more than 10,000 donors was subjected to chromatography involving Sephadex G25 to separate ethanol from the IgG molecule as it was thought that lyophilization in the presence of ethanol (used for the manufacture of intramuscular immunoglobulin) damaged the IgG molecule and therefore caused adverse reactions when such preparations were administered intravenously. The resulting immunoglobulin solution was then freeze-dried and formulated as a lyophilized preparation. This preparation was clearly highly infective as all 12 immunodeficient recipients in the initial clinical trial developed NANBH from a single batch (2).

An investigation of the manufacturing procedures for immunoglobulin preparations at BPL was undertaken, and it was observed that the intramuscular immunoglobulin preparation derived from the same Cohn fraction II paste, as the infective experimental IVIG preparation had not been associated with any cases of hepatitis transmission (R. S. Lane, personal communication). It was therefore suggested that the reason for the infectivity of this experimental IVIG preparation could have been an absence of a virucidal finishing step, and it was speculated that lyophilization in the presence of ethanol could have been virucidal for the NANBH virus. Alternatively, the Sephadex G25 chromatography column may have been contaminated by the NANBH virus, perhaps from previous experimental IVIG manufacturing cycles. It was considered that the likelihood of contamination of the column was unlikely, since the Sephadex was decontaminated using a concentrated sodium hydroxide solution after the immunoglobulin solution derived from Cohn fraction II was passed through it. However, this possibility could not be completely excluded, and it was also suggested that the cold ethanol fractionation procedure itself probably had only weak virucidal activity since the final product in this particular preparation procedure had infected all the individuals receiving it. Finally, as intramuscular immunoglobulin preparations are formulated as aqueous preparations and stored for variable periods prior to administration, it is possible that some viruses may have a reduced stability in the aqueous phase. No further studies were carried out at BPL, but these reports were followed by further reports of NANBH transmission involving IVIG preparations in which an adsorption chromatography step was used (Table 2).

TRANSMISSION OF NON-A, NON-B HEPATITIS BY IVIG PREPARATIONS INVOLVING PURIFICATION BY DEAE SEPHADEX

In 1985, it was reported that an experimental IVIG preparation manufactured at a pilot plant by the Baxter Healthcare Corporation transmitted NANBH (3). The starting material for this IVIG preparation was plasma derived from donors screened for HBsAg. As with the previous episode, cold ethanol fractionation was performed on a large plasma pool, but instead, DEAE Sephadex chromatography was used to purify the IgG molecule in as nondamaging a form as possible. The IgG molecule was eluted and albumin then added as a stabilizer. This was followed by freeze-drying so that the experimental IVIG preparation could be formulated as a lyophilized preparation prior to clinical use.

Seven of 16 patients developed NANBH in the initial clinical evaluation (3,4), and, as in the previous episode, it was speculated that the absence of a virucidal finishing step (used in the production of intramuscular immunoglobulin preparations)—i.e., freeze-drying of the IgG solution in the presence of ethanol—could have been the explanation for infectivity. Contamination of the DEAE Sephadex chromatography material (due to reuse), as an explanation for the infectivity of the experimental IVIG preparation to be infective, was excluded as the chromatography material was discarded after each chromatographic purification procedure (J. A. Hooper, personal communication). Contamination by HCV containing material elsewhere in the pilot plant could have been an explanation, but no specific evidence for this was ever discovered (J. A. Hooper, personal communication). Another possible explanation was the contamination of the albumin stabilizer, as this was derived from human plasma. However, this explanation was considered to be unlikely in view of the routine pasteurization of albumin preparations, their excellent safety record regarding transmission of viral infections, and the absence of evidence that there had been any problems with pasteurization of the batch of albumin used as a stabilizer for the infective IVIG batches. As with the BPL episode, no final cause for the transmission of NANBH (which was subsequently shown to be due to HCV, see below) was ever identified, but, interestingly, a subsequent preparation manufactured in a large-scale fractionation facility using similar technology was shown to be free of hepatitis transmissions during initial studies (see below).

The above episode was followed by further reports involving a licensed IVIG preparation manufactured by Kabi called Gammonativ (5–7,10). This preparation was used widely in Sweden and in Norway, as initial clinical trials to evaluate tolerance in patients with primary hypogammaglobulinemia had suggested that it had a very low adverse reaction rate. Gammonativ was manufactured by a similar method to the experimental IVIG preparation manufactured at the Baxter pilot plant (described above). Plasma was obtained from donors screened for HBsAg, and cold ethanol fractionation was performed on a large plasma pool. DEAE Sephadex chromatography was used to purify the IgG molecule, and an albumin stabilizer was added following which the IVIG preparation was formulated in a lyophilized form. However, 16 of 77 patients developed NANBH in the best-documented of the initial trials (7), and other patients were also known to be infected by this IVIG preparation (5,6,10) (also personal communication, L. Hammarstrom). The possible explanations for infectivity by an NANBH virus (also subsequently shown to be HCV; see below) were thought to be similar to those suggested for the experimental IVIG preparation described above from the Baxter pilot plant, but, as with other IVIG preparations, no final conclusion was reached regarding the explanation for the infectivity of the IVIG preparations.

NANBH TRANSMISSION BY IVIG AND ANTI-D PREPARATIONS FOR INTRAVENOUS ADMINISTRATION, NOT INVOLVING COLD ETHANOL FRACTIONATION

Another NANBH transmission episode associated with an experimental IVIG preparation occurred in Finland at approximately the same time as the NANBH transmission described above was observed in association with Gammonativ therapy. Eight patients were studied in a clinical trial of an IVIG preparation manufactured by the Finnish Red Cross Blood Transfusion Service (FRC BTS). However, this preparation was manufactured using plasma as the starting material instead of a fraction derived from cold ethanol fractionation. In the FRC BTS manufacturing procedure, plasma was passed down a DEAE Sephadex column, and four of the recipients developed NANBH (9), which was later found to be due to HCV in two patients using the polymerase chain reaction (PCR) to detect HCV RNA (F. Davidson and P. L. Yap, unpublished observations). No specific cause for the NANBH transmission by FRC BTS IVIG was identified, but it was speculated that the cause might be similar to the possibilities proposed above for the two other IVIG preparations involving DEAE Sephadex, associated with NANBH transmission (G. Myllyla, personal communication).

In 1991 and 1994, two further episodes of NANBH transmission that had occurred between 1977 and 1979 were reported (13,45), although one of the episodes had been previously reported but not generally known (12). These episodes involved anti-rhesus D (anti-D) immunoglobulin preparations for intravenous administration instead of standard IVIG preparations derived from unselected donations. Anti-D preparations are used to prevent hemolytic disease of the newborn and have traditionally been made by cold ethanol fractionation and formulated as an aqueous immunoglobulin solution for intramuscular use only. Most anti-D preparations have been manufactured on a relatively small scale due to the difficulty in obtaining large volumes of donor plasma with raised levels of specific antibodies and the lower patient demand for such hyperimmune preparations, compared with IVIG preparations. However, the yield of anti-D antibodies in the final product with cold ethanol fractionation was usually low (46), and alternative methods for increasing the yield of anti-D in fractionation processes have been sought.

In 1973, Hoppe et al. published a method that avoided cold ethanol fractionation and instead involved using plasma as a starting material and separating IgG from other plasma proteins with an ion exchange chromatography column (47). The IgG in the subsequent eluate was found to be very pure and in an unmodified state so that it could be administered intravenously without any immediate adverse reactions after formulation as a lyophilized preparation. Of more importance was the high yield of specific anti-D IgG from the Hoppe process, and it became an attractive alternative to cold ethanol fractionation for the manufacture of hyperimmune anti-D immunoglobulin preparations on a small (47–49) or large (50) scale. This process (or processes using a similar methodology) appeared to be adopted by only a small number of manufacturers located in Hamburg (47), East Germany (48), Ireland (49), and Canada (Winnipeg Rhesus Institute) (50), and it was suggested that anti-D administered intravenously was superior to anti-D administered by the intramuscular route, since anti-D levels were raised immediately (51). Initial studies suggested that the process was safe and did not mention hepatitis as an adverse reaction in recipients of immunoglobulin preparations manufactured by this method (47,48,50,51).

In 1979, several cases of NANBH were observed in East Germany following administration of anti-D IgG (12) manufactured by the Hoppe method (47,48). Unfortunately, information about this episode became generally available only in 1991, when it was shown that the NANBH was due to HCV (45,52), but a retrospective investigation of the outbreak revealed two hyperimmune anti-D plasma donors who had developed acute hepatitis following the initial administration of erythrocytes from a rhesus D-positive individual with an inapparent hepatitis to increase the levels of anti-D antibodies in the donor plasma. Plasma from the infected hyperimmune donors was included in different anti-D immunoglobulin batches manufactured by the Hoppe method. Interestingly, an episode of transmission of hepatitis B by deliberate hyperimmunization with red cells had been previously reported in 1978. In this episode, red blood cells from a single donor were used for the stimulation of red cell antibodies in 32 volunteers; HBsAg or anti-HBs became detectable in 28 of the 32 volunteers, demonstrating the hazards of alloimmunization of plasma donors in using red cells to boost specific antibody levels in plasma destined for immunoglobulin preparations (53).

The East German immunoglobulin preparation had been derived from small plasma pools of 10 donors by DEAE-Sephadex chromatography followed by precipitation with a final concentration of 25% ethanol and sterile filtration (45,48). The small pool of hyperimmune plasma prior to chromatography and the inclusion of plasma from anti-D donors who had recently developed acute hepatitis are likely to have resulted in a high titer of HCV in the starting plasma pool, and it is likely that the ethanol precipitation step after DEAE-Sephadex chromatography was insufficiently virucidal to ensure safety in the end product. The final formulation of the anti-D preparation was in a lyophilized form; this may have been important in stabilizing the HCV virions prior to intravenous administration. All these factors may have important differences compared with conventional anti-D immunoglobulin preparations derived from cold ethanol fractionation which are formulated as aqueous solutions and have never been reported to be associated with hepatitis transmission (see below). Such preparations are also formulated for intramuscular use only, but it is unlikely that the route of administration was relevant since HCV can be spread by needlestick injuries (54). In addition, it is believed that the chromatography material was used repeatedly rather than discarded after such production procedure, thus spreading the HCV contamination to anti-D batches not involving the two HCV-infected anti-D plasma donors (J. Löwer, personal communication).

A large number of cases of HCV transmission by anti-D in Ireland in 1977–1978 were also reported in 1994 (13). In 1977, jaundice had been reported in six recipients of Irish anti-D, but it had been concluded that this was community acquired NANBH (55). However, in 1993 a retrospective study of HCV-infected blood donors highlighted a number of female donors whose only risk factor was anti-D administration (13). A further intensive screening of 60,000 recipients of anti-D in Ireland for anti-HCV and for HCV RNA by PCR indicated that all of the many hundreds of HCV-infected recipients had received anti-D manufactured by the Hoppe method (48) in Ireland (49) in 1977–1978.

Small plasma pools (approximately 1.5 L in volume) had been used in the chromatographic purification procedure to separate IgG from other plasma proteins, and the eluted IgG was then lyophilized (49). The anti-D was licensed for intravenous administration and was used routinely in Ireland. A retrospective investigation of hyperimmune donors to the anti-D plasma pool revealed that one anti-D donor had been anti-HCV positive in 1977. Sequencing studies of an archive sample from the suspect anti-D plasma donor, one of the implicated anti-D immunoglobulin batches and the HCV-infected anti-D recipients, revealed an almost identical HCV sequence at NS-5, a polymorphic part of the HCV genome (56). As with the East German incident, it is probable that the titer of HCV would also have been high in the initial plasma pool for anti-D manufacture, due to its small size. The ethanol precipitation step (49) was unlikely to have been sufficiently virucidal to ensure the anti-D preparation was safe, and it is possible that there may have been a small number of cases of HCV transmission by Irish anti-D after the 1977–1978 episode relating to a separate source of HCV contamination of the starting plasma pool (J. Power, E. Lawlor, personal communication).

In summary, HCV infection appeared to be transmitted by IVIG preparations derived from unscreened plasma if freeze-drying in the presence of ethanol did not occur, suggesting that this might be a specific viral inactivation procedure. Three of the above transmission episodes used a product of cold ethanol fractionation, suggesting that incubation in ethanol is not reliable as a virus inactivation procedure despite the well-known safety record of immunoglobulin preparations for intramuscular use derived from cold ethanol fractionation. Five of the implicated preparations used chromatography for the purification of IgG, suggesting that the process could not be relied upon to completely remove virus or to partition IgG from infective virus; in these transmission episodes the lack of a specific virucidal finishing step was the most likely explanation rather than contamination of equipment, chromatography material, or stabilizer. All the preparations were lyophilized, suggesting that the storage in the liquid phase may inactivate contaminating viruses, and the lyophilization may have helped preserve the infectivity of the contaminating HCV virions. Finally, the two episodes of transmission by anti-D preparations demonstrated that the infectivity of IVIG preparations was not simply due to the higher doses of IgG administered since the amount of IgG administered in the anti-D preparations was relatively small.

NANBH TRANSMISSION BY IVIG PREPARATIONS INVOLVING A PH 4/MILD PEPSIN FINISHING STEP

Many other different approaches were used in the 1960s and 1970s for the development of immunoglobulin preparations safe for intravenous use. One approach was the incorporation of a pH4 finishing step in the absence or presence of low concentrations of porcine pepsin after cold ethanol fractionation; this produced an IVIG preparation with a very low adverse rate (57) that also seemed to be free of hepatitis transmission (58–61). However, in 1989 NANBH transmission was reported to be associated with an IVIG preparation manufactured by the Scottish National Blood Transfusion Service

(SNBTS IV IgG) in which pH4 incubation with low concentrations of pepsin was used in the manufacturing process (8). This was of particular interest since this pH4–treated IVIG preparation had previously been shown to not transmit NANBH (58). This preparation had some important differences from the six immunoglobulin preparations for intravenous use associated with NANBH described above. The donors had been screened for anti-HIV as well as HBsAg, and although cold ethanol fractionation was used, there was no subsequent chromatographic finishing step, a pH4 incubation step substituting for chromatography. Sucrose was used as a stabilizer, and the preparation was formulated in a lyophilized form (8).

This transmission episode also differed from other NANBH episodes as only one specific SNBTS IV IgG batch was involved, the previous 109 batches of this preparation not having been associated with transmission of hepatitis. Furthermore, of the 34 recipients of the batch, only four developed NANBH, and the liver enzyme abnormalities were transient in three of those four (8), suggesting that the NANBH virus (subsequently shown to be HCV) may have been in very low concentrations and possibly near the limit of infectivity compared with the IVIG preparations described above associated with NANBH. Surprisingly, subsequent batches of SNBTS IV IgG (62) did not transmit NANBH despite an unchanged IVIG manufacturing procedure, and it was speculated that this transmission episode could have been due to a failure of good manufacturing practice (GMP) near the terminal stages of the manufacturing procedure, leading to contamination of this particular IVIG batch (8). Unfortunately, an extensive investigation by the manufacturer did not reveal any specific GMP failures (63), so there was no final conclusion as to the cause of the NANBH transmission. Nonetheless, in view of the experimental data that incubation at pH4 is virucidal (see below), it could be concluded that whereas all the above six episodes of NANBH transmission had been due to a lack of a virucidal step for HCV (prior to the introduction of anti-HCV screening of plasma donors), if contamination of the IVIG with HCV-containing plasma (or plasma fractions) occurred after the virucidal finishing step, then HCV transmission could still occur.

TRANSMISSION OF HCV BY IVIG FOLLOWING THE INTRODUCTION OF HCV SCREENING

Following the different episodes of NANBH associated with IVIG preparations in the 1980s, some of the manufacturers involved attempted to develop safer IVIG preparations. Production of one of the experimental IVIG preparations associated with NANBH in the Baxter pilot plant was transferred to a large-scale manufacturing facility, and an extensive prospective study of liver enzymes in patients who had received the IVIG preparation produced in a large-scalae manufacturing facility did not indicate any transmission of NANBH (64). This IVIG preparation (Gammagard) was therefore licensed for clinical use and was widely used in many different countries as it was accepted to be free of viral transmission.

In 1989 HCV was discovered (23), and as soon as first-generation anti-HCV screening assays (containing a single HCV antigen) became available, they were applied to stored sera from previously conducted prospective studies of NANBH. In an analysis of donor-recipient relationships in a multicenter transfusion-transmitted virus study it was shown that an anti-HCV positive donor was associated with 81% of hepatitis C cases and that this proportion of cases might have been prevented had these screening assays been available in the 1970s, when these studies were originally conducted (65). The later retrospective application of a second-generation anti-HCV screening assay (containing additional HCV antigens) to this same cohort and a correction for background transaminitis showed that second-generation assays on blood donors would have prevented 93% of cases of NANBH transmission. Similar findings were shown in a prospective study conducted in Barcelona (66). Immediately prior to the introduction of anti-HCV screening, the incidence of NANBH in Barcelona was 9.6%. One year after the exclusion of anti-HCV-positive blood donors, the incidence in recipients of blood transfusion had fallen to 1.9%, an 80% reduction attributed to anti-HCV testing.

Screening for HCV infection was therefore carried out routinely for blood donors, and in 1991 anti-HCV screening was incorporated into the screening of plasma donors, but the value of this procedure for such donors was extensively debated. Some experts considered that anti-HCV screening of plasma donors would provide an additional measure of safety to recipients of blood products (67,68); others expressed concern regarding a change in the safety of IVIG preparations (69,70). In particular it was suggested that while the basis for the safety of IVIG (and intramuscular immunoglobulin) preparations was unknown, it could be hypothesized that anti-HCV screening could lead to the removal of unidentified neutralizing anti-HCV antibodies from the plasma pool used for the manufacture of IVIG. Experiments were therefore performed to assess viral safety in a chimpanzee model, and it appeared that screening of plasma donors, using a first-generation anti-HCV enzyme immunoassay did not result in an IVIG preparation that was infectious for HCV (71). When second-generation anti-HCV tests then became available, they were incorporated into the routine screening of plasma donors.

In 1994 it was reported that HCV was transmitted by some batches of Gammagard (14,15) used in a number of different countries. This was completely unexpected, and the donors in this episode had been screened for HBsAg, anti-HIV, anti-HCV (by a second-generation anti-HCV test) and for a raised alanine aminotransferase level. The plasma pool used for fractionation was very large, and cold ethanol fractionation was used followed by DEAE Sephadex purification, the addition of an albumin stabilizer, and lyophilization. Attempts were made to identify the cause of HCV transmission, and it was suggested that as the only change had been the introduction of anti-HCV screening, the removal of anti-HCV antibodies in the starting plasma pool may have removed neutralizing antibodies for HCV and altered the partitioning characteristics of HCV in the manufacturing process of Gammagard so that infective HCV virions that had previously been partitioned into fractions that had been discarded following cold ethanol fractionation now appeared in the fraction rich in IgG used for chromatography and subsequent IVIG formulation. It was noted that infective batches may have only occurred after the introduction of a second-generation anti-HCV EIA since HCV PCR batches appeared only then (72,73), and it was suggested that the first-generation anti-HCV EIA may have only partially removed anti-HCV antibodies, since this screening test was estimated to have only detected just over half of all HCV-infected blood donors due to its using only one HCV antigen for screening, compared with the second-generation test, which had more HCV antigens in it and which would have resulted in the removal of almost all HCV infected blood donors (74).

By this time, it became possible to use sequencing techniques in an attempt to study the variant of HCV present in the infective Gammagard batches and in some of the recipients who had developed HCV infection. Amplification of HCV RNA using the polymerase chain reaction (PCR) was followed by sequencing of amplified HCV cDNA at the NS-5 part of the HCV genome, as described above for the Irish episode, and it was possible to demonstrate that an HCV variant present in the batch that appeared to have infected almost all the English patients receiving it was also present in the English HCV-infected recipients (19). As second-generation anti-HCV tests are very effective (see above), it could be speculated that the donor (or donors) who may have been missed by second-generation anti-HCV EIA (and hence contaminating the plasma pool) may have been in the initial stages of HCV infection prior to the development of anti-HCV antibodies. This would have resulted in free HCV virons rather than HCV in the form of an immune complexes in the plasma pool used for Gammagard manufacture, and this, together with the loss of possible neutralizing anti-HCV antibody (which would have been derived from the plasma donation of other anti-HCV positive donors, prior to the introduction of second generation screening, discussed above) and the lack of any specific virucidal finishing step, may have caused some of the Gammagard batches to become infective for HCV. Additionally, it is known that individuals at the time of primary HCV infection may have levels of HCV as high as 10^8 (75), which is much higher than the levels found in individuals with chronic HCV infection where the HCV virions may also be of low infectivity due to complexing with anti-HCV antibodies (74).

VIRUSES POTENTIALLY TRANSMISSIBLE BY IVIG PREPARATIONS

Lipid-Enveloped Viruses

Hepatitis C

In 1992, following the identification of HCV as the causative virus in NANBH associated with coagulation factor concentrate therapy (26), the PCR for the detection of HCV RNA was used to investigate whether HCV could also be the implicated virus in IVIG-associated NANBH and to assess if PCR could be used to identify infective batches of IVIG. As described above, many studies have confirmed that HCV is also the causative virus in NANBH associated with IVIG therapy (Table 2). In a detailed longitudinal study based on stored serum samples (24), of the 33 patients with IVIG-associated NANBH studied, HCV RNA could be detected in 15 who were HCV RNA–negative prior to the development of NANBH after administration of implicated IVIG batches. In eight of the nine patients in whom no sample was available for PCR testing prior to IVIG therapy, HCV RNA could be detected after IVIG therapy with IVIG batches implicated in NANBH transmission. In six patients who were HCV PCR–negative prior to IVIG therapy, samples were repeatedly HCV PCR–positive up to 8 years after implicated IVIG batches were administered, suggesting that once HCV infection occurs in this patient category, it persists.

Samples were available from patients prior to the administration of implicated or suspected IVIG batches, and nine patients were HCV PCR–positive before IVIG therapy, suggesting that some patients previously exposed to blood products (including fresh-frozen plasma) might have asymptomatic HCV infection. In this particular study, an unexpected finding was that exposure to an experimental IVIG batch in 1978–1979, manufactured in Sweden, was identified as the possible source of their HCV infection (J. Bjorkander, personal communication); in these patients samples obtained prior to 1979 and stored frozen till testing by PCR were HCV PCR–negative. In the remaining five patients, a definite source of exposure to HCV could not be identified, but blood or platelet transfusions were present as risk factors. Four patients were HCV PCR–negative after IVIG therapy with batches implicated in NANBH transmission, but, surprisingly, three patients became HCV PCR–positive despite the absence of symptoms suggestive of NANBH, and HCV RNA could not be detected in four patients who had definite NANBH after IVIG therapy. These results are relevant when considering the interpretation of published data on NANBH associated with IVIG therapy.

The same study attempted to assess if PCR could identify infective IVIG batches. Three of the IVIG preparations that were implicated in the various episodes of IVIG associated NANBH (3,7,8) were studied by HCV PCR; both batches of the experimental IVIG preparation implicated in NANBH and manufactured at the Baxter Pilot Plant (3) and six of the 14 batches of Gammonativ strongly suspected to transmit NANBH had detectable HCV RNA by PCR (7). However, the implicated batch of SNBTS IV IgG (8) and a further nine batches of this preparation that were manufactured at the same time but not implicated in NANBH transmission, were negative for HCV RNA, supporting the suggestion (see above) that HCV was present at a very low level in this transmission episode.

These results have been supported more recently by data obtained from the recent Gammagard outbreak, described above. In Spain (20), France (21), and Sweden (22), multiple genotypes and subtypes have been identified in patients with HCV infection following the administration of Gammagard, and many of these genotypes are present in more than one patient and in patients from different countries, confirming that the probable source of infection was one or more Gammagard batches common to one or more country. However, further studies by our group (Blake et al., manuscript in preparation) and in Sweden (22) have been able to identify only three different HCV genotypes present in possibly implicated batches of Gammagard, confirming the observation made above that HCV PCR–negative batches might still be capable of transmitting HCV infection.

More recently, attention has focused on partitioning of HCV during fractionation. These studies have either employed PCR to study the elimination of HCV or used a suitable model virus such as Bovine viral diarrhea virus (BVDV) to study both inactivation and elimination. Yei et al. reported that in an experimental IVIG batch manufactured from HCV antibody-positive donations, the resultant immunoglobulin contained detectable HCV RNA and that the fractionation process eliminated 4.7 $\log_{10}$ virus (detected by PCR), indicating that the fractionation process did not result in the complete removal of all HCV virions (77). In another study, Louie et al. investigated the removal of BVDV during the manufacture of IVIG preparations by modeling manufacturing procedures at a laboratory (100-ml) scale. This group observed an overall clearance of >3.5 $\log_{10}$ with no evidence of inactivation of BVDV during any of the fractionation steps. The majority of the virus was lost by fractionation into fraction III, a fraction not used for IVIG production (78). Lower levels of partitioning of BVDV have been reported, where only 0.9 $\log_{10}$ were cleared over the entire cold ethanol treatment stage (79). As described above, the presence or absence of anti-HCV antibody in the starting plasma pool may affect partitioning of HCV during the IVIG manufacturing procedure (72,73).

These results emphasize that the ultimate safety of IVIG as far as HCV is concerned depends on a virus inactivation step after cold ethanol fractionation specific for HCV, such as treatment with solvent detergent (80) or incubation at a low pH, which has been shown to be a particularly powerful means of inactivating lipid-enveloped model viruses (81,82) (see below).

Human immunodeficiency virus

In 1985, it became clear that the human immunodeficiency virus (HIV) could be transmitted by human coagulation factor concentrates, and there was concern that HIV could also be transmitted by IVIG preparations. The possibility of transmission of a retrovirus was raised by Webster and Lever, who reported that 1 of the 12 patients found to have HIV infection after receiving an experimental IVIG preparation in 1983 had also developed a progressive demyelinating disease of the spinal cord. Since demyelination of the spinal cord has not been seen in more than 200 patients with XLA or CVI, the possibility that the experimental IVIG preparation also transmitted a retrovirus was raised (84).

Before 1985 IVIG preparations were also derived from the plasma of donors who were not screened for antibody to HIV. As a result, there were numerous reports of patients who had apparently seroconverted for HIV after receiving IVIG or intramuscular immunoglobulin preparations. However, in extensive follow-up studies, none of these recipients who had passively acquired anti-HIV antibody developed any evidence of HIV infection (85). Subsequently, it was demonstrated that fractionation procedures used to manufacture IVIG preparations (modeled on a laboratory scale) are highly effective in inactivating and removing HIV from the starting plasma (86,87). In addition, the role of pH4 incubation (81–83,88) and incubation in the liquid phase in inactivating HIV was also demonstrated (86). Since the routine introduction of HIV antibody screening of all blood donors in 1985, there have been no reports of HIV transmission by IVIG preparations, which confirms the safety of current fractionation procedures with respect to HIV and the importance of HIV antibody screening of blood donors.

Hepatitis G

A new virus described either as hepatitis G virus (HGV) (89) or GBV-C (90) has been shown to cause persistent infection in humans. HGV has an RNA genome and is similar to hepatitis C virus (HCV) and other flaviviruses in its genome organization (91). The clinical significance of infection with HGV remains uncertain, but HGV RNA sequences have been detected by PCR in the plasma from a proportion of individuals with acute, fulminant hepatitis (92), although its causative role has been questioned (93). However, active infection with HGV can also be detected in a suprisingly high proportion of the general population. For example, 1.7% of nonremunerated blood donors in whom infection is presumably asymptomatic were HGV PCR–positive (89), which has prompted the concern that HGV infection may be transmitted by blood products such as factor VIII and IX concentrates and immunoglobulin preparations, in view of the similarity between HGV and HCV.

There are few data available regarding blood product safety at present, but we have recently developed a nested PCR to amplify the highly conserved 5' noncoding region of HGV and found that HGV RNA was present in factor VIII and IX concentrates prior to the institution of heat treatment, but also in batches of an IVIG preparation that had previously been shown to transmit HCV. However, when we tested the recipients of this IVIG preparation, none of them showed evidence of HGV, suggesting that while HGV RNA might be present in IVIG preparations, the batches received by these individuals were unlikely to be infective (94). More research is clearly needed, but these preliminary results are particularly relevant since it has proved difficult hitherto to develop a practical screening test to identify donors who might transmit HGV infection by serological techniques. However, it is likely that manufacturing procedures that are virucidal for HCV are also virucidal for HGV, and if an effective screening procedure cannot be developed, in vitro and in vivo evidence of partitioning and inactivation of HGV during the manufacture of IVIG preparations will be required.

Hepatitis B

Hepatitis B virus (HBV) has been shown to be transmitted by coagulation factor concentrates, and there have also been occasional incompletely documented reports of HBV transmission by intramuscular immunoglobulin preparations (see above). There are also two previous anecodotal reports of HBV transmission by intravenous immunoglobulin preparations. In the first report, an experimental gammaglobulin preparation was obtained from the supernatant of Cohn fraction II and was administered intravenously to 15 patients, most of whom were critically ill. Three patients were not critically ill and two, both with hypogammaglobulinemia, developed hepatitis later shown to be associated with the Australia antigen, and in retrospect these patients were infected with HBV (95). Unfortunately, this transmission incident was reported only in abstract form, although it was subsequently suggested that Cohn fractionation had not been used (personal communication to A. M. Prince by G. L. Gitnick).

Acute hepatitis B infection following intravenous immunoglobulin was also reported in 1976 (94). In the report of a single case, 2.5 g of gammavenin, an IVIG preparation based on pepsin treatment after cold ethanol fractionation, was administered daily for 6 days. Higher concentrations of pepsin were used than those used in combination with pH4 incubation (81,82), and the resulting IgG molecule in the IVIG preparation would have been partially fragmented. This observation suggests that if the HBV infection was caused by the gammavenin therapy, then the concentration of pepsin used in the manufacturing process for this IVIG preparation may have been insufficient to ensure viral safety as far as HBV was concerned.

Since these two reports, there have been no other reports of HBV transmission by IVIG preparations, presumably due to the combination of HBsAg screening, the presence of sufficient levels of anti-HBs in the plasma pool used for fractionation, the efficacy of cold ethanol fractionation in virus partitioning and removal, and viral inactivation steps such as solvent-detergent, pH4, or heat treatment in inactivating HBV. However, it is possible that some HBV mutants may not be susceptible to anti-HBs-mediated neutralization and may not be detected by HBsAg screening. Such mutants may become more common with increased vaccination against HBV, and it is conceivable that HBV infections could develop in recipients of IVIG preparations in which cold ethanol fractionation or a method of virus inactivation suitable for HBV was not involved in the manufacturing procedure. It is therefore important to exclude infection with hepatitis B in patients with unexplained hepatitis, and in such patients additional tests such as the measurement of HBV DNA or tests for hepatitis B infection other than the measurement of HBsAg should be considered, since some HBV mutants may not be detected by HBsAg screening alone.

Non-Lipid-Enveloped Viruses

There have also been reports that human coagulation factor concentrates might transmit non-lipid-enveloped viral pathogens such as the hepatitis A virus (HAV) (97,98), but unfortunately there are no specific data regarding the safety of IVIG preparations with respect to nonenveloped viruses other than the absence of reports of transmission of such viruses. Another non-lipid-enveloped virus, parvovirus B19, has also been transmitted by coagulation factor concentrates (99), and there was one case of a patient suffering from bone marrow aplasia in the 12 cases of NANBH associated with IVIG in 1983 (84), raising the possibility of parvovirus B19 transmission. However, parvovirus B19 DNA could not be detected in a stored sample from this patient when tested subsequently by PCR (F. Davidson et al., unpublished data), suggesting that parvovirus B19 infection was not the cause of bone marrow aplasia in this particular patient. Only one study has investigated IVIG preparations for parvovirus B19 DNA, and in a study of 10 IVIG batches, all were found to be negative (99).

Various mechanisms are likely to be important in ensuring the safety of IVIG preparations for non-lipid-enveloped viral pathogens. First, neutralizing antibodies are present in IVIG preparations and could neutralize viruses in the starting plasma pool and during IVIG manufacturing procedures, or neutralize viruses in the final product. Such antibodies could also provide protection to the recipients in the form of passive humoral immunity. However, to establish the mechanism of neutralization as a viral inactivation procedure, further validation data and batch control procedures by IVIG manufacturers would be required. Second, clearance of viral contaminants by cold ethanol fractionation may occur by physical partitioning over the various precipitation steps, and inactivation of such viruses may occur in the presence of various reagents, such as ethanol, used in the fractionation procedure or during freezing and/or thawing of cold ethanol fractions, as with lipid-coated viruses. Finally, it is possible that some loss of virus infectivity may occur during freeze-drying, but there are few published data on this aspect. Continued awareness of the possibility of transmission of new non-lipid-enveloped viruses is therefore required.

New Emerging Viruses

The emergence, discovery, and worldwide spread of HIV and HCV and their threat to the health of recipients of blood and blood products have focused attention on the importance of donor selection criteria, serological screening, and effective and well-validated viral inactivation procedures. However, there are many viruses that are a potential threat to human populations worldwide, and many factors are involved in their emergence, including global travel, changing behavior patterns, and human population growth. The viruses may demonstrate rapid genomic change; this is particularly true of single-stranded RNA viruses (100).

Hemorrhagic fever viruses (101) are among the most pathogenic examples of the new emerging viruses, and the rapid spread and high mortality associated with such viral infections have been captured graphically by Preston in *The Hot Zone*, a description of various episodes of Marburg and Ebola virus infection (102). Another potential threat, as yet unrealized, may arise from xenotransplantation where a transplant from an animal to a human may lead to a new human infectious disease. Transplants from baboons to humans have been proposed, and this is particularly dangerous since it is well established that many new emerging viral infections have their origins in other species. Examples include the simian immunodeficiency viruses found in African non-human primates, two of which (HIV-1 and HIV-2) have crossed into humans and are responsible for millions of cases of AIDS, and the human T-cell lymphotropic viruses (HTLV-1 and HTLV-2) which appear to have arisen by cross-species transmission of the related simian T-cell lymphotropic virus (STLV). The potential threat from xenotransplantation is magnified by the likelihood that the xenotransplant recipient would be immunosuppressed and less likely to clear viruses contaminating the transplanted organ.

At present the risk of new emerging viruses to the viral safety of IVIG preparations would seem to be unquantifiable and very low, but this may not be a problem that can be contained simply by exclusion of plasma collection from identifiable high-risk areas for the emerging virus infections. First, air travel can rapidly transport individuals harboring various diseases, and while they themselves may not be eligible to be blood donors, they may unknowingly spread the infection to other individuals who may themselves donate blood. Second, diseases may be spread by imported animals, typically primates, as exemplified by the near public health disaster when an Ebola virus outbreak occurred at a primate facility in Reston, Virginia (102). Several individuals were infected with the Reston Ebola virus but fortunately did not succumb to the disease and did not spread the disease to others. Third, the most insidious emerging viruses are unlikely to be those such as Ebola or Marburg virus disease, which have immediate and dramatic effects (and are likely to lead to donor self-exclusion for health reasons), but viruses such as the retroviruses that have an extended clinical latency following infection and are therefore difficult to identify in the absence of demonstrable clinical symptomatology.

The safety of IVIG preparations as far as new emerging viral infections are concerned is unlikely to be based on the availability of a screening test since in many cases the tests are still in the research category or are not widely available. While neutralizing antibody may be present in individuals who have recovered from the viral infection, as has been demonstrated for Lassa fever (103), it is unlikely that sufficient neutralizing antibody will be present in the plasma pool for IVIG manufacture or to provide passive immunity to recipients. Reliance for viral safety will therefore need to be placed on viral partitioning procedures, such as cold ethanol fractionation, and also on viral inactivation procedures, as described below. Inactivation procedures that remove or inactivate a wide range of viruses would be particularly desirable such as UV irradiation or the use of viral filtration or a combination of different methods.

In summary, although the risk from the new emerging viruses is speculative and cannot be quantified at present, clinicians treating patients with IVIG should be aware of this remote possibility and unexpected novel infections in IVIG recipients should be carefully investigated. Should a novel infection occur, records of the plasma source or of fractionation intermediates should be sufficiently detailed that donors can ultimately be traced retrospectively, should it prove necessary.

FACTORS RELEVANT TO THE VIRAL SAFETY OF IVIG PREPARATIONS

Many factors are relevant to the viral safety of IVIG preparations (Table 3). Some of the factors, such as donor exclusion criteria and donor screening for relevant viral infections, are important for all blood products whereas other factors, such as the specific viral inactivation steps, are relevant only to IVIG preparations. Some factors may be of critical importance, such as the nature of the viral inactivation procedure whereas other factors such as the final formulation may be relevant only if there is residual viral contamination of the IVIG preparation. Not all IVIG manufacturers carry out the procedures shown in Table 3. For instance, at least one manufacturer of an intravenous anti-D preparation does not use cold ethanol fractionation in the manufacturing procedure (50), and the testing of final IVIG batches by PCR for HCV RNA is only a regulatory requirement in the U.S., and only for intramuscular immunoglobulin preparations where there is no virucidal step in the manufacturing procedure.

Efficacy of Blood or Plasma Donor Screening

All blood and plasma collecting organizations have exclusion criteria in an attempt to identify high-risk donors for viral infection. However, high-risk donor exclusion is not fully effective, as shown by the continued detection of HIV- and HCV-infected donors who have not undergone self-deferral. The reasons for this are complex (105), but this may be a significant source of viral contamination. Attempts are also made to assess the general health; such screening procedures are important in reducing the viral load in the plasma pool used for IVIG manufacture. Nonetheless, such screening procedures can never be completely effective, as donors can be viremic prior to the development of either clinical symptoms, as in the case of HAV and parvovirus B19 infection, or prior to the development of antibodies that can be detected by a serological test, as in the case of HIV and HCV. A reduction of the viral load by partitioning and specific viral inactivation procedure are therefore of critical importance in ensuring IVIG safety.

Attempts have been made to calculate the residual risk of plasma pool contamination by viruses such as HCV and HIV, after donor exclusion criteria are taken into account. For HCV, there has been a major improvement in the detection of anti-HCV infection in blood and plasma donors, with the introduction of second-generation, multiantigen anti-HCV testing (104), and it has been estimated that the second-generation anti-HCV test is 93% sensitive (65). Nonetheless, there is no doublt that for HCV, donations may be collected from individuals with HCV infection during the so-called window period prior to the development of HCV antibody (106,107). Such window donations may be highly viremic and contain 10^8 copies/ml (75) or higher (106) of HCV virions compared with individuals in the chronic phase of HCV infection, who have titers of 10^2-10^7 copies/ml (108). However, not only are window donations particularly important due to the much higher titer, but there is also evidence that HCV complexed to antibody may be much less infectious (76).

Another source of possible HCV contamination of the plasma pool used for IVIG manufacture is the failure of the screening laboratory to detect all anti-HCV positive donations. The various causes of such failures include methodological differences in screening tests among different manufacturers, inadequate control of testing, problems with sample handling, and identification and improper test performance or calculations

(109). While there have been no published reports of laboratory errors leading to a failure to detect HCV-infected donors, it is possible that two anti-HCV-positive donors may not have been detected initially in the United Kingdom due to a failure of automated equipment (J. Barbara, personal communication).

One further aspect relates to the occurrence of different genotypes of HCV (110). Although all the known HCV genotypes can be detected by the current second- and third-generation anti-HCV tests, it should be noted that such tests are all based on antigens derived from one genotype, type HCV-1, and there is indirect evidence that common genotypes such as HCV-3 may be less easily detected (111,112).

Ideally, an alternative method of detection of HCV-infected donors prior to seroconversion or of chronically HCV-infected seropositive donors would be desirable. The testing of blood donors for raised alanine aminotransferase (ALT) levels was originally introduced in 1986 and 1987 as a method for detecting NANBH, in the absence of a specific serological test. However, in a recent detailed analysis, the yield, predictive value, and cost-effectiveness of ALT screening of blood donors was found to have declined dramatically with the introduction of routine anti-HCV testing, particularly of second-generation screening; it has therefore been suggested that ALT screening should be discontinued (113). Although PCR is a promising methodology and has been shown to be potentially applicable to the screening of viral contaminants (99), numerous practical obstacles preclude the routine use of PCR as a donor screening method for HCV.

Similar calculations of the risk of an HIV-infected donation contaminating the plasma pool, despite current anti-HIV testing assays, have also been made. A recent study in the U.S. calculated that one donation in every 360,000 was made during the window period, confirming that the risk of contaminating the plasma pool by screened blood is very small (114) primarily because of the sensitivity of the current anti-HIV enzyme immunoassays. This risk may theoretically be reduced further with HIV antigen testing, although this remains to be proven.

A small but significant problem is also likely to be associated with laboratory errors in anti-HIV testing. Two cases were recently reported where transcription errors during anti-HIV screening led to the release and transfusion of blood from HIV-positive blood donors. Increased automation and computerization of record keeping should make such errors less likely, but the risk of error during the testing, distribution, or administration of blood donations should not be overlooked (115). This would presumably also apply to plasma donations destined for fractionation.

In summary, there is an extremely low residual risk of HIV contamination of plasma pools due to the effectiveness of anti-HIV screening (116). The residual risk of HCV contamination is probably at least 1 log order of magnitude higher (117), and HCV will remain the main concern regarding viral safety of IVIG preparations as far as the starting plasma pool is concerned. The use of PCR at this stage for the detection of HCV RNA may therefore be an important way of increasing the viral safety of IVIG preparations (see below).

Methods of Virus Partitioning or Inactivation Used in IVIG Manufacture

Many of the improvements in the viral safety of blood products have arisen from the introduction of viral inactivation steps (Table 4). However, the importance of partitioning of viruses should not be underestimated. In virtually all IVIG manufacturing procedures

Table 4 Methods of Viral Partitioning or Inactivation Used in the Production of IVIG Preparations

Cold ethanol fractionation ethanol	Has weak virucidal activity—main importance is in partitioning of virus into waste fractions as demonstrated for HBV, HIV, and HCV.
Downstream purification	Usually chromatographic procedure. This is not considered a virucidal step but it may assist in the partitioning of viruses.
Finishing step	Solvent-detergent Heat treatment pH4/pH4.25 β-propriolactone + UV Antibody-mediated virus neutralization Viral filtration UV irradiation
Postfill storage	Some viruses may have reduced infectivity in liquid phase, especially in acid pHs.

this is achieved by cold ethanol fractionation, and the term "virus partitioning" is to be preferred to "virus elimination" or "virus removal," since the virus may partition into other fractions that could be used for other blood products. The term "inactivation" is also preferred, since viral RNA (or DNA) can be still detectable by PCR despite major reductions in infectivity (118).

There are four basic approaches used to establish the efficacy of a viral inactivation procedure. First, the protein that is being purified needs to be assessed for structural and functional integrity, as some viral inactivation procedures can damage proteins so that there is an increased incidence of adverse reactions or reduced efficacy on administration to patients. Second, the effectiveness of the inactivation procedure should be evaluated by adding ("spiking") a known amount of virus into the starting plasma pool or the intermediate fraction and reassaying for the virus following the inactivation procedure. Third, animal studies can be undertaken, although these are used less nowadays due to the expense and concerns about the relevance of animal models. Finally, clinical trials can be undertaken that include infectious disease surveillance of recipients, who are ideally previously unexposed to the virally inactivated material.

A number of different methods have been employed for virus inactivation (and elimination) and there are summarized in Tables 5 and 6. A number of processes used in plasma fractionation, such as cold ethanol fractionation and antibody-mediated neutralization precipitation, are relevant for viral safety. Although these processes are difficult to validate and are not controlled for virus removal, they are discussed in detail due to their importance. For IVIG preparations, two main methods have been used: incubation at pH4 (or pH4.25), and solvent-detergent treatment; these are also discussed in detail below. One method (β-propiolactone treatment) is used by only one manufacturer for IVIG and is no longer used for clotting factors due to recent problems with HIV transmission (120) and is therefore not discussed in detail.

Use of model viruses

The evaluation of virus inactivation methods is a complex subject (119), but due to the difficulties of obtaining and introducing high titers of pathogenic viruses into an IVIG manufacturing facility, model viruses are used (Table 5). Viruses may be chosen either because, like HIV, they are potential contaminants of the plasma pool used for IVIG manufacture (and are therefore relevant viruses) or because they have certain physico-chemical properties (and are therefore model viruses). Model viruses provide an assurance that any virus will be removed or inactivated to some degree by the virucidal process. To some extent, all viruses are "model" viruses in that they are grown in the laboratory, but it should be noted that small-volume experiments using model viruses are often employed to evaluate virucidal procedures. For instance, inactivation data with HIV and various model viruses have been obtained from small-volume experiments (typically about 20 ml). As the manufacturing process is operated on a very much larger scale, such model experiments may therefore not fully reflect routine manufacturing procedures for IVIG preparations.

It is clearly important that, where possible, relevant model viruses be used in validation studies as only HIV and HAV, of the viruses known to be transmitted by blood, can be cultured reliably in vitro. Although primate models can be used for HBV and HCV, these models are used less frequently than before due to the shortage and cost of such animals and doubts about the full relevance of the data obtained. Where model viruses are used, it is important that consideration be given to the process being studied. For instance, there may be differences in the susceptibility of different strains of the same model virus, and the choice of viral strain will depend on the virus inactivation or removal methodology being investigated; e.g., heat-resistant virus strains should be used to validate heat treatment processes, and small viruses should be selected to validate filtration methods (see below).

The choice of the model virus to use is not straightforward. HCV is currently classified as a flavivirus and model flaviviruses such as yellow fever virus have been used, as have pestiviruses such as BVDV (see above) or hog cholera virus. Sindbis, a togavirus, has also been used, and it is still unclear as to whether one model virus can be used for the investigation of all inactivation procedures or whether the choice of virus depends on the inactivation step being studied. Semliki Forest virus, a togavirus that

Table 5 Some Factors Relevant to the Use of Model Viruses to Study Viral Inactivation

All but one of the reported episodes of HCV transmission by IVIG used production methods that did not have a specific viral inactivation step

In vitro validation of viral inactivation steps are now required by regulatory bodies prior to clinical studies

Viruses used can either be defined as relevant (e.g., HIV) or model, for viruses which cannot be cultured in vitro (e.g., HBV, HCV)

Data are required for enveloped and nonenveloped viruses (e.g., HAV)

A shortage of animals and doubts about validity of animal models have hampered animal studies with HBV and HCV

Investigations of viral inactivation for important viruses other than HIV depend on the use of model viruses

A wide range of model viruses should be used, and it is essential that model viruses selected take account of process being validated—e.g., heat-resistant model viruses for heat treatment processes and small viruses for filtration

Virus strain should be selected carefully—e.g., two different BVDV strains show different resistance to heat treatment at 37 °C; HAV strains may show similar variability in properties

Reliable and reproducible viral culture methods for model viruses are needed

Table 6 Summary of Viral Inactivation Methods

Antibody-mediated virus neutralization
    present in all IVIG preparations but difficult to quantify for viruses that are neutralized by
        antibodies in the donor population
    relevant for HBV, HAV, parvovirus B19
    potentially expensive and difficult to control and validate on an industrial manufacturing
        scale
Treatment with pH4 or pH4.25
    not generally considered as a viral inactivation procedure
    includes pepsin at trace concentrations in some IVIG preparations
    enveloped viruses (HCV, HIV) readily inactivated
    acid-resistant, nonenveloped viruses, e.g., poliovirus not inactivated
    temperature and incubation time at pH4 may be relevant
    usually combined with freeze-dried final product formulation that may stabilize virus
β-Propriolactone treatment (+ UV irradiation)
    used for manufacture of IVIG (one manufacturer)
    βPL process active against HCV and lipid enveloped model viruses (pseudorabies,
    vesicular stomatitis virus) and HAV
    limited effect on SV40
Solvent-detergent treatment
    inactivates lipid-enveloped viruses (HIV, HBV, HCV)
    solvent-detergent mixture removed at end of process by chromatography
    excellent safety record for coagulation factor concentrates
    not designed to inactivate non-lipid-enveloped viruses such as HAV, B19
Pasteurization in the presence of stabilizers
    used for many coagulation factor concentrations and one IVIG preparation
    potential for increasing adverse reaction rate
    excellent safety record for coagulation factor concentrates but isolated cases of viral
        transmission still occur (HBV, HCV, B19)
    stabilizers for IgG may also stabilize viruses
Viral filtration
    filters of different sizes are available that could remove viruses while allowing IgG
        molecule to pass through
    currently under investigation for coagulation factors
    initial results promising but more research is needed
UV irradiation
    experimental method under evaluation at present
    capable of inactivating a wide range of viruses
    may be particularly relevant for viruses that are not inactivated by treatment with solvent-
        detergent or incubation at low pH

---

has been used as a model virus for HCV, has been reported to be more resistant than BVDV to incubation at pH4 in the presence of low concentrations of pepsin, but this property is also strain-dependent. Even where a virus transmitted by blood products can be cultured, such as HAV, there may be difficulties with studying the kinetics of viral inactivation. For instance, first, to culture HAV the wild-type strain needs to be adapted to laboratory conditions. Second, when studying the viral safety of immunoglobulin preparations, the presence of neutralizing antibody may interefere with spiking experiments and even make the study impractical. Third, it may be difficult to culture HAV to a sufficient titer for experimental use.

Cold ethanol fractionation

Cold ethanol fractionation was first described by Cohn and co-workers in 1946 (32), and since then there have been many variants such as the Kistler-Nitschmann process (33). The main contribution of cold ethanol fractionation to the viral safety of IVIG preparations is probably based on the partitioning and subsequent removal of viruses during each precipitation step; in support of this concept, a reduction in the levels of HBsAg (121) and HIV (86,87) during cold ethanol fractionation have previously been demonstrated.

During cold ethanol fractionation, inactivation in the presence of processing reagents such as ethanol or inactivation of viruses during freezing and/or thawing of cold ethanol fractions may also occur. However, the incubation in ethanol probably has a minor effect of viral inactivation as shown for HIV (122) and presumably other lipid-enveloped viruses. In view of the long-established and proven safety record of intramuscular immunoglobulin and IVIG preparations (with the exceptions described above) derived from cold ethanol fractionation, it is likely that cold ethanol fractionation will remain an essential part of manufacturing processes ensuring the safety of IVIG in the foreseeable future.

Antibody-mediated virus neutralization

IVIG preparations contain a wide spectrum of antiviral antibodies that reflects the range of antibodies in the donor population. There is relatively little known about the importance of most of these antibodies to viral safety, but the relevance and significance of neutralizing antibodies was recently demonstrated by the report that screening for HCV-infected donors using an anti-HCV EIA had the paradoxical effect of decreasing the viral safety of IVIG, suggesting that the loss of HCV antibodies from the plasma pool used for IVIG manufacture either removed neutralizing activity or could have changed the partitioning characteristics of HCV during plasma fractionation (see above).

The existence of neutralizing antibodies for HCV in donor plasma has been hotly debated, as the majority of HCV-infected individuals have persistent infection despite the presence of multiple antibodies that are reactive with HCV antigens, suggesting that neutralizing antibodies have a minimal role in viral clearance. However, in a study where a chimpanzee was deliberately infected with HCV, and sera obtained at variable periods after infection were mixed with acute-phase infection serum—i.e., viremic serum prior to the development of anti-HCV antibodies—it was shown that a serum obtained 11 years after infection had no neutralizing effect, whereas a serum obtained 2 years after infection was able to neutralize the presumed infecting HCV strain. Although these sera differed markedly in their neutralizing response, they both contained antibodies against nonstructural and structural HCV proteins including the envelope antigen. In an attempt to explain these results, an analysis of sequential viral isolates was undertaken and showed that significant genetic divergence of the HCV strain had occurred, beginning early in the course and persisting throughout. Further, different strains were recovered from different champanzees, given the same acute-phase inoculum, consistent with the early presence of quasispecies as outlined above (123).

In addition, neutralization of HCV has been examined using an in vitro model, and, using inhibition of in vitro HCV replication as the end point, it has been demonstrated that serum from a chronically infected patient was able to neutralize the original infecting inoculum for a period of 5 years, but not thereafter. Virus isolated from this patient later in his course was not neutralized by serum obtained early in this course but was neutralized by serum obtained 1 year after the later isolation (124).

These studies therefore suggest that neutralizing antibody responses do occur but are highly strain-specific and may therefore have little protective activity in the HCV-infected individual. When plasma is pooled, as during the course of IVIG manufacture, neutralizing antibodies from many anti-HCV-positive individuals are present so that all strains of HCV could theoretically be neutralized. However, because of a lack of understanding of the precise nature of neutralizing antibodies for HCV and the incorporate of anti-HCV screening into routine blood and plasma collection, it is unlikely that there could be a reversion to the situation prior to 1991, when blood and plasma collection centers did not screen at all for HCV.

The situation concerning HAV and parvovirus B19 and other potential or unidentified nonlipid-enveloped viruses is complex. However, the safety of IVIG preparations with respect to nonenveloped viruses (and indeed enveloped viruses) is likely to benefit from the presence of neutralizing antibodies present throughout the IVIG manufacturing process. Such antibodies could theoretically neutralize virus in the plasma pool, during processing, and in the final product, and, in addition, provide protection to the recipients by providing passive immunity. The relevance of this is exemplified by the regulatory requirement that all batches of immunoglobulin preparations must contain at least 0.5 IU of anti-HBsAg antibody per gram immunoglobulin. This requirement is based on the observation that early batches of intravenous immunoglobulin contained small amounts of HBsAg in the form of immune complexes (125) and that an excess of anti-HBs could prevent HBV transmission caused by coagulation factors (126). However, to establish neutralization as a well-defined viral inactivation (or elimination) step, further validation data are required.

Treatment at pH4 (or pH4.25)

The incubation of the immunoglobulin solution during IVIG manufacture at pH4 (or pH4.25 in the case of one IVIG manufacturer) in the presence or absence of low concentrations of pepsin is a widely used procedure after cold ethanol fractionation. Incubation at acid pH was originally introduced to reduce adverse reactions to intravenously administered IgG (57) but has since been shown to inactivate a wide range of viruses, including enveloped viruses such as HIV and HCV (78,81–83). However, some nonenveloped viruses such as poliovirus appear to be acid-resistant and are not inactivated (81). It is noteworthy that there has been only one reported case of transmission of HCV associated with an IVIG preparation with a pH4 finishing step compared with IVIG preparations in which chromatographic steps were involved, and in this particular episode the cause of transmission was thought to be due to a GMP failure (63).

Precise details for the acid incubation conditions are not available from IVIG manufacturers, who may well differ in their acid incubation procedures. However, it should be noted that there are differences in the inactivation rate of viruses at pH4 depending on the time and temperature of incubation. One IVIG manufacturer formulates the IVIG preparations in the liquid form at pH4.25 with a holding period of 21–24 days at 21–27 °C, thus maximizing the viral inactivating effect of acid incubation.

Heat treatment

The use of heat treatment as a method of virus inactivation has been utilized for albumin solutions, which are usually treated at 60 °C for at least 10 h, a form of virus inactivation usually described as liquid pasteurization. Albumin solutions are generally regarded as being free of viral transmission, but there have been few formal trials of viral safety reported, possibly because such developments preceded major concerns about the viral safety of blood products. Coagulation factor concentrates are subjected to a variety of viral inactivation procedures. Among the methods used are either liquid pasteurization or dry heat treatment; a great deal of evidence is available that both forms of heat treatment inactivate a wide range of viruses present in coagulation factor concentrates. Nonetheless, there are case reports of HBV, HCV, and parvovirus B19 transmission following administration of heat-treated coagulation factor concentrates, indicating that some viruses may not be totally inactivated, and possibly indicating that it is essential to minimize the virus load in the plasma pool used for fractionation.

Heat treatment has not been widely applied to IVIG preparations, as heating can affect the IgG molecule and potentially increase the adverse reaction rate. Also, until recently, viral transmission was not considered to be as serious a problem with IVIG preparations as with coagulation factor concentrates. Nonetheless, one IVIG manufacturer has developed a process for liquid pasteurization, which does not denature the IgG molecule, involving heating at 60 °C for 10 h, in the presence of sorbitol as a stabilizer. HIV and various model viruses were shown to be inactivated by this procedure (127), and a recent clinical trial has demonstrated that there was no increase in the adverse reaction rate or difference in efficacy when the liquid-pasteurized IVIG preparation was compared with two other, widely used, licensed IVIG preparations (128).

The possibility of dry heat treatment of IVIG preparations has been raised, as this can be performed in the final container in which the IVIG is formulated, thus permitting the viral inactivation step to be the very last stage in the IVIG production process (129). Dry heat treatment at 100 °C was suggested as this could be added to existing licensed IVIG preparations without little or no increase in cost, but would be able to improve viral safety. However, data were subsequently reported about the functional integrity of the IgG molecule, aggregation, and anticomplementary activity after heating at 80 °C for 72 h, a heating regimen commonly used for coagulation factor concentrates. It was found that heat treatment resulted in aggregation and a functional impairment of the IgG molecule. Caution was also expressed about the efficacy of heat treatment even at 100 °C as a method of viral inactivation (130).

This is clearly an area for future development, since heat treatment could act as a second viral inactivation step in combination with other procedures and with a different spectrum of viruses that could be inactivated, but further development work is required. Long-term studies of virus safety and to exclude the development of antibodies against neoantigens in the IgG molecule (resulting from heat treatment) in nonimmunodeficient recipients of pasteurized IVIG will also be required to assess if this procedure is as safe as incubation at acid pH or solvent detergent treatment.

Solvent-detergent treatment

The treatment of coagulation factor concentrates with a nonvolatile solvent and a detergent has been shown to inactivate lipid-enveloped viruses (131). Following completion of the virus inactivation step, the mixture of solvent and detergent must be removed, usually by chromatography. This method has been used for many coagulation factor concentrates, and no cases of HIV, HBV, or HCV transmission appear to have been reported in association with this method. The use of solvent-detergent treatment has recently been extended to IVIG preparations, but there are as yet relatively few clinical data about safety and efficacy. However, one study of an IVIG preparation, derived from Cohn fractionation II, treated with low concentrations of pepsin at pH4.4 and solvent-detergent, showed that the IVIG preparation was well tolerated; trough serum IgG levels were comparable with two other IVIG preparations, suggesting the half-life of the IgG molecule was unaffected (80).

Treatment with β-propiolactone

One IVIG manufacturer has used β-propiolactone (βPL) in combination with ultraviolet light to activate the βPL. This IVIG preparation has been available for many years and has been demonstrated to be clinically efficacious, but it has been reported that βPL may result in some modifications to the IgG molecule with a slightly reduced half-life in vivo (132). More recently, the efficacy of βPL in inactivating HIV in plasma was questioned (133), but data about the efficacy of viral inactivation for IVIG manufacture were subsequently reported (79). Although this process can inactivate nonlipid-coated viruses such as HAV, it has not been widely used due to technical difficulties in utilizing βPL in the routine production of IVIG.

Other methods of viral partitioning or inactivation

There are a number of other methods for partitioning or inactivation of potentially contaminating viruses.

Chromatography. Chromatographic methods such as the use of columns containing ion exchange resins like DEAE-Sephadex have been investigated extensively in the manufacture of blood products as methods for purifying various proteins such as IgG (134) from plasma with a high yield and little or no change in the native structure. On first sight, the case for the introduction of adsorption chromatography would seem to be an attractive one, but, as described above, all but one of the HCV transmission incidents seem to have been associated with this purification procedure. The reason for this may lie in the need for a very high efficiency of virus removal. For instance, at a virus particle concentration of 10^5/ml (a concentration that could be present in a plasma pool if there was one "window" donation in 1000 negative donations), an efficiency of >99.9999% is required on every occasion that the chromatography column was being used. Because of the costs of the columns, there is a temptation to reuse chromatography material (50), and the efficacy and reliability of decontamination becomes critical.

The concept that a chromatographic method can be considered a method for partitioning the virus from the protein being purified is therefore a controversial one, but in practical terms it is a process that is difficult to validate and control on a large scale, and minor differences in physicochemical properties of viruses can have a major influence, which makes the effectiveness of chromatography difficult to extrapolate from validation studies. The presence or absence of antibodies may influence the effectiveness of chromatography, and this method is now not generally regarded as a viral partitioning or inactivation method by regulatory authorities.

Nonetheless, there are data indicating that chromatography can effectively remove viral contaminants during the manufacture of immunoglobulin preparations. Zoltan and Padvelskis studied the ability of various ion exchange resins to remove HBsAg from a plasma sample containing a very high HBsAg concentration. It was shown that some ion exchange resins could remove more than 4 $\log_{10}$ HBsAg particles (135).

These studies were extended to an investigation of whether ion exchange chromatography could remove HBV infectivity from an intravenous immunoglobulin preparation using an animal model. Plasma with high levels of HBV was purified by ion exchange chromatography, and the IgG from this procedure was evaluated for viral safety by administration to two experimental chimpanzees and one control chimpanzee (which receiv!ed HBV-containing plasma prior to processing). It was found that ion exchange chromatography could reduce the HBsAg level from 200 ng/ml to <1 ng/ml. The two experimental chimpanzees did not develop hepatitis, unlike the control chimpanzee, indicating that ion exchange chromatography might have a role in virus removal for HBV-contaminated plasma (136).

Filtration. The possibility of removing viruses by filtration is an attractive one since it can be used in combination with other physicochemical inactivation processes such as pH4 incubation or solvent-detergent treatment and near the terminal stages of IVIG production, thus reducing the likelihood of contamination at a late stage in the manufacturing process. A membrane with a mean pore size of 100 nm is required to reliably remove HIV, whereas a much smaller pore size, 20 nm, is required to reliably remove HCV, as the size of this virus has been estimated to be 30–38 nm in diameter (137). The use of filters has been successfully demonstrated for the removal of HCV (137) and HIV (138).

Unfortunately, there are many difficulties with introducing membrane filtration as a virus-removing step. The process is difficult to control as it is dependent on the characteristics of the filter used, the composition of the solution being processed, and the fluid flow characteristics near the membrane surface. The pores in the membrane may vary in size, and the larger pores in a filter of a defined mean size could theoretically let viruses larger than the mean pore size through. However, there is a multilayered structure to some of the membranes (138), with up to 100 or more layers. As each layer may filter about 15% of the virus, such multilayered filters can be very efficient.

There are, however, some disadvantages to membrane filtration. It is important to demonstrate that the viruses are removed by the filter and not to the gel layer at the filter surface or simply absorbed to the matrix or to protein material fouling the filter. Aggregation of viruses may also affect the level of virus removed by the filter. Despite much research, the properties of filters remains complex, and quality control and validation are therefore difficult. The flow of fluids through pores is related to the pore radius, and a filter with a suitable size may reduce fluid flow rate, making this technology greatly impractical on a large scale. Finally, the membranes that are available for viral filtration are expensive, and this technology is unlikely to become widely used in the near future.

Ultraviolet irradiation. Ultraviolet (UV) irradiation was first used during World War II for the sterilization of pooled plasma. However, in recent years UV irradiation has been superseded by other methods of sterilization. More recently, the use of UV irradiation during the production of IVIG preparations has been investigated using model viruses by Hart and co-workers, who found that UV treatment only altered one characteristic of the IgG molecule—the percentage of aggregates in the IVIG preparation. The UV doses used were effective on a dry-heat-resistant virus, vaccimia; Semliki Forest virus, a model virus for HCV, was also inactivated. Two other model viruses (poliovirus 2 and T4 phage), which were nonenveloped and nonacid-labile, were also inactivated, and UV irradiation would therefore seem to be particularly relevant to processes where the viral safety of an IVIG preparation is dependent upon pH4 incubation or treatment with solvent detergent (139). This is clearly an inactivation method with potential as an additional step in combination with existing methods.

PROCEDURES THAT MIGHT IMPROVE THE VIRAL SAFETY OF IVIG PREPARATIONS

PCR

There are various procedures that are not routinely used by IVIG manufacturers that might improve the safety of IVIG preparations (Table 3). The testing of plasma pools for evidence of viral infection by measuring antibodies to HIV and HCV and HBsAg have been performed for many years. However, while a sample from an HIV-infected donor can be diluted 100–10,000 fold and still be positive in the anti-HIV enzyme immunoassay and similarly for HBsAg, the same is not true for HCV. There has therefore been the suggestion that plasma pools destined for fractionation should be investigated for the presence of HCV RNA by PCR, as the concentration of HCV RNA is likely to be higher than in the final product, and HCV RNA has previously been detected in plasma pools (140). Also, the testing of the plasma pools by PCR would be a useful additional test of the anti-HCV screening of donors in case an unknown failure had occurred during donor screening (109); the European regulatory authorities have proposed that plasma pools should be tested for HCV RNA. In addition, some manufacturers are in favor of testing plasma pools, since they could be discarded if found to be PCR-positive before any blood products manufacturing procedures are carried out. It is also possible to test other so-called intermediate products in IVIG manufacture, but the decision as to which samples to test, other than plasma pool samples from the IVIG manufacturing procedure, is at present controversial.

In contrast, the Food and Drug Administration (FDA) in the U.S. has requested the routine introduction of PCR testing for HCV in all IVIG preparations that do not have a well-documented virus inactivation procedure in their manufacturing process, following the recent transmission of HCV infection by an IVIG preparation. This approach is an attractive one, since coagulation factor concentrates have been shown to contain HCV RNA (141) and immunoglobulin batches have been shown to contain HCV RNA in them (142). PCR testing could therefore act as a criterion for product release. However, a blood product could be PCR-positive and yet not be infective. This is not surprising, since infectivity depends on the presence of more than just RNA and DNA, and viral enzymes and proteins may be important in the infectivity process. These viral enzymes and proteins may be denatured during the virus inactivation procedure used in blood product manufacture and yet have no effect on the results of the PCR test (118). In addition, PCR is a technically demanding test, and false-negative and false-positive PCR results are possible. At present, all PCR testing kits are designated as being for research use only, and standardized, reproducible, highly sensitive PCR kits are urgently needed. Nonetheless, it is likely that PCR testing will be introduced in some form or another for a range of relevant viruses over the next few years by manufacturers of IVIG preparations as a criterion for proceeding with fractionation and/or product release.

Multiple Inactivation Steps

The idea that multiple, well-quantified inactivation steps might increase the safety of IVIG procedures has been discussed for many years for coagulation factor concentrates in order to allow the inactivation of a range of viruses or higher quantities of viruses. For instance, solvent-detergent treatment does not inactivate nonlipid-coated viruses and may not be adequate to ensure complete viral safety in IVIG preparations that are not based on cold ethanol fractionation as an initial partitioning step (50) compared with IVIG preparations derived from cold ethanol fractionation (80). It is therefore possible that one or more IVIG manufacturers may in the future use solvent-detergent treatment as an additional virus inactivation step (after incubation at acid pH). However, as these two procedures appear to have a similar spectrum of viruses inactivated (143), there might not be an increase in the viral safety of the doubly inactivated IVIG preparation.

The Paul-Ehrlich Institute in Germany has attempted to codify and quantify requirements for viral inactivation (144). They have issued guidelines that state that manufacturing procedures must include virus inactivation and removal procedures that give a 10 log removal of encapsulated viruses and a 6 log removal for nonencapsulated viruses. There must also be two stages each effecting a titer reduction of 4 logs or greater for encapsulated viruses, and one corresponding stage of this order of magnitude must be supplied for nonencapsulated viruses.

There have been a number of criticisms of these guidelines. These include the observation that the need for two reduction steps for nonenveloped viruses has not been scientifically proven, and the reasons for two reduction steps for enveloped viruses of 10 logs should not be extended to all plasma products. Of more relevance, reduction factors of 10 logs cannot be absolutely proven, e.g., for HIV; there would need to be at least 2000 donors with the highest HIV RNA titers per plasma pool of 1000 L to justify this degree of virus removal or inactivation. Finally, HIV is the only clinically relevant virus used in validation studies, and model viruses are used instead. Each model virus has advantages and disadvantages, and the choice of model viruses and their use in validation studies needs to be flexible. As a result, although the guidelines were issued in 1994, they have remained controversial and have not yet been adopted by the regulatory authorities in Europe or the U.S. Nonetheless, as the concept of more than one inactivation procedure being carried out is being applied to coagulation factor concentrates (145), it may be incorporated by one or more manufacturers to IVIG preparations (80).

In Vitro Infectivity Assays

The study of the viral safety of blood products depends on the availability of in vitro infectivity assays. Unfortunately, for HCV the only animal models available is the use of primates, and such experiments have not significantly helped our understanding of factors that affect HCV infectivity (71,146). The availability of an in vitro infectivity assay for HIV has helped greatly in studying the effects of various methods of viral inactivation on HIV, and a similar model for HCV would be highly desirable. There has been much work in this area over the past few years, and it appears that it may now be possible to culture HCV, albeit at low levels of infection (147). Progress can therefore be expected in the area of in vitro infectivity assays which would be complementary to data on HCV RNA measured by PCR and model viruses for HCV.

CONCLUSIONS

It is now clear that HCV can be transmitted by IVIG preparations in a manner similar to HCV transmission by human coagulation factor concentrates. Although the number of patients infected by HCV has been very small in relation to the total number of patients treated with IVIG, it should be noted that there are occasional anecdotal reports of possible additional cases of hepatitis after IVIG therapy (16,148), but it is important to distinguish such episodes from previous reports of the passive transmission of anti-HCV antibodies found in patients receiving IVIG preparations prior to the introduction of HCV screening (149–151) and possible nosocomial infections (152,153). As patients with HCV infection may have normal ALT levels (154,155), it is essential that HCV PCR be used for investigating patients with suspected NANBH after IVIG therapy, particularly if they suffer from a primary (156) or secondary immunodeficiency. HCV PCR testing of IVIG batches is probably only of value where HCV transmission by IVIG is suspected (157,158); careful batch and infusion records are essential for definitely linking IVIG batch with patients (19,56).

This analysis of HCV transmission by IVIG preparations confirms that cold ethanol fractionation is of critical importance in ensuring the viral safety of IVIG preparations, as shown by the high rate of HCV infection of anti-D recipients manufactured by the Hoppe method. Virucidal finishing steps are essential (Table 6) since most of the episodes of HCV transmission by IVIG preparations have involved a chromatographic procedure as a finishing step, and the data to date suggest that IVIG preparations manufactured by such procedures should be followed by the incorporation of specific procedures that are known to be virucidal in IVIG manufacture. It is not generally appreciated that such virucidal procedures should be capable of being defined, controlled, and validated within the manufacturing process, and whereas several other factors such as chromatography may also contribute to virus safety, they were not designed for this purpose and are therefore not particularly relevant to viral safety. The need for more than one virucidal procedure in the same manufacturing process remains controversial.

While it is likely that anti-HCV screening may improve the safety of blood products by decreasing the titer of anti-HCV in the starting plasma pool for fractionation, second- or (third-) generation anti-HCV screening is not completely effective in removing plasma donation infective for HCV and would not detect the viremic plasma donor at the time of primary HCV infection. The introduction of plasma pool screening for HCV and other relevant viruses may therefore be very important. The role of PCR screening of the final IVIG product seems less clear, since PCR positivity may not necessarily correlate with infectivity. Further studies are also required to fully define the margin of safety of IVIG preparations with respect to nonlipid-enveloped viruses, in particular by studying the relevance of steps such as neutralization by antibodies against such viruses.

It is also noteworthy that all the IVIG preparations associated with HCV transmission have been formulated as lyophilized preparations. While this step has been introduced to ensure stability of the IgG molecule prior to the administration of the IVIG preparation, it may have had the unfortunate side effect of stabilizing any HCV virions present in the final product. It is known that HIV virions are less stable in the liquid phase, particularly at room temperature, and it is possible to speculate that this may also apply to HCV virions, since both HIV and HCV are single-stranded RNA viruses.

While the focus of this overview has been mainly on previous episodes of HCV transmission by IVIG, the importance of general factors that contribute to blood product safety, such as high standards of GMP and careful clinical trials, should not be forgotten (159,160). If failures of GMP are responsible for sporadic NANBH transmission episodes, then routine anti-HCV screening of plasma donors may also increase safety by reducing the possibility of contamination of fractionated products by plasma infective for HCV within the fractionation facility. Finally, although there is no evidence of viruses other than HCV being transmitted, the possibility of transmission of new emerging or novel viruses and a degree of vigilance with careful IVIG batch recording and collection of representative blood samples from regular IVIG recipients would be desirable to ensure that any new episodes of viral transmission by IVIG are rapidly recognized and investigated.

ACKNOWLEDGMENTS

I thank Peter Foster for many helpful suggestions and comments, and Bob Perry, Bruce Cuthbertson, and Fraser Leslie for many useful discussions on blood product safety. I also thank June MacLeod and Barbara Caine for bibliographic assistance, and Sandra Sneddon for assisting with manuscript preparation.

REFERENCES

1. Lane RS. Non-A non-B hepatitis from intravenous immunoglobulin. Lancet 1983; ii:974–975.
2. Lever AML, Webster ADB, Brown D, Thomas HC. Non-A non-B hepatitis occurring in agammaglobulinaemic patients after intravenous immunoglobulin. Lancet 1984; ii:1062–1064.
3. Ochs HD, Fischer SH, Virant FS, Lee MI, Kingdon HS, Wedgewood RJ. Non-A non-B hepatitis and intravenous immunoglobulin. Lancet 1985; i:404–405.
4. Ochs HD, Fischer SF, Virant FS, et al. Non-A, non-B hepatitis after intravenous immunoglobulin. Lancet 1986; i:323.
5. Weiland O, Mattson L, Glaumann H. Non-A non-B hepatitis after intravenous gammaglobulin. Lancet 1986; i:976–977.
6. Hammarstrom L, Smith CIE. IgM production in hypogammaglobulinaemia patients during non A, non B hepatitis. Lancet 1986; i:743.
7. Bjorkander J, Cunningham-Rundles C, Lundin P, Olsson R, Soderstrom R, Hanson LA. Intravenous immunoglobulin prophylaxis causing liver damage in 16 of 77 patients with hypogammaglobulinaemia or IgG subclass deficiency. Am J Med 1988; 84:107–111.
8. Williams PE, Yap PL, Gillon J, Crawford RJ, Galea G, Cuthbertson B. Transmission of non-A, non-B hepatitis by pH4 treated intravenous immunoglobulin. Vox Sang 1989; 57:15–18.
9. Suomela H. Inactivation of viruses in blood and plasma products. Transfus Med Rev 1993; 7:42–57.
10. Bjoro K, Froland SS, Yan Z, Samdal HH, Haaland T. Hepatitis C infection in patients with primary hypogammaglobulinaemia after treatment with contaminated immune globulin. N Engl J Med 1994; 331:1607–1611.
11. Lockner D, Bratt G, Lindborg A, Tornebohm E. Acute unidentified hepatitis in a hypo-

gammaglobulinaemic patient on intravenous gammaglobulin successfully treated with interferon—case report. Acta Med Scand 1987; 221:413–415.

12. Renger FG, Frank KH, Reimann W, et al. Erste Ergebnisse zur Virushepatitis C als Klinisch and immunologisch definierbare Form der non-A, non-B-Hepatitiden. Med Aktuell 1979; 11:518–519.

13. Power JP, Lawlor E, Davidson F, et al. Hepatitis C viraemia in recipients of Irish intravenous anti-D immunoglobulin. Lancet 1994; 334:116–117.

14. Outbreak of hepatitis C associated with intravenous immunoglobulin administration—United States, October 1993–June 1994. MMWR 1994; 43:505–509.

15. Pawlotsky J-M, Bouvier M, Deforges L, Dural J, Bierling P, Dhumeaux D. Chronic hepatitis C after high dose intravenous immunoglobulin. Transfusion 1994; 34:86–87.

16. Quinti I, Pandolf F, Paganelli R, et al. HCV infection in patients with primary defects of immunoglobulin production. Clin Exp Immunol 1995; 102:11–16.

17. Taliani G, Guerra E, Rosso R, et al. Hepatitis C virus infection in hypogammaglobulinaemic patients receiving long-term replacement therapy with intravenous immunoglobulin. Transfusion 1995; 35:103–107.

18. Schiano TD, Bellary SV, Black M. Possible transmission of hepatitis C virus infection with intravenous immunoglobulin. Ann Intern Med 1995; 122:802–803.

19. Healey CJ, Sabharwal NK, McOmish F, et al. Outbreak of acute hepatitis C following the use of anti-HCV screened intravenous immunoglobulin therapy. Gastroenterology 1996; 110:1120–1126.

20. Echevarria JM, Leon P, Dimingo CJ, et al. Laboratory diagnosis and molecular epidemiology of an outbreak of hepatitis C virus infection among recipients of a human intravenous gammaglobulin in Spain. Transfusion 1996; 36:725–730.

21. Lefrere J-J, Martinot-Peignoux M, Mariotti M, et al. Infection by hepatitis C virus through contaminated intravenous immune globulin gammagard: results of a national prospective inquiry. Transfusion 1996; 36:394–397.

22. Widal A, Zhang Y-Y, Andersson-Gare B, Hammarstrom L. At least six different hepatitis C virus strains found in swedish and Danish patients with gammagard associated hepatitis C. Transfusion (in press).

23. Choo QI, Kuo G, Weiner AJ, Overby IR, Bradley DW, Houghton M. Isolation of a cDNA clone derived from a blood borne non-A, non-B viral hepatitis genome. Science 1989; 244:359–362.

24. Yap PL, McOmish F, Webster ADB, et al. Hepatitis C virus transmission by intravenous immunoglobulin. J Hepatol 1994; 21:455–460.

25. Kuo G, Choo Q-L, Alter HJ, et al. An assay for circulating antibodies to a major etiologic virus of human non-A, non-B hepatitis. Science 1989; 244:362.

26. Manucci PM. Clinical evaluation of viral safety of coagulation factor VIII and IX concentrates. Vox Sang 1993; 64:197–203.

27. Propert SA. Hepatitis after prophylactic serum. Br Med J 1938; 2:677–678.

28. Anonymous. Hepatitis following administration of human serum. (Editorial.) Ann Intern Med 1943; 19:368–371.

29. Neefe JR, Stokes J Jr, Reinhold JG, Lukens FDW. Hepatitis due to the infection of homologous blood products in human volunteers. J Clin Invest 1944; 23:836–856.

30. Murray R, Ratner F. Safety of immune serum globulin with respect to homologous serum hepatitis. Proc Soc Exp Biol Med 1953; 83:554–555.

31. Pennell RB. The distribution of certain viruses in the fractionation of plasma. In: Hartmann FW, Lo Grippo GA, Mateer JG, Barron J, eds. Hepatitis Frontiers. London: Churchill J&A, 1957:297–310.

32. Cohn EJ, Strong LE, Hughes WL Jr, et al. Preparation and properties of serum and plasma proteins. IV. A system for the separation into fractions of the proteins and lipoprotein components of biological tissues and fluids. J Am Chem Soc 1946; 68:459–475.

33. Kistler P, Nitschmann H. Large scale production of human plasma fractions. Vox Sang 1962; 7:414–424.

34. Cockburn WC, Harrinton JA, Zeitlin RA, Morris D, Campa FE. Homologous serum hepatitis and measles prophylaxis. Br Med J 1951; 2:6.

35. Janeway CA. Clinical use of blood derivatives. JAMA 1948; 138:859.

36. Keusch GT, Olsson RA, Troncale FJ. Asymptomatic hepatitis in adults given gamma-globulin for prophylaxis. Arch Intern Med 1969; 124:326–329.

37. Petrilli FL, Crovari P, de Flora S. Hepatitis B in subjects treated with a drug containing immunoglobulins. J Infect Dis 1977; 135:252–258.

38. John TJ, Ninan GT, Rajagopalan MS, et al. Epidemic hepatitis B caused by commercial human immunoglobulin. Lancet 1979; i:1074.

39. Tabor E, Gerety R. Transmission of hepatitis B by immune serum globulin. Lancet 1979; ii:1293.

40. de Silva LC, Sette H, Antonacio F, Lopes JD. Commercial gammaglobulin (CGG) as a possible vehicle of transmission of HBsAg in familial clustering. Rev Inst Med Trop Sao Paulo 1977; 19:352–354.

41. Dioguardi N, de Franchis R. Hepatitis B surface antigen in commercial gammaglobulin. Lancet 1975; ii:816.

42. Berg R, Bjorling H, Berntsen K, Espmark A. Recovery of Australia antigen from human plasma products separated by a modified Cohn fractionation. Vox Sang 1972; 22:1–13.

43. Leveque P, Dronet J, Schmitt Lauesler R, North ML, Amouch P, Magras J. HBs antigen in human plasma fractions. Vox Sang 1975; 28:1–8.

44. Hoofnagle JH, Gerety RJ, Thiel J, Barker LF. The prevalence of hepatitis B surface antigen in commercially prepared plasma products. J Lab Clin Med 1976; 88:102–113.

45. Dittmann S, Roggendorf M, Durkop J, Weise M, Lorbeer B, Deinhardt F. Long term persistence of hepatitis C virus antibodies in a single source outbreak. J Hepatol 1991; 13:323–327.

46. Bowman JM, Friesen AD. Anti-D immunoglobulin and immune thrombocytopenia—a problem of ethics in blood transfusion practice. Vox Sang 1989; 56:136–137.

47. Hoppe HH, Mester T, Henning W, Krebs HJ. Prevention of Rh-immunisation. Modified production of IgG anti-Rh for intravenous application by ion-exchange chromatography (IEC). Vox Sang 1973; 25:308–316.

48. Tesar V. The production and properties of human immunoglobulin G-anti-D (Halle). Gesundheitswesen 25:741–745.

49. Cunningham CJ. Production of human immunoglobulin anti-D (Rho) for intravenous administration for a national Rh prophylaxis programme. Biochem Soc Transfus 1980; 8:178–179.

50. Friesen AD, Bowman JM, Bees WCH. Column ion exchange chromatographic production of human immune serum globulin for intravenous use. Vox Sang 1985; 48:201–212.

51. Bowman JM. The advantages of intravenous Rh-immune globulin. Clin Obstet Gynaecol 1982; 25:341–347.

51. Walsh TJ, O'Riordan JP. A review of the production and clinical use of intravenous anti-D immunoglobulin. Irish Med J 1982; 75:243–244.

52. Roggendorf, Lu M, Fuchs K, et al. Variability of the envelope regions of HCV in European isolates and its significance for diagnostic tools. Arch Virol 1993; 7(S7):27–39.

53. Rinker J, Galambos JT. Prospective study of hepatitis B in thirty-two inadvertently infected people. Gastroenterology 1981; 81:686–691.

54. Sodeyama T, Kiyosawa K, Urushihara A, Matsumoto A, Tanaka E, Furutas, et al. Detection of hepatitis C virus marker and hepatitis C-virus genomic-RNA after needle stick accidents. Arch Intern Med 1993; 153:1565–1572.

55. Expert Group of the Blood Transfusion Service Board. Report. Stationary Office Publication 1538. Dublin 1995.

56. Power JP, Lawlor E, Davidson F, Holmes EC, Yap PL, Simmonds P. Molecular epidemiology of an outbreak of infection with hepatitis C virus in recipients of anti-D immunoglobulin. Lancet 1995; 345:1211–1213.

57. Barandun S, Kistler P, Jennet F, Isliker H. Intravenous administration of human gammaglobulin. Vox Sang 1962; 7:157–174.

58. Leen CLS, Yap PL, Neill G, McClelland DBL, Westwood A. Serum ALT levels in patients with primary hypogammaglobulinaemia receiving replacement therapy with intravenous immunoglobulin or fresh frozen plasma. Vox Sang 1986; 50:26–32.

59. Rousell RH, Good RA, Piofsky B, Schiff RI. Non-A, non-B hepatitis and the safety of intravenous immune globulin. pH 4.2: a retrospective survey: preliminary communication. Vox Sang 1988; 54:6–13.

60. Gutteridge CN, Veys P, Newland AC. Safety of intravenous immunoglobulin for treatment of autoimmune thrombocytopenia. Acta Haematol 1988; 79:88–90.

61. Imbach P, Perret BA, Babington R, Kaminski K, Morell A, Heiniger HJ. Safety of intravenous immunoglobulin preparations: a prospective multicenter study to exclude the risk of non-A, non-B hepatitis. Vox Sang 1991; 61:240–243.

62. Yap PL. Supply of blood products. Br Med J 1991; 302:1538.

63. Foster PF, McIntosh RV. Current safety of clotting factor concentrates. Arch Pathol Lab Med 1990; 114:1188.

64. Lee ML, Courter SG, Tait D, Kingdon HS. Long term evaluation of intravenous immune globulin preparation with regard to non-A, non-B hepatitis safety. In: Zuckerman AJ, ed. Viral Hepatitis and Liver Disease. New York: Alan R Liss, 1988:596–599.

65. Aach RD, Stevens CE, Hollinger FB, et al. Hepatitis C virus infection in post-transfusion hepatitis. N Engl J Med 1991; 325:1325–1329.

66. Esteban JI, Gonzalez A, Hernadez JM, et al. Open prospective efficacy trial of anti-HCV screening of blood donors to prevent post-transfusion hepatitis. In: Hollinger FB, Lemon SM, Margolis HS, eds. Viral Hepatitis and Liver Disease. Baltimore: Williams and Wilkins, 1991:441.

67. Habibi B, Garetta M. Screening for Hepatitis C Virus antibody in plasma for fractionation. Lancet 1990; 335:855–856

68. Schiff P, Kemp A. Safety of IVIG made from HCV-antibody screened plasma. Lancet 1991; 338:1076

69. Finlayson JS, Tankersley DL. Anti-HCV screening and plasma fractionation: the case against. Lancet 1990; 335:1274–1275

70. Thomas DP. Immunoglobulins and hepatitis C virus. Lancet 1990; 335:1531–1532

71. Biswas RM, Nedjar S, Wilson LT, Mitchell FD, Snoy PJ, Finlayson JS, Tankersley DL. The effect on the safety of intravenous immunoglobulin of testing plasma for antibody to hepatitis C. Transfusion 1994; 34:100–104

72. Yu MW, Mason BL, Guo ZP, Tankersley DL, Nedjar S, Mitchell FD, Biswas RM. Hepatitis C transmission associated with intravenous immunoglobulins. Lancet 1995; 345:1173–1174

73. Nubling CM, Willkommen H, Löwer J. Hepatitis C transmission associated with intravenous immunoglobulins. Lancet 1995; 345:1174

74. Takano S, Nakamura K, Kawai S, Yokosuka O, Satomura Y, Omata M. Prospective assessment of donor blood screening for antibody to hepatitis C virus by first- and second-generation assays as a means of preventing post-transfusion hepatitis. Hepatology 1996; 23:708–712

75. Alter H, Sanchez-Pescador R, Urdea MS, Wilber JC, Lagier RJ, Di Bisceglie AM, Shih JW, Neuwald PD. Evaluation of branched DNA signal amplification for the detection of hepatitis C virus RNA. Journal of Viral Hepatitis 1995; 2:121–132

76. Hijikata M, Shimizu YK, Kato H, et al. Equilibrium centrifugation studies of hepatitis C virus: evidence for circulating immune complexes. J Virol 1993; 67:1953–1958.

77. Yei S, Yu MW, Tankersley DL. Partitioning of hepatitis C virus during Cohn Oncley fractionation of plasma. Transfusion 1992; 32:824–828.

78. Louie RE, Galloway CJ, Dumas ML, Wong MF, Mitra G. Inactivation of hepatitis C virus on low pH intravenous immunoglobulin. Biologicals 1994; 22:13–19.

79. Dichtelmuller, Rudnick D, Breuer B, Ganshirt KH. Validation of virus inactivation and removal for the manufacturing procedure of two immunoglobulins and a 5% serum protein solution treated with β-propiolactone. Biologicals 1993; 21:259–268.

80. Ebeling F, Baer M, Hormila P, et al. Tolerability and kinetics of a solvent-detergent-treated intravenous immunoglobulin preparation in hypogammaglobulinaemia patients. Vox Sang 1995; 69:91–94.

81. Reid KG, Cuthbertson B, Jones ADL, McIntosh RV. Potential contribution of mild treatment at pH4 to the viral safety of human immunoglobulin products. Vox Sang 1988; 55:75–80.

82. Kempf C, Jentsch P, Poirier B, et al. Virus inactivation during production of intravenous immunoglobulin. Transfusion 1991; 31:423–427.

83. Hamalanen E, Suomela H, Ukkonen P. Virus inactivation during intravenous immunoglobulin production. Vox Sang 1992; 63:6–11.

84. Webster ADB, Lever AML. Non-A, non-B hepatitis after intravenous immunoglobulin. Lancet 1986; i:322.

85. Centers for Disease Control. Safety of therapeutic immunoglobulin preparations with respect to transmission of human T-lymphocyte virus type I/lymphadenopathy associated virus infection. MMWR 1986; 35:231–232.

86. Mitra G, Wong MF, Mozen MM, Mcdougal FS, Levy JA. Elimination of infectious retroviruses during preparation of immunoglobulin. Transfusion 1986; 36:394–397.

87. Wells MA, Wittek AE, Epstein JS, et al. Inactivation and partition of human T-cell lymphotrophic virus, type III, during ethanol fractionation of plasma. Transfusion 1986; 26:210–213.

88. Kempf C, Barre-Sinoussi F, Morgenthaler J-J, Germann D. Inactivation of human immunodeficiency virus (HCV) by low pH and pepsin. J AIDS 1991; 4:828–830.

89. Linnen J, Wages J, ShangKeck ZY, et al. Molecular cloning and disease association of hepatitis G virus: a transfusion transmissible agent. Science 1996; 271:505–508.

90. Simons JN, Pilot-Matias TJ, Learly TP, et al. Identification of two flavivirus-like genomes in the GH hepatitis agent. Proc Natl Acad Sci USA 1995; 92:3401–3405.

91. Leary T, Muerhoff AS, Simons JN, et al. Sequence and genomic organization of GBV-C: a novel member of the Flaviviridae associated with human non-A-E hepatitis. J Med Virol 1996; 48:60–67.

92. Yoshiba M, Okamoto H, Mishiro S. Detection of the GBV-C hepatitis virus genome in serum from patients with fulminant hepatitis of unknown aetiology. Lancet 1995; 346:1131–1132.

93. Kao JH, Chen PJ, Chen DS. GBV-C in the aetiology of fulminant hepatitis. Lancet 1996; 347:120.

94. Jarvis LM, McOmish F, Hanley JP, Yap PL, Ludlam CA, Simmonds P. Low transfusion rate of hepatitis G virus/GBV-C to haemophiliacs and other recipients of plasma products. Lancet 1996; 348:1352–1355.

95. Winters RE, Gitnick GL. Australia antigen related hepatitis transmitted by gamma-globulin. Gastroenterology 1971; 60:732.

96. Nakamura S, Sato T. Acute hepatitis B after administration of gammaglobulin. Lancet 1976; i:487.

97. Manucci PM. Outbreak of hepatitis A among Italian patients with haemophilia. Lancet 1992; 339:819.

98. Lawlor E, Graham S, Davidson F, et al. Hepatitis A transmission by factor IX concentrates. Vox Sang 1996; 71:126–128.

99. McOmish F, Yap PL, Jordan A, Hart H, Cohen BJ, Simmonds P. Detection of parvovirus B19 in donated blood: a model system for screening of polymerase chain reaction. J Clin Microbiol 1993; 31:323–328.

100. Holland JJ. Evolving virus plagues. Proc Natl Acad Sci USA 1996; 93:545–546.

101. Le Guenno B. Emerging viruses. Sci Am 1995; Oct.:30–37.

102. Preston R. The Hot Zone. New York: Random House, 1994.

103. Jahrling PB, Peters CJ, Stephen EL. Enhanced treatment of Lassa fever by immune plasma combined with ribavarin in cynomolgus monkeys. J Infect Dis 1984; 149:420–427.

104. Kleinman S, Alter H, Busch M, et al. Increased detection of hepatitis C virus (HCV)-infected blood donors by a multi-antigen HCV enzyme immunoassay. Transfusion 1992; 32:805–813.

105. Dodd RY. Viral contamination of blood components and approaches for reduction of infectivity. Immunol Invest 1995; 24:25–48.

106. Vrielink H, van der Poel CL, Reesink HW, Zaaijer HL, Lelie PN. Transmission of hepatitis C virus by anti-HCV-negative blood transfusion. Vox Sang 1995; 68:55–56.

107. Kitchen AD, Wallis PA, Gorman AM. Donor-to-donor and donor-to-patient transmission of hepatitis C virus. Vox Sang 1996; 70:112–113.

108. Bresters D, Mauser-Bunschoten EP, Reesink HW, et al. Sexual transmission of hepatitis C virus. Lancet 1993; 342:210–211.

109. Sazama K. Existing problems in the testing for infectious disease. Immunol Invest 1995; 24:131–146.

110. Simmonds P, Holmes EC, Cha TA, et al. Classification of hepatitis C virus into six major genotypes and a series of subtypes by phylogenetic analysis of the NS-5 region. J Gen Virol 1993; 74:2391–2399.

111. McOmish F, Chan SW, Dow BC, et al. Detection of three types of hepatitis C virus in blood donors: investigation of type-specific differences in serologic reactivity and rate of alanine aminotransferase abnormalities. Transfusion 1993; 33:7–13.

112. Dhaliwal SK, Prescott LE, Dow BC, et al. Influence of viraemia and genotype upon serological ractivity in screenikng assays for antibody to hepatitis C virus. J Med Virol 1996; 48:184–190.

113. Busch MP, Korelitz JJ, Kleinman SH, et al. Declining value of alanine aminotransferase in screening of blood donors to prevent posttransfusion hepatitis B and C virus infection. Transfusion 1995; 35:903–910.

114. Lackritz EM, Satten GA, Aberle-Grasse J, et al. Estimated risk of transmission of the human immunodeficiency virus by screened blood in the United States. N Engl J Med 1995; 333:1721–1725.

115. Linden JV. Error contributes to the risk of transmissable disease. Transfusion 1994; 34:1016.

116. Schreiber GB, Busch MP, Kleinman SH, Korelitz JJ. The risk of transfusion-transmitted viral infections. N Engl J Med 1996; 334.

117. Riggert J, Schwartz DWM, Uy A, et al. Risk of hepatitis C virus (HCV) transmission by anti-HCV-negative blood components in Austria and Germany. Ann Hematol 1996; 72:35–39.

118. Hart H, McOmish F, Hart WG, Yap PL, Simmonds P. A comparison of PCR with an infectivity assay for HIV-1 titration during virus inactivation of blood products. Transfusion 1993; 33:838–841.

119. Minor PD. Meeting report. Meeting of the acceptance criteria for virus validation studies. Biologicals 1995; 23:107–110.

120. Arzneimittelkommission. Informationen. Beriplex HS 250 und 500. Arzneimittel Pharmazeutische Zeitung 1994; 139:2192–2193.

121. Schroeder BD, Mozen MM. Australia antigen, distribution during cold ethanol fractionation of human plasma. Science 1970; 168:1462–1464.

122. Henin Y, Marechal V, Barre-Sinoussi F, Chermann J-C, Morgenthaler J-J. Inactivation

and partition of human immunodeficiency virus during Kistler and Nitschmann fractionation of human blood plasma. Vox Sang 1988; 54:78–83.

123. Farci P, Alter HJ, Govindarajan S, et al. Lack of protective immunity against reinfection with hepatitis C virus. Science 1992; 258:135–140.

124. Shimizu YK, Yoshikura H, Hijikata M, Iwamoto A, Alter HJ, Purcell RH. Neutralising antibodies against hepatitis C virus and the emergence of neutralization escape mutant viruses. J Virol 1994; 68:1494–1500.

125. Hoofnagle JH, Waggoner JG, Hepatitis A and B virus markers in immune serum globulin. Gastroenterology 1980; 78:259–263.

126. Tabor E, Aronson DL, Gerety R. Removal of hepatitis B infectivity from factor IX complex by hepatitis B immune-globulin. Lancet 1980; ii:68–70.

127. Uemura Y, Uriyu K, Hirao Y, et al. Inactivation and elimination of viruses during the fractionation of an intravenous immunoglobulin preparation: liquid heat treatment and polyethylene glycol fractionation. Vox Sang 1989; 56:155–161.

128. Zuhrie SR, Webster ADB, Davias R, Fay ACM, Wallington TB. A prospective controlled crossover trial of a new heat-treatment intravenous immunoglobulin. Clin Exp Immunol 1995; 99:10–15.

129. Rubinstein AI, Rubinstein DB, Tom W. Terminal 100C dry heat treatment of intravenous immunoglobulin preparations to assure sterility. Vox Sang 1994; 66:295–296.

130. Matejschuk P, Harrison P, More JE. Dry heat treatment of intravenous immunoglobulin—some practical considerations. Vox Sang 1995; 68:255–257.

131. Horowitz MS, Rooks C, Horowitz B, Hilgartner M. Virus safety of solvent-detergent treated anti-haemophilic factor concentrate. Lancet 1988; ii:186–189.

132. Morell A, Schurch B, Ryser D, Hoger F, Skvaril F, Barandum S. In vivo behaviour of gamma globulin preparations. Vox Sang 1980; 38:272–283.

133. Norley SG, Lower J, Kurth R. Insufficient inactivation of HIV-1 in human cryo poor plasma by beta-propiolactone: results from a highly accurate virus detection method. Biologicals 1993; 21:251–258.

134. Baumstark JS, Laffin RJ, Bardawil WA. A preparative method for the separation of 7S gamma globulin from human serum. Arch Biochem Biophys 1994; 108:514–522.

135. Zolton RP, Padvelskis JV. Evaluation of an ion-exchange procedure for removal of hepatitis type B comtamination from human gamma globulin products. Vox Sang 1984; 47:114–121.

136. Zolton PR, Padvelskis JV, Kaplan PM. Removal of hepatitis B virus infectivity from human gamma-globulin prepared by ion-exchange chromatography. Vox Sang 1985; 49:381–389.

137. Yuasa T, Ishikawa G, Manabe-S-i, Sekiguchi S, Takeuchi K, Miyamura T. The particle size of hepatitis C virus estimated by filtration through microporous regenerated cellulose fibre. J Gen Virol 1991; 72:2021–2024.

138. Hamamoto Y, Harada S, Kobayashi S, et al. A novel method for removal of human immunodeficiency virus: filtration with porous polymeric membranes. Vox Sang 1989; 56:230–236.

139. Hart H, Reid K, Hart W. Inactivation of viruses during ultraviolet light treatment of human intravenous immunoglobulin and albumin. Vox Sang 1993; 64:82–88.

140. Simmonds P, Zhang LQ, Watson HG, et al. Hepatitis C quantification and sequencing in blood products, haemophiliacs, and drug users. Lancet 1990; 336:1469–1472.

141. Garson JA, Preston FE, Makris M, et al. Detection by PCR of hepatitis C virus in factor VIII concentrates. Lancet 1990; 335:1473.

142. Yu MYW, Mason BL, Tankersley DL. Detection and characterization of hepatitis C virus RNA in immune globulins. Transfusion 1994; 34:596–602.

143. Hart H, Hart WG, Foster PR. Virus inactivation in intravenous immunoglobulin: a comparison with S/D treatment of factor VIII. Transfus Med 1945; 5:41.

144. Paul Ehrlich Institute, Langen, Germany. Bundesanzelger 1994; 101:9243–9244.

145. Biesert L, Lemon S, Goudeau A, Suhartono H, Wang LR, Brede HD. Viral safety of a new highly purified factor VIII (octate). J Med Virol 1996; 48:360–366.

146. Iwarson S, Wejstal R, Ruttimann E. Non-A, non-B hepatitis associated with the administration of intravenous immunoglobulin—transmission studies in chimpanzees. Serodiagn Immunother 1987; 1:261–266.

147. Nakajima N, Hijikata M, Yoshikura H, Shimizu YK. Characteristics of long term culture of hepatitis C virus. J Virol 1996; 70:3325–3329.

148. Quinti I, Sacco G, el Salman D, et al. Intravenous immunoglobulin may still infect patients. Br Med J 1994; 308:856.

149. Horst H-A, Schmitz N, Glinike C, Loffler H, Lanfs R. Seroconversion for hepatitis C virus antibody in bone marrow recipients treated with immune globulin. N Engl J Med 1991; 325:132–133.

150. Ward KN, Morgan G, Ashworth K, Bremner J, O'Callaghan A, Teo CG. Spurious outbreak of HCV in bone-marrow recipients treated with cytomegalovirus immunoglobulin. Lancet 1992; 340:1290–1291.

151. Dodd LG, McBride JH, Gitnick GL, Howantiz PJ, Rodgerson NO. Prevalence of non-A, non-B hepatitis/hepatitis C virus antibody in human immunoglobulins. Am J Clin Pathol 1992; 97:108–113.

152. Bruce Dull H. Syringe transmitted hepatitis: a recent episode in historical perspective. JAMA 1961; 176:413–418.

153. Mitsui T, Iwano K, Masuko K, et al. Hepatitis C virus infection in medical personnel after needlestick accident. Hepatology 1992; 16:1109–1114.

154. Healey CJ, Chapman RWG, Fleming KA. Liver histology in hepatitis C infection: a comparison between patients with persistently normal or abnormal transaminases. Gut 1995; 37:274–278.

155. Rossini A, Gazzola GB, Ravaggi A, et al. Long-term follow-up of and infectivity in blood donors with hepatitis C antibodies and persistently normal alanine aminotransferase levels. Transfusion 1995; 35:108–111.

156. Webster ADB, Brown D, Franz A, Dusheiko G. Prevalence of hepatitis C in patients with primary antibody deficiency. Clin Exp Immunol 1996; 103:5–7.

157. Dammacco F, Sansonno D, Beardsley E, Gowans EJ. Failure to detect hepatitis C virus (HCV) genome by polymerase chain reaction in human anti-HCV positive intravenous immunoglobulins. Clin Exp Immunol 1993; 92:205–210.

158. Lafrere JJ, Mariotti M, Trepo C, et al. Testing for HCV-RNA in commercial intravenous immunoglobulins. Lancet. 1993; 341:834–835.

159. Cuthbertson B, Perry RJ, Foster PR, Reid KG, Crawford RJ, Yap PL. Factors influencing the viral safety of intravenous immunoglobulin. J Infect 1987; 15:125–133.

160. Zuck TF. Current good manufacturing practices. Transfusion 1995; 35:955–966.

7
Alternative Methods for the Administration of Intravenous Immunoglobulin

Martin L. Lee
School of Public Health, University of California, Los Angeles, California

INTRODUCTION

Historically, the goal in the production of immunoglobulin concentrates was to formulate a safe and efficacious product that could be administered by the intravenous route, as opposed to the painful and less advantageous intramuscular approach. Most manufacturers have formulated a product which is concentrated at about 5% (weight by volume), and can usually be administered at rates on the order of 4 ml/kg of body weight per hour. As a result, a 400 mg/kg infusion would require about 2 h to administer. This brief chapter will review attempts not to only reduce the time of the infusion by both increasing the rate of administration and concentration (and thus reducing the volume), but also to examine other administration routes of IVIG for specialized indications.

REDUCED ADMINISTRATION TIMES

As noted above, the average time to administer a dose of 400 mg/kg is about 2 h. Of course, in various autoimmune disorders for which doses of 1–2 g/kg are routine (see various other chapters in this book), the infusion time will be proportionally higher. These intervals pose a problem for the patient and create difficulties for the treating investigator in their ability to serve a significant number of individuals. They may also have an important impact on the cost of treatment.

A reduction in the administration time may be accomplished either by increasing the infusion rate, increasing the concentration of IVIG (utilizing less diluent in the case of a lyophilized preparation), or a combination of the two. In the early clinical trials in patients with primary immunodeficiency syndromes, attempts to increase the rate of administration beyond 4 ml/kg/h were met with limited success due to infusion rate-related adverse reactions (1). Subsequently, more carefully controlled approaches were able to tolerize the patient to a greater extent, and these have been documented in isolated published reports (2,3). From experiments in 16 primary immunodeficient patients receiving 170 infusions, it became clear that an infusion time of 30 min for a 400 mg/ kg dose could be achievable if a 10% solution was administered at 8 ml/kg/h. The rate of systemic reactions, e.g., chills or fever, was 12.4%, not substantially different from that expected with a standard infusion protocol.

We have recently summarized a series of studies conducted in the U.S., Luxembourg, and Sweden, which systematically examined the ability to safely reduce IVIG infusion times (4).

In the U.S. component of the trial, 27 primary immunodeficient patients were placed on a monthly regimen where the goal after 10 monthly infusions was to achieve a 30-min infusion time using a 10% concentration and an infusion rate of 8 ml/kg/h. (Initially, the concentration was increased, followed by a gradual increase in the rate.) Twenty-six of the 27 subjects (96%) were successfully infused over 30 min for at least two consecutive infusions. (Indeed, eight of the patients were infused at a rate in excess of 8 ml/kg/h). The one failure was an individual who had a prior history of reactions to IVIG preparations (who because of study enrollment criteria should not have been entered in the trial). Systemic adverse reactions occurred in 10.1% (of 276 infusions) and included flushing, backache, and nausea. Only one event (GI distress/backache) was classified as severe. Not surprisingly, the frequency of reactions occurred early in the study regimen and gradually tapered off as patients became accustomed to the increasing IVIG infusion concentration and, to a lesser extent, the rate.

The Luxembourg and Swedish sites enrolled a total of 38 patients with the majority presenting with nonimmunodeficient syndromes such as idiopathic thrombocytopenia purpura (ITP), chronic lymphoctyic leukemia (CLL), multiple myeloma, various autoimmune disorders, and bone marrow transplantation. As with the U.S. cohort, almost all subjects reached the minimal infusion time with a systemic reaction rate on the order of 10% (although only one of the Swedish patients reported any reaction at all [localized pain]). It is interesting to note that the administration of IVIG under these conditions had no effect on the average peak IgG level achieved.

While these trials demonstrate that a very short infusion time is achievable in various types of patients requiring IVIG, it should be kept in mind that all but one studied subject had had no prior reactions to this product. Thus, the use of such regimens should be considered primarily in the better candidates—e.g., chronic IVIG users and younger patients.

ALTERNATIVE ROUTES OF ADMINISTRATION

Intraperitoneal Administration

Intraperitoneal administration of IVIG has been successfully administered for the prophylaxis and treatment of peritoneal infections after major abdominal surgery. A total dose of 10 g of a 5S IgG preparation was utilized (5).

Intrathecal Administration

The treatment of bacterial meningitis by the intravenous use of immunoglobulin is hindered because of the blood-brain barrier, although high doses administered over very brief intervals have the potential to overcome this problem. The intrathecal use of IVIG has been considered based on an experimental rabbit model of meningitis (6). However, the use of IVIG under these conditions is limited by the volume that may be delivered (no more than 10 ml in adults), which in turn limits the total dose (7). This approach can therefore offer only supplemental treatment, at best.

A single case report has been presented in the literature involving the use of a hyperimmune IgM product (8). This preparation was chosen as it contained reasonably high titer antibodies against the isolate of echovirus recovered from an infected patient. Using both intrathecal and intravenous administration of IVIG, sterilization of the cerebrospinal fluid was achieved, but the virus was not eliminated from the central nervous system tissue. The patient ultimately died. On the other hand, Kondoh et al. (9) reported marked improvement with intrathecally administered IgG after a poor response to IVIG in a 7-year-old patient with echovirus 11 infection. This patient also received intrathecal α-interferon and was reported to be well at a 21-month follow-up examination.

Intraventricular Administration

Similarly, IVIG has been administered intraventricularly for the treatment of meningoencephalitis with varying degrees of success (10–14). Erlendsson and colleagues initially reported the successful treatment of enterovirus encephalitis in a patient with X-linked agammaglobulinemia (10). Treatment utilized placement of an Ommaya reservoir in a lateral ventricle with subsequent injection (138 mg given over 5 days followed by 5.6 g over 15 days) of concentrated (6%) IVIG.

Two further cases using a similar method were reported by the same group with successful resolution in one of the subjects and mixed results in the second (12). McKinney et al. reported substantial improvement in 6 of 12 agammaglobulinemic patients with chronic enteroviral meningoencephalitis given a different IVIG preparation through a reservoir device placed intraventricularly (11). On the other hand, Misbah and colleagues were unsuccessful in their one reported case and have recommended the use of intraventricular Ig only in those patients whose clinical condition deteriorates while receiving high-dose IVIG (13).

Oral Administration

Surprisingly, after oral administration of IVIG, studies have shown that fragments of IgG could be found in feces and, furthermore, that these fragments were functional (15,16). This finding has potential significance in two particular groups of patients: premature, low-birth-weight neonates, and individuals undergoing bone marrow transplantation (BMT). In both situations, the absence of protective immunoglobulins in the gastrointestinal tract can lead to significant viral and bacterial infection.

A randomized, placebo-controlled study has been reported in 25 premature low-birth-weight neonates infected with rotavirus; 14 received oral doses of 500 mg IVIG four times daily for 7 days, while the remainder were given placebo (17). Infectious symptoms as well as disease duration were significantly reduced in the active treatment group.

Similarly, the prophylactic use of IVIG in BMT patients administered both orally (at 50 mg/kg/day for 28 days post-BMT) and intravenously (500 mg/kg every 2 weeks) resulted in only two cases of hemorrhagic gastroenteritis (18).

Subcutaneous Administration

Recently, IVIG has been administered subcutaneously in patients with primary immunodeficiency syndromes to reduce the risk of infection introduced by repeated connections to permanent indwelling catheters. Webb et al. reported the treatment of two hypogammaglobulinemic patients by means of an implantable subcutaneous catheter (19). More than 90 infusions were given by this method without complications. The obvious suggestion for use in the home care setting was made. This report was followed by several more, indicating the safety, adequate pharmacokinetics, and effectiveness of this route of administration, particularly in the home environment (20–22).

CONCLUSIONS

Clearly some success has been achieved in administering IVIG by other than the intravenous route for specialized circumstances. However, because the data are limited and the delivery methods are not those recommended by the manufacturers, caution should be exercised in this regard.

REFERENCES

1. Ochs HD, Lee ML, Fischer SH, Kingdon HS, Wedgwood RJ. Efficacy of a new intact immunoglobulin preparation (Gammagard) in primary immunodeficient patients. Clin Ther 1988; 9:512–522.
2. Porter N, Stiff P. A clinical trial of rapid infusion of 10% intravenous immunoglobulin. Oncology Nursing Society Meeting, 1990, Washington, D.C. Abstract.
3. Schiff R, Sedlak D, Buckley R. Rapid infusion of Sandoglobulin in patients with primary humoral immunodeficiency. J Allergy Clin Immunol 1991; 88:61–67.
4. Lee ML, Dicato M, Smith TF, et al. Clinical evaluation of the safety of an intravenous immunoglobulin preparation given at increasing rates of administration and increased concentrations. Submitted.
5. Eckert P. Immunoglobulin determination in serum and peritoneal secretion during the postoperative period. In: Doenicke A, Steinbereithner K, eds. Immunology in Anaesthesiology and Intensive Care. Vienna, Munich, Berne: Maudrich Verlag, 1982:125–127.
6. Gigliotti F, Lee D, Insel RA, Scheld WM. IgG penetration into the cerebrospinal fluid in a rabbit model of meningitis. J Infect Dis 1987; 156:394–398.
7. Delire M. Immunoglobulins: Rationale for the Clinical Use of Polyvalent Intravenous Immunoglobulins. Petersfield, U.K.: Wrightson Biomedical Publishing, 1995:72–73.
8. Hadfield MG, Seidlin M, Houff SA, Adair CR, Markowitz SM, Straus SE. Echovirus meningomyeloencephalitis with administration of intrathecal immunoglobulin. J Neuropath Exp Neurol 1985; 44:520–529.
9. Kondoh H, Kobayashi K, Sugio Y, Hayashi T. Successful treatment of echovirus meningoencephalitis in X-linked agammaglobulinemia by intrathecal and intravenous injection of high titre gammaglobulin. Eur J Paedratr 1987; 146:610–612.
10. Erlendsson K, Swartz T, Dwyer JM. Successful reversal of echovirus encephalitis in X-linked hypogammaglobulinaemia by intraventricular administration of immunoglobulin. N Engl J Med 1985; 312:351–353.
11. McKinney RE, Katz SL, Wilfert CM. Chronic enteroviral meningoencephalitis in agammaglobulinemic patients. Rev Infect Dis 1987; 9:334–356.

12. Dwyer JM, Erlendsson K. Intraventricular gamma-globulin for the management of enterovirus encephalitis. Pediatr Infect Dis J 1988; 7:S30–S33.

13. Misbah SA, Spickett GP, Ryba PCJ, et al. Chronic enteroviral meningoencephalitis in agammaglobulinemia: case report and literature review. J Clin Immunol 1992; 12:266–270.

14. Roberton DM, Jack I, Joshi W, Law F, Hosking CS. Failure of intraventricular gamma-globulin and α interferon for persistent encephalitis in congenital hypogammaglobulinemia. Arch Dis Child 1988; 63:948–952.

15. Blum PM, Phelps DL, Ank BJ, Krantman JH, Steihm ER. Survival of oral human immune serum globulin in the gastrointestinal tract of low birth weight infants. Pediatr Res 1981; 15:1256–1260.

16. Losonky GA, Johnson JP, Winkelstein JA, Yolken RHA. Oral administration of human serum immunoglobulin in immunodeficient patients with viral gastroenteritis. A pharmacokinetic and functional analysis. J Clin Invest 1985; 76:2362–2367.

17. Barnes GL, Doyle LW, Hewson PH, et al. A randomized trial of oral gammaglobulin in low-birth-weight infants infected with rotavirus. Lancet 1982; 1:1371–1373.

18. Tutschka PJ, Copelan EA, Klein JP. Bone marrow transplantation for leukemia following a new busulfan and cyclophosphamide regimen. Blood 1987; 70:1382–1388.

19. Webb DB, Kendra JR, Gross E, Stamatakis JD. Infusion of intravenous immunoglobulin via implantable subcutaneous catheter. Lancet 1991; 337:1617–1618.

20. Gardulf A, Hammarstrom L, Smith CIE. Home treatment of hypogammaglobulinemia with subcutaneous gammaglobulin by rapid infusion. Lancet 1991; 338:162–166.

21. Waniewski J, Gardulf A, Hammarstrom L. Bioavailability of gammaglobulin after subcutaneous infusions in patients with common variable immunodeficiency. J Clin Immunol 1994; 14:90–97.

22. Gardulf A, Anderson V, Bjorkander J, et al. Subcutaneous immunoglobulin replacement in patients with primary antibody deficiencies: safety and costs. Lancet 1995; 345:365–369.

8

IVIG in Bone Marrow Transplantation

Maurice J. Wolin
Chiron Therapeutics, Emeryville, California

Robert Peter Gale
Salick Health Care, Inc., Los Angeles, California

INTRODUCTION

Intravenous immunoglobulin (IVIG) is widely used in bone marrow transplantation to modify or prevent CMV, decrease graft-versus-host disease (GvHD), prevent infections other than CMV, and treat posttransplant autoimmune disorders. Here, we review relevant data in auto- and allotransplants.

CYTOMEGALOVIRUS INFECTION AND RELATED INTERSTITIAL PNEUMONIA

Risk of CMV Infection

CMV infection is a serious complication of allotransplants. Infection results from activation of latent CMV infection in the recipient, donor bone marrow, transfused blood products, or combinations thereof (1,2). Transplant recipients who are CMV-seropositive have a greater risk of infection than those who are CMV-seronegative: 50–70% vs. 20–30%.

CMV disease is a frequent consequence of CMV infection. Pneumonia develops in 30–50% of persons with CMV infection; case mortality exceeds 50% (3–5). Other forms of CMV disease include hepatitis, enteritis, and retinitis. Although CMV enteritis is relatively common, others are rare.

Prevention of CMV-Pneumonia

Transfusion of CMV-Seronegative Blood
Current efforts are aimed at preventing CMV infection. The most important is to avoid transfusing untested or CMV-seropositive blood products to CMV-seronegative recipients.

Infection rates in CMV-seronegative patients receiving only CMV-seronegative blood and a CMV-seronegative graft are 0–6% (6–8). Table 1 shows CMV infection rates in allotransplant recipients with different CMV-seropositive states.

Table 1 CMV Infection Rates in Allotransplant Recipients

	Donor −	Donor +
Recipient −	0–6%	62%
Recipient +	50–70%[a]	50–70%

[a]Unstudied but assumed to be similar to donor +.

Treatment of CMV-Seropositive Recipients

There are two approaches to treating or preventing CMV-seropositive recipients. The first is to give anti-CMV therapy at the first evidence of CMV infection. CMV infection is typically documented by assays of cells from bronchoalveolar lavage, blood, urine, or throat cultures. In two studies, ganciclovir significantly reduced CMV disease (primarily CMV pneumonia) in persons with documented CMV infection (9,10).

Another approach is to treat all CMV-seropositive recipients whether or not they develop CMV infection. Three trials of ganciclovir (10–12) showed significantly less CMV disease (primarily CMV pneumonmia) compared with controls but no increase in survival. This discrepancy is attributed to the toxicity of ganciclovir—predominately due to delayed granulocyte recovery.

IVIG-based therapies. In some studies, IVIG was used instead of ganciclovir to prevent CMV disease in CMV-seropositive patients. These studies indicate significantly less CMV infection and a moderate decrease in CMV disease compared to control (Table 2). Mortality was not impacted by the use of IGIV.

Studies of IVIG in CMV prophylaxis. In one study, CMV-seronegative patients were randomized to receive IVIG or placebo (14). There was less CMV disease (but not CMV infection) in persons receiving IVIG. In another study of CMV-seropositive and -negative people (15), there was significantly less CMV disease in both groups. Like the previous study, CMV infection rates were similar. Persons receiving IVIG also had less acute GvHD and less gram-negative sepsis. The fact that GvHD was less in

Table 2 IVIG Studies for Prevention of CMV Disease

Reference	CMV infection treatment/control	CMV disease treatment/control	GvHD	Survival
O'Reilly, 1983 (13)	0%/50%	0%/30%	No difference	No difference
Winston, 1987 (14)	21%/46%	18%/46%	Less	No difference
Sullivan, 1990 (15)		22%/13%	Less. Also decreased risk of bacterial infection, requirement for platelets	No difference
Winston, 1993 (12)	7%/9%	No cases	Less	No difference

CMV-seronegative subjects receiving IVIG suggests an immune-modulating effect independent of its effect in CMV infection and CMV disease.

In studies of CMV-IVIG (an IVIG preparation with high titers of anti-CMV antibodies), patients had significantly less CMV infection. However, the incidence of CMV disease and survival are similar (6,7,16).

Treatment of CMV Disease

Once CMV disease develops it is difficult to treat. The most serious complication is CMV pneumonia mortality, of 65-85%. In controlled studies, ganciclovir failed to improve survival. In contrast, IVIG or CMV-IVIG combined ganciclovir resulted in improved survival (17-22).

IGIV is also used in the other CMV-related diseases like retinitis and enteritis. Its effectiveness alone or in combination with ganciclovir is unproven.

MODIFYING GRAFT-VERSUS-HOST DISEASE

GvHD occurs in 40-50% of allotransplant recipients and is even more common in recipients of alternative donor transplants. Drugs used to modify or prevent GvHD include cyclosporine, methotrexate, and corticosteroids. IVIG given to prevent CMV infection significantly decreases GvHD, even in CMV-seronegative recipients (14,15).

TREATMENT OF PLATELET-REFRACTORY PATIENTS

Platelet refractoriness is common after auto- and allotransplants; most transplant recipients need platelet transfusions. IVIG reduces the numbers of platelet transfusions given to allotransplant recipients (15). This might be explained by less GvHD and infections. However, it is also possible that IVIG decreases or prevents immunization to or destruction of allogeneic platelets (this is discussed in more detail in Chapter 21).

IVIG IN OTHER TRANSPLANTED DISEASES

Aplastic Anemia

Persons with aplastic anemia receiving allotransplants followed by IVIG have better survival than those not receiving IVIG. The reason for this is uncertain but it seems to be a consequence of less GvHD, CMV-interstitial pneumonia, and hepatic veno-occlusive disease of the liver (see below) (23).

Hepatic Veno-Occlusive Disease

Persons with leukemia receiving allotransplants have a 5% risk of developing veno-occlusive disease of the liver (24,25). In persons receiving conditioning with total body radiation, this risk is significantly decreased in those also receiving IGIV. The reason for this is uncertain.

SUMMARY

IVIG is central to managing of recipients of allogeneic bone marrow transplants. People who are CMV-seropositive have a lower risk of CMV-related disease like pneumonitis; other complications like veno-occlusive disease and GvHD are also lessened. For patients with CMV-disease, therapy with IVIG and ganciclovir is most effective, but does not increase survival. The mechanism of action of IVIG in allograft recipients is unknown and likely multifactorial.

What are possible future directions of IVIG in transplants? The use of IVIG in CMV prevention and treatment is likely to decrease because of the increasing use of prophylaxis ganciclovir . In contrast, the use of IVIG for immune modulation is likely to increase. GvHD prevention is an especially interesting area.

REFERENCES

1. Myers J. Prevention of cytomegalovirus infection after marrow transplantation. Rev Infect Dis 1989; 11 (suppl 7):s1691–s1705.
2. Meyers J, Flournoy N, Thomas E. Risk factors for cytomegalovirus after human marrow transplantation. J Infect Dis 1986; 153:478–488.
3. Neiman P, Wasserman P, Wentworth B, et al. Interstitial pneumonia and cytomegalovirus as complications of human marrow transplantation. Transplantation 1973; 15:478–485.
4. Neiman P, Reeves W, Ray G, et al. A prospective analysis of interstitial pneumonia and opportunistic viral infection among recipients of allogeneic bone marrow grafts. J Infect Dis 1977; 136:754–767.
5. Myers J, Spencer H, Watts J, et al. Cytomegalovirus pneumonia after human marrow transplanation. Ann Intern Med 1975; 82:181–188.
6. Bowden R, Sayers M, Flournoy N, et al. Cytomegalovirus immune globulin and seronegative blood products to prevent primary cytomegalovirus infection after marrow transplantation. N Engl J Med 1986; 314:1006–1010.
7. Bowden R, Fisher L, Rogers K, et al. Cytomegalovirus (CMV)-specific intravenous immunoglobulin for the prevention of primary CMV infection and disease after marrow transplant. J Infect Dis 1991; 164:483–487.
8. Miller W, McCullough J, Balfour H, et al. Prevention of cytomegalovirus infection following bone marrow transplantation: a randomized trial of blood product screening. Bone Marrow Transplant 1991; 7:227–234.
9. Einsele H, Ehninger G, Steidle M, et al. Polymerase chain reaction to evaluate antiviral therapy for cytomegalovirus disease. (See comments.) Lancet 1991; 338:1170–1172.
10. Goodrich J, Bowden R, Fisher L, et al. Prevention of cytomegalovirus disease after allogeneic marrow transplant by ganciclovir prophylaxis. Ann Intern Med 1993; 118:173–178.
11. Atkinson K, Downs K, Golenia M, et al. Prophylactic use of ganciclovir in allogeneic bone marrow transplanation; absence of clinical cytomegalovirus infection. Br J Hematol 1991; 79:57–62.
12. Winston DJ, Ho WG, Bartoni K, et al. Intravenous immunoglobulin and CMV-seronegative blood products for prevention of CMV infection and disease in bone marrow transplant recipients. Bone Marrow Transplant 1993; 12:283–288.
13. O'Reilly RJ, Reich L, Gold J, et al. A randomized trial of intravenous hyperimmune globulin for the prevention of cytomegalovirus (CMV) infections following marrow transplantation: preliminary results. Transplant Proc 1983; 15:1405–1411.
14. Winston DJ, Ho WG, Lin CH, et al. Intravenous immune globulin for prevention of cytome-

galovirus infection and interstitial pneumonia after bone marrow transplantation. Ann Intern Med 1987; 106:12–18.

15. Sullivan KM, Kopecky KJ, Jocom J, et al. Immunomodulatory and antimicrobial efficacy of intravenous immunoglobulin in bone marrow transplantation. (See comments.) N Engl J Med 1990; 323:705–712.

16. Myers J, Leszczynski J, Zaia J. Prevention of cytomegalovirus infection by cytomegalovirus immunoglobulin after marrow transplantation. Ann Intern Med 1983; 98:442–446.

17. Reed E, Bowden R, Dandliker P, et al. Treatment of cytomegalovirus pneumonia with ganciclovir and intravenous cytomegalovirus immunoglobulin in patients with bone marrow transplants. Ann Intern Med 1988; 109.

18. Emanuel D, Cunningham I, Jules-Elysee K, et al. Cytomegalovirus pneumonia after bone marrow transplantation successfully treated with the combination of ganciclovir and high dose intravenous immune globulin. Ann Intern Med 1988; 109:777–782.

19. Schmidt G, Kovacs A, Zaia J, et al. Ganciclovir/immunoglobulin combination therapy for the treatment of human cytomegalovirus-associated interstitial pneumonia in bone marrow allograft recipients. Transplantation 1988; 46:905–907.

20. Ljungman P, Englehard D, Link H, et al. Treatment of interstitial pneumonitis due to cytomegalovirus with ganciclovir and intravenous immune globulin: experience of European Bone Marrow Transplant Group. Clin Infect Dis 1992; 14:831–835.

21. Reed E, Bowden R, Dandliker P, et al. Treatment of cytomegalovirus (CMV) pneumonia in bone marrow transplant (BMT) patients with ganciclovir and CMV immunoglobulin. Blood 1987; 70(suppl 1):313a.

22. Bratanow N, Ash R, Turner P, et al. Ganciclovir and intravenous immunoglobulin in the treatment of serious cytomegalovirus infections in thirty-one allogeneic bone marrow transplant patients. Blood 1987; 70(suppl 1):302A.

23. Passweg JR, Horowitz MM, Atkinson KA, Barrett AJ, Gale RP, Gratwohl A, Jacobsen N, Klein JP, Ljungman P, Rowlings PA, Schaefer UW, Vossen JM. Influence of protected isolation on outcome of allogeneic bone marrow transplantation for leukemia. Bone Marrow Transplant (submitted).

24. Jones R, Lee K, Beschorner W, et al. Venocclusive disease of the liver following bone marrow transplantation. Transplantation 1987; 44:779–783.

25. McDonald G, Hinds M, Fisher L, et al. Veno-occlusive disease of the liver and multiorgan failure after bone marrow transplantation: a cohort study of 355 patients. Ann Intern Med 1993; 188:255–267.

9

Use of Intravenous Immunoglobulins for the Prevention and Treatment of Viral Infections in Solid Organ Transplantation

Jeffrey A. DesJardin and David R. Snydman
New England Medical Center and Tufts University School of Medicine, Boston, Massachusetts

INTRODUCTION

Numerous factors including more careful selection of candidates, advances in surgical technique, better regulation of immunosuppressive therapy, and better strategies to prevent and treat infectious complications have led to improvements in graft and patient survival in recipients of solid organ transplants (1). Despite these advances, infection remains a major barrier to success. Specifically, the human herpes group viruses [cytomegalovirus (CMV), Epstein-Barr virus (EBV), herpes simplex virus 1 and 2 (HSV-1, HSV-2), human herpes virus 6 (HHV-6), varicella zoster virus (VZV)], hepatitis B (HBV), and hepatitis C (HCV) virus, and rarely, human immunodeficiency virus (HIV) constitute an important group of microbial pathogens that affect patients undergoing solid organ transplantation (2). Patients are at greatest risk of infection from these agents in the 2–6 months following transplantation (3,4).

These viruses, most notably CMV, may contribute to morbidity and mortality by several mechanisms. They directly cause a variety of clinical syndromes, due to either primary infection or reactivation. In addition, these immunomodulating viruses create a state of immunosuppression, which predisposes the transplant recipient to superinfection with opportunistic bacteria, parasites, or fungi. Also, a role for some of these viruses in the production of acute and chronic allograft injury has been suggested. Finally, herpes group viruses may contribute to the pathogenesis of certain forms of malignancy, such as that seen in EBV-associated posttransplant lymphoproliferative disease (PTLD) (2). Thus, in view of the potential adverse impact these pathogens may have on the outcome of solid organ transplantation, it is not surprising that the recognition, prevention, and treatment of these viral infections have become an important area of focus in the transplant field. In this regard, immunoglobulins have been increasingly utilized in the battle against viral infections complicating solid organ transplantation. Unselected immunoglobulins, CMV-specific immunoglobulin (CMVIG), HBV immunoglobulin (HBIG), and VZV immunoglobulin (VZIG) have been shown, to varying degrees, to be clinically useful in the prevention of viral infections in immunosuppressed patients. This chapter will review the expanding role intravenous (IV) immunoglobulins play in the prevention and treatment of viral infections in solid organ transplant recipients.

USE IN CYTOMEGALOVIRUS INFECTION

Prevention of Cytomegalovirus Disease

Cytomegalovirus is the single most important opportunistic pathogen following solid organ transplantation; symptomatic CMV infection occurs in 8%, 29%, 25%, and 39% of kidney, liver, heart, and heart-lung transplantation recipients, respectively (5). Prevention of CMV infection and disease requires a combination of strategies including the prevention of acquisition of CMV from blood products or the donor organ (if possible), the use of specific antiviral chemotherapy, and passive immunization using IV immunoglobulins (6).

The administration of IV immunoglobulins is the only successful immunological strategy for preventing CMV disease. Standard immunoglobulin preparations differ in their manufacturing process, donor pool sources, and IgG compositions even among lots of the same preparation. By contrast, CMVIG has five to eight times the titer of neutralizing antibody, and there is little lot-to-lot variation permitted by the manufacturing standards (6). These agents have proved to be safe, and the incidence of adverse effects related to immunoglobulins or CMVIG is less than 5%. Manifestations are usually mild and self-limited. The most frequent side effects encountered in clinical trials of transplant patients include headache, myalgias, nausea, back pain, fever, and chills and are often related to infusion rates. Anaphylaxis may occur in patients with selective IgA deficiency. There have been reports of contamination of some immunoglobulin preparations with HCV. However, all currently manufactured preparations require the screening of the plasma pools for antihepatitis C antibody, the removal of such pools for immunoglobulin production, and the use of an additional viral inactivation step (7).

Several randomized controlled trials have evaluated the efficacy of both standard immunoglobulin and CMVIG for the prevention of CMV disease in renal transplant patients. The specific details of these studies are presented in Table 1. Standard immunoglobulins and CMVIG have been shown to prevent or attenuate CMV disease in most (8–10,12) but not all (11), trials in renal transplant patients. The investigation by Snydman and others (10) not only revealed a significant reduction in CMV disease in patients receiving CMVIG, but also a reduction in the rate of severe CMV disease inclusive of complicating invasive opportunistic fungal and parasitic infections. The effects of CMVIG on graft survival and mortality in renal transplantation are not as clear. When taken together, the results from the original randomized study from Snydman et al. (10), an open-label extension of that trial (13), and an analysis of patients participating under an FDA-approved treatment IND (14) document a consistent trend for decreased graft loss and mortality in patients treated with CMVIG. Conti and others were able to document a significant improvement in graft survival at 1 year in patients treated with standard immunoglobulin when compared to historical controls (89% vs. 61%) (12). Based on several of these studies, CMVIG is now FDA-licensed for use in renal transplant recipients who are seronegative for CMV (R–) and who receive a kidney from a CMV seropositive donor (D+) (15).

Other studies have also specifically examined the efficacy of standard immunoglobulin or CMVIG as preemptive therapy in renal transplant patients. Preemptive therapy of CMV infection involves the administration of therapy to a subgroup of high-risk patients [i.e., patients receiving antithymocyte globulin (ATG) or OKT3 monoclonal antibodies (OKT3)], but prior to the appearance of disease (16). When used as preemptive therapy, Metselaar and others were able to prevent fatal CMV disease with CMVIG (17), while Steinmuller et al. demonstrated a reduction in symptomatic infection with standard immunoglobulin (18).

Although these immunoglobulins are relatively expensive, they have been shown to be cost-effective in the setting of renal transplantation. Tsevat and coinvestigators calculated $29,800 per year of life gained for renal transplant recipients at risk of primary CMV disease (19). Such cost savings are comparable with other accepted medical therapies.

Randomized trials have also evaluated the efficacy of standard immunoglobulin and CMVIG in liver and other solid organ transplants. These trials are summarized in Table 2. In liver transplant recipients, standard immunoglobulin does not appear to reduce the incidence of CMV infection or disease (20). Snydman and co-workers demonstrated a significant reduction in severe CMV disease and in the number of fungal and parasitic infections with CMVIG in a trial of all serostrata of liver transplant recipients, although the subset of D+/R- liver transplant recipients did not appear to benefit (21). However, a subsequent analysis of that study (22) and an earlier study (23) did reveal some reduction in CMV disease in D+/R- recipients given CMVIG. As in renal transplantation, the data on the effects that immunoglobulins have on graft survival and mortality in liver transplantation are not certain. In one study, 1-year graft survival was improved with the use of CMVIG when compared to placebo recipients, although these results did not reach statistical significance (22). Data in two studies demonstrated weak statistical trends in improvement in survival (21,24). The use of standard immunoglobulin with acyclovir as preemptive therapy in high-risk liver transplant patients receiving OKT3 did not reduce the incidence of CMV infection (24), although the incidence of HSV, EBV, and fungal infections were reduced with such therapy.

The randomized trials to date of patients with other transplanted organs (e.g., heart, lung, or pancreas) have not revealed significant benefit from either standard immunoglobulins or CMVIG (25–27). However, aspects of each study may explain the lack of beneficial effects with immunoglobulin prophylaxis. In the study by Boland and others, the time of administration of the first dose of CMVIG was relatively late—7 days after transplantation (25). Bailey et al. used a standard immunoglobulin preparation which, as stated above, has lower anti-CMV antibody than CMVIG (26). Dunn et al. used a CMVIG-containing regimen in which the CMVIG was only given for 1 week rather than the typical duration of administration of several weeks used in many other studies (27). Clearly, more randomized controlled trials are needed to better define the effect of immunoglobulins on heart, lung, or pancreas transplantation.

Two meta-analyses also offer some insight as to the efficacy of standard immunoglobulins or CMVIG in the prevention of CMV disease in solid organ transplantation. A meta-analysis by Glowacki and Smaill revealed a reduction in the incidence of symptomatic CMV disease in the group receiving immunoglobulin as compared to the untreated group [odds ratio (OR) 0.59 (95% CI: 0.42–0.77)] (28). Although no apparent advantage was demonstrated comparing the use of CMVIG over standard immunoglobulin in this meta-analysis, bone marrow and solid organ transplant patients were pooled

Table 1 Randomized Trials of Intravenous Immunoglobulins as Prophylaxis Against CMV Infection in Kidney Transplant Recipients

Organ transplanted	Reference	Study type	No. of patients (treatment/ control)	CMV status[a]	Prophylactic regimen	Pertinent outcomes (treatment vs. control)	Mortality (treatment vs. control)
Kidney	Gregor et al., 1986 (8)	Primary and secondary prophylaxis; randomized, non-placebo-controlled	24/24	R+ and R− (donor status not stated)	Hyperimmune serum 0.1 g/kg biweekly day 0, 1, and q 3 weeks for 6 months vs. no treatment	Reduction in clinical symptoms of CMV disease in patients on cyclosporin (0% vs. 17%) but not CMV infection. No reduction in severity of illness or CMV infection in patients on Azathioprin/ATG.	Not reported
	Fassbinder et al., 1986 (9)	Primary and secondary prophylaxis; randomized	42/34	R+ and R− (donor status not stated)	10 g CMV hyperimmune globulin (Cytotect) days 0, 18, 38, 58, 78 vs. standard immunoglobulin (Intraglobulin) over same interval	No difference in frequency of primary or secondary CMV infections. Decrease in severity of symptoms of primary infection in patients receiving hyperimmune globulin.	No fatal cases in either group
	Snydman et al., 1987 (10)	Primary prophylaxis; randomized, non-placebo-controlled	24/35	All D+/R−	CMV immune globulin (MA Public Health Biological Laboratories) 150 mg/kg within 72 h of transplantation, 100 mg/kg at 2 and 4 weeks; 50 mg/kg at weeks 6, 8, 12, 16 vs. no treatment	No significant difference in overall rates of CMV viremia, viral isolation, or seroconversion. Reduction in CMV disease (21% vs. 60%). Reduction in rate of fungal or parasitic infections (0% vs. 20%).	No significant difference (4% vs. 14%)
	Kasiske et al., 1989 (11)	Primary and secondary prophylaxis; randomized, non-placebo-controlled	15/13	Mixture of D+/ R−; D+/R+; D−/R−; D−/ R+	Polyvalent immune globulin (Gamimune-N) 500 mg/ kg within 48 h of transplantation and weekly for 12 weeks vs. no treatment	No significant difference in incidence or severity of CMV infection.	Not reported

Reference	Study design	No.	Serostatus[a]	Regimen	Results	Mortality
Metselaar et al. 1989 (17)	Primary and secondary prophylaxis; preemptive therapy—patients received ATG for rejection; double-blind, randomized, placebo-controlled	19/20	Mixture of D+/R−; D+/R+; D−/R−; D−/R+	Anti-CMV immunoglobulin (Cytotect) 100 mg/kg on day of ATG treatment and on days 7, 14, 35, 56, and 77 vs. albumin over same interval	No significant difference in incidence of CMV isolation, viremia, or disease.	No deaths in treated group (0% vs. 20%)
Steinmuller et al., 1990 (18)	Secondary prophylaxis; preemptive therapy—patients had received ATG or OKT3 for ≥7 days posttransplant or rejection treatment within first 2 weeks; randomized, non-placebo-controlled	16/18	Mixture D+ and D−; all R+	Immunoglobulin (Sandoglobulin) 500 mg/kg every 2 weeks for 3 doses, then 250 mg/kg every 2 weeks for 2 doses vs. no treatment	Reduction in number of patients with symptomatic infection (12% vs. 39%). Significant reduction in number of days febrile, number of days hospitalized secondary to CMV, and number of complications due to CMV.	No patients in either group died of CMV infection
Conti et al., 1994 (12)	Primary prophylaxis; randomized	27/24	All D+/R−	Conventional immunoglobulin 500 mg/kg within 48 h of transplant and 1 week after, then 250 mg/kg every week for 5 doses vs. low-dose IV ganciclovir 2.5 mg/kg/day on days 1–21 vs. historical controls	Both immunoglobulin and ganciclovir groups had decreased incidence of CMV syndrome vs. historical controls (22% vs. 21% vs. 39%). Immunoglobulin and ganciclovir groups had less incidence invasive CMV disease vs. historical controls (4% vs. 0% vs. 20%).	No significant difference (0% vs. 0% vs. 13%)

[a]Donor CMV seropositive (D+); recipient CMV seropositive (R+). Donor CMV seronegative (D−); recipient CMV seronegative (R−).

Table 2 Randomized Trials of Intravenous Immunoglobulins as Prophylaxis Against CMV Infection in Liver and Other Solid Transplant Recipients

Organ transplanted	Reference	Study type	No. of patients (treatment/ control)	CMV status[a]	Prophylactic regimen	Pertinent outcomes (treatment vs. control)	Mortality (treatment vs. control)
Liver	Saliba et al., 1989 (23)	Primary prophylaxis; randomized, non-placebo-controlled	22/12	Mixture D+ and D−; all R−	CMV hyperimmune globulin 250 mg/kg day 0, then 125 mg/kg every 10 days until third month vs. no treatment	Significant decrease in rate of CMV disease in D+/R− group (27% vs. 86%). No significant effect in D−/R− group.	Not reported
	Cofer et al., 1991 (20)	Primary and secondary prophylaxis; double-blinded, randomized, placebo-controlled	25/25	Mixture of D+/R−; D+/R+; D−/R−; D−/R+	Immunoglobulin (Sandoglobulin) 500 mg/kg on postop days, 1, 7, 14, 21, 28, 42, 56, 70, 84 vs. albumin at same interval	No significant difference in incidence of CMV infection or disease. (Note: no D+/R− patients in treatment arm.)	Not reported
	Stratta et al., 1992 (24)	Primary and secondary prophylaxis; preemptive therapy—all patients had received OKT3 for a minimum of 4 days; randomized, non-placebo-controlled	50/50	Mixture of D+/R−; D+/R+; D−/R−; D−/R+	Immunoglobulin (Gammagard) 0.5 mg/kg on days 1, 3, 5 after OKT3 and weekly for 3 weeks plus oral acyclovir (400 mg 5 times daily) for 3 months vs. no treatment	Significant reduction in the incidence of HSV infections (12% vs. 32%) and EBV infections (0% vs. 10%). Significant reduction in number of fungal infections (22% vs. 42%). No effect on incidence of CMV infection.	Trend toward improved mortality (10% vs. 22%)

	Snydman et al., 1993 (21)	Primary and secondary prophylaxis; double-blinded, randomized, placebo-controlled	69/72	Mixture of D+/R−; D+/R+; D−/R−; D−/R+	CMV immunoglobulin (MA Public Health Biological Laboratories) 150 mg/kg within 72 h of transplant and at weeks 2, 4, 6, 8, then 100 mg/kg at weeks 12, 16 vs. albumin at same interval	No significant reduction in CMV disease. Significant reduction in severe CMV disease (12% vs. 26%). No reduction in CMV disease or severe CMV disease in high-risk group (D+/R−). Significant reduction in incidence of invasive fungal disease (7% vs. 18%).	No significant difference (17% vs. 25%)
Heart or Kidney	Boland et al., 1993 (25)	Primary prophylaxis; randomized, non-placebo-controlled	14/14	All D+/R−	CMV hyperimmune globulin (Cytotect) 1 ml/kg at 1, 2, 3, 5, 7 weeks post-transplant vs. no treatment	No influence on incidence of CMV infection or on incidence or severity of CMV disease.	Not reported
Heart, Lung, or Kidney	Bailey et al., 1993 (26)	Primary prophylaxis; randomized	11/10	All D+/R−	Immune globulin (Gamimune) 300 mg/kg within 72 h of transplant then every 2 weeks for 10 weeks plus acyclovir 800 mg orally 4 times daily vs. acyclovir alone	No significant difference in incidence of CMV infection or disease.	No significant difference (9% vs. 0%)
Kidney, Kidney-Pancreas, Pancreas, or Liver	Dunn et al., 1994 (27)	Primary and second prophylaxis; patients either posttransplant or post any rejection therapy; randomized	133/133	Mixture of D+/R−; D+/R+; D−/R−; D−/R+	Immunoglobulin (Minnesota CMV immune globulin or Sandoglobulin) 100 mg/kg on days 1, 4, 7 plus ganciclovir 5 mg/kg every 12 h for 7 days vs. acyclovir 800 mg orally or 400 mg IV 4 times daily for 12 weeks postop or 6 weeks after any antirejection therapy	Higher incidence of CMV disease in immune globulin/ganciclovir group (32% vs. 21%). Higher incidence of CMV disease in D+/R− subgroup receiving immune globulin/ganciclovir (55% vs. 25%).	No significant difference (14% vs. 10%)

aDonor CMV seropositive (D+); recipient CMV seropositive (R+). Donor CMV seronegative (D−); recipient CMV seronegative (R−).

together, thus combining two separate pathogenic processes. When the use of immuno-prophylaxis in solid organ transplants was analyzed separately, the adjusted OR was 0.47 (95% CI: 0.27–0.82) with pooled data from the CMVIG studies. For the standard immunoglobulin studies the adjusted OR was 0.66 (95% CI: 0.3–1.5) and was not statistically significant from 1.0 ($P = .32$) (29). This subgroup analysis suggests that CMVIG may be superior to standard immunoglobulin in preventing CMV disease. Wittes and colleagues have recently performed a meta-analysis to evaluate the efficacy of CMVIG for the prevention of CMV infection in bone marrow and solid organ transplant recipients (30). Among solid organ transplant recipients, CMVIG prophylaxis reduced the risk of CMV infection or seroconversion as compared to untreated patients [OR 0.53 (95% CI: 0.33–0.84), $P < .005$]. The use of CMVIG was also effective in preventing severe CMV disease [OR 0.40 (95% CI: 0.22–0.75), $P < .005$] and CMV-related death [OR 0.35 (95% CI: 0.16–0.74), P < .001]. All measures showed strong, statistically significant beneficial effects of CMVIG.

IV immunoglobulins have been used to prevent CMV disease in solid organ transplantation by combining them with antiviral agents. Several retrospective trials have noted varying degrees of effectiveness of CMVIG plus an antiviral agent in renal (31), liver (32), lung (33), and heart (34) transplant recipients. However, only a few prospective comparative trials exist that have examined the efficacy of such combination therapy. Nicol and colleagues prospectively treated 73 high-risk (D+/R–) renal transplant recipients with CMVIG plus low-dose oral acyclovir and compared these patients to non-D+/R– patients who received acyclovir alone (35). Graft survival was significantly improved at 1 and 3 years compared to the group that received acyclovir alone. Stratta and others compared the combination of standard immunoglobulin plus oral acyclovir with untreated controls in a randomized trial involving liver transplant recipients who received OKT3 (24). They concluded that combination prophylaxis was effective in preventing HSV, EBV, and fungal infections but had no effect on the incidence of severity of CMV infections. Bailey et al. evaluated standard immunoglobulin plus acyclovir to acyclovir alone in D+/R– heart, lung, or kidney transplant patients (26). In this randomized trial, no significant difference in the incidence of CMV infection or disease was demonstrated. In combined pancreas-kidney transplant recipients, Stratta et al. consecutively assigned patients to receive one of four treatment regimens: standard immunoglobulin plus oral acyclovir, IV ganciclovir plus oral acyclovir, standard immunoglobulin plus IV ganciclovir then oral acyclovir, or CMVIG plus IV ganciclovir then oral acyclovir (36). No differences in the incidence, timing, or severity of symptomatic CMV infections could be demonstrated among the four groups. Of note, however, only six of the 82 patients were considered high-risk (D+/R–). Dunn and coinvestigators compared standard immunoglobulin or CMVIG plus ganciclovir to acyclovir alone in 266 solid organ transplant recipients (kidney, liver, pancreas, or kidney-pancreas) (27). The incidence of CMV disease was actually higher in the combination group. However, as noted above, the short duration of combination treatment, only 7 days, makes this study difficult to compare to others. Despite the limitations of the available data, prophylactic strategies using CMVIG and an antiviral agent appear to offer an advantage over monotherapy in preventing serious CMV disease in high-risk (D+/R–) patients and in those receiving antilymphocyte preparations.

In general, the results from the available trials and meta-analyses indicate that immunoglobulins are efficacious in preventing CMV disease in solid organ transplants, and CMVIG appears to be more beneficial than standard immunoglobulins. The data to date are more consistent for renal transplants, and perhaps liver transplants, than with other solid organ transplants, especially within the high-risk (D+/R–) group. In addition, combination therapy with CMVIG and an antiviral agent appears to be more beneficial than monotherapy in high-risk patients. The overall effects of CMVIG on various outcomes in kidney and liver transplantation are summarized in Table 3.

Despite these apparent advantages, the exact use of IV immunoglobulin therapy in the prevention of CMV disease in solid organ transplantation remains to be determined. The optimal dose, duration of therapy, and mechanism of action all need further clarification. Current prophylactic approaches using immunoglobulins, either with or without antiviral agents, vary significantly among transplant programs. This variation reflects the relative lack of large multicenter randomized trials and the fact that small, single-center studies are frequently difficult to interpret. Moreover, inherent differences in the type of solid organ transplanted should be considered, since prophylaxis found to be effective for one type of solid organ transplant may not necessarily apply to another. Until more data are collected, the use of immunoglobulins in solid organ transplantation will continue to vary depending on the potential risk of infection in the recipient, the type of solid organ transplanted, and the specific regimen utilized by the transplant center.

Treatment of Established Cytomegalovirus Disease

Immunoglobulins have also been used in solid organ transplantation in combination with an antiviral agent to treat established CMV disease. However, only limited data in solid organ transplant patients exist. The basis for immunoglobulin use in such patients has been extrapolated from animal models and the experience with treating CMV pneumonitis in bone marrow transplant recipients. In animal models, CMV antibody infusions combined with ganciclovir are more effective for the treatment of CMV disease than either modality alone, especially in CMV pneumonia models (37,38). The use of ganciclovir in combination with immunoglobulins for the treatment of CMV pneumonia has been validated in at least two trials of allogeneic bone marrow transplant recipients. Reed and coinvestigators were able to show an improvement in survival with CMVIG in combination with ganciclovir as compared to historical controls (52% vs. 15%) (39). Emanuel and others also showed a survival benefit with ganciclovir and standard immunoglobulin compared to either treatment alone (70% vs. 0%) (40). As

Table 3 Summary of Effects of CMVIG in Kidney and Liver Transplantation

Effect	Kidney	Liver
Reduction	+	?
Primary CMV disease	+	+
Severity of CMV disease	+	+
Frequency of severe disease	+	+
Fungal opportunistic disease	+	+
Severe CMV disease in OKT3-treated patients	+	+
Increase		
Graft survival	+	?
Patient survival	+	?

stated above, no randomized controlled trials examining the role of combination treatment with ganciclovir plus immunoglobulin exist for the treatment of established CMV disease in solid organ transplant patients. George and colleagues retrospectively evaluated their experience with the use of combination treatment in orthotopic liver transplant recipients (41). They were able to demonstrate a shorter duration of intubation among recipients of combination treatment and a trend toward reduced survival at 1 year. Together, the above data provide some support for the use of combination treatment for severe CMV disease in solid organ transplant recipients, and such therapy is recommended by many experts (42).

PREVENTION OF HEPATITIS B INFECTION IN ORTHOTOPIC LIVER TRANSPLANTATION

Hepatitis B hyperimmune globulin (HBIG) is derived from plasma donors who have been stimulated by immunization with hepatitis B vaccine and is available in the U.S. as an intramuscular agent (43). An IV formulation is available in Europe and has been used as passive immunoprophylaxis to prevent recurrent HBV infection in hepatitis B surface antigen (HBsAg)-positive patients who receive an orthotopic liver transplant. Liver transplantation in patients with cirrhosis or hepatitis caused by HBV is complicated by high rates of HBV infection of the transplanted liver (44). Nonrandomized studies have suggested a benefit of long-term therapy with HBIG in preventing HBV recurrence (45,46). More recently, Samuel and the investigators of the European Concerted Action on Viral Hepatitis Study discovered that frequent, long-term therapy with high doses of HBIG significantly reduced the recurrence of HBV infection compared to short-term (3 months) therapy or no therapy (47) (Fig. 1). Despite the absence of a licensed indication, administration of HBIG, either intramuscularly or by slow IV infusion, has become standard for the prevention of HBV recurrent in HBsAg-positive patients who undergo orthotopic liver transplant. However, the optimal dosage, route of administration, and duration of therapy are unclear.

PREVENTION OF VARICELLA ZOSTER VIRUS INFECTION

Varicella zoster hyperimmune globulin contains high titers of antibody to VZV. Studies in immunosuppressed children at risk for primary VZV infection have shown that the administration of VZIG within 96 h of exposure reduces the incidence of morbidity associated with chickenpox (48). Although there are no controlled studies evaluating the use of VZIG in solid organ transplantation, its use is recommended in immunosuppressed adults—including solid organ transplant recipients, who are believed to be susceptible to VZV and have had significant exposure (49). Currently, VZIG is only available in the U.S. as an intramuscular agent. However, certain standard IV immunoglobulins have been shown to achieve VZV titers equivalent to those achieved with VZIG (50). Therefore, administration of IV immunoglobulin may be useful as prophylaxis in patients with known exposure to VZV and who are at risk for primary infection (51). Neither VZIG nor standard IV immunoglobulin has been shown to be effective in the treatment of established VZV infection (25).

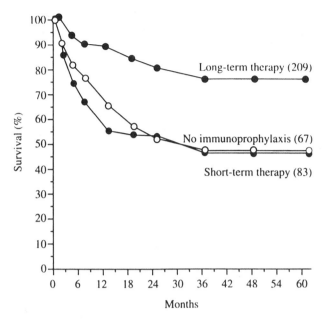

Figure 1 Actuarial survival according to duration of passive prophylaxis with anti-HBsAg immunoglobulin. Survival in the group given long-term therapy was significantly better than in either of the other groups ($P < .001$). Values in parentheses denote numbers of patients. (From Ref. 47 with permission of *The New England Journal of Medicine*. Samuel et al. Liver transplantation in European patients with the hepatitis B surface antigen. N Engl J Med 1993; 329:1842–1847. Copyright 1993, Massachusetts Medical Society.)

PREVENTION OR TREATMENT OF POSTTRANSPLANT LYMPHOPROLIFERATIVE DISORDER

The therapy of EBV-associated PTLD is generally disappointing, and there are no prospective or controlled trials evaluating different treatment regimens for this disease. For established PTLD, immunosuppressive therapy is usually reduced, antiviral agents are often employed, and radiotherapy or cytotoxic chemotherapy is utilized in select cases (53). An intriguing use for immunoglobulins in solid organ transplantation would be for the prevention or treatment of PTLD. A situation analogous to PTLD occurs in a rare but fatal congenital disease associated with male phenotypic expression, known as Duncan's syndrome (54). These individuals have a selective immunodeficiency that renders them susceptible to fatal infectious mononucleosis occasionally accompanied by acquired agammaglobulinemia or progression to lymphoma (55). The use of monthly IV immunoglobulins, which contain antibody to the EBV viral capsid antigen, has been generally successful in preventing disease in these kindreds (56). The use of such a strategy in preventing PTLD, especially in transplant recipients at risk for primary EBV infection, may warrant clinical investigation. In addition, an anecdotal report using combination treatment consisting of immunoglobulin plus α-interferon suggests a role for the use of immunoglobulins in the treatment of established EBV-associated PTLD (57). An additional report noted the effectiveness of CMVIG and ganciclovir for the treatment of EBV-associated disease in a renal transplant recipient (58). Of interest, the authors further noted that the CMVIG contained not only high titers of CMV antibodies but also high titers of antibodies to EBV early antigen, EBV nuclear antigen, and EBV viral capsid antigen.

CONCLUSIONS

Intravenous immunoglobulins clearly have an established role in solid organ transplantation, although many questions remain. The use of immunoglobulins, specifically CMVIG, in preventing CMV disease in high-risk renal transplant patients has been verified by randomized trials and now by meta-analysis. This benefit holds true for liver transplant recipients as well, although the efficacy of such therapy in other solid organ transplant recipients is less clear. In addition, the use of CMVIG in combination with an antiviral agent for prophylaxis in high-risk patients has become routine in many transplant centers. Similarly, the use of CMVIG plus antiviral therapy is commonly used for the treatment of established CMV disease. The use of HBIG is the standard of care for liver transplant recipients at risk for HBV recurrence. Standard IV immunoglobulin in solid organ transplant may be useful for susceptible patients with exposures to VZV when VZIG is not readily available. Finally, a future role for IV immunoglobulins in the prevention and treatment of PTLD has been postulated. The discrepancies in the existing data and the prospects for future use of IV immunoglobulins in solid organ transplantation should be further explored through carefully designed and controlled trials.

REFERENCES

1. Dummer JS, Ho M, Simmons RL. Infections in solid organ transplant recipients. In: Mandell GL, Bennett JE, Dolin R, eds. Principles and Practice of Infectious Diseases. New York: Churchill Livingstone, 1995:2722–2732.
2. Rubin RH. Infection in the organ transplant recipient. In: Rubin RH, Young LS, eds. Clinical Approach to Infection in the Compromised Host. New York: Plenum Press, 1994:629–705.
3. Rubin RH, Wolfson JS, Cosimi AB, et al. Infection in the renal transplant recipient. Am J Med 1981; 70:405–411.
4. Winston DJ, Emmanouilides C, Busuttil RW. Infections in liver transplant recipients. Clin Infect Dis 1995; 21:1077–1091.
5. Ho M. Advances in understanding cytomegalovirus infection after transplantation. Transplant Proc 1994; 26(suppl 1):7–11.
6. Hibberd PL, Snydman DR. Cytomegalovirus infection in organ transplant recipients. Infect Dis Clin North Am 1995; 9:863–877.
7. Siber GR, Snydman DR. Use of immune globulins in the prevention and treatment of infections. Curr Clin Top Infect Dis 1992; 12:208–256.
8. Greger B, Vallbracht A, Kurth J, et al. The clinical value of CMV prophylaxis by CMV hyperimmune serum in the kidney transplant patient. Transplant Proc 1986; 18:1387–1389.
9. Fassbinder W, Ernst W, Hanke P, et al. Cytomegalovirus infection after renal transplantation: effect of prophylactic hyperimmunoglobulin. Transplant Proc 1986; 18:1393–1396.
10. Snydman DR, Werner BG, Heinze-Lacey B, et al. Use of cytomegalovirus immune globulin to prevent cytomegalovirus disease in renal-transplant recipients. N Engl J Med 1987; 317:1049–1054.

11. Kasiske BL, Heim-Duthoy KL, Tortorice KL, et al. Polyvalent immune globulin and cytomegalovirus infection after renal transplantation. Arch Intern Med 1989; 149:2733–2736.

12. Conti DJ, Freed BM, Gruber SA, et al. Prophylaxis of primary cytomegalovirus disease in renal transplant recipients. Arch Surg 1994; 129:443–447.

13. Snydman DR, Werner BG, Tilney NL, et al. Final analysis of primary cytomegalovirus disease prevention in renal transplant recipients with a cytomegalovirus-immune globulin: comparison of the randomized and open-label trials. Transplant Proc 1991; 23:1357–1360.

14. Werner BG, Snydman DR, Freeman R, et al. Cytomegalovirus immune globulin for the prevention of primary CMV disease in renal transplant patients: analysis of usage under treatment IND status. The treatment IND study group. Transplant Proc 1993; 25:1441–1443.

15. Nightingale SL. From the food and drug administration. JAMA 1990; 264:168.

16. Rubin RH. Preemptive therapy in immunocompromised hosts. N Engl J Med 1991; 324:1057–1059. Editorial.

17. Metselaar HJ, Rothbarth PH, Brouwer RML, et al. Prevention of cytomegalovirus-related death by passive immunization. Transplantation 1989; 48:264–266.

18. Steinmuller DR, Novick AC, Streem SB, et al. Intravenous immunoglobulin infusions for the prophylaxis of secondary cytomegalovirus infection. Transplantation 1990; 49:68–70.

19. Tsevat J, Snydman DR, Pauker SG, et al. Which renal transplant patients should receive cytomegalovirus immune globulin: a cost-effectiveness analysis. Transplantation 1991; 52:259–265.

20. Cofer JB, Morris CA, Sutker WL, et al. A randomized double-blind study of the effect of prophylactic immune globulin on the incidence and severity of CMV infection in the liver transplant recipient. Transplant Proc 1991; 23:1525–1527.

21. Snydman DR, Werner BG, Dougherty NN, et al. Cytomegalovirus immune globulin prophylaxis in liver transplantation. A randomized, double-blind, placebo-controlled trial. Ann Intern Med 1993; 119:984–991.

22. Snydman DR, Werner BG, Dougherty NN, et al. A further analysis of the use of cytomegalovirus immune globulin in orthotopic liver transplant patients at risk for primary infection. Transplant Proc 1994; 26(suppl 1):23–27.

23. Saliba F, Arulnaden JL, Gugenheim J, et al. CMV hyperimmune globulin prophylaxis after liver transplantation: a prospective randomized controlled study. Transplant Proc 1989; 21:2260–2262.

24. Stratta RJ, Shaefer MS, Cushing KA, et al. A randomized prospective trial of acyclovir and immune globulin prophylaxis in liver transplant recipients receiving OKT3 therapy. Arch Surg 1992; 127:55–64.

25. Boland GJ, Ververs C, Hene RJ, et al. Early detection of primary cytomegalovirus infection after heart and kidney transplantation and the influence of hyperimmune globulin prophylaxis. Transplant Int 1993; 6:34–38.

26. Bailey TC, Ettinger NA, Storch GA, et al. Failure of high-dose oral acyclovir with or without immune globulin to prevent primary cytomegalovirus disease in recipients of solid organ transplants. Am J Med 1993; 95:273–278.

27. Dunn DL, Gillingham KJ, Kramer MA, et al. A prospective randomized study of acyclovir versus ganciclovir plus human immune globulin prophylaxis of cytomegalovirus infection after solid organ transplantation. Transplantation 1994; 57:876–884.

28. Glowacki LS, Smaill FM. Use of immune globulin to prevent symptomatic cytomegalovirus disease in transplant recipients—a meta-analysis. Clin Transplant 1994; 8:10–18.

29. Snydman DR. Use of immune globulin to prevent symptomatic cytomegalovirus disease in transplant recipients—a meta-analysis. Clin Transplant 1995; 9:490–491. Letter.

30. Wittes J, Kelly A, Plante K. Meta-analysis of CMV-IG studies for the prevention and treatment of CMV-infection in transplant patients. Transplant Proc 1996. In press.

31. Carrieri G, Jordan ML, Shapiro R, et al. Acyclovir/cytomegalovirus immune globulin com-

bination therapy for CMV prophylaxis in high-risk renal allograft recipients. Transplant Proc 1995; 27:961–963.

32. Stratta RI, Shaefer MS, Cushing KA, et al. Successful prophylaxis of cytomegalovirus disease after primary CMV exposure in liver transplant recipients. Transplantation 1991; 51:90–97.

33. Maurer JR, Snell G, deHoyos A, et al. Outcomes of lung transplantation using three different cytomegalovirus prophylactic regimens. Transplant Proc 1993; 25:1434–1435.

34. Valenza M, Czer LSC, Shi-Hui P, et al. Combined antiviral and immunoglobulin therapy as prophylaxis against cytomegalovirus infection after heart transplantation. J Heart Lung Transplant 1995; 14:659–665.

35. Nicol DL, MacDonald AS, Belitsky P, et al. Reduction by combination prophylactic therapy with CMV hyperimmune globulin and acyclovir of the risk of primary CMV disease in renal transplant recipients. Transplantation 1993; 55:841–846.

36. Stratta RJ, Taylor RJ, Bynon JS, et al. Viral prophylaxis in combined pancreas-kidney transplant recipients. Transplantation 1994; 57:506–512.

37. Rubin RH, Lynch P, Pasternak MS, et al. Combined antibody and ganciclovir treatment of murine cytomegalovirus-infected normal immunosuppressed BALB/c mice. Antimicrob Agent Chemother 1989; 33:1975–1979.

38. Stals FS, Wagenaar SS, Bruggeman CA. Generalized cytomegalovirus (CMV) infection and CMV-induced pneumonitis in the rat: combined effect of 9-(1,3-dihydroxy-2-propoxymethyl) guanine and specific antibody treatment. Antiviral Res 1994; 25:147–160.

39. Reed EC, Bowden RA, Dandliker PS, et al. Treatment of cytomegalovirus pneumonia with ganciclovir and intravenous cytomegalovirus immunoglobulin in patients with bone marrow transplants. Ann Intern Med 1988; 109:783–788.

40. Emanuel D, Cunningham I, Jules-Elysee K, et al. Cytomegalovirus pneumonia after bone marrow transplantation successfully treated with the combination of ganciclovir and high-dose intravenous immune globulin. Ann Intern Med 1988; 109:777–782.

41. George MJ, Snydman DR, Werner BG, et al. Use of ganciclovir plus cytomegalovirus immune globulin to treat CMV pneumonia in orthotopic liver transplant recipients. Transplant Proc 1993; 25(suppl 4):22–24.

42. Martin M, Snydman DR, Rubin RH, et al. Question-and-answer session. High-risk transplantation. Transplant Proc 1994; 26(suppl 1):31–32.

43. Immunization Practice Advisory Committee. Hepatitis B virus: a comprehensive strategy for eliminating transmission in the United States through universal childhood vaccination. Recommendations of the immunization practices advisory committee (ACIP). MMWR 1991; 40(RR-13):1–25.

44. Starzl TE, Demetris AJ, van Thiel D. Liver transplantation. N Engl J Med 1989; 321:1092–1099.

45. Samuel D, Bismuth A, Mathieu D, et al. Passive immunoprophylaxis after liver transplantation in HBsAg-positive patients. Lancet 1991; 337:813–815.

46. Muller R, Gubernatis G, Farle M, et al. Liver transplantation in HBs antigen (HBsAg) carriers: prevention of hepatitis B virus (HBV) recurrence by passive immunization. J Hepatol 1991; 13:90–96.

47. Samuel D, Muller R, Alexander G, et al. Liver transplantation in European patients with the hepatitis B surface antigen. N Engl J Med 1993; 329:1842–1847.

48. Zaia JA, Levin MJ, Preblud SR, et al. Evaluation of varicella-zoster immune globulin: protection of immunosuppressed children after household exposure to varicella. J Infect Dis 1983; 147:737–743.

49. Centers for Disease Control. Varicella-zoster immune globulin for the prevention of chickenpox. Recommendations of the immunization practices advisory committee. Ann Intern Med 1984; 100:859–865.

50. Paryani SG, Avin AM, Koropchak CM, et al. Comparison of varicella zoster antibody titers in patients given intravenous immune serum globulin or varicella zoster immune globulin. J Pediatr 1984; 105:200–205.
51. Winston DJ. Use of intravenous immunoglobulin in viral infections. In: Stiehm ER, moderator. Intravenous immunoglobulins as therapeutic agents. Ann Intern Med 1987; 107:367–382.
52. Stevens DA, Merigan TC. Zoster immune globulin prophylaxis of disseminated zoster in compromised host: a randomized trial. Arch Intern Med 1980; 140:52–54.
53. Basgoz N, Preiksaitis JK. Post-transplant lymphoproliferative disorder. Infect Dis Clin North Am 1995; 9:901–923.
54. Bar RS, DeLor CJ, Clausen KP, et al. Fatal infectious mononucleosis in a family. N Engl J Med 1974; 290:363–367.
55. Purtilo DT, Sakamoto K, Barnabel V, et al. Epstein-Barr virus-induced diseases in boys with the X-linked lymphoproliferative syndrome (XLP): updated on studies of the registry. Am J Med 1982; 73:49–56.
56. Sullivan JL, Byron KS, Brewster FE, et al. X-linked lymphoproliferative syndrome. Natural history of the immunodeficiency. J Clin Invest 1983; 71:1765–1768.
57. Taguchi Y, Purtilo DT, Okano M. The effect of intravenous immunoglobulin and interferon-alpha on Epstein-Barr virus-induced lymphoproliferative disorder in a liver transplant recipient. 1994; 57:1813–1815.
58. Delone P, Corkill J, Jordan M, et al. Successful treatment of Epstein-Barr virus infection with ganciclovir and cytomegalovirus hyperimmune globulin following kidney transplantation. Transplant Proc 1995; 27(suppl 1):58–59.

10

Intravenous Immunoglobulin Use in the Newborn Infant: Treatment and Prevention of Infection

Rajam S. Ramamurthy

University of Texas Health Science Center, San Antonio, Texas

INTRODUCTION

Protection from disease by bolstering the natural defenses of the human body has kindled the interest of mankind for decades. The Chinese sought to counter the deadly smallpox through inoculation of the patient with material from smallpox lesions. Jenner in England in 1796 injected material from cowpox scabs to modify the virulent smallpox. These crude experiments were frequently disastrous. From these early beginnings to the present, where targeted immunoglobulins are emerging for various infections, it has been an incredible march through painstaking laboratory and clinical investigations. The neonate may be considered physiologically immunodeficient, and the preterm infant severely deficient. Therefore, it is understandable that immunotherapy is a tempting option in neonatal infections.

Prior to 1940, our understanding and capability of using immunotherapy were limited by the unavailability of a purified version of the antibodies that were safe and efficacious. The earlier preparations were harvested from animals. These hyperimmune gammaglobulins were larger molecules that could not be used intravenously and had to be given in large volumes intramuscularly (1). The risk of anaphylaxis and serum sickness was considerable. The small muscle mass and the large volume of the injection limited use of these in newborn infants.

In 1940 Cohn and Oncley fractionated pooled serum and separated gamma globulins from other serum proteins (2). Cohn fraction II contains about 90% IgG. The preparation known as standard gammaglobulin (SGG) was used intramuscularly in large volumes, and, when used intravenously, this produced severe reaction due to the presence of protein aggregates. Early attempts at treating neonates with gammaglobulins were enlightening. In 1963 Amer et al. published their experience with monthly gammaglobulin administration to preterm infants and demonstrated limited protection (3). They concluded that the expense and the invasiveness of the injections did not warrant routine use. Steen et al., in 1960 (4), and Diamond et al., in 1966 (5), studied the effect of prophylactic gammaglobulin in preterm infants and concluded that they did not modify the infectious morbidity or mortality. Thus, for a number of years, immunoglobulin therapy for infants was not a practical option.

In the mid-1970s, modified fractions of pooled plasma, pH treatment, and chemical modification of IgG reduced protein aggregation. Anaphylactic reactions were reduced. Kistler and Nitschmann modified the Cohn-Oncley fractionation method and obtained preparations not only safe from viruses, but free of protein aggregates (6). At the present time, there are several safe intravenous preparations of human immunoglobulins. In order to understand the benefits and limitations of immunoglobulins in the therapeutic armamentarium of neonatal infections, it is necessary to understand the host defense mechanisms at the disposal of the infant.

GENERAL SCHEMA OF HOST DEFENSE

The myriad of interactions involved in immune defense, the voluminous literature concerning the direct and indirect evidence of immune responses, and the speculations regarding as yet unproven interactions are dealt with to a certain extent in other chapters in this book. In this chapter only information that will enhance the understanding of immune mechanisms in the young infant will be mentioned. The immune function in this age group is intimately interconnected with the developmental stage of the fetus and newborn infant. The relevance of this information lies in the potential for developing strategies for the diagnosis, treatment, and prevention of infectious diseases in the newborn.

NONSPECIFIC HOST DEFENSE IN THE NEWBORN INFANT

Host defense may be envisioned as nonspecific, specific, and injurious to the host. The interaction of nonspecific host defense involving the macrophages and phagocytes and the specific responses of B and T cells and the complement system are all intricately woven together; deficiencies in one will affect the other. In addition, in the age group we are concerned with, the stage of development of each system is an additional variable. Most infectious agents are effectively cleared by the resident macrophages in the local tissue. When the quantity or virulence of the infectious agent is high, recruitment of phagocytes from other sites is activated (Fig. 1). The phagocytes adhere to the vascular endothelium; they deform and exit the vascular compartment and migrate to the site of infection. The phagocytes are attracted to the site by release of the chemotactic factors of the complement system, C3a and C5a (7).

In limited studies in humans it has been shown that alveolar macrophages are fewer in number at birth and increase rapidly after birth in healthy but not in the sick infants. Also, the pool of polymorphonuclear leukocytes (PMNs) and their precursors are rapidly depleted in the newborn infant in the presence of infection. The rate at which phagocytes reach the site of infection is also slower compared to adults (8). Elegant experiments have shown that in the newborn the phagocytes do not deform well, the adherence to cell surface is decreased, they do not bind chemotactic factors, and, therefore, the movement toward the site of injury is impaired. The life-span of the polymorphonuclear leukocytes is also short compared to adults. The role of antibodies in this process is indirect. The bacterial coating with antibodies is shown to activate the complement factors C3a and C5a, called the chemotactic factors, which attract the phagocytes to the site.

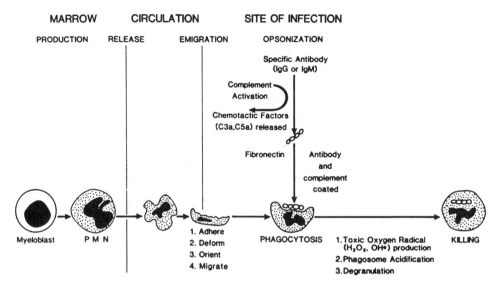

Figure 1 Defense mechanism against group B streptococcus. Source: Wilson, CB. Immuniological basis for increased susceptibility of the neonate to infection. J. Pediatr. 1986; 108:2.

Once the cells reach the target organism, they may engulf it without any enhancement. On the other hand, the more virulent organisms must be prepared by a coating of complement and antibodies prior to phagocytosis. There are several studies that have shown that under ideal laboratory conditions, the PMNs from neonates engulf bacteria just as well as adult PMNs. However, in the presence of deficiency of opsonins or with heavy inoculum of organisms, the neonatal cells are shown to be less efficient (9). The role of antibodies in this process is very apparent. Without antibody coating of the bacteria, there will be no phagocytosis of the more virulent bacteria. The fetus is dependent on the mother for the supply of antibodies, which does not occur in significant quantities until the 34th week of gestation. Even when infected, most neonates do not make detectable type-specific antibodies to group B *Streptococcus* (GBS) and other bacteria. This may be due to the developmental immaturity of the B lymphocytes and the T lymphocytes that facilitate the process. Antibodies and complement do not kill bacteria in the absence of phagocytes.

Following phagocytosis the bacteria must be killed. Within the cell there is an increase in oxygen consumption caused by enhanced glucose utilization by the hexose monophosphate pathway (HMP). Products of reduction of molecular O_2—namely, superoxide anion, the precursor of hydrogen peroxide, and hydroxyl radical—are all important in the killing. The nitroblue tetrazolium test (NBT) is a screening method for the measurement of HMP activity. The data related to this in the newborn are inconsistent—some showing normal, and others decreased, NBT reaction (10). In the newborn, chemiluminescence, which correlates with the production of hydroxyl radical, is decreased (11). In summary, PMNs from neonates kill bacteria less efficiently. This may be due to the high density of bacteria that overwhelm the phagocytes, delayed influx of PMNs from the pool, or the immaturity of the intracellular mechanisms that kill the bacteria. There is a direct role of antibodies which are essential for the killing. Most neonatal investigations in this area have focused on GBS infection. Monoclonal antibodies against GBS have significantly reduced mortality in rat models. The effect seems to be related to whether the infusion is given prior to the bacterial inoculum. This has not been studied in human newborn infants. Infusion of leukocytes in severely ill infants with leukocyte depletion has yielded controversial results in the few published studies (12).

Cellular defense in viral and intracellular pathogenic infections is more dependent on availability of opsonins and specific immunity. Virus replication occurs intracellularly, which may be prevented by cytotoxic or noncytotoxic mechanisms. Interferon produced by macrophages, fibroblasts, and nonimmune lymphocytes in response to viral challenge produces noncytotoxic viral killing. Specifically sensitized lymphocytes produce gamma interferon with similar capabilities. Monocytes and PMNs may ingest extracellular virus and effectively clear them. Monocytes, lymphocytes, and, to a certain extent, PMNs also may lyse virus-infected cells in the presence of specific antibody by a process known as antibody-dependent cell-mediated cytotoxicity (ADCC). To a small extent, cell-mediated cytotoxicity may operate in the absence of specific antibody by natural killer cells. It may be surmised that specific cytotoxic T lymphocytes are necessary for ultimate eradication of infection. In the newborn, primary infection of the mother presents a larger inoculum of virus as well as lack of the IgG antibodies that have not come from the mother. Studies have also shown that alpha and beta interferon are normal, whereas gamma interferon is markedly reduced (13). The role of immunoglobulins in the therapy of viral infections is just emerging. In vitro experiments show that protection occurs only when immune intervention precedes viral challenges. As in GBS infection, maternal antibody level appears to be critical in viral infections.

Unlike pyogenic bacteria that can be engulfed and killed, intracellular organisms such as toxoplasma, *Chlamydia, Salmonella, Listeria,* and *Mycobacterium* tuberculosis may actually be protected within the cell. In these infants, T lymphocytes, monocytes, and macrophages play a critical role (14). Resolution of infection and establishment of protective immunity depend on the interaction between macrophages and T lymphocytes. The interaction leads to the production of a series of interrelated hormone-like mediators known as cytokines, lymphokines, and interleukins. After killing, the microbial products, namely antigens, are then displayed on the surface of macrophages in association with class II major histocompatibility epitopes. Lymphokine-dependent cellular immunity appears to be the principal mechanism in the ability of the host to resist infection with intracellular pathogens. Antibody appears to play a very small role. Although antimicrobial therapy is available for many of these pathogens, immunological enhancement of host defense would also be beneficial. Interleukin-2 and gamma interferon produced through recombinant DNA methods are proving useful in HIV infections.

SPECIFIC HOST DEFENSE

The specific host defense involves two mechanisms: production of specific antibodies from B cells, and cell-mediated or the T-cell system. The developmental aspects of these systems and information pertaining to the newborn infant alone will be elucidated here (15–18). In the human fetus, the immune responsiveness begins in the 8th to 12th week of gestation. The progenitor stem cells are located in the yolk sac, liver, and the bone marrow. Granulocytes are noted in the fetal liver about the eighth week of gestation. By 5 months, the bone marrow demonstrates increased activity. By 15–18 weeks of gestation, the number of immunoglobulin-bearing lymphocytes approaches that seen in adults.

The progenitor cells destined to become B cells, influenced by an undefined anatomical area (well-recognized site in birds called the bursa of Fabricius), populate thymic-independent areas in the lymph node. These cells can be identified by their surface markers. The B lymphocytes' first interaction with antigen is referred to as primary immune response. Some of the B cells will mature into plasma cells that produce the antibodies or immunoglobulins. Other B cells become memory cells. The predominant class of antibody produced is IgM, which begins 5–7 days following exposure to antigen, reaches peak levels by 7–10 days, and falls to baseline at 14 days. The production of IgG antibodies occurs later, around 7–10 days; reaches higher levels than IgM by 14 days; and drops to baseline by 21 days. Upon a second exposure to the same antigen, the memory carried by the B cells results in a quick IgG response in 3–5 days that is severalfold higher than the primary response. The IgM production coincides with IgG, but reaches a much lower peak level than IgM primary response and drops within a week. The above statements are true in general. However, newborn infants born at different stages of gestation may not have the ability to respond to antigenic stimuli in the same manner. This is an important consideration in immunizing the premature infant. The experience with vaccines in the newborn is dealt with in a separate chapter.

MATERNAL ENDOWMENT OF IMMUNOGLOBULINS TO THE FETUS

The ability of the fetus to develop without being rejected despite carrying 50% of the genes that are foreign to the mother is largely attributed to the placental membrane barrier. Animals that have several layers of placental membranes, such as the horse, receive negligible amounts of immunoglobulins transplacentally and receive a lot more from colostrum. The human fetus receives significant amounts transplacentally, and the colostral immunoglobulins are not absorbed from the GI tract in any significant quantity. Transfer across the placenta is an active process by virtue of a receptor located on the FC portion of the immunoglobulin (19). Thus, the fetus receives a rich endowment of preformed antibodies of the IgG class from the mother, a composite reflection of her encounters with the microbial world. At the same time, the newborn at birth is immunologically deficient in those antibodies that the mother does not supply. Applying this to exogenous preparations of immunoglobulins that are made from pooled plasma from the population, it is conceivable that they may not contain antibodies to organisms not prevalent in that population. IgG immunoglobulins are the only type that cross the placenta by virtue of their low molecular weight. The others do not. IgA immunoglobulin is found in abundance in the breast milk and provides local protection at the mucous membrane of the lungs and intestines. They are not absorbed into the circulation (20).

In adults, IgG constitutes 75% of the total circulating pool of immunoglobulin. There are four subclasses of IgG1: 1, 2, 3, and 4. IgG constitutes 60–70% of the total IgG, IgG2 20%, IgG3 4–8%, and IgG4 1.4–2%. IgG2 crosses the placenta more slowly. Antibodies to protein antigens, such as tetanus and diphtheria toxoids, are found predominantly in the IgG1 subclass. The majority of antibodies against capsular polysaccharide of highly virulent organisms such as *Haemophilus influenzae, Streptococcus pneumoniae*, and group B streptococci are of the IgG2 subclass, which does not cross the placenta very well. IgG4 is found with IgE in the membranes of mast cells, which contain the histamine and heparin granules and may play a protective role. IgM forms 10% of the immunoglobulins. It is a macroglobulin and is a pentamer of IgG molecules. IgM is the earliest immunoglobulin to be produced in response to an infection, does not cross the placenta, and serves as a diagnostic marker for intrauterine infections. IgD is present in very small quantities, 0.2% in adult serum, and its role is not very clear. IgE constitutes about 0.004% of the total serum immunoglobulin in adults. IgE binds with allergens at the F_{Ab} region and to mast cells at the F_c portion, and induces release of histamine in allergic reactions.

Most of the immunoglobulin present in cord serum is IgG obtained from the mother (Fig. 2). There is little or no IgM or IgA, as these do not cross the placenta. This means that the opsonins and bactericidal antibodies that are so necessary to protect against encapsulated organisms, particularly of the gram-negative variety, are not available to the fetus. The type of IgG that comes form the mother is also variable. The low-molecular-weight antibodies against measles that are found in abundance in maternal serum are readily transferred, whereas antibodies against pertussis come in much smaller quantities. Larger macroglobulins are not transferred. The passively transferred IgG has a half life of 20–30 days and is at its lowest level around 2–4 months of age. The newborn infant, who is exposed to several antigens, begins to make immunoglobulins in the same sequence as that seen in a primary immune response. IgM levels reach those of the adult by 1 year of age, IgG by 5–6 years, and IgA by 10 years. The effect of maternal antibodies on immunization of the newborn will be dealt with more completely elsewhere in this chapter.

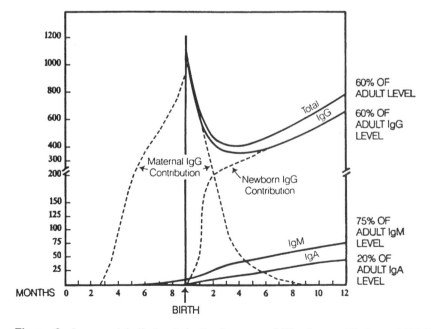

Figure 2 Immunoglobulin levels in the first year of life. *Source*: Wedgwood RJ, Davis SD, Ray CG, eds. Infections in Children. Philadelphia: Harper & Row, 1982.

The other component of specific response to infection is known as cell-mediated immunity. From the progenitor stem cell, the lymphopoietic cells enter the thymus gland via the bloodstream at about the eighth week of gestation and differentiate into lymphocytes. The thymus gland is derived from the epithelium of the fourth pharyngeal pouches by the sixth week of gestation. A hormone, thymosin, may be operative in the generation of lymphocytes. The lymphocytes that emerge from the thymus acquire new surface antigen markers, which may be antigen recognition units. The lymphocytes travel via lymphatics and the bloodstream, and populate very specific areas in the lymph nodes called "thymic-dependent" areas and the periarterial areas of the spleen. These pools of lymphocytes have a very long life. The whole complex is referred to as the T cell system (21). The DiGeorge syndrome, presenting with hypocalcemia and repeated viral and fungus infections, is explained by the development of the thymus and parathyroid glands from the same third and fourth pharyngeal pouch (17). If a newborn infant presents with hypocalcemia not explained on the basis of other problems, an evaluation of thymic-dependent immunity would be in order. Cellular immunity must be active in the fetus, as the phytohemagglutinin (PHA) test that stimulates the thymic cells is positive from about 14 weeks. Also, maternal lymphocytes that enter the fetal circulation should mount a graft-versus-host reaction, if they were not rejected by a competent system in the fetus that rejects them.

HOST RESPONSE INJURIOUS TO THE HOST

If antigen persists, there may be continued and maximal host response, which may be injurious to the host such as seen in autoimmune disorders. For the most part, the fetus does not have a tertiary response, but it is present in certain situations like Rh incompatibility or intrauterine infection such as syphilis.

In summary, the fetus unchallenged in utero may be considered immunologically pristine. However, it is capable of producing immunoglobulins when challenged. The response is still not as vigorous as seen in later life. Passive transfer of IgG immunoglobulins to the fetus occurs in significant quantities only after 34 weeks of gestation. Despite the levels of IgG which in full-term newborns are equal to or even slightly higher than maternal levels, they may lack those components necessary for protection against virulent pathogens that produce disease in this age group. Lastly, viral infections causing devastating disease in this age group are more likely to be helped by preexisting immunoglobulin.

POTENTIAL FOR IMMUNOGLOBULIN THERAPY
IN THE NEWBORN INFANT

Early use of intramuscular immunoglobulin was mostly intended for viral infections. Availability of intravenous immunoglobulins (IVIG) opened the door for both therapeutic and prophylactic use.

In 1980, Sidiropoulous studied IVIG in 82 infants with clinical evidence of sepsis (22). Thirty-five of these had proven sepsis. Fifteen infants received only antibiotics, and 20 were given antibiotics plus IVIG. Term infants were given 1 g and preterms 0.5 g daily for 6 days. Four out of 15 died in the non-IVIG group (26%), compared to 2 of 20 in the treated group (10%). This difference was not statistically significant.

When preterm infants were separated, four of nine in the untreated and one of 13 in the treated group died ($P = .04$). Convinced of the efficacy of this limited trial, the study was stopped, and IVIG therapy was instituted for all septic infants. This led to a very interesting study using IVIG in pregnant women (23). Women at 27–36 weeks of gestation at risk of infection (fever, chorioamnionitis, prolonged rupture of membranes) were assigned to one of three groups. Twenty-four women received only antibiotics, 16 received antibiotics and a single infusion of 12 g of IVIG (low dose), and 11 received antibiotics and 120 g of IVIG (high dose). There was no increase in cord IgG in the low-dose group compared to controls. There was a threefold rise in the high-dose group. There was no difference in the incidence of infection in all three groups below 32 weeks' gestation. There was a difference in neonatal infections in the over 32 weeks' gestation group. The numbers were too small to obtain statistical significance.

In 1986, Chirico et al. reported from Italy their experience with infants < 1500 g and < 34 weeks' gestation who were randomly assigned to receive IVIG or no therapy within 24 h of life (24). Sandoglobulin preparation 0.5 g/kg weekly for 1 month was given. A second group of infants weighing > 1500 g but receiving intensive care were also randomly assigned to receive the product during the period they were receiving intensive care. The groups were comparable in birth weight, gestational age, Apgar score, maternal factors such as duration of rupture of membranes, etc., and the initial symptomatology in the neonate. There was a significant difference between the treated and untreated groups in the incidence of infection, particularly septicemias in the infants < 1500 g. There was no difference in the incidence of infection or mortality in the infants with birth weight > 1500 g. There was no difference in the incidence of necrotizing enterocolitis (NEC), pneumonia, or urinary tract infection (UTI). The therapy was more effective in preventing generalized than localized infections. They also measured serum IgG levels and specific antibody levels to GBS serotype III, *Escherichia coli*, and cytomegalovirus (CMV) and found that the half-life of the administered antibodies was about 11 days. No side effects were observed.

Another study comes from Haque et al. (25), who looked at three groups of infants, 50 in each group. Group A received Intraglobulin (a preparation from West Germany), within 2–4 h of delivery. Group B received it on both day 1 and 8, and group C served as a control. With one injection the serum IgG levels increased to 500 mg/dl and stayed high on day 8, when they were measured. With the second dose, the level went about 1600 g. The authors concluded that prophylaxis was encouraging.

A more recent study from Christensen and colleagues in Utah evaluated the safety of administering IVIG (26). They used the Gamimune (Miles, Inc.) preparation. Twenty preterm infants were studied who were < 7 days of age and < 2000 g at birth. They were randomly assigned to receive 750 mg/kg body weight of IVIG. The controls received an albumin infusion. There were no differences in heart rate, respiratory rate, temperature, or urine output, or in the serum electrolytes, liver function tests, or routine blood count. The serum IgG level peaked at 1400 mg/dl with a level of 900 mg/dl after 24 h and still remained above 600 mg at 8 days of age. There were no documented infections in the group of infants studied.

PROPHYLACTIC USE OF INTRAVENOUS IMMUNOGLOBULIN

The immune deficiency of the preterm infant, the relentless decline of passively acquired maternal antibodies, and the dangerously low levels reached by 4–15 weeks of age all make the prophylactic use of IVIG in the newborn infant an attractive possibility. In one double-blind controlled study, one injection of 500 mg/kg of lyophilized IVIG (Sandoglobulin) was infused over a 2-h period (27). Albumin 5 mg/kg was used in the control infants. There were 372 IVIG and 381 albumin recipients. At study entry the serum IgG concentration was related to gestational age. The IgG level remained significantly higher in the IVIG group for 8 weeks. The change in IgG level after the infusion did not correlate with gestational age. There was no difference in the incidence of sepsis or timing of the occurrence of sepsis. Sepsis occurred after the fifth day after the study entry. Multiple infections occurred in three instances in the controls, and four instances in the IVIG group. It is interesting to note that of the 89 episodes of sepsis reported, 66 were due to *Staphylococcus epidermidis*. Twenty of these were confirmed by two blood cultures, and 46 by one blood culture. This raised the concern about the IVIG preparation having antibodies against the infecting organism.

The two large multicenter studies that have produced conflicting results bear close scrutiny. In the first multicenter double-blind placebo-controlled study (28), 577 infants (of 588 randomized) who completed the protocol were analyzed. The infants weighed between 500 and 1750 g and were stratified in 250-g increments in birth weight. A lyophilized, highly purified preparation of IVIG obtained by Cohn fractionation and ion exchange adsorption was used (Gammagard, Baxter Healthcare, Hyland Division). Five hundred milligrams per kilogram body weight IVIG were given by slow infusion over a period of 30 min. The first dose was administered at 3–7 days of age, again at 1 week, and subsequently every 14 days for a total of five infusions or until discharge from the hospital. The control infants received 5 mg/kg albumin. Serum IgG levels were measured prior to each infusion and a week after the infusion (Fig. 3). IgG levels were comparable between groups prior to the infusions and steadily declined in the placebo group, while the trough Ig level at each point tested in the IVIG group was higher than the preinfusion level. There was a significantly lower incidence of infections in the IVIG group. The infusions were well tolerated by the patients. There was a significant reduction in the number of hospital days in the infants with infection. Coagulase-negative infections were the most frequent in the IVIG (34%) and in the control group (31%).

The second large multicenter trial (29) involved 2416 infants stratified by 500-g increments in birth weight. The study was done in two phases: 1218 infants were included in phase 1 (595 were given IVIG, and 623 were given placebo). Study infants received 500 mg/kg IVIG (lyophilized human immunoglobulin, Sandoglobulin, Sandoz Pharmaceuticals). Infants < 1000 g were given 900 mg/kg, and those between 1000 and 1500 g were given 700 mg/kg, to maintain serum level of 700 mg/dl. The infusions were given every 2 weeks until the infants reached 1800 g or were discharged. Five percent albumin solution was used as placebo. In phase 2, 1198 infants were assigned—609 to IVIG and 589 to no infusion. Entry occurred at 44 ± 25 h after birth.

Adverse reactions were noted in < 1% of cases in the form of transient tachycardia or rise in blood pressure. Baseline serum immunoglobulin levels and subsequent trough values following the infusions showed that in the IVIG group immunoglobulin trough levels exceeded 700 mg/dl at all points checked. In the control group the target level of IgG was maintained in only 18 of these infants. The IVIG group had significantly higher levels when compared to the placebo group.

During phase 1, 11.6% of the immune globulin group and 16.4% of the albumin group had septicemia. In phase 2, the incidence of septicemia increased to 19.2% in IVIG and 18.2% in the control groups. When the data were combined, 15.5% of

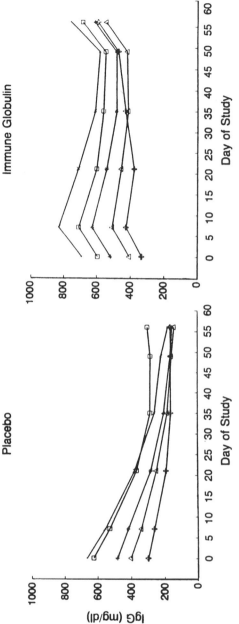

Figure 3 Mean serum IgG levels at enrollment, before each infusion was given, and 1 week after the final infusion, according to birth-weight category, in the placebo group and the immune globulin group. The birth-weight categories are denoted as follows: crosses, 500–750 g; triangles, 751–1000 g; asterisks, 1001–1250 g; squares, 1251–1500 g; and X's 1501–1750 g. Immune globulin or placebo was first given on day 0 of the study. *Source:* Baker CJ et al. Intravenous immunoglobulin for the prevention of nosocomial infection in low-birth-rate neonates. New Engl J Med 1992; 327:216.

IVIG and 17.2% of controls had septicemia. This difference was not statistically significant. Infants weighing 501–1000 g at birth had more infections than those with a birth weight of 1000–1500 g, regardless of treatment received. There was also no difference noted in the rate of second infections, those with a diagnosis of probable sepsis, average length of hospital stay, or time interval to the first episode of infection. IVIG also had no specific effect on gram-negative, *Candida*, or fungal infections. It is important to note that there were fewer infections due to group B *Streptococcus*,—two in the IVIG group compared to 12 in the control group ($P < .01$). Necrotizing enterocolitis was seen in 22% of all septic episodes.

The conflicting results in these two large multicenter trials are intriguing. The incidence of infection in the Gammagard study, 35% in IVIG and 24% in placebo, is much higher than that reported in the Sandoglobulin study (19% and 17%, respectively). The patient profile and the antibody profiles of the immunoglobulin preparations may account for the disparity between the studies. The overall incidence of group B streptococcal sepsis and gram-negative sepsis in the centers that participated in the latter study in phases 1 and 2 is interesting. This background incidence that is shown to naturally wax and wane (30) in nurseries is very important when different treatment modalities are instituted and the incidence of infection is used as a variable. Other studies involving smaller numbers of patients also have not shown a benefit of IVIG in reducing infections. Others using different study designs giving a single dose of Sandoglobulin to raise IVIG levels in infants with birth weight between 500 and 2000 g have also not shown a beneficial effect (31,32). The very high incidence of coagulase-negative staphylococcal (CNS) infection in all the studies raises the issue of the antibody titers to CNS in IVIG preparations.

IMMUNOGLOBULIN THERAPY FOR SPECIFIC INFECTIONS IN THE NEWBORN INFANT

Coagulase-Negative Staphylococcal Infection

In a recent survey of pathogens isolated from blood cultures taken from neonates in our hospital between 1977 and 1994, coagulase-negative staphylococci were found to be the most common isolates (33). This commensal organism, long regarded as a nonpathogen, has become well recognized as a potential pathogen, especially in the preterm infant (34). CNS rapidly colonize newborns (35) and are a major cause of septicemia, pneumonia, and infections associated with indwelling intravenous catheters and ventricular shunts, and pneumonia associated with chronic endotracheal intubation (36). In adults, it has been shown that one species of CNS, *Staphylococcus epidermides* has emerged as a major cause of all biomaterial-associated infections (37). In the very low-birth-weight infant, who has prolonged hospitalization, endotracheal intubation, and central venous catheters, the risk of infection is very high. These infections are difficult to treat because of multiple drug resistance to these organisms.

Seventy premature neonates with a mean gestation of 30.5 ± 2.8 weeks and a mean birth weight of 1320 ± 310 g were followed over a 2-month period to evaluate polymophonuclear leukocyte (PMN) function (38). Luminal-dependent chemiluminescence microassay was used to assess PMN function. There were 33 episodes of serious infections in 23 infants (32.9%), and coagulase-negative staphylococci were implicated in 12 (52%). Twenty of the 23 infants had depressed PMN function.

The sera of the CNS-infected infants were tested by an enzyme-linked immunosorbent assay (ELISA) for antibody levels against their own infecting strains of CNS. Sera were also collected from CNS-uninfected infants matched for sex, birth weight, and gestational age. At a mean postnatal age of 5 days, the mean ELISA value for the infected infants was only 45% of the mean value for the uninfected controls, which suggests that low antibody levels to CNS could predispose these infants to infection with CNS. Multiple serum samples were collected through their hospital stay. Each serum sample was tested by ELISA for antibody activity against its own infecting microorganism. Results indicated that infants mounted a specific antibody response against their homologous microorganism including CONS. The mean ELISA values for those in the IVIG group for sera collected on days 12, 24, 39, and 54 almost doubled and were 79–89% of the uninfected control infant values. For those receiving placebo, the mean values remained lower and were 47–64% of the uninfected control infants values through day 39, but by day 54 were almost twice that of uninfected controls, indicative of an immune response against the infecting microorganism. The findings suggest that the immunoglobulin preparation used (Gammagard®) has a high titer of CNS antibodies. The analysis was done to evaluate the adequacy of antibody levels, but not the efficacy of prophylaxis to prevent infection. These studies suggest that the neonate is prone to CNS infections because of inadequate phagocyte function, as well as low antibody levels. Further studies are needed to evaluate the efficacy of exogenous immunoglobulin to prevent colonization and infection.

Group B Steptococcal Infection

IVIG utilization has been studied more extensively in the treatment of neonatal GBS infection than any of the other bacterial infections in the newborn. Baker et al. in 1976 showed that newborn babies with a deficiency of antibody to GBS have an increased risk of developing GBS sepsis and meningitis (39). Fisher et al. showed in rat models that passively acquired antibody levels drop appreciably in 6–8 h following infection, and no antibody was detected 24 h following the infection (40). For IVIG to be effective, the preparation must contain sufficient opsonic antibodies. There is lot-to-lot variability in antibody levels. Also, antigen-binding assays such as ELISA do not discriminate effectively between low and high levels, and other methods may be needed to measure antibody levels. It may be necessary to monitor levels of opsonic antibodies during therapy to ensure adequate levels. Gloser et al. produced a GBS hyperimmune preparation that contained a 14-fold higher concentration of specific antibodies than Sandoglobulin (40). Sandoglobulin was also found to have considerable lot-to-lot variation in antibody titers. The hyperimmune preparation contained antibodies to the type-specific antigen of all five types of GBS. Human studies using these hyperimmune preparations are lacking. Christensen et al. have shown that mothers of GBS-infected infants show an abnormality in switching from IgM to IgG production. While the IgM antibodies protect the mother, they do not cross the placenta and therefore cannot afford protection to the neonate. Christensen et al. have shown that infusion of a high dose of nonspecific antibodies could lead to a decrease in survival time of specific antibodies already present in the baby (42).

IVIG given to pregnant women showed that mothers who received a low dose, 12 g, had a significant rise in IgG level and that the level tripled with the administration of 120 g (23). The infants born to low-dose mothers had no change in IgG level, while in the high-dose group those infants born prior to 32 weeks showed no change,

Table 1 Pharmacokinetics of IVIG in Neonates

Author	Sample size	Dose	Meat BWT	Kinetics
Weisman	5	0.5 g/kg	2.5 kg	Vd = 69 ml/kg Clearance = 4.2 ml/kg/day Alpha $t_{1/2}$ = 11.3 days Beta $t_{1/2}$ = 30.7 days
Chirico	35	0.5 g/kg	1.1 and 2.2 kg	Combined $t_{1/2}$ = 10 days
Noya	8 9	0.5 g/kg 0.75 g/kg	0.75–1.5 kg	Beta $t_{1/2}$ = 22 days
Kyllonen	49	0.5–1.3 g/kg	0.6–1.5 kg	Beta $t_{1/2}$ = 17 days initial dose = 23 days final dose = 16 days < 1 kg initial dose = 28 days > 1.5 kg initial dose
	43	Endogenous (maternal)		Beta $t_{1/2}$ = 33 days
Roderman	13 7	1 g/kg 0.5 g/kg	< 1.5 kg < 1.5 kg	Nonseptic = 17.1 days Septic = 13 days
Noya	21	0.5, 0.75, 1.0 g/kg	0.75–1.5 kg	Beta $t_{1/2}$ = 33 days

Source: Kliegman RM, Clapp D.W. Rational Principles for Immunoglobulin Porophylaxis and Therapy of Neonatal Infections. Clin Perinatol 1991; 18:313.

but those born after 32 weeks had high levels compared to controls. There was a tendency toward decreased infection in the high-dose group, but the numbers were too small to draw definitive conclusions. The two large multicenter collaborative studies have not conclusively proven that IVIG therapy will change the incidence or mortality of neonatal sepsis significantly. Overall, most recent studies (Table 1) have demonstrated a beneficial effect of IVIG for reducing the incidence of nosocomial bacterial infection in the low-birth-weight infants.

IVIG for Other Neonatal Infections

Newborn infants remain highly susceptible to bacterial infections with K_1 *E. coli* strains. K_1 capsular antibody would provide protection against this organism. However, these antibodies are of the IgM class and do not cross the placenta. IgG antibodies to K_1 in IVIG preparations would be theoretically useful. Recently, human monoclonal IgM antibody against the lipid A domain of endotoxin has been demonstrated to reduce the mortality from gram-negative bacteremia (30% vs. 49%) and from gram-negative bacterial septic shock (33% vs. 57%) (43). An IgM-enriched IVIG preparation containing 30 mg IgM, 30 mg IgA, and 190 mg IgG/5 ml given at 5 ml/kg dose on 4 consecutive days to neonates with sepsis showed a decrease in mortality compared to standard therapy with only antibiotics (33% vs. 20% survival, respectively). The preparation has high antibody titers to gram-negative organisms and endotoxins, but may not be useful in gram-positive infections. Thus, the treatment of neonatal sepsis with intravenous immunoglobulins requires further clinical studies.

IVIG for Respiratory Syncytial Virus Infection

Respiratory syncytial virus (RSV) is a major cause of lower respiratory tract infection in children. The peak age of hospitalization for RSV bronchiolitis or pneumonia is 2–5 months of age. Primary RSV infection occurs in children less than a year of age. By 2 years of age, 95% of children will have serological evidence of RSV infection. Children with underlying pulmonary disease and those who are immunocompromised are at greater risk for serious disease.

Naturally acquired immunity to RSV is incomplete. Repeated infections are common; however, the severity is much less after the primary infection. Animal studies have shown that polyclonal and monoclonal antibodies against both F and G glucoproteins of the virus confer passive protection. Cell-mediated immunity appears to be important, especially in the recovery phase and in limiting virus shedding. There is one report of treating RSV-infected infants with IVIG containing high RSV titers of neutralizing antibodies (44), which resulted in a significant reduction in nasal RSV shedding. A more recent study showed a significant reduction in the number of RSV infections and significantly reduced hospital days in infants who received a high dose of hyperimmune globulin against RSV (45). The success of immunoprophylaxis in high-risk infants has led to the development of specific monoclonal antibodies against RSV. The monoclonal antibodies are directed against specific epitopes of the virus, and a much higher concentration of IVIG can be given in a small volume. These preparations are currently under investigation.

CONCLUSION

In conclusion, the use of intravenous immunoglobulins for the treatment of early-onset neonatal sepsis has not been proven. The benefit of prophylactic use of IVIG for prevention of late-onset sepsis has shown varying results. The differences in the two large multicenter trials is puzzling, although it may be related to antibody levels in the different preparations studied. A fact to consider is the very high incidence of coagulase-negative staphylococcal infections reported in almost all of the series with large numbers of patients. CNS antibody titers are available for one IVIG preparation (Gammagard), but not for other commercially available preparations. These and other organisms that are unique in the neonatal period may require an IVIG preparation with adequate antibody titers against these organisms.

IVIG is well tolerated by even the smallest infants when caution is exercised with the rate of infusion. The use of IVIG specifically targeted toward respiratory syncytial virus is yet another landmark therapeutic advance in neonatal medicine. Attention to the current infectious problems in neonatal intensive care units, particularly infections with coagulase-negative staphylococcus, will be beneficial to the smallest and the sickest of the neonates.

REFERENCES

1. Stiehm ER, Ashida E, Kim KS, et al. Intravenous immunoglobulins as therapeutic agents. Ann Intern Med 1987; 107:367–382.

2. Berkman SA, Lee ML, GAle RP. Clinical uses of intravenous immunoglobulins. Semin Hematol 1988; 25:140–158.

3. Amer J, Ott E, Ibbott FA, et al. The effect of monthly gamma-globulin administration on morbidity and mortality from infection in premature infants during the first year of life. Pediatrics 1963; 32:4–9.

4. Steen JA. Gamma globulin in preventing infections in premature infants. Arch Pediatr 1960; 77:291–294.

5. Diamond EF, Porugganan HB, Choi, HJ. Effect of prophylactic gamaglobulin administration on infection morbidity in premature infants. Ill Med J 1966; 130:668–670.

6. Ugazio AG, Duse M, Notarangelo LD. Intravenous immunoglobulin and immunodeficiency in children. Curr Opin Pediatr 1989; 1:5–12.

7. Wilkinson PC. Leukocyte locomotion and chemotaxis. Effects of bacteria and viruses. Rev Infect Dis 1980; 2:1618.

8. Bankhurst AD, Mosito T, Williams RC. Studies of human cord blood and adult lymphocyte interactions with in vitro immunoglobulin production. J Clin Invest 1979; 64:990.

9. Wright WC, Ank BJ, Herbert J, Stiehm ER. Decreased bactericidal activity of luekocytes of stressed newborn infants. Pediatrics 1975; 56:579.

10. Belanti JA, Cantz BE, Maybee DA. Defective phagocytosis by newborn leukocytes: a defect similar to that of chronic granulomatous disease. Pediatr Res 1969; 3:376. Abstract.

11. Driscoll MS, Thomas VL, Ramamurthy RS, Casto DT. Longitudinal evaluation of polymorphonuclear leukocyte chemiluminescence in premature infants. J Pediatr 1990; 116:429–434.

12. Lawlenti F, Ferro R, Isacchi G, et al. Polymorpholeucocyte transfusion for treatment of sepsis in the newborn infant. J Pediatr 1981; 98:118–123.

13. Bryson YJ, Winter HS, Gard SE, Fischer TJ, Stiehm ER. Deficiency of immune interferon production by leukocytes of normal newborns. Cell Immunol 1980; 55:191.

14. Wilson CB. Immunologic basis for increased susceptibility of the neonate to infection. J Pediatr 1986; 180:1.

15. Stiehm R, Fulginiti VA. Pediatric Immunologic Diseases. Philadelphia: W. B. Saunders, 1973.

16. Lawton AR, Self KS, Royal SA, Cooper MD. Ontogeny of B lymphocytes in the human fetus. Clin Immunol Immunopathol 1972; 1:84.

17. Hong R, Gatti RA, Rathbun J, Good RA. The second and third pharyngeal pouch syndrome. A developmental anomaly of thyroid gland and thymus. N Engl J Med 1970; 282:470.

18. August CS, Berkel AI, Merler E. Onset of the lymphocyte function in the developing human fetus. Pediatr Res 1971; 5:539.

19. Gitlin D, Kumate J, Urrusti J, et al. The selectivity of the human placenta in the transfer of plasma proteins. J Clin Invest 1964; 43:1938.

20. Tomasi TB, Grey HM. Structure and function of immunoglobulin A. Prog Allergy 1972; 16:81.

21. Bellanti JA, ed. Immunology. Philadelphia: W. B. Saunders, 1971.

22. Sidiropoulos D. Immunoglobulin therapy in preterm neonates with perinatal infections. In: Morell A, Nydegger UE, eds. Clinical Use of Intravenous Immunoglobulins. London: Academic Press, 1986:159.

23. Sidiropoulos D, Boehme U, Von Muralt G, et al. Immunoglobulin supplementation in prevention or treatment of neonatal sepsis. Pediatr Infect Dis 1986; 5:S193–S194.

24. Chirico G, Rondini G, Plebani A, et al. Intravenous gamma globulin therapy for prophylaxis of infection in high-risk neonates. J Pediatr 1987; 110:437–442.

25. Haque KN, Zaidi MH. IgM-enriched intravenous immunoglobulin therapy in neonatal sepsis. Am J Dis Child 1988; 142:1293–1296.

26. Christensen RD, Hardman T, Thorton J, Hill HR. A randomized double blind placebo controlled investigation of the safety of intravenous immune globulin administration to preterm neonates. J Pediatr 1994; 125:922–930.

27. Weisman LE, Stoll BJ, Kueser TJ, et al. Intravenous immune globulin prophylaxis of late-onset sepsis in premature neonates. J Pediatr 1994; 125:922–930.
28. Baker CJ. Neonatal IVIG Collaborative Study Group. Multicenter trial of intravenous immunoglobulin (IVIG) to prevent late-onset infection in preterm infants: preliminary results. Pediatr Res 1989; 25:275A.
29. Fanaroff AA, Korones SB, Wright E: A controlled trial of intravenous immune globulin to reduce nosocomial infections in very-low-birth-weight infants. N Engl J Med 1994; 330:1107–1113.
30. Pyati SP, Pildes RS, Ramamurthy RS, Jacobs N. Decreasing mortality in neonates with early onset group B streptococcal infection: reality or artifact. J Pediatr 1981; 98:625–627.
31. Magny JF, Bremard-Oury C, Brault D, et al. Intravenous immunoglobulin therapy for prevention of infection in high-risk premature infants: report of a multicenter, double-blind study. Pediatrics 1991; 88:437–443.
32. Kinney J, Mundorf L, Gleason C, et al. Efficacy and pharmacokinetics of intravenous immune globulin administration to high-risk neonates. Am J Dis Child 1991; 145:1233–1238.
33. Ramamurthy RS, Kumara V. Seventeen year survey of bacterial isolates from blood cultures in the newborn nursery. Abstr J Perinatol 1996.
34. Eriksson M, Melen B, Myrback K-E, Winbladh B, Zetterstrom R. Bacterial colonization of newborn infants in a neonatal intensive care unit. Acta Paediatr Scand 1982; 71:779–783.
35. Brook I, Martin WJ. Bacterial colonization in intubated newborns. Respiration 1980; 40:323–328.
36. Brook I, Martin WJ. Bacterial colonization in incubated newborns. Respiration 1980; 40:323–328.
37. Dankert J, Hogt AH, Feijen J. Biomedical polymers: bacterial adhesion, colonization and infection. CRC Crit Rev Biocompat 1986; 2:219–301.
38. Driscoll MS, Thomas VL, Ramamurthy RS. Polymorphonuclear leukocyte function and antibody levels in premature infants with coagulase-negative staphylococcal infections. Southern Society for Pediatric Research, 1989. Abstract J-PM-0022.
39. Baker CJ, Kasper DL. Correlation of maternal antibody deficiency with susceptibility to neonatal group B streptococcal infection. N Engl J Med 1976; 294:753–756.
40. Fisher GW, Hemming VG, Hunter KW, et al. Intravenous immunoglobulin in the treatment of neonatal sepsis: therapeutic strategies and laboratory studies. Pediatr Infect Dis 1986; Suppl 5:8171.
41. Gloser H, Bachmayer H, Helm A. Intravenous immunoglobulin with high activity against group B streptococci. Pediatr Infect Dis 1986; Suppl 5:8176.
42. Christensen KK, Christensen P. Intravenous gamma-globulin in the treatment of neonatal sepsis with special reference to group B streptococci and pharmacokinetics. Pediatr Infect Dis 1986; 5:5189.
43. Ziegler EJ, Fisher CJ, Sprung CI, et al. Treatment of gram negative bacteremia and septic shock with HA-1A human monoclonal antibody against endotoxin. N Engl J Med 1991; 324:429.
44. Groothuis JR. Prophylactic administration of respiratory syncytial virus immune globulin to high-risk infants and young children. N Engl J Med 1993; 329:1524–1530.
45. Groothuis JR. Respiratory syncytial virus in children with bronchopulmonary dysplasia. Pediatrics 1988; 82:199–203.

11

Use of Intravenous Immunoglobulins in High-Risk Surgical Procedures and in Posttrauma Patients

Giorgio Zanetti and Michel-Pierre Glauser
University Hospital, Lausanne, Switzerland

INTRODUCTION

Despite improvements in postoperative supportive care and the development of new potent anti-infective agents, infection remains a major cause of mortality and morbidity among patients admitted to intensive care units after surgery or severe trauma. For instance, nosocomial pneumonia occurs in 7–30% of these patients (1); it is associated with mortality rates of 28–37% in recent series and lead to prolonged hospitalization duration for patients who survive (2). Another striking example of this problem is sepsis due to gram-negative bacteremia, whose mortality varies from 20% to 40% (3), reaching 50–75% in the case of development of septic shock (4,5). Several causes concur to the prevalence and the severity of infection in surgical and trauma patients: environmental factors, leading to selection of virulent and resistant micro-organisms; more aggressive surgical procedures in patients with more advanced underlying conditions; use of numerous devices, such as intravascular catheters, required for postoperative management; and alterations of immune defenses. The hope to diminish these alterations by administrating intravenous immunoglobulins (IVIG) has motivated several trials, in an attempt to prevent or to treat postoperative and posttrauma infection. In this chapter, we will first briefly review the rationale for use of IVIG, and then discuss the results of available trials.

RATIONALE FOR USE OF IVIG

Several authors have reported on immune dysfunctions in surgical and trauma patients. Obviously, one major impairment of host defenses is surgical or traumatic alteration of anatomical barriers. In addition, acquired deficiencies have been described in both cellular and humoral immunity. Diminished levels of IgG, IgA, and IgM have been reported after trauma and after major elective surgical procedures (6,7). In burned patients, the marked fall of the serum level of IgG is attributed to increased loss and catabolism of proteins, in addition to abnormal Ig synthesis, as suggested by impaired polyclonal response to mitogenic factors (7–10). The postulated significance of low Ig levels in critically ill patients is supported by the observation that favorable outcome in patients who develop a septic complication is correlated with the level of antibodies directed against the causative organism (11). Other authors have reported abnormally high levels of Ig in some settings, such as children with head trauma (12) or patients with esophageal cancer (13), but have suggested that it could be correlated to a less efficient specific response against a given pathogen.

Dysfunction of polymorphonuclear neutrophils (PMN) are also described after surgery, trauma, or thermal injury and include impairment of chemotaxis (14), of adhesion (15), of phagocytosis (16), and of intracellular killing (17). Besides primary defects of PMN function, one can postulate that opsonization is also less efficient due to reduced levels of Ig and to consummation of complement factors that have been shown to occur in burned patients (18). Based on these findings, passive immunotherapy with IVIG may be motivated by an attempt to restore normal levels of antibodies directed against common organisms and to enhance PMN function.

Several concerns regarding efficacy and safety of IVIG must be kept in mind, however. First, much evidence suggests that surgery and trauma induce a state of immunodeficiency that is not restricted to acquired hypo- or dysgammaglobulinemia and impaired PMN function. For instance, it is also postulated that function of monocytes and T lymphocytes might be altered (6,7,10,19–23). Accordingly, IVIG administration could only partly restore such functions if at all. Second, many of the above-mentioned observations have been made in studies including small numbers of patients and need to be confirmed, in particular using immunological monitoring methodologies as developed recently. Third, one has to consider the possibility of harmful effects when manipulating the immune system with IVIG. For instance, IVIG could block phagocytic cells by nonspecific binding to Fc receptors. Such a mechanism could be useful in immune diseases but harmful for the defense against pathogens. Fourth, the hypothetical benefit of IVIG administration would probably depend on the amount of antibodies directed against a given organism in a given preparation, and might then be inconsistent, depending on lot-to-lot variability. It can then be concluded that the results of clinical studies need to be analyzed carefully, and that marginal efficacy could be difficult to reproduce.

CLINICAL TRIALS WITH IVIG

Passive immunotherapy has been tested in surgical and trauma patients using three approaches: administration of nonspecific immunoglobulins; administration of hyperimmune preparations, i.e., preparations containing high levels of immunoglobulins directed against organisms selected for their frequency or high virulence, or against their toxins; and, more recently, the use of monoclonal antibodies, also directed against epitopes of selected pathogens. The endotoxin of gram-negative bacteria is the target that has been most often chosen for hyperimmune preparations or monoclonal antibodies. In this chapter, we will review only studies using nonspecific IVIG for prevention (prophylactic use) or treatment (therapeutic use) of infections in surgical and trauma patients.

Studies with Prophylactic Use of IVIG

IVIG has been given prophylactically in high-risk patients in seven main studies (Table 1). In the study of Duswald and colleagues (24), 2.5 g IVIG had no protective effect when compared to placebo in 150 patients after thoracic or abdominal surgery. In a double-blind study, Glinz et al. randomized 150 patients with mechanical ventilation for more than 24 h duration to receive IVIG (12 g on days 0, 5, and 12 after admission to the ICU) or albumin (25). They observed a significant decrease in the incidence of pneumonia (28/76 vs. 43/74), but this was not accompanied by a difference in mortality, in mortality due to infection, or in infections other than pneumonia. Similar results have been reported in a larger, blinded, randomized study completed by the Intravenous Immunoglobulin Collaborative Study Group in 352 patients at high risk of infection after predefined surgical procedures (26). In this three-arms-blinded, controlled trial, authors compared albumin to a standard IVIG preparation (400 mg/kg) and to a hyperimmune preparation containing higher titers of immunoglobulins directed against the core portion of the endotoxin of gram-negative bacteria. The number of patients in whom infection developed was significantly lower in the group receiving standard IVIG than in the group receiving placebo (36/109 patients vs. 53/112 respectively, $P = .03$), as was the incidence of pneumonia (15 vs. 30, respectively, $P = .04$). IVIG also accounted for a significant reduction of the number of days spent in ICU and of the total days spent in the hospital. Hospital mortality did not differ between groups, however. In contrast to standard IVIG, the hyperimmune preparation had no detectable prophylactic effect on infection, a difference that could not be explained but that might be related to a smaller repertoire of specific antibodies in the hyperimmune IVIG, since 300 donors had been selected for its preparation compared to 10,000–30,000 for the preparation of standard IVIG.

Cafiero and co-workers reported an efficacy of IVIG plus antibiotics in preventing overall infections, as compared with antibiotics alone in 80 high-risk patients undergoing surgery for colorectal cancer (27). This study is hampered by methodological problems, however; high-risk patients have been selected according to a scoring system that has not been sufficiently validated, using delayed hypersensitivity skin test and electrophoretic profile of serum proteins. In addition, definitions of infections were questionable in that study. The results of this study may hardly be taken into account.

IVIG administration for prevention of infection has also been tested in burned patients. None of the three published studies have reported beneficial effect, however (28–30). Although these studies included only a small number of patients, there is no evidence to support the administration of IVIG in burned patients or to perform further studies.

Studies with Therapeutic Use of IVIG

Data are scarce regarding the use of IVIG to treat established infections in surgical and trauma patients (Table 2). In an unblinded, randomized clinical trial with 104 surgical ICU patients, Just and colleagues administered an IgG- and IgM-containing IVIG preparation in conjunction with antibiotics as soon as an infection was suspected (31). Control patients received antibiotics alone. The overall mortality in the two groups did not differ, nor did the mortality attributed to infection. IVIGs were reported to be effec-

Table 1 Studies with Prophylactic Use of IVIG

Author (Ref.)	Year of publication	Setting	Number of patients	Blinded	Result
Duswald (24)	1980	Thoracic or abdominal surgery	150	No	No benefit
Glinz (25)	1985	Trauma patients with mechanical ventilation	150	Yes	Reduction in acquired pneumonia
IICSG[a] (26)	1992	Surgical ICU	352	Yes	Reduction in acquired pneumonia, hospitalization duration
Cafiero (27)	1992	Patients with colorectal cancer	80	No	Reduction in postoperative infection (doubtful)
McManus (28)	1988	Burned patients	24	Yes	No benefit
Munster (29)	1987	Burned patients	20	Yes	No benefit
Waymack (29)	1989	Burned patients	50	Yes	No benefit

[a]IICSG: Intravenous Imunoglobulin Collaborative Study Group.

Table 2 Studies with Therapeutic Use of IVIG

Author (Ref.)	Year of publication	Setting	Number of patients	Blinded	Result
Just (31)	1986	Infected surgical patients	104	No	No benefit
Jesdinsky (32)	1987	Patients with fibrinopurulent peritonitis	288	No	No benefit
Dominioni (33)	1991	Patients with sepsis score $\geq$ 20	62	Yes	Reduction in mortality

tive in patients classified as "high-risk"; this result should be considered cautiously, however, since it was obtained in only one of several subgroups that were defined in a post hoc analysis. Jesdinsky et al. performed a multicenter, unblinded, randomized controlled trial among 288 patients with fibrinopurulent peritonitis (32). One hundred forty-five patients received 10 g IVIG over 5 days, and 143 were not treated with IVIG. The study failed to demonstrate any efficacy of IVIG.

In a double-blind, multicenter study by Dominioni et al., 62 surgical patients with septic score of 20 or greater (according to a scoring system that has not been widely validated) were randomized to receive either IVIG (0.4 g/kg on days 1 and 5) or albumin (33). Overall mortality was significantly lower in the IVIG-treated group (38%) than in the control group (67%), as was the mortality attributed to septic shock (7% vs. 33%, respectively). In addition, higher IgG levels were correlated with survival in the IVIG-treated patients. However, the small sample size, the lack of precise definition of infection, and the absence of data regarding the adequacy of antibiotic treatment in that study once again preclude any definitive conclusion on the administration of IVIG to treat infection in surgical patients.

CONCLUSION

Up to now, data are not sufficient to support the routine administration of IVIG in surgical and trauma patients. Available trials clearly do not justify their widespread use to treat established infections. In prophylactic use, as reported, IVIG diminished the incidence of nosocomial pneumonia in two studies and did not in one study, while its efficacy was doubtful in a fourth study. However, none of these studies suggesting efficacy demonstrated reduction of mortality, and only one study has reported an impact on hospitalization duration. Thus, given the elevated cost of IVIG, its real indication remains controversial. Advances in understanding the impact of surgery and trauma on immunity will perhaps help to define in what subgroups of patients IVIG could be of more clear-cut benefit.

REFERENCES

1. Pennington JE. Nosocomial respiratory infections. In: Mandell GL, Douglas RG, Bennett JE, eds. Principles and Practice of Infectious Diseases. New York: Churchill Livingstone, 1995: 2599–2607.
2. Dal Nogare AR. Nosocomial pneumonia in the medical and surgical patient. Med Clin North Am 1994; 78(5):1081.
3. Bryan CS, Reynolds KL, Brenner ER. Analysis of 1186 episodes of gram-negative bacteremia in non-university hospitals: the effects of antimicrobial therapy. Rev Infect Dis 1983; 5:629–638.
4. Ziegler EJ, McCutchan JA, Fierer J, et al. Treatment of gram-negative bacteremia and shock with human antiserum to a mutant Escherichia coli. N Engl J Med 1982; 307:1225–1230.
5. Calandra T, Glauser MP, Schellekens J, Verhoef J, Swiss-Dutch J5 Immunoglobulin Study Group. Treatment of gram-negative septic shock with human IgG antibody to Escherichia coli J5: a prospective, double-blind, randomized study. J Infect Dis 1988; 158:312–319.
6. Grob P, Holch M, Fierz W, et al. Immunodeficiency after major trauma and selective surgery. Pediatr Infect Dis 1988; 7(5):S37–S42.

7. McRitchie DI, Girotti MJ, Rotstein OD, Teodorczyk-Injeyan JA. Impaired antibody production in blunt trauma. Arch Surg 1990; 125:91–96.

8. Munster AM, Hoagland HC, Pruitt BA. The effect of thermal injury on serum immunoglobulins. Ann Surg 1970; 172:965–969.

9. Moran K, Munster AM. Alterations of the host defense mechanism in burned patients. Surg Clin North Am 1987; 67:47–56.

10. Ninneman JL, Condie T. Lymphocyte response following thermal injury: the effect of circulating immunosuppressive substances. JBCR 1981; 2:196–199.

11. McGowan JE Jr, Barnes WM, Finland MB. Bacteremia at Boston City Hospital: occurrence and mortality during 12 selected years (1935–1972) with special reference to hospital-acquired cases. J Infect Dis 1975; 132:326–341.

12. Wilson NW, Wu YP, Petersen B, Bastian JF. Immunoglobulins and IgG subclasses in children following severe head injury. Intens Care Med 1994; 20:508–510.

13. Saito T, Kuwahara A, Shimoda K, et al. Enhanced immunoglobulin levels correlate with infectious complications after surgery in esophageal cancer. J Surg Oncol 1991; 46:3–8.

14. Warden GD, Mason AD, Pruitt BA. Evaluation of leukocyte chemotaxis in vitro in thermally injured patients. J Clin Invest 1974; 54:1001–1004.

15. Christou NV, Tellado JM. In vitro polymorphonuclear neutrophil function in surgical patients does not correlate with anergy but with "activating" processes such as sepsis or trauma. Surgery 1989; 106:718–724.

16. Inoue T, Obata M, Mishima Y. Polymorphonuclear leukocyte function and serum opsonic activity in surgical patients. Surg Today 1992; 22:233–243.

17. Grogan JB, Miller RR. Impaired function of polymorphonuclear leukocytes in patients with burns and other trauma. Surg Gynecol Obstet 1973; 137:784.

18. Bjornson AB, Altemeier WA, Bjornson S, et al. Host defense against opportunist microorganisms following trauma. I. Studies to determine the association between changes in humoral components of host defense and septicemia in burned patients. Ann Surg 1978; 188(1):93.

19. Ferrera JJ, Peterson RD, Hester R, et al. Inhibition of lymphocyte blastogenesis caused by suppression of interleukin-2 receptor sites after thermal injury. J Burn Care Rehabil 1989; 10:119–124.

20. Howard RJ, Simmons RL. Acquired immunologic deficiencies after trauma and surgical procedures. Surg Gynecol Obstet 1974; 139:771–782.

21. Faist E, Mewes A, Strasser T, et al. Alteration of monocyte function following major injury. Arch Surg 1988; 123:287–292.

22. Markewitz A, Faist E, Weinhold C, et al. Alterations of cell-mediated immune response following cardiac surgery. Eur J Cardio-Thor Surg 1993; 7:193–199.

23. Wakefield CH, Carey PD, Foulds S, et al. Changes in major histocompatibility complex class II expression in monocytes and T cells of patients developing infection after surgery. Br J Surg 1993; 80:205–209.

24. Duswald KH, Müller K, Seifert J, Ring J. Wirksamkeit von i.v. Gammaglobulin gegen backterielle Infektionen chirurgischer Patienten. Muench Med Wschr 1980; 122:832–836.

25. Glinz W, Grob JP, Nydegger UE, et al. Polyvalent immunoglobulins for prophylaxis of bacterial infections in patients with multiple trauma. Intens Care Med 1985; 11:288–294.

26. Intravenous Immunoglobulin Collaborative Study Group. Prophylactic intravenous administration of standard immune globulin as compared with core-lipopolysaccharide immune globulin in patients at high risk of postsurgical infection. N Engl J Med 1992; 327:234–240.

27. Cafiero F, Gipponi M, Bonalumi U, et al. Prophylaxis of infection with intravenous immunoglobulins plus antibiotic for patients at high risk for sepsis undergoing surgery for colorectal cancer: results of a randomized, multicenter clinical trial. Surgery 1992; 112:24–31.

28. McManus AT, Missavage AE, McManus WF, et al. Intravenous immune globulin does not prevent infections nor alter mortality in seriously burned patients. In: Immunocompromised

Host Society. Fifth International Symposium on Infections in the Immunocompromised Host. Noordwijkerhout, Netherlands, 1988:161.

29. Munster AM, Moran KT, Thupari J, et al. Prophylactic intravenous immunoglobulin replacement in high-risk burn patients. J Burn Care Rehabil 1987; 8:376–380.
30. Waymack JP, Jenkins ME, Alexander JW, et al. A prospective trial of prophylactic intravenous immune globulin for the prevention of infection in severly burned patients. Burns 1989; 15(2):71–76.
31. Just HM, Metzger M, Vogel W, Pelka R. Einfluss einer adjuvanten immunoglobulintherapie auf Infectionen bei Patienten einer operativen Intensiv-Therapie-Station. Klin Wochenschr 1986; 64:245–256.
32. Jesdinsky HJ, Tenpel G, Castrup HJ, Seifert J. Cooperative group of additional immunoglobulin therapy in severe bacterial infections: results of a multicenter randomized controlled trial in cases of diffuse fibrinopurulent peritonitis. Klin Wochenschr 1987; 65:1132–1138.
33. Dominioni L, Dionigi R, Zanello M, et al. Effects of high-dose IgG on survival of surgical patients with sepsis score of 20 or greater. Arch Surg 1991; 126:236–240.

12

Intravenous Gammaglobulin Regimen for HIV-Infected Children: Infection Prophylaxis and Immunomodulation

Arye Rubinstein
Albert Einstein College of Medicine, Bronx, New York

HISTORICAL OVERVIEW OF IV GAMMAGLOBULIN TREATMENT FOR PEDIATRIC HIV INFECTION

Polyvalent intravenous gammaglobulin (IVIG) preparations have been used for many years to prevent bacterial and viral infections in hypo- or agammaglobulinemic patients. In 1978 we encountered an infant who became the first confirmed case of HIV infection. The infant and a subsequently identified cluster of HIV-infected children presented with a curious constellation of recurrent bacterial infections, sepsis, and abnormal specific antibody responses in the face of hypergammaglobulinemia (1–3). This pattern of humoral immune defect was reminiscent of the Nezeloff syndrome (3). Therefore, in 1979, before AIDS was discovered, we treated these patients with 200 mg/kg body weight monthly IVIG regimen as recommended for congenital B-cell defects. Subsequently, a variety of IVIG regimens have been utilized in controlled and uncontrolled studies.

By 1983 the syndrome of HIV infection and its associated immune aberrations had become well recognized in children. It became evident that in HIV-infected children the humoral immunodeficiency was often accompanied by autoimmune phenomena and T-cell aberrations. We therefore modified our IVIG treatment plan to address these additional immune pathologies. The new regimen consisted of a higher dose of IVIG (300 mg/kg) administered in shorter intervals of 2 weeks. This regimen has been used by us to the present (4–14).

Following our reports on the use of IVIG, several additional small uncontrolled trials utilizing lower doses of IVIG have confirmed the reduction of infectious complications by its periodic use (15–17). In 1988 the National Institutes of Child Health and Human Development (NICHD) embarked on a multicenter, placebo-controlled randomized trial of monthly 400 mg/kg IVIG (18–22). Following closure of the blinded trial, open-label IVIG was offered to all children (21). The NICHD studies by and large confirmed our results. The higher dose with the shorter interval between treatments, as utilized by us, appeared, however, to provide added benefit, albeit at a higher cost.

The purpose of this review is to analyze the clinical and immunological data from the various IVIG trials and to offer recommendations for improved treatment regimens.

RATIONALE FOR USE OF IVIG IN HIV-INFECTED CHILDREN

Both adults and children with HIV infection display immunological dysfunction. The hallmark of HIV infection in adults is T-cell depletion and impaired cell-mediated immunity. In general, adults have formed anamnestic antibody responses to a wide array of pathogens prior to their HIV infection, and retain a reasonable complement of B cells. In contrast, the majority of peri-/prenatally HIV-infected children typically exhibit signs of B-cell dysfunction prior to the development of overt T-cell dysfunction (1–3,7–11,23–29). The deficits in humoral immunity during the neonatal period may further be exacerbated by the transplacental transfer of dysfunctional antibody from the HIV-infected mother. In adults the risk of bacterial infections and abnormal B-cell function (30–32) increases with depletion of CD4 cells and is highest among those with CD4 counts < $200/mm^3$ (30); so pregnant women at this stage of disease will also confer poor passive antibody immunity to their fetuses.

Most HIV-infected children exhibit hypergammaglobulinemia with an increased number of B cells (1,2,8,23,24). Only a small percentage are hypogammaglobulinemic; these patients have the worst prognosis. Abnormal antibody responses are noted in both patient groups: primary and secondary antibody responses to neoantigens such as tetanus toxoid (5) or bacteriophage OX174 are diminished with a poor IgM-to-IgG antibody switch (2). Immunization with a pneumococcal vaccine with antigens capable of eliciting B- and T-cell responses has resulted in poor antibody responses to both (2), suggesting that the B-cell abnormalities in these infants are the result of intrinsic B cell defects as well as of abnormalities in the T-cell compartment. Although not all HIV-1-infected infants have a prominent B-cell defect early in life (33), most lose their antibody responses with time. Therefore, children who have received live measles vaccine may later on in life succumb to measles infection (26).

This lack of protection from infection correlates with the absence of anamnestic antibody responses, and with low-affinity/avidity antibodies in antigen excess (2,9,10). Most prominent are the decreased in vitro proliferative lymphocyte responses to pokeweed mitogen (PWM), staphylococcal Cowan A, and to antigens (12–14,27–29). PMW-driven gammaglobulin antibody secretion in vitro is diminished even in the presence of normal T cells (7), suggesting an intrinsic B-cell defect. This B-cell unresponsiveness may be due to the predominance of terminally differentiated B cells, leaving only a minority of virgin B cells that can still respond to mitogens and antigens. The inordinate B-cell activation was ascribed to chronic infections, to various HIV-1 proteins (31–34) and/or to loss of negative feedback for B cells. We have documented a diminished downregulation of in vitro immunoglobulin secretion by suppressor T cells (7) in HIV-infected children. Deregulation of humoral immunity is often accompanied by formation of autoantibodies to platelets, neutrophils, and anticoagulants (35). Thus, clinically, the humoral immunodeficiency presents with severe and recurrent bacterial infections. Additionally, autoimmune thrombocytopenia, neutropenia, and anemia are common. Both the in vivo and in vitro evidence for B-cell dysfunction provide the rationale for early institution of IVIG therapy in HIV-infected infants and children.

RESULTS OF CLINICAL TRIALS OF IVIG

Clinical Observations: Effect on Infectious Complication

Although the criteria for institution of treatment and the regimen for IVIG administration have varied, most investigators have observed a reduction in febrile episodes and infection rates (4–17,36). In our first cohort of 12 children on IVIG with a prior septic episode, no additional serious bacterial infections occurred between 1980 and 1983. In an expansion of this study from 1983 to date, a regimen of biweekly 300 mg/kg was utilized in over 100 children (4–14), resulting in significant reduction in minor and serious bacterial infection and hospital admissions over a period of 4–10 years (14). In fact, almost all long-term survivors (> 10 years) from our original patient cohort identified between 1979 and 1985 belong to the IVIG-treated group. A significant decrease in bacterial and viral infections would not be expected to occur in HIV-infected children solely due to passage of time. The beneficial effect on infectious complications must therefore be attributed to the IVIG protocol. The randomized NICHD double-blind, placebo-controlled multicenter trial which compared IVIG at 400 mg/kg every 28 days to IV albumin in 372 HIV-infected children confirmed most of our findings. However, IVIG in this study significantly prolonged the time free from serious laboratory-proven bacterial or clinically diagnosed serious infections only in children with entry CD4 lymphocyte counts > 200/ml (18). Using our regimen, no such distinction could be noted, probably due to the higher doses of IVIG employed (14). Further analysis of the NICHD study revealed that this decrease in the rate of serious bacterial infections, minor bacterial infections, viral infections, and acute care hospitalization was maintained for 3 years (19,21). This decrement in infections was observed regardless of trimethoprim-sulfamethoxazole prophylaxis.

Following closure of the NICHD trial, open-label IVIG was offered to all children on study. This enabled the evaluation of the effect of IVIG treatment in patients who had received albumin placebo during the original study. In this study (21), neither IVIG nor three-times-weekly trimethoprim-sulfamethoxazole separately or in combination decreased the risk for sinusitis (21,22). Again, such correlation was noted, presumably because of the lower IVIG dose; penetration of immunoglobulin into loculated spaces may require higher and more frequent dosing of IVIG.

Immunomodulatory Effects of IVIG

Effect on Serum HIV Antigens

We have observed a decrease in serum p17, p24, gp41, and gp120 levels in 14 treated patients (unpublished data; 37). Hague et al. (36) noted in four children with high serum p24 levels that serum p24 became undetectable during IVIG treatment; in only one did it again become detectable during follow-up. Since these IVIG preparations did not contain intrinsic anti-p24 antibody activity, IVIG must have indirectly decreased serum p24 levels by reducing viral replication probably via immunomodulation.

Effect on Circulating Immune Complexes (CIC)

Using both the Raji cell assay and the C1q assay for immune complex (CIC) quantitation, we could not detect a significant reduction of CIC in six patients receiving 300 mg IVIG/kg at 4-week intervals. In contrast, in 50 patients receiving 300 mg/kg IVIG biweekly, a significant ($P < .01$) cumulative decrease of CIC occurred (9,10,14). Similarly, Schaad et al. (17) noted a lower mean CIC level in IVIG-treated patients.

Serum LDH Levels

A characteristic LDH isoenzyme pattern can identify the source of the enzyme. Isomorphic elevations (LDH isoenzyme 1 over 2 < unity) are characteristic for B-cell hyperproliferation and B-cell neoplasia (38) in HIV-infected children and adults. Serum LDH levels were shown by us also to reflect B-cell lymphoproliferation and disease activity (5). We have noted a significant decrease in elevated LDH levels in 64% of IVIG-treated patients (5,6), presumably resulting from control of excessive B-cell proliferation.

Effect on In Vitro Lymphocyte Mitogenic Responses

In contrast, the effect on in vitro lymphocyte proliferative responses to phytohemagglutinin (PHA) and to PWM detected by us was minimal. PHA responses increased in 10 of 14 treated patients as compared to 3 of 27 control patients during the same study period (4,6). This improvement was transient, however, and must be confirmed in larger scale studies.

Effect on CD4 Cell Counts

In 1984 we first reported an increase in CD4 cell count in 14 patients after treatment with IVIG. In an expanded study, a 10% increase in cell counts occurred in 43% of al patients in the first year of IVIG treatment (14). This benefit was, however, minimal by the end of the fourth year of treatment. In the NICHD study, the rates of CD4+ cell count decline were measured using age-adjusted regression analysis, confirming a cumulative significant slowing of the decline by 13.5 cells/ml/month (20). In contrast to our observations (14), this beneficial effect of IVIG on slowing CD4+ cell decline did not translate into reduced mortality (20).

Effect on Suppressor T Cells

Although HIV-infected children also have markedly elevated CD8+ cell counts, these cells may not be functionally intact as suggested by decreased in vitro CD8 T-cell suppression of PWM-driven immunoglobulin secretion (7), uncontrolled polyclonal hypergammaglobulinemia, and the abundance of autoimmune phenomena. Reduced PWM-driven IgG secretion in vitro normalized in five of six children studied following 1 year of high-dose IVIG treatment, with restoration of in vitro concanavalin-A-stimulated generation of suppressor T cells (7).

MECHANISMS OF ACTION OF IVIG IN PEDIATRIC HIV INFECTION

The multifactorial mechanisms of action of IVIG will be discussed only as they pertain to its observed immunomodulatory effects in HIV-infected children.

Direct Effects

IVIG contains a pool of specific antibodies that react with a wide spectrum of bacteria and viruses. This quality of IVIG is important for its use in congenital and acquired agammaglobulinemic patients and may be responsible for the reduced infections in pediatric HIV-infected patients treated with IVIG. We noted in one patient who experienced recurrent pneumococcal sepsis on IVIG that the lot of IVIG used contained a low titer of antibodies to this infectious agent (unpublished data). Preference should therefore be given to IVIG with high-titer antibodies to streptococcal pneumonia and *Hemophilus influenzae* B bacteria.

Indirect Effects

A reduced rate of infections may reduce lymphocyte activation and thereby decrease viral replication. Similarly, the removal of CIC by IVIG may decrease cellular activation as well as immunosuppression by CIC in antigen excess, both of which are present in HIV-infected children. These indirect effects may be responsible for the observed preservation of CD4 cell counts, the decrease in serum LDH levels, the decrease in HIV serum antigens, and improvement in suppressor T-cell function. In one study, the CD4 sparing effect of IVIG treatment persisted even in patients experiencing serious infections (20). We have also reported reductions in serum β2 microglobulin (39), neopterin (40), and tumor necrosis factor levels (41)—all markers of lymphocyte activation and HIV disease activity. These findings suggest that IVIG may act by inhibition of the effector functions of activated T cells, ultimately reducing the release of injurious cytokines.

Other mechanisms of action of IVIG have been postulated, including serving as a source of anti-idiotypic antibodies and of soluble CD4+, CD8+, HLA class I and class II molecules, etc. None of these have yet been evaluated in IVIG-treated AIDS patients.

DOSING OF IVIG: HIGH VERSUS LOW DOSE

Several studies in a variety of immunodeficient states have suggested an advantage of high-dose and shorter interval treatment regimens. For example, patients with congenital agammaglobulinemia (XLA) who received high-dose IVIG (400–600 mg/kg every 3 weeks) showed a significant increase in trough serum IgG levels and decrease in the incidence of pneumonias as compared to patients treated by lower dose IVIG (42). Improvement of pulmonary functions in XLA patients with chronic lung disease was noted preferentially in those receiving high doses of IVIG replacement (43,44). Supraphysiological levels of immunoglobulin neutralize complement neoantigens (45) and inhibit formation of the membranolytic attack complex from activated C3b and C4b fragments (46), and high-dose IVIG has been shown to suppress in vitro cytokine-dependent human T-cell proliferation (47).

The interval of IVIG dosing may also have important consequences. In HIV-infected children, IVIG administered at 4-week intervals resulted only in a transient decline of CIC, while 2-week intervals induced a sustained marked reduction in CIC (14). Clinically, in HIV-infected children the 400 mg monthly dose did not reduce the rate of sinusitis (22) as compared to the 300 mg biweekly dose.

In summary, higher doses of IVIG regimens appear to have clinical and immunological advantages (14). Therefore, new regimens utilizing higher doses and shorter intervals merit further evaluation despite increased cost and issues of compliance.

CRITERIA FOR INSTITUTION OF IVIG TREATMENT

Entry criteria must be adjusted according to the IVIG regimen used. The NICHD study suggested that beneficial effects were observed mainly in children with entry CD4+ counts of >200 cells/ml (19), indicating this regimen be reserved only for children with such CD4+ cell counts. Results from ACTG 051 study designed to evaluate IVIG infection prophylaxis in a more severely ill population of children with AIDS showed no added benefit by IVIG at 400 mg/kg monthly doses (48). Nonetheless beneficial responses were noted by us in more advanced pediatric AIDS cases (14). IVIG should thus be considered also for this group of patients.

We recommend the following entry criteria for HIV+ children receiving IVIG biweekly at 300 mg/kg:

1. A history of one or more serious bacterial infections such as meningitis, sepsis, or pneumonia with positive bacterial culture or with prompt response to antibiotic treatment.
2. Three or more recurrent "minor" bacterial infections such as otitis, pharyngitis, bronchitis, urinary tract infection, or recurrent febrile episodes without specific organ manifestations (FUO).
3. No history of prior bacterial infection, but abnormal in vitro lymphocyte mitogenic responses to PWM and to staphylococcal Cowan A and poor antibody responses to current vaccinations or to phage OX174 immunization.

FUTURE DIRECTIONS

Newer IVIG treatment regimens should be designed and evaluated for HIV+ patients in early stages as well as for those with advanced disease. Doses up to 500 mg/kg biweekly may be of greater benefit. The IVIG treatment will certainly be complemented in the near future by spiking IVIG preparations with specific monoclonal antibodies to HIV antigens. Such specific immunotherapies can be optimized only if developed against the background of a generic IVIG treatment with maximal benefits for this patient population.

REFERENCES

1. Rubinstein A, Sicklick M, Gupta A, Bernstein L. Acquired immunodeficiency with reversed T4/T8 ratios in infants born to promiscuous and drug addicted women. JAMA 1983; 249:2352–2356.
2. Bernstein L, Ochs H, Wedgwood RJ, Rubinstein A. Defective humoral immunity in pediatric AIDS. J Pediatr 1985; 107:353–357.
3. Rubinstein A. AIDS in infants. Am J Dis Child 1983; 137:825–827. Editorial.
4. Rubinstein A, Sicklick M, Bernstein L, Silverman B. Treatment of AIDS with intravenous gammaglobulin. Pediatr Res 1984; 18:264A.
5. Silverman B, Rubinstein A. Serum LDH levels in adults and children with AIDS and ARC. Possible indicator of B cell lymphoproliferation and disease activity. Effect of intravenous gammaglobulin on enzyme levels. Am J Med 1985; 78:728–735.

6. Calvelli TA, Rubinstein A. Intravenous gammaglobulin in infant AIDS. Pediatr Infect Dis 1986; 5:S207–S210.

7. Gupta A, Novick B, Rubinstein A. Restoration of suppressor T cell functions in children with AIDS following intravenous gammaglobulin treatment. Am J Dis Child 1986; 140:146.

8. Rubinstein A. Pediatric AIDS. Curr Probl Pediatr 1986; 16:361–409.

9. Ellaurie M, Calvelli TA, Rubinstein A. Human immunodeficiency virus (HIV) circulating immune complexes in infected children. AIDS Res Human Restroviruses 1990; 6:1437–1441.

10. Ellaurie M, Calvelli TA, Rubinstein A. Immune complexes in pediatric human immunodeficiency virus infection. Am J Dis Child 1990; 144:1207–1209.

11. Ellaurie M, Burns ER, Bernstein L, Shah K, Rubinstein A. Thrombocytopenia and HIV in children. Pediatrics 1988; 82:905–908.

12. Calvelli TA, Rubinstein A. Intravenous gammaglobulin in pediatric HIV infection. Treatment rationale and effects. Immunol Today 1992; Part 1; 4(3):1–5.

13. Calvelli TA, Rubinstein A. Intravenous gammaglobulin in pediatric HIV infection. Treatment rationale and effect. Immunol Today 1992; Part 2; 4(4):1–8.

14. Rubinstein A, Calvelli T, Rubinstein R. Intravenous gammaglobulin for pediatric HIV-1 infection. Effects on infectious complications, circulating immune complexes and CD4 cell decline. Ann NY Acad Sci 1993; 693:151–157.

15. Siegal FP, Oleske JA. In: Morell A, Nydegger UE, eds. Clinical Use of Intravenous Immunoglobulin. New York: Academic Press, 1986:373–384.

16. Pahwa S. Intravenous immune globulin in patients with AIDS. J Allergy Clin Immunol 1989; 84:625–631.

17. Schaad UB, Gianella-Borrador A, Perret B, Imbach P, Morell A. Intravenous immune globulin in symptomatic pediatric HIV infection. Eur J Pediatr 1988; 147:300–303.

18. NICHD IVIG Collaborative Group. Efficacy of intravenous immunoglobulin for the prophylaxis of serious bacterial infections in symptomatic HIV-infected children. N Engl J Med 1991; 325:73–80.

19. Moffenson LM, Moye J, Bethel J, et al. Prophylactic intravenous immunoglobulin in HIV-infected children with CD4+ counts of 0.20×10^9/L or more. Effect on viral, opportunistic and bacterial infections. JAMA 1992; 268:483–488.

20. Moffenson LM, Bethel J, Moye J, et al. Effect on intravenous immunoglobulin on CD4+ lymphocyte decline in HIV-infected children in a clinical trial of IVIG infection prophylaxis. J AIDS 1993; 6:1103–1113.

21. Moffenson LM, Moye J, Korelitz J, et al. Crossover of placebo patients to intravenous immunoglobulin confirms efficacy of prophylaxis of bacterial infections and reduction of hospitalizations in HIV-infected children. Pediatr Infect Dis J 1994; 13:477–484.

22. Moffenson LM, Korelitz J, Pelton S, et al. Sinusitis in children infected with human immunodeficiency virus: clinical characteristics, risk factors and prophylaxis. Clin Infect Dis 1995; 21:1175–1181.

23. Bernstein L, Krieger B, Novick B, Rubinstein A. Bacterial infection in the AIDS of children. Pediatr Infect Dis 1985; 4:472–475.

24. Calvelli TA, Rubinstein A. Pediatric HIV infection: a review. Immunodefic Rev 1990; 2:83–127.

25. Borkowsky W, Steele C, Grubman S, et al. Antibody responses to bacterial toxoids in children infected with HIV. J Pediatr 1986; 110:563–569.

26. Krasinski K, Borkowsky W. Measles and measles immunity in children infected with HIV. JAMA 1989; 261:2512–2516.

27. Borkowsky W, Rigaoud M, Krasinski K, Morre T, Laurence R, Pollack H. Cell-mediated and humoral immune responses in children infected with HIV during the first four years of life. J Pediatr 1992; 12:371–375.

28. Johnson J, Hebel R, Shinaberry R. Lymphoproliferative responses to mitogens and antigens in HIV infected children. AIDS Res Human Retroviruses 1991; 7:781–786.

29. Chirmule N, Lesser M, Gupta A, Ravipati M, Kohn N, Pahwa S. Immunological characteristics of HIV-infected children: relationship to age, CD4 counts, disease progression, and survival. AIDS Res Human Retroviruses 1995; 11(10):1209–1219.

30. Hirschtick RE, Glassroth J, Jordan MC, et al. Bacterial pneumonia in persons infected with HIV. N Engl J Med 1995; 333:845–851.

31. Schnittman SM, Lane HC, Higgins SE, et al. Direct polyclonal activation of human B-lymphocytes by the AIDS virus. Science 1986; 233:1084–1086.

32. Yarchoan R, Redfield RR, Broder S. Mechanism of B cell activation with AIDS and related disorders. J Clin Invest 1986; 78:439–447.

33. Blanche S, Le Deist F, Fischer A, et al. Longitudinal study of 18 children with perinatal LAV/HTLV-III infection: attempt at prognostic evaluation. J Pediatr 1986; 109:965–970.

34. Chirmule NB, Kalyanarama V, Oyaizu N, Pahwa S. Inhibitory influences of envelope glycoproteins of HIV-1 on antigen specific responses. J AIDS 1988; 1:425–430.

35. Burns ER, Krieger BZ, Bernstein L, Rubinstein A. Acquired circulating anticoagulants in children with AIDS. Pediatrics 1988; 82:763–765.

36. Hague RA, Yap PL, Mok JY, et al. Intravenous immunoglobulin in HIV infection: evidence for efficacy of treatment. Am J Dis Child 1989; 68:1146–1150.

37. Ellaurie M, Calvelli T, Rubinstein A. Reduction of HIV-1 antigens in the serum of HIV-infected children following treatment with IVIG. Blood 1987. Abstract.

38. Jacobs DS, Robinson RA, Clarke GM, Tucker JM. Clinical significance of the isomorphic pattern of the isoenzymes of serum lactate dehydrogenase. Ann Clin Lab Sci 1977; 7:411–421.

39. Ellaurie M, Rubinstein A. Beta-2 microglobulin concentrations in pediatric human immunodeficiency virus infection. J Pediatr Infect Dis 1990; 9:807–809.

40. Ellaurie M, Calvelli T, Rubinstein A. Neopterin levels in pediatric HIV infection as predictor of disease activity. J Pediatr Infect Dis 1992; 11:286–289.

41. Ellaurie M, Rubinstein A. Tumor necrosis factor in pediatric HIV-1 infection. AIDS 1992; 6:1265–1268.

42. Liese JG, Wintergerst U, Tympner KD, Belohradsky BH. High versus low-dose immunoglobulin therapy in the long-term treatment of X-linked agammaglobulinemia. Am J Dis Child 1992; 146:335–339.

43. Roifman CM, Levison H, Gelfand EW. High-dose versus low-dose intravenous immunoglobulin in hypogammaglobulinemia and chronic lung disease. Lancet 1987; 1:1075–1077.

44. Ochs HD, Fischer SH, Wedgwood RJ, et al. Comparison of high-dose and low-dose intravenous immunoglobulin in patients with primary immunodeficiency disease. Am J Med 1989; 76:78–82.

45. Bacchi VF, Maillet F, Berlan L, Kazatchkine MD. Neutralizing antibodies against C3NeF in intravenous immunoglobulin. Lancet 1992; 340:63–64.

46. Basta M, Kirshbom P, Frank MM, Fries LS. Mechanism of therapeutic effect of high-dose intravenous immunoglobulin: attenuation of acute, complement-dependent immune damage in a guinea pig model. J Clin Invest 1989; 84:1974–1981.

47. Amran D, Renz H, Lack G, Bradley K, Gelfand EW. Suppression of cytokine dependent human T-cell proliferation by intravenous immunoglobulin. Clin Immunol Immunopathol 1994; 73:180–186.

48. Spector SA, Gelber RD, McGrath N, et al. A controlled trial of intravenous immune globulin for the prevention of serious bacterial infections in children receiving zidovudine for advanced human immunodeficiency virus infection. N Engl J Med 1994; 331(18):1181–1187.

13

Use of Intravenous Immune Globulin in Adults with HIV Disease

David J. Rechtman

PharmaMedical Consultants International, Missoula, Montana

INTRODUCTION

Intravenous immunoglobulin (IVIG) was originally developed for the treatment of primary immune deficiencies that result in a state of hypogammaglobulinemia. The product was initially viewed as a simple replacement therapy. As time progressed, however, it became clear that through one mechanism or another, the product could be used to treat some immunologically mediated disease conditions, notably idiopathic thrombocytopenic purpura (ITP) (1).

As these initial explorations of the uses of IVIG were taking place, the AIDS epidemic was making itself felt in the United States and Western Europe. At first the epidemic seemed to involve mostly adults, and the nature of the opportunistic infections they were getting indicated that the immune deficit was a T-cell problem. In fact, many patients were found to be hyperglobulinemic, so the concept of IVIG therapy in adult AIDS patients was not widely considered.

As the epidemic spread and more females of childbearing potential were affected, there was an increase in the incidence of children born already infected with HIV. It was soon noted that B-cell function in these children was also deficient. The details of IVIG use in the pediatric population infected with HIV is discussed in detail in the next chapter. The impact of these observations on physicians caring for adults was that it sensitized them to the fact that B-cell function could be compromised in patients infected with HIV.

It was noted that a subset of patients with HIV were subject to a higher incidence of certain bacterial infections, and that recurrences of these infections were also common in some of these patients. This gave rise to the speculation that, despite the hyperglobulinemia that most patients exhibited, there was a functional deficit in antibody response in some patients with HIV (2,3). This speculation was later borne out by several investigations showing decreased in vitro responsiveness to challenge (4).

Once a B-cell component was seen in at least some patients, it became reasonable to investigate the use of IVIG in the treatment of these patients. At the same time, ITP was being associated with AIDS and IVIG had already been investigated as a treatment for ITP in other contexts. Despite this, the picture is much less clear in terms of the use of IVIG in adults than it is in children. This is partially due to a dearth of published trials in this patient cohort, partly to the methodological problems in most of the published trials, and partly due to the apparently conflicting results of what has been published. Another factor is the confusion inherent in the concept of "use of IVIG in adults with HIV disease." More precise definition of what is being treated is required.

Unlike the situation in pediatrics, there is no large, randomized, blinded study of the use of IVIG as therapy in adults with AIDS. Most of the studies reported to date are small and many are unblinded, with an observation arm rather than placebo as the control. What studies exist also tend to focus on the use of IVIG to treat differing aspects of the overall disease spectrum.

USE IN ITP

There have been a number of studies published on the use of IVIG in the treatment of idiopathic (immune) thrombocytopenic purpura (ITP). ITP was the earliest autoimmune phenomenon to be treated with IVIG and arose from the serendipitous observation that a patient with both primary immunodeficiency and ITP, who was treated for the former with IVIG, saw resolution of the latter condition as well (1). It was thus natural that IVIG would be tried in HIV-related cases of ITP.

Two regimens have been used in most published studies. The earliest regimen investigated was 0.4 g/kg given daily over 5 days. A later modification of this regimen delivered the total dose of 2 g/kg over a 2-day period in equal doses of 1 g/kg daily. There did not appear to be any significant difference in response rate between the regimens. Mean time to response may have been somewhat shorter in patients receiving the shorter regimen.

Almost without exception the published data indicate a beneficial effect seen with IVIG (Table 1). The benefit, however, was short-lived. As long as the patients continued to receive IVIG, they showed an increased platelet count. Upon withdrawal of IVIG therapy, however, this benefit was noted to wane. A review by Hoffman et al. (5) indicated an overall response rate of 88% for HIV-infected patients treated for thrombocytopenia with IVIG.

The consensus apparent in the published literature is that IVIG is indicated in the treatment of adults with HIV who need rapid short-term increase in platelets. Such would be the case in very low platelet counts with active or threatened bleeding or prior to invasive procedures such as dental extraction or splenectomy.

In similar fashion IVIG may have a role in other cytopenias related to HIV infection. Gottlieb and Deutsch (15) reported a case of red cell asplasia which was the initial manifestation of HIV disease and which responded to 1 g/kg IVIG daily for 2 days.

USE TO ALTER NATURAL HISTORY

There is far less consensus and far fewer available data on the question of the use of IVIG in adults to decrease the incidence of infection or to alter the course of the underlying disease. A number of small studies and uncontrolled series have been published.

Table 1 Summary of Published Outcomes When Using IVIG to Treat HIV-Associated ITP

Authors	No. pts. treated	Dose	Duration	Outcome
Ellis and Flegg (6)	1	0.4 mg/kg (sic)	5 days	Short-term resolution
Beard and Savage (7)	5	0.4 g/kg	5 days	Short-term resolution
Pollack et al. (8)	3	0.4 g/kg	5 days	Short-term resolution
		1 g/kg	2 days	
Landonio et al. (9)	17	0.4 g/kg	5 days	Short-term resolution, responded to retreatment. Sustained response in 4/17
Lim et al. (10)	5	0.4 g/kg	5 days	Short-term resolution 4/5
Rarick et al. (11)	5	1 g/day	2 days	Short-term resolution 4/5 Long-term resolution 1/5
Drenaggi et al. (12)	4	0.4 g/kg (4)	5 days	No response 2/4
		0.2 g/kg (1)	1 day	Short-term resolution 2/4 and 1/1
Rarick et al. (13)	14	1 g/kg	2 days + day 15	Short-term resolution
Jahnke et al. (14)	12	1 g/kg	2 days/week × 4 weeks	Short-term resolution

One of the earliest studies was reported by Silverman and Rubinstein (16) in 1985. They reported on 17 adults of whom six received IVIG therapy. Of these, four had a diagnosis of pneumocystis carinii pneumonia and had elevated LDH levels. The remaining two adults had Kaposi's sarcoma and normal LDH levels. Of the four with PCP, all had an initial decrease in LDH following initiation of IVIG therapy. Two had relapses of elevated LDH and subsequently died. The remaining four patients were stable.

The authors postulated that LDH elevation might be an indicator of increased B-cell metabolism and hence of disease activity in some patients with HIV. They noted the lower LDH levels following IVIG therapy and an apparent correlation with improved outcome. No overall survival comparisons with the nontreated patients are made, and it is difficult to determine the presence or magnitude of any beneficial effects exerted by IVIG on the adults.

A single case was reported by Parkin et al. (17) in 1987. These investigators had observed that of 87 patients with AIDS they had seen at their institution about one-quarter had serious bacterial or pyogenic infections, sometimes recurrent. By this time functional hypogammaglobulinemia in the face of actual hyperglobulinemia had been noted in patients with AIDS. The investigators therefore treated a patient with recurrent bacterial infections of the respiratory tract with 0.3 g/kg IVIG biweekly, and reported resolution of pulmonary symptoms. This report represents a single case, and little can be concluded from it on its own merits.

Building on these and other observations from the pediatric sphere, Yap and Williams (18) postulated in 1988 that there might be a role for IVIG therapy in patients with recurrent bacterial infections, who had thus demonstrated functional hypogammaglobulinemia. They therefore undertook a modified crossover study of six adults (19). The patients were selected based on a history of recurrent infection unresponsive to antibiotic therapy. IVIG was given at a dose of 0.2 g/kg every 3 weeks. End points were antibiotic use and hospital days over the 6-month trial period compared with the same data obtained retrospectively for the 6 months prior to initiation of IVIG therapy. Patients thus served as their own controls. In the setting of HIV disease the passage of time would be expected to worsen rather than improve the clinical situation, thus obviating one of the major objections to this type of study design. The authors reported a significant ($P < .05$) reduction in both antibiotic use and hospitalization while the patients were on IVIG. Of course, this was not a randomized controlled trial, the control data were gathered retrospectively, and the numbers are small. Nevertheless, the results are suggestive of a possible benefit.

In 1990 Brunckhorst et al. (20) reported on a randomized trial of 40 patients in either stages WR2B-4B (7 pts) or WR5-6 (13 pts). Patients were randomized either to IVIG 0.2 g/kg fortnightly or to observation. Patients were followed for opportunistic infection, hospitalization, and mortality. In the more advanced disease group three patients receiving IVIG died, while in the observation group 13 patients died. This difference was statistically significant ($P < .004$). Overall there were nine OIs in the treatment group and 14 in the observation group ($P = $ NS). There was also a trend toward decreased hospitalization. No differences were noted between groups among the patients with less advanced disease. The authors attributed the difference in mortality to less severe OIs. No data, however, were provided with regard to bacterial infection, and it is possible that IVIG therapy reduced the rate of primary or complicating secondary bacterial infections in the treatment group, thereby improving survival. The actual reason for the results remains purely speculative.

Akutsu et al. (21) reported on an attempt to influence the course of HIV disease per se with IVIG in an asymptomatic hemophiliac. They treated the patient with 0.2 g/kg every other week for 5 weeks. They reported an increase in CD4 counts (313–414/μl). Following treatment there was a decline, and a second course provided similar results. No further data were provided. Given an N of one and a patient who was asymptomatic, it is hard to make very much of these results, and to this author's knowledge no other larger studies have reproduced these results.

In 1990 Schrappe-Bacher et al. (22) reported on the results of a 12-month trial of IVIG. Thirty patients had been randomized to either IVIG 0.4 g/kg every other week or to an albumin placebo. This represents the first and apparently only double-blinded trial of IVIG in adults. Patients with ARC or WR-5 disease were eligible. Clinical status was measured by an index consisting of fever, diarrhea, night sweats, fatigue, oral candidiasis, and mucosal or cutaneous herpes simplex. Patients received treatment for 26 weeks and were followed up for an additional 26 weeks. There was no difference in progression to AIDS in the two groups (four placebo, three treatment). There was a significant difference ($P < .05$) in symptom score by the technique used by the authors. This difference consisted almost entirely of improvement in fatigue and fever in the treatment group. No other differences were noted. Again, although the authors noted the reports of others on increased bacterial infections in patients with AIDS, they did not follow or report on these in their trial. It is tempting to speculate if a reduction in such infections was responsible for the decrease in fever and fatigue reported in this study for the IVIG group.

In 1993 Kiehl et al. (23) reported on a randomized, unblinded trial in which 48 patients were randomized to receive IVIG while 46 were randomized to observation. This represents the largest randomized trial of IVIG in adults. Patients with CDC-IV disease were enrolled. Primary end points were infection and death; hospitalization and febrile days were also followed. Patients in the treatment arm received IVIG 0.4 g/kg initially and then 0.2 g/kg every 21 days. Treatment was continued for 17 weeks among patients with AIDS and for 16 weeks for patients with ARC. The authors report that there was a statistically significant reduction in the incidence of infection in the IVIG group (7 treatment, 20 control: $P < .001$). They do not specifically define whether they are referring to opportunistic or bacterial infections. Fever and diarrhea were both reduced in the IVIG group as compared to the controls ($P = .029$ and $P = .01$, respectively). Among patients with AIDS there was also a significant reduction in hospital days, most of which were secondary to infection (median 13 control, 4 IVIG: $P = .004$) There was a trend toward reduced mortality from infection in the IVIG group, but the difference was not statistically significant (8 control, 1 IVIG: $P = .09$). There was a trend toward reduced mortality from infection in the IVIG group, but the difference was not statistically significant (8 control, 1 IVIG, $P = .09$). There was no difference in overall mortality between the groups.

Rogna et al. (24) published a paper in 1988 on the combination of plasmapheresis and IVIG replacement in HIV-positive patients of various disease stages. Patients received from one to three courses of treatment. A course consisted of one pheresis a week for 5 weeks, each followed by infusion of 15 g IVIG. Each plasmapheresis course was followed by five weekly infusions of 15 g IVIG. The authors report marked improvement in clinical condition including weight gain, decreased night sweats, pruritis, and anorexia. Chronic staphylococcal pharyngitis and vaginitis resolved in one patient as did chronic *Candida* esophagitis and herpes genitalis in another.

A paper published by De Simone et al. (25) in 1991 represents the only random-ized trial of IVIG in the context of simultaneous treatment with AZT. Thirty patients were randomized to receive either 0.5 g/day AZT or 0.5 g/day AZT and 0.4 g/kg IVIG daily for 3 days followed by 0.6 g/kg every 4 weeks. The study patients were treated for 1 year. End points included type and severity of infections, lymphocyte marker changes, platelet counts, and incidence of OI. The authors reported that patients receiv-ing AZT alone were significantly more likely to experience an OI during the course of the trial than those receiving AZT and IVIG ($P < .01$) There also appeared to be fewer fevers of unknown origin in the combined treatment group, although precise figures and statistics were not provided. No changes in lymphocyte subsets were noted; how-ever, an increase in platelet count was seen in the combination treatment group com-pared to a no change or net decrease in the AZT-alone group.

There have been reports of trials of IVIG in mixed cohorts of children and adults, usually hemophiliacs, which have produced similar results (26,27) to those discussed above.

USE FOR SPECIFIC THERAPY OF INFECTION

There have also been some isolated reports of the use of IVIG in HIV-infected adults as treatment for specific opportunistic infections. Liesveld et al. (28) report a case of a patient diagnosed with anemia secondary to parvovirus B19. The patient was treated with IVIG 0.4 g/kg daily for 5 days. The patient recovered and upon subsequent re-lapse was retreated with good response and continued on maintenance IVIG monthly.

Stogner et al. (29) reported a case of measles pneumonia which responded to a combination of Ribavirin and IVIG.

In contrast Morgello and Simpson (30) reported that a case of CMV-associated demyelinated polyneuropathy did not respond to high-dose IVIG, despite its reported efficacy in other neuropathies. Similarly Jacobson et al. (31) reported the failure of a CMV hyperimmune IVIG to alter the course of CMV-associated retinitis.

CONCLUSIONS

Thus the role of IVIG in the treatment of adults with HIV disease remains unclear. In large part its suitability depends on what it is one wishes to treat. It seems clear from the literature that the treatment of the immune thrombocytopenia associated with HIV disease with IVIG is appropriate in the context of the need for a rapid response of rela-tively limited duration.

Examples are for dental or other invasive procedures or where there is serious risk of spontaneous hemorrhage. Other treatment modalities are more appropriate for long-term control.

While there are a variety of theoretical rationales for expecting IVIG to be use-ful in patients with HIV infection (32), there is little if any evidence that commercial IVIG has any role in attempts to modify the course of HIV disease itself. What studies exist, limited though they may be in terms of numbers, designs, or reporting, lend little support to the concept that IVIG affects the underlying disease per se. This is not nec-essarily the case for HIV hyperimmune IVIG derived from infected individuals. Such products are not currently commercially available and are beyond the scope of this chapter.

There does, however, seem to be evidence from the literature that IVIG may decrease the incidence of secondary bacterial infections in HIV-infected patients. It may also improve symptoms such as fever and fatigue even when the patient is receiving antiviral chemotherapy. Whether the cost justifies the benefit is questionable for the population at large. The approach of limiting use of IVIG to patients who have demonstrated an inability to deal with secondary bacterial infections is reasonable based on existing data. Only large, well-designed trials will provide an ultimate answer as to its utility even in this setting.

Finally, IVIG may be used in patients with HIV to treat infections for which it is useful in patients without HIV such as parvovirus B19. As the reports from Morgello and Simpson (30) and Jacobson et al. (31) show, however, CMV infection may be less responsive to IVIG in these patients than in those uninfected with HIV.

REFERENCES

1. Imbach P, A'Puzzo V, Hirt A, et al. High dose intravenous gamma globulin for idiopathic thrombocytopenic purpura in childhood. Lancet 1981; 1:1228–1231.
2. Sjamsoedin-Visser EJM, Heijen CJ, Zegers BJM, et al. Defect in B cell function in HTLV-III/LAV positive hemophilia patients. Blood 1987; 69:1388–1393.
3. Rubinstein A, Sicklick M, Gupta A, et al. Acquired immunodeficiency with reversed T4/T8 ratios in infants born to promiscuous and drug addicted mothers. JAMA 1983; 249:2350–2356.
4. Bernstein LJ, Ochs HD, Wedgwood RJ, et al. Defective humoral immunity in pediatric acquired immune deficiency syndrome. J Pediatr 1985; 107:352–357.
5. Hoffman DM, Caruso RF, Mirando T. Human immunodeficiency virus-associated thrombocytopenia. DICP 1989; 23:157–160.
6. Ellis M, Flegg P, Alderson D. Use of intravenous normal immunoglobulin in high doses as a possible safer alternative to oral steroids in managing HIV associated immune thrombocytopenic purpura [letter]. J Infect 1986; 13(3): 312–313.
7. Beard J, Savage GF. High-dose intravenous immunoglobulin and splenectomy for the treatment of HIV-related immune thrombocytopenia in patients with severe hemophilia. Br J Haematol 1988; 68:303–306.
8. Pollack AN, Janinis J, Green D. Successful intravenous immune globulin therapy for human immunodeficiency virus associated thrombocytopenia. Arch Intern Med 1988; 148:695–697.
9. Landonino G, Galli M, Nosari A, et al. HIV-related severe thrombocytopenia in intravenous drug users: prevalence, response to therapy in a medium term follow-up, and pathogenic evaluation. AIDS 1990; 4:29–34.
10. Lim SG, Lee CA, Kernoff PBA. The treatment of HIV associated thrombocytopenia in hemophiliacs. Clin Lab Haematol 1990; 12:237–245.
11. Rarick MU, Burian P, De Guzman N, et al. Intravenous immune globulin use in patients with human immunodeficiency virus–related thrombocytopenia who require dental extraction. West J Med 1991; 155:610–612.
12. Drenaggi D, Petrelli E, Cagnoni G, et al. Therapy with immunoglobulin of the HIV infection related idiopathic thrombocytopenia. Allergol Immunopathol 1991; 19:157–159.
13. Rarick MU, Montgomery T, Groshen S, et al. Intravenous immunoglobulin in the treatment of human immunodeficiency virus–related thrombocytopenia. Am J Hematol 1991; 38:261–266.

14. Jahnke L, Applebaum LA, Sherman PA, et al. An evaluation of intravenous immunoglobulin in the treatment of human immunodeficiency virus–associated thrombocytopenia. Transfusion 1994; 34:759–764.

15. Gottlieb F, Deutsch J. Red cell aplasia responsive to immunoglobulin therapy as initial manifestation of human immunodeficiency virus infection. Am J Med 1992; 92:331–333.

16. Silverman BA, Rubinstein A. Serum lactate dehydrogenase levels in adults and children with acquired immune deficiency syndrome (AIDS) and AIDS-related complex: possible indicator of B cell lymphoproliferation and disease activity. Am J Med 1985; 78:728–736.

17. Parkin JM, Rowland-Hill RJ, Shaw KE, et al. Pyogenic infection in patients with AIDS and a possible role for IVIG in treatment of functional hypogammaglobulinemia. Vox Sang 1987; 52:173.

18. Yap PL, Williams PE The treatment of human immunodeficiency virus infected persons with intravenous immunoglobulin. J Hosp Infect 1988; 12(suppl D):35–46.

19. Williams PE, Thompson C, Yap PL, et al. Controlled study of intravenous IgG therapy for HIV-infected adults with recurrent bacterial infections. Vox Sang 1991; 60:126–127.

20. Brunkhorst U, Sturner M, Willers H, et al. Efficacy of intravenous immunoglobulins in patients with advanced HIV-1 infection. A randomized clinical study. Infection 1990; 18:28–32.

21. Ahkutsu Y, Mori K, Suzuki S, et al. High dose intact-immunoglobulin treatment for HIV-infected asymptomatic carrier with hemophilia. Tohoku J Exp Med 1990; 160:95–96.

22. Schrappe-Bacher M, Rasokat H, Bauer P, et al. High-dose intravenous immunoglobulins in HIV-1 infected adults with AIDS-related complex and Walter Reed 5. Vox Sang 1990; 59(suppl):3–14.

23. Kiehl M, Stoll R, Domschke W. Intravenose Immungloulinsusstitution bei patienten mit ARC und AIDS (WR3-6). Immun Infekt 1994; 22:53–55.

24. Rogna S, Puppo F, Stagnaro R, et al. Plasma exchange plus immunoglobulins for the treatment of hypergammamlobulinaemic patients with AIDS and AIDS-related complex (ARC). Cancer Detect Prevent 1988; 12:273–276.

25. De Simone C, Tzantzoglou S, Santini G, et al. Clinical and immunological effects of combination therapy with intravenous immunoglobulins and AZT in HIV-infected patients. Immunopharm Immunotoxicol 1991; 13:447–458.

26. Wintergerst U, Niinivaara-Kreuzer G, Notheis K, et al. High-dose intravenous immunoglobulins in the treatment of adolescent and adult HIV-infected hemophiliacs. Clin Invest 1994; 72:122–126.

27. Wagner N, Bialek R, Radinger H, et al. Intravenous immunoglobulin in HIV infected hemophiliac patients. Arch Dis Child 1992; 67:1267–1271.

28. Liesveld JL, Weissbach NE, Shafer JA, et al. In vitro erythroid effects of a human stem cell factor in a case of human immunodeficiency virus related chronic parvovirus B19 induced anemia. Hematol Pathol 1993; 7:23–32.

29. Stogner SW, King JW, Black-Payne C, et al. Ribavirin and intravenous immune globulin therapy for measles pneumonia in HIV infection. South Med J 1993; 86:1415–1418.

30. Morgello S, Simpson DM. Multifocal cytomegalovirus demyelinative polyneuropathy associated with AIDS. Muscle Nerve 1994; 17:176–182.

31. Jacobson MA, O'Donnell JJ, Rousell R, et al. Failure of adjunctive cytomegalovirus intravenous immune globulin to improve efficacy of ganciclovir in patients with aquired immunodeficiency syndrome and cytomegalovirus retinitis: a phase I study. Antimicrob Agents Chemother 1990; 34:176–178.

32. De Simone C, Antonaci S, Chirigos M, et al. Report of the symposium on the use of intravenous gammaglobulin in adults infected with the human immunodeficiency virus. J Clin Lab Anal 1990; 4;313–317.

14

Treatment of Primary Immunodeficiency Diseases with Gammaglobulin

Richard I. Schiff
Miami Children's Hospital, Miami, Florida

INTRODUCTION

The first routine indication for the use of gammaglobulin was for the treatment of a primary immunodeficiency, Bruton's or X-linked agammaglobulinemia. Prior to that, immune serum globulin had been used to prevent several infectious diseases, including measles, tetanus, and diphtheria, but the discovery in 1952 by Ogden Bruton (1) that some patients with recurrent infections lacked the ability to make immunoglobulins led to the rapid establishment of gammaglobulin replacement as the standard of care. Acceptance was so rapid that in 1957, when the British Medical Research Council planned a study of the use of gammaglobulin in the treatment of immunodeficiency, they concluded that the use of a placebo control would be unethical (2). Hence, the most widely accepted use of gammaglobulin has never been subjected to a double-blind, placebo-controlled trial. The efficacy in numerous open-label studies has been so clear that few would question its use in any of the severe primary immune deficiencies, though controversies exist regarding the need for gammaglobulin replacement in incomplete immunodeficiency states such as polysaccharide antibody deficiency.

CLINICAL USES OF INTRAMUSCULAR AND INTRAVENOUS GAMMAGLOBULIN

Immunodeficiency Syndromes

The first congenital immunodeficiency disease was recognized in 1952 when Bruton described a child who lacked the gammaglobulin fraction in his serum (1). Since then, a large number of other defects have been identified which have been classified based on whether they primarily involve antibody formation by B cells, cellular immunity under the control of T cells, or a combination of the two (3) (Table 1). Most patients with T-cell defects also have a defect in antibody formation; T cells provide help for the B cells, without which production of specific antibody is blunted or absent. Therapy

Table 1 Classification of the Primary Immunodeficiency Diseases (Lymphocyte Disorders)

Designation	Associated features
Predominantly B-cell disorders	
X-linked agammaglobulinemia	Susceptible to enteroviral infections
Hyper-IgM syndrome	Neutropenia, thrombocytopenia, opportunistic infections
Common variable immunodeficiency	Malignancy, autoimmune disease. T-cell defects common
IgA deficiency	Increased incidence of allergy, autoimmune disease
Antibody deficiency with normal Ig's	
X-linked lymphoproliferative syndrome	Antibody deficiency, malignancy
IgG subclass deficiency	May or may not have associated antibody deficiency
Transient hypogammaglobulinemia	Incidence of infections variable
Primary T-cell disorders	
DiGeorge syndrome	Craniofacial anomalies, cardiac defects, hypocalcemia. B-cell function may also be reduced in complete form
Combined B- and T-cell defects	
Severe combined immune deficiency (SCID)	Failure to thrive; opportunistic infections
Cartilage hair hypoplasia	Short-limbed dwarfism
Purine nucleoside phosphorylase deficiency	Hemolytic anemia, neurological complications
MHC class II deficiency	Intractable diarrhea, failure to thrive
Reticular dysgenesis	Granulocytopenia, thrombocytopenia
Receptor defects CD3, CD8	
Other combined defects	
Wiskott-Aldrich syndrome	Eczema, thrombocytopenia, opportunistic infections, lymphoreticular malignancies
Ataxia telangiectasia	Ataxia, recurrent sinopulmonary infections, lymphoreticular malignancies
Chronic mucocutaneous candidiasis	Some have antibody deficiency. Increased incidence of disseminated fungal and viral infections
Leukocyte adhesion defect type I	Neutrophil and NK defects predominate

Table 2 Characteristics of the Humoral Antibody Deficiency Syndromes

Infectious complications		
Infection	Infectious agents	
Recurrent pneumonia	Bacterial	*Streptococcus pneumoniae*
Sinusitis		*Haemophilus influenzae*
Recurrent otitis		Streptococcus
Conjunctivitis		Meningococcus
Pharyngitis/tonsilitis		Pseudomonas
Adenitis		Campylobacter
Pyoderma		Mycoplasma
Meningitis		Ureaplasma
Sepsis		
Persistent diarrhea	Viral	Enterovirus (echo, polio)
Chronic urethritis		Rotavirus
Septic arthritis		
Osteomyelitis	Protozoal	*Giardia lamblia*
Pyoderma gangrenosum		*Cryptosporidium*
Viral meningoencephalitis		*Pneumocystis carinii*
Viral hepatitis		
Noninfectious complications		
Malignancy	Non-Hodgkin's lymphoma	
	Adenocarcinoma of stomach, ovary, colon	
	Squamous cell carcinoma of cervix, vagina, skin	
	Thymoma	
Autoimmune	Idiopathic thrombocytopenia	
	Hemolytic anemia	
	Neutropenia	
	Arthritis	
	Primary biliary cirrhosis	
	Alopecia	
	Pernicious anemia	
	Guillain-Barré syndrome	
Other associated complications	Malabsorption	
	Inflammatory bowel disease	
	Gastritis	
	Splenomegaly	
	Nodular lymphoid hyperplasia	

(Adapted from Refs. 4–5,6,9,10.)

with gammaglobulin is therefore appropriate whenever there is a defect in immunoglobulin production, regardless of whether T-cell function is normal.

The clinical manifestations of the antibody deficiency syndromes are shown in Table 2. As would be expected, infectious complications are the most prominent. In a review of 103 patients with common variable immunodeficiency (CVID), all had serious or recurrent infections and 22% had developed chronic lung disease (4). Infection was the cause of death or a major factor in 13 of the 23 patients who had died. Although bacterial pneumonia, sinusitis, and otitis are the most common infections, patients with defective antibody synthesis are susceptible to a wide variety of infections, including those induced by viruses, protozoa, and fungi (4–6). Recurrent respiratory infections led to the diagnosis of immune deficiency in 26 of 30 children; diarrhea of infectious cause was the second most common manifestation, occurring in 17 of the patients (6). Many of the children suffered from growth failure secondary to chronic lung disease or malabsorption. Patients with normal T-cell function are not thought to be highly susceptible to viral and protozoal infections, yet some organisms cause serious morbidity and mortality, such as enteroviruses in patients with X-linked agammaglobulinemia; and hepatitis, rotavirus, *Giardia lamblia*, and *Cryptosporidium* in all forms of antibody deficiency. The effectiveness of gammaglobulin has not been proven in all these infections, particularly gastrointestinal infections and malabsorption. Oral gammaglobulin was shown to be of some benefit in neonates with rotavirus infection (7), but the titer of antirotavirus antibody in IVIG is low; when cow colostrum with higher titers was used, a greater clinical effect was observed (8). Thus, it is important to consider that replacement of antibodies in the peripheral blood does not ensure control of infections, particularly in the gastrointestinal tract, the central nervous system, or in areas of chronic infection. Gammaglobulin cannot help with T-cell defects and is of limited benefit in the control of other complications, such as autoimmune disease and malignancy.

Noninfectious complications in patients with antibody deficiency are nearly as common and frequently are devastating, particularly in adults (Table 2). Fifteen of 103 primarily adult patients with CVID developed malignancies, either lymphoma (8), adenocarcinoma of the stomach, ovary, or colon; or squamous-cell carcinoma of the vagina, cervix, or skin (4). Autoimmune disease is common in both adults and children (4,6,9,10). Hematological disorders such as thrombocytopenia or hemolytic anemia are most frequently seen, but arthritis, chronic active hepatitis, Guillain-Barré syndrome, sprue, and endocrinopathies occur far more commonly than in patients with normal immunity. Some patients, particularly those with CVID, develop lymphoid hypertrophy with splenomegaly, adenopathy, and lymphoid nodular hyperplasia of the gastrointestinal tract and lungs (4,11). The relationship of the lymphoid hypertrophy to the development of lymphoid malignancy is not clear, but some are associated with Epstein-Barr virus (EBV) infection and progress to lymphoproliferative disease. Treatment with IVIG may decrease the degree of hyperplasia and obviate the need for splenectomy or biopsies of the lung (11), but there are no data to suggest that treatment can prevent the development of malignancy. Similarly, although very high doses of IVIG are used to treat a variety of autoimmune disorders (12,13), it is unlikely that replacement of gammaglobulin has any effect on the development or course of these diseases.

Clinical Trials of IM and IV Gammaglobulin

The use of gammaglobulin to treat patients with hypogammaglobulinemia was rapidly adopted (14) after the initial report of Bruton (1) demonstrated that replacement therapy would reduce the incidence of infections and thereby decrease the morbidity and mortality associated with the immune deficiency. The purpose was simple: to provide antibodies against a variety of pathogens to neutralize toxins, directly kill microorganisms, and enhance phagocytosis. Therapy was largely empiric and based on the observation that IgG levels below 200 mg/dl were associated with a higher incidence of infections. Though these early trials were uncontrolled, the perception of clinical benefit was so great that in 1956, when the British Research Medical Council decided to do a prospective study, they felt it unethical to include a placebo control (2). All subsequent studies evaluated variations in dose or different preparations, but the use of antibody replacement for immune deficiency has never been subjected to a blinded, placebo-controlled study. The only form of gammaglobulin available at the time was suitable only for intramuscular administration, and thus the dose was limited to approximately 100 mg/kg/month.

Experimental forms of IVIG were available in Europe (15) and Australia (16) in the late 1960s and in the United States in the early 1970s (17). Initially, the intravenous preparations were compared to intramuscular gammaglobulin either directly or to an historical control period (17–21). In an early study, 20 patients were treated with a modified immune serum globulin prepared by reduction and alkylation (18). Mild adverse events, including nausea, flushing, fever, headache, and muscle cramps, were common, but no catastrophic reactions occurred. While treated with 150 mg/kg/month of the intravenous preparation, the patients had only 0.103 acute infections per month compared to 0.295 infections per month while receiving the intramuscular gammaglobulin.

A 2-year crossover study of the same modified immune serum globulin in 34 immunodeficient patients treated monthly with 100 mg/kg did not show a difference in the incidence of infections between the intramuscular and intravenous preparations (17), but all of the patients favored the IV form despite a high incidence of "phlogistic" reactions such as fever, chills, nausea, vomiting, backache, and headache. The incidence of these reactions decreased significantly when maltose was added to prevent aggregation of the IgG molecules (22). The lack of improvement with IVIG was not surprising since the dose was the same for both forms of gammaglobulin. When the intravenous dose was increased to 300 mg/kg/month of Sandoglobulin, there was a substantial reduction in the incidence of infections compared to the historical period when the patients were treated with 100 mg/kg intramuscularly (19). Similar benefits were seen in a study in England using the same dose of Intraglobin-F (21). A dramatic decrease in the number of infections, or days with fever, in bed, or in hospital, was observed in 23 children treated with 150–300 mg/kg every 3 weeks compared to the historical period of intramuscular gammaglobulin (23). The children seldom had IgG levels over 100 mg/dl on IM therapy, but averaged more than 500 mg/dl on IV therapy. Even though the IV gammaglobulin was more expensive, they were able to show an overall cost savings because of the decreased hospitalizations and need for antibiotics. Intravenous gammaglobulin also led to clinical improvement compared to plasma therapy, even when the dose was only 150 mg/kg, but the benefits were greater when patients were treated with 500 mg/kg/month (20).

Other studies have indicated benefit of IVIG, though none of these have included a placebo control (24–29). A variety of preparations have been studied. Although it is considered desirable that the IgG in IVIG be maintained in its "native" state, there has been no evidence to show greater benefit of native IVIG preparations compared to chemically modified preparations (25). Chemically modified products have shown good clinical efficacy, despite lacking IgG3 (24); indeed, the lack of IgG3 did not seem to prevent clinical benefit even when used to treat patients with specific IgG3 subclass deficiency and chronic inflammatory chest disease (26).

DETERMINATION OF DOSE

The optimal dose of gammaglobulin for the treatment of patients with immunodeficiency diseases has never been determined in a blinded, controlled trial. The initial recommendation of 100 mg/kg/month was determined empirically (14) based on the observation that if the serum IgG level was raised by 200 mg/dl, invasive bacterial infections could be prevented. This could be achieved by giving a loading dose of 300 mg/kg followed by monthly injections of 100 mg/kg, usually in weekly divided doses. This was the maximum that could be given intramuscularly, and it was not until intravenous forms of gammaglobulin were available that higher doses could be employed.

The British Medical Research Council compared 25 mg/kg/week to 50 mg/kg/week using the intramuscular preparation, or immune serum globulin (ISG), and showed a small but statistically significant difference in favor of the higher dose, especially with regard to diarrhea and pneumonia (2). However, immunological studies were limited in 1969, and the inclusion of patients with T-cell defects and other complex immunologic disorders made interpretation of the results difficult.

During the subsequent 15 years, several studies compared intramuscular to intravenous gammaglobulin given at a higher dose. Nolte and co-workers reported a significant improvement in patients given 150 mg/kg intravenously compared to 100 mg/kg given IM (18). The incidence of acute infections decreased from 0.295 per month to only 0.103. Similar benefits were seen in a multicenter study of 21 patients given intravenous gammaglobulin at 300 mg/kg every 3 weeks for 1 year compared to the patients' historical control period when treated with intramuscular gammaglobulin at 100 mg/kg/month (19). Eighteen of the patients showed significant improvement, and overall the number of sick days decreased from 834 to 258 ($P < .001$) and the number of days on antibiotics from 3249 to 1829. The improvement was most evident during the second 6 months of the study. The number of days hospitalized increased from 14 to 35, but 28 days were attributed to one patient.

The majority of studies comparing two doses of intravenous gammaglobulin have shown clinical benefit at the higher dose, but the finding has not been universal. In an open study comparing 100 mg/kg/month to 400 mg/kg/month for 1 year in patients with primary defects of humoral immunity (30), there was no difference in the incidence of infections or use of antibiotics between the two groups. The lack of benefit may have been due to the short duration of the study or the presence of chronic sinopulmonary disease that could not be cleared with either gammaglobulin or antibiotics. There was no improvement in a study of 16 patients treated for 6 months with 100 mg/kg/month then treated for an additional 6 months with a dose calculated to maintain the trough IgG concentration over 200 mg/dl (24). However, the calculated doses were only 150–300 mg/kg, and the increase in serum concentration was modest, which could account for the lack of clinical improvement. Sorensen and Polmar also observed that increasing the dose to 200 mg/kg in order to maintain the IgG levels over 400 mg/dl did not decrease the incidence or severity of infections (31).

Other studies have shown significant benefit at higher doses (20,32–34). A dose of intravenous gammaglobulin of 500 mg/kg/month was better than 150 mg/kg, which was significantly better than a retrospective period when 12 children with primary immunodeficiencies had been treated with plasma (20). The total number of days with clinical disease decreased from 284 while on plasma to 218 while receiving 150 mg/kg and to 108 while receiving 500 mg/kg. The effects were not significant for pneumonia, sinusitis, and arthritis. They also noted an improvement in pulmonary function while the children received the higher dose of IVIG. In another study of 12 children and adults, improvement was noted even in patients who had chronic sinopulmonary disease (32,33). Patients were infused with either 200 mg/kg or 600 mg/kg for 6 months and then crossed over to the alternative dose. Data were analyzed relative to the serum concentration of IgG. When the level of IgG was less than 500 mg/dl, there were 16 major infections, compared to only three when the level was greater than 500 mg/dl. The incidence of minor infections, primarily upper respiratory infections, was similarly decreased from 31 to 12 in a 6-month period. Finally, Liese and his co-workers in Germany retrospectively analyzed the incidence of infections in 29 patients treated since 1965 (34). They noted that patients treated with high-dose intravenous gammaglobulin at 400 mg/kg or more every 3 weeks showed a significant decrease in the incidence of pneumonia and days hospitalized compared to 200 mg/kg intravenously or 100 mg/kg given intramuscularly. Improvement was particularly evident if treatment with high dose began before the patient was 5 years of age. Since this was a retrospective study, it did not consider improvements in diagnosis or antibiotic therapy that occurred over those 27 years; however, importantly, no episodes of meningitis, sepsis, or chronic pulmonary disease developed in any patient who started treatment with high-dose IVIG before age 5.

Thus, although no controlled comparison studies have been done, there is evidence that many patients will have fewer infections if treated with high doses of IVIG, generally 400 mg/kg/month or enough to maintain the trough serum IgG concentration over 500 mg/dl. Patients who are started early in life, before serious infections and chronic lung disease develop, will show the greatest benefit. Higher doses of IVIG may be of particular benefit in patients with X-linked agammaglobulinemia for the prevention and treatment of echovirus meningoencephalitis. However, not every study has shown an advantage of using higher doses, and thus the decision regarding dose must be individualized based primarily on clinical course rather than levels of IgG.

SPECIAL CONSIDERATIONS

Pregnancy

Women with antibody deficiency who are receiving intravenous gammaglobulin should continue infusions throughout pregnancy (35–37). The risk of infection, especially in women with underlying lung disease, far outweighs any possible consideration of adverse reactions. Additionally, the infused IgG crosses the placenta so that the infant is born with normal serum concentration of IgG and decreased risk of infection in the first months of life (38,39). The number of pregnant women treated with ISG or IVIG is too small to accurately determine benefit or to detect a minor change in fetal wastage; however, the incidence of infection during pregnancy was decreased, and most investigators have considered the infusions to be beneficial (35–37,40,41). IVIG also has been given to women with recurrent pregnancy loss secondary to antiphospholipid antibodies and lupus anticoagulant (42,43) with an improvement in overall outcome (see Chapter 35 for greater detail).

There are no published reports of adverse events related to infusions of IVIG during pregnancy; however, anecdotally several woman have aborted within hours to days of receiving gammaglobulin. One woman experienced an acute reaction during the infusion, and the onset of uterine contractions may have been secondary to prostaglandins and other mediators released during the reaction. In the other situations there was not a close association of abortion and the infusion of IVIG, and the loss of the fetus may have been related to the overall health of the mother. Special care should be taken to avoid adverse reactions during the infusions, especially in women with a prior history of reactions to gammaglobulin, but the gammaglobulin therapy should be continued.

Since the fetus derives its IgG from the mother, the transfer of IgG to the baby, plus the increase in intravascular volume in the mother, usually necessitates an increase in the dose of IVIG to maintain adequate serum levels (37,39,41,44). Not all of the IVIG preparations have been evaluated, but since the currently available preparations are unmodified, the Fc portion of the molecule can interact with receptors appropriately and the IgG should cross the placenta normally.

Chronic Enteroviral Meningoencephalitis

Patients with antibody deficiency are unusually susceptible to infection with hepatitis viruses and the enteroviruses. Chronic enteroviral meningoencephalitis (CEM) occurs primarily in patients with X-linked agammaglobulinemia, although some patients with common variable immunodeficiency have developed similar infections (45). The majority of infections have been caused by the ECHO viruses, although several infections with Coxsackie viruses have occurred. Infections are usually manifest by slow progressive neurological deterioration with loss of developmental milestones, seizures, memory loss, ataxia, paresthesias, and lethargy or coma. Some patients additionally have developed a dermatomyositis-like syndrome with edema, rash, and contractures (46). The majority of patients developing these syndromes were either untreated or receiving intramuscular gammaglobulin, but some were receiving standard doses of IVIG. Even with aggressive therapy the disease is usually fatal.

Specific antibodies were shown to inhibit the growth of echovirus 5 in one patient (47), suggesting that the disease could be treated if patients were given adequate doses of gammaglobulin. Mease and co-workers reported a cure of one patient with high-dose IVIG (48), but their patient later relapsed. Although some patients have cleared their central nervous system (CNS) of virus with high doses of IVIG alone, most have required direct instillation of gammaglobulin into the ventricles via an Ommaya reservoir (49). Using a combination of high-dose IVIG and the direct application into the CNS, most patients can at least clear their spinal fluid of the virus.

Early diagnosis and institution of therapy is crucial, for although the disease may be arrested, there is little improvement in the neurological state once damage has occurred. Though some investigators have suggested monitoring patients with regular lumbar punctures, careful observation and neurological assessment with psychometric testing may be adequate. Once the disease is suspected, spinal fluid must be obtained for culture and PCR testing for enterovirus. Multiple evaluations may be necessary, since the virus may not be readily detected. If the virus can be isolated, individual lots of IVIG should be screened to find one with high titers of specific antibody. The dose of IVIG has not been determined with certainty, but should be adequate to maintain the trough level of IgG in the range of 600–1000 mg/dl above baseline (49). Usually at least 400 mg/kg every 2–3 weeks is required. The amount of gammaglobulin to be instilled into the Ommaya reservoir has not been determined precisely, but 2–10 ml of a 5%, 6%, or 10% solution can be safety infused with minimal side effects. The IVIG preparations having low pH should not be used, because the ventricular fluid has little buffer capacity and little is known of the effects of rapidly changing the pH in the ventricles. Initially the gammaglobulin should be injected daily, then several times a week, and then with decreasing frequency based on normalization of the ventricular fluid and results of viral cultures. Some patients may go into prolonged remission, but others require intermittent therapy for many years (49,50).

ADVERSE REACTIONS TO INTRAVENOUS GAMMAGLOBULIN

Anaphylactic and Anaphylactoid Reactions

Although the safety and risks of IVIG are discussed elsewhere in this volume, some problems are particularly relevant to patients with immune deficiency diseases. Soon after attempts were made to administer gammaglobulin intravenously, it became apparent that immune deficiency patients were more susceptible to anaphylactoid or phlogistic reactions. Barandun and his colleagues diluted the 16% ISG 10-fold and infused it into normal volunteers and patients with a variety of immunodeficiency diseases (15). Forty-eight of 55 normal volunteers tolerated the infusions given over a 90- to 120-min period. Under the same conditions 14 of 15 immunodeficient patients experienced early signs of flushing, nausea, and shivering, followed by a rise in temperature to 38 or 39°C. Two of the patients suffered more severe, anaphylactoid reactions. When the infusions were discontinued until the reactions subsided, the patients were able to tolerate infusions of the remainder of the gammaglobulin without further reactions. In some as yet unexplained manner the patients were desensitized by the reaction. Barandun believed that the IgG was spontaneously fixing complement and releasing mediators to cause the reactions. Treatment of the gammaglobulin with enzymes, ultracentrifugation, or low pH to reduce the anticomplementary activity reduced but did not eliminate the reactions.

The mechanisms of these adverse reactions still are not understood (51). The incidence of reactions decreased significantly when sugars such as maltose were added to the preparations (22), presumably because sugars and amino acids such as glycine decrease the tendency of IgG to aggregate. Despite the improved quality of the gammaglobulin preparations currently available, between 5% and 15% of immunodeficient patients experience adverse reactions. For most patients the incidence of adverse reactions is rate-dependent, and slowing the infusion or interrupting the infusion until the reaction subsides makes it possible to infuse the complete dose. For others, pretreatment with aspirin, acetaminophen, diphenhydramine, or corticosteroids is required (52–54). Reactions are more frequent during the initial infusions. Once infections are controlled and the patients have adequate levels of IgG, the incidence of phlogistic or anaphylactoid reactions decreases.

True anaphylactic reactions are rare. Patients who are completely IgA-deficient may have severe reactions if infused with plasma or IVIG that contains IgA (55–58). The presence of IgG anti-IgA antibodies does not always predict these reactions (57,59), which may be life-threatening. In some cases the epitope on the IgA molecule that the antibody is directed against may determine the severity of the ensuing reaction (60). The rapid onset and severity of the reactions in these patients are suggestive of true anaphylaxis, which is mediated by IgE. Indeed, several CVID patients who completely lacked IgA and had a history of severe reactions to infusions of IVIG were shown to have IgE anti-IgA antibodies (57). Patients with selective IgA deficiency are not candidates for therapy with IVIG, in part because of the risk of anaphylactic reactions, but primarily because the IVIG does not have appreciable quantities of IgA and that present is not secreted onto the mucosal surfaces where it is needed. Patients with CVID have a more global immune defect and should be treated with IVIG even if they are completely IgA-deficient; these patients can be treated with IVIG preparations that have sufficiently low IgA concentrations, such as Gammagard-SD (58), though they should always be infused under circumstances where severe reactions can be rapidly treated.

Hepatitis C

The risk of transmission of hepatitis C and other viral agents by gammaglobulin is discussed in detail in another chapter. The question has been raised whether patients with immune deficiency are particularly susceptible to infection with hepatitis C or if the disease is more severe in these patients (61,62). The first report of non-A, non-B hepatitis associated with infusions of intravenous gammaglobulin was that of Lane from the Blood Products Laboratory in England (63). Twelve hypogammaglobulinemic patients developed hepatitis consistent with non-A, non-B hepatitis; more specific testing was not available in 1983. Two of the patients were mildly icteric for a short period, and the others had mild elevations in aminotransferase levels that persisted for more than 10 months (63,64). However, upon follow-up 3 years later, at least six of the patients showed signs of progressive disease (65). Five still had very high ALT levels, one of whom complained of lethargy and had a large tender liver. One patient died of sepsis secondary to bone marrow failure that occurred shortly after the onset of the hepatitis. Several patients had evidence of cirrhosis on biopsy.

Shortly after the initial report, Ochs and his colleagues reported seven cases of non-A, non-B hepatitis that occurred in 16 immune-deficient patients during evaluation of experimental lots of IVIG produced by Hyland Therapeutics (66). Two years after the study began, one patient developed edema, ascites, and jaundice accompanied by an increase in aminotransferase levels. That patient later died of coronary artery disease and had a grossly cirrhotic liver. Six additional patients were found to have elevated aminotransferase levels but were asymptomatic. The remaining nine patients were not affected at that time. One of the differences between the two groups was that none of the patients who became affected had previously received IVIG; it is possible that passively administered antibody protected the patients who had been treated with IVIG prior to entering the study. On follow-up in 1986, two of the patients who were initially normal had developed mild but progressive rise in aminotransferases, though they were asymptomatic (67). Five of the original seven patients remained asymptomatic although they continued to have fluctuating ALT levels. One of the patients had micronodular cirrhosis detected on serial liver biopsies.

The most severe outbreak of non-A, non-B hepatitis prior to 1993 was related to infusion of Gammonativ, made by KabiVitrum in Sweden (61,62,68). This was the first outbreak of hepatitis from IVIG prepared by a large commercial source. The first report was that of Weiland and co-workers at the Karolinska Institute in 1986 (68). They reported four patients who developed elevated transaminases; one complained of feeling tired, and another developed joint pain, lethargy, and dark urine. The other two were asymptomatic. Two of the patients were healthy volunteers who received the IVIG in a study of the product's half-life. They did not have progressive disease noted on biopsy. The other two patients received the IVIG as replacement therapy for hypogammaglobulinemia, and both had evidence of progressive cirrhosis on biopsy. These two groups differed in the amount of IVIG they received, and both of the immune-deficient patients had received other forms of gammaglobulin prior to receiving Gammonativ. Thus, it could not be concluded that the more severe disease in the patients with hypogammaglobulinemia was related to the underlying immune deficiency.

In 1988 Björkander and colleagues in New York and Göteborg, Sweden, reported another, larger outbreak of non-A, non-B hepatitis in 16 of 77 immunodeficient patients treated with Gammonativ (61). Twelve of the patients were symptomatic and five died, with hepatitis being the cause of death in two and a contributing factor in three. The other patients had persistent elevation in transaminases, though they were asymptomatic at the time of the report. The livers of four of the eight patients who underwent biopsy showed signs of chronic active hepatitis with various degrees of inflammation.

Additional cases of hepatitis C caused by Gammonativ were reported in 1994 by Bjøro and co-workers (62). Seventeen of 20 Norwegian immunodeficient patients who had received Gammonativ between 1982 and 1986 were seropositive for hepatitis C RNA. All 15 liver biopsies showed portal inflammation, bile duct damage, and focal necrosis. In six patients there was cirrhosis. Two patients died of liver failure, and the others had persistently abnormal aminotransferases. None of the patients had a good response to therapy with interferon.

Three years after the episode of hepatitis in Sweden was reported, Williams, Yap, and others at the Edinburgh and South East Scotland Blood Transfusion Service reported four cases of non-A, non-B hepatitis related to therapy with a pH 4–treated IVIG prepared at the Blood Transfusion Center (69). Two of the patients had mild symptoms of hepatitis, and the other two were asymptomatic. One of the patients had persistent elevation of aminotransferases and evidence of chronic active hepatitis on biopsy. Thirty additional patients who were treated with the same IVIG preparation remained seronegative and asymptomatic. This same group had previously retrospectively analyzed their patients in 1986, after the reports of hepatitis in Sweden, and found no evidence of transmission of hepatitis by their product at that time (70).

The outbreak of hepatitis C associated with Gammagard in 1994 is the largest and the only one associated with a gammaglobulin preparation licensed for use in the United States (71). Nearly all of the cases occurred between October 1993 and June 1994 and were associated with multiple lots of the gammaglobulin used in the United States and throughout the world. Thus far there has been no publication of the long-term consequences of this episode of hepatitis; not all of the patients were immunodeficient, and some comparison may thus be possible. Although many of the patients were initially reported to be asymptomatic or minimally affected, several cases of chronic active hepatitis and death have been unofficially reported. Even in the patients who are clinically well, longer follow-up will be necessary before the full effects are known.

Based on the initial reports of non-A, non-B hepatitis (61–63,65–67), it would appear that the course of the disease is more severe in patients with immunodeficiency than in immunologically normal individuals. However, factors other than the immunological state of the patients must be considered. The incidence and severity in these reports, particularly in the cases associated with Gammonativ, were extraordinarily high. This suggests that the degree of contamination must have been very high. If this rate of infection were extrapolated to other IVIG products, there would be tens of thousands of cases of hepatitis C reported. Retrospective (70,72,73) and prospective (73,74) evaluations of patients receiving IVIG have not revealed evidence of symptomatic infection. Thus, although there is a very high incidence of progressive disease in these patients with immunodeficiency, it is not clear whether the cause is related to a lack of host defense or because they received large doses of heavily contaminated IVIG and thus were infected with very large amounts of virus.

METHODS OF ADMINISTRATION

Alternative Methods of Administration

Until the early 1980s in the United States, the only form of IgG that was available for clinical use was given intramuscularly. The amount given was limited by pain, and the amount absorbed was reduced by proteolysis. Plasma therapy was used as an alternative (75). Plasma had the theoretical benefit of providing IgA and IgM as well as the IgG, but the short half-life of those severely limited the degree of replacement. The amount of plasma that could be infused limited the ability to give large quantities of IgG, but the major problem with plasma therapy was the transmission of hepatitis. Thus, alternatives were sought that would allow large quantities of IgG to be given safely. In 1980 Berger and co-workers reported the use of a pump to give large quantities of immune serum globulin subcutaneously (76). Patients infused themselves at home, usually overnight. Patients achieved higher levels of IgG with fewer side effects and had fewer infections (76,77). Although subcutaneous infusion has been largely supplanted by IVIG, it remains a viable alternative for the rare patient who cannot tolerate IVIG or, since it allows the use of the less expensive immune serum globulin, for patients who cannot afford IVIG.

Rapid Infusion

The infusion rates used in the early trials were conservative, largely because the high incidence of phlogistic or anaphylactoid reactions that occurred when immunodeficient patients were infused with gammaglobulin intravenously (15). It still is not known why patients with immunodeficiency are more susceptible to these reactions than normal volunteers, but the incidence is higher during initial treatments and is rate-dependent. In the first clinical trials the 5% solution of IgG was infused starting at 0.01 cc/kg/min and increasing at 15- 30-min intervals to a maximum of 0.08 cc/kg/min. This regimen became the standard; similar rates were used in nearly all of the clinical trials and were the recommended rates when the IVIG was licensed for general use. Some patients cannot attain these rates unless they are pretreated with steroids, aspirin, acetaminophen, or diphenhydramine. However, many patients can be infused more rapidly than the rates recommended in the package inserts. In a study of 16 patients infused with 12% Sandoglobulin, six were able to attain rates > 15 mg/kg/min—nearly five times the standard rates (78). Seven of the patients completed the infusion of 400 mg/kg in less than 30 min, and four were infused within 15 min. These patients were selected because they had a long history of tolerating infusions of IVIG without adverse reactions, but even in this selected population three of the patients had to withdraw because of adverse reactions at the higher rates. Similar results were obtained in a study of 27 immunodeficiency patients infused with Gammagard (79).

In some centers patients are routinely infused at rapid rates, completing their infusions in less than 30 min. However, these patients are all selected because they are known to tolerate IVIG without difficult and are infused in a setting where adverse reactions can be managed by experienced personnel. It is not appropriate to begin patients at high rates or infuse at home or in a setting where emergency medical care is not readily available. For patients who can tolerate high infusion rates, the social impact of receiving IVIG can be greatly reduced.

Home Therapy

Infusions of IVIG result in a day lost from work or school every 3 or 4 weeks. In an effort to reduce the impact of this essential therapy, Ashida and Saxon first reported home infusions of IVIG by self-administration in 1986 (80). Seven patients were selected who had no history of adverse reactions to IVIG, had good venous access, and were in good health. Infusions were given using an Auto Syringe to control rates, and all patients were able to complete the study. Others reports similar success with home infusions (81–83). In each of these, patients were selected who did not have a history of adverse reactions; most could infuse without using a pump, which further reduced the cost of the infusions (81). Patients were instructed in starting intravenous lines and gave themselves at least one infusion while observed in the clinic. Advantages of home infusions include less time lost from work or school, decreased cost, ability to give the infusions more frequently, thereby maintaining a higher mean IgG concentration, and improved self-image (81,82). In a quality-of-life assessment, most patients felt that home therapy was preferable (84).

In these studies patients started their own intravenous lines and supervised the infusions. In practice, many patients have had the infusions done by home care nurses, which expands the population who can get home therapy, but decreases the cost savings. IVIG obtained through home care agencies is frequently more expensive than that obtained through hospitals, so the cost differential is not always as great as would be predicted. Another potential problem is that the patients are not evaluated as often, and medical problems may go unrecognized; however, that same problem exists when patients are treated in infusion centers where they are not seen by a physician.

The decision to treat a patient at home must be individualized. For some, the decreased loss of time from work or school is a major issue. For others, who have more unstable disease, closer follow-up is more important and ultimately will result in less illness and therefore greater productivity. At a minimum, patients who are selected for home care should (1) have a history of tolerating IVIG infusions without adverse effects; (2) demonstrate stability and responsibility and, when the patient is a child, have a stable home situation and a parent who can take responsibility; and (3) be instructed in starting the infusions, adjusting the infusion rates, and treating reactions. Emergency medications should be available and patients should not infuse themselves when home alone. Regular follow-up visits must be scheduled to be sure that problems do not go unrecognized for long periods. The use of home care nurses provides additional support and measure of safety but significantly increases the cost. With proper selection of patients and adequate preparation, many patients can safely be infused at home and enjoy a better quality of life.

SUMMARY

Treatment of primary immunodeficiency diseases was the initial induction and remains the best-defined use of IVIG. All immune-deficient patients who have a defect in specific antibody production, regardless of immunoglobulin levels or T-cell function, are candidates for therapy with gammaglobulin. The dose and timing of infusions have been determined empirically and through uncontrolled studies, but the predominance of evidence suggests that higher doses, sufficient to maintain serum IgG concentrations at least 400–600 mg/dl, are more efficacious than the lower doses used initially. However, since patients differ in the catabolic rate of IgG, presence of chronic infections, and other factors that have not yet been elucidated, the dose for any patient should be individualized based on clinical response rather than an arbitrary serum concentration. Higher doses of IVIG may be necessary in patients with X-linked agammaglobulinemia to treat or prevent enteroviral infections. Numerous studies have demonstrated the need to begin therapy early, before the onset of serious infections and the development of chronic disease. The use of IVIG for partial or transient immunodeficiency states, such as IgG subclass deficiency, polysaccharide antibody deficiency, and transient hypogammaglobulinemia of infancy, is poorly defined and controversial. However, it is not appropriate to withhold therapy in a patient with a significant immune defect who is clinically well, because the first infection might be life-threatening. Though expensive, IVIG has been shown to be cost-effective by reducing the need for antibiotics, hospitalizations, and time lost from work or school. For some patients the social impact of IVIG therapy can be further reduced by giving the infusions at home, but at the cost of less frequent evaluations, which could allow medical problems to increase in severity. An alternative may be to give infusions rapidly in a center where patients can be closely observed. Ultimately, the dose, schedule, and infusion program must be tailored to best meet the needs of the individual patient.

REFERENCES

1. Bruton OC. Agammaglobulinemia. Pediatrics 1952; 9:722–728.
2. Medical Research Council. Hypogammaglobulinaemia in the United Kingdom. Lancet 1969; 1:163–168.
3. WHO Scientific Group. Primary immunodeficiency diseases: report of a WHO scientific group. Clin Exp Immunol 1995; 99:1–24.
4. Cunningham-Rundles C. Clinical and immunologic analyses of 103 patients with common variable immunodeficiency. J Clin Immunol 1989; 9:22–33.
5. Stiehm ER, Chin TW, Haas A, Peerless AG. Infectious complications of the primary immunodeficiencies. Clin Immunol Immunopathol 1986; 40:69–86.
6. Hausser C, Virelizier J, Buriot D, Griscelli C. Common variable hypogammaglobulinemia in children. Am J Dis Child 1983; 137:833–837.
7. Barnes GL, Hewson PH, McLellan JA et al. A randomised trial of oral gammaglobulin in low-birth-weight infants infected with rotavirus. Lancet 1982: 1792–512.
8. Hilpert H, Brussow H, Mietens C, Sidoti J, Lerner L, Werchau H. Use of bovine milk concentrate containing antibody to rotavirus to treat rotavirus gastroenteritis in infants. J Infect Dis 1987; 156:158–166.
9. Conley ME, Park CL, Douglas SD. Childhood common variable immunodeficiency with autoimmune disease. J Pediatr 1986; 108:915–922.
10. Preston SJ, Buchanan WW. Rheumatic manifestations of immune deficiency. Clin Exp Rheumatol 1989; 7:547–555.
11. Knutsen AP, Merten DF, Buckley RH. Colonic nodular lymphoid hyperplasia in a child with antibody deficiency and near normal immunoglobulins. J Pediatr 1981; 98:420–423.

12. Schwartz SA. Intravenous immunoglobulin (IVIG) for the therapy of autoimmune disorders. J Clin Immunol 1990; 10:81–89.

13. Ronda N, Hurez V, Kazatchkine MD. Intravenous immunoglobulin therapy of autoimmune and systemic inflammatory diseases. Vox Sang 1993; 64:65–72.

14. Janeway CA, Rosen RS. The gamma globulins. IV. Therapeutic uses of gamma globulin. N Engl J Med 1966; 275:826–831.

15. Barandum S, Kistler P, Jeunet F, Isliker H. Intravenous administration of human gamma-globulin. Vox Sang 1962; 7:157–174.

16. Simons MJ, Schumacher MJ, Fowler R. Intravenous gamma globulin therapy of immuno-globulin deficiency diseases. Aust Paediatr J 1968; 4:127–133.

17. Ammann AJ, Ashman RF, Buckley RH, et al. Use of intravenous gammaglobulin in anti-body imunodeficiency: results of a multicenter controlled trial. Clin Immunol Immunopathol 1982; 22:60–67.

18. Nolte MT, Pirofsky B, Gerritz GA, Golding B. Intravenous immunoglobulin therapy for antibody deficiency. Clin Exp Immunol 1979; 36:237–243.

19. Cunningham-Rundles C, Siegal FP, Smithwick EM, et al. Efficacy of intravenous immuno-globulin in primary humoral immunodeficiency disease. Ann Intern Med 1984; 101:435–439.

20. Bernatowska E, Madalinski K, Janowicz W, et al. Results of a prospective controlled two-dose crossover study with intravenous immunoglobulin and comparison (retrospective) with plasma treatment. Clin Immunol Immunopathol 1987; 43:153–162.

21. Garbett ND, Currie CC, Cole PJ. Comparison of the clinical efficacy and safety of an intra-muscular and an intravenous immunoglobulin preparation for replacement therapy in idio-pathic adult onset panhypogammaglobulinaemia. Clin Exp Immunol 1989; 76:1–7.

22. Ochs HD, Pirofsky B, Rousell RH, et al. Safety and patient acceptability of intravenous immune globulin in 10% maltose. Lancet 1980; 2:1158–1159.

23. Galli E, Barbieri C, Cantani A, Solano A, Longhi MA, Businco L. Treatment with gammaglobulin preparation for intravenous use in children with humoral immunodeficiency: clinical and immunologic follow-up. Ann Allergy 1990; 64:147–150.

24. Schiff RI, Rudd C, Johnson R, Buckley RH. Use of a new chemically modified intravenous IgG preparation in severe primary humoral immunodeficiency: clinical efficacy and attempts to individualize dosage. Clin Immunol Immunopathol 1984; 31:13–23.

25. Steele RW, Augustine RA, Tannenbaum AS, Charlton RK. A comparison of native and modified intravenous immunoglobulin for the management of hypogammaglobulinemia. Am J Med Sci 1987; 293:69–74.

26. Bernatowska-Matuszkiewicz E, Pac M, Skopcynska H, Pum M, Eibl MM. Clinical efficacy of intravenous immunoglobulin in patients with severe inflammatory chest disease and IgG3 subclass deficiency. Clin Exp Immunol 1991; 85:193–197.

27. European Group for Immunodeficiencies. Intravenous gammaglobulin for immunodeficiency: report from the European Group for Immunodeficiencies (EGID). Clin Exp Immunol 1986; 65:683–690.

28. Williams P, White A, Wilson JA, et al. Penetration of administered IgG into the maxillary sinus and long-term clinical effects of intravenous immunoglobulin replacement therapy on sinusitis in primary hypogammaglobulinemia. Acta Otolaryngol 1991; 111:550–555.

29. Robertson DM, Hosking CS. The long term treatment of childhood hypogammaglobulinaemia in Melbourne with intravenous gammaglobulin, 1972–1985. Dev Biol Stand 1987; 67:273–280.

30. Ochs HD, Fischer SH, Wedgwood RJ, et al. Comparison of high-dose and low-dose intra-venous immunoglobulin therapy in patients with primary immunodeficiency diseases. Am J Med 1984; 76:78–82.

31. Sorensen RU, Polmar SH. Efficacy and safety of high-dose intravenous immune globulin therapy for antibody deficiency syndromes. Am J Med 1984; 76:83–90.

32. Roifman CM, Levison H, Gelfand EW. High-dose versus low-dose intravenous immuno-globulin in hypogammaglobulinemia and chronic lung disease. Lancet 1987; 1:1075–1077.

33. Gelfand EW, Reid B, Roifman CM. Intravenous immune serum globulin replacement in hypogammaglobulinemia. A comparison of high- versus low-dose therapy. Monogr Allergy 1988; 23:177–186.

34. Liese JG, Wintergerst U, Tympner KD, Belohradsky BH. High- vs low-dose immunoglo-bulin therapy in the long-term treatment of X-linked agammaglobulinemia. Am J Dis Child 1992; 146:335–339.

35. Sacher RA, King JC. Intravenous gamma globulin in pregnancy: a review. Obstet Gynecol 1988; 44:25–34.

36. von Muralt G, Sidiropoulos D. Experience with intravenous immunoglobulin treatment in neonates and pregnant women. Vox Sang 1986; 51:22–29.

37. Sorenssen RU, Tomford JW, Gyves MT, Judge NE, Polmar SH. Use of intravenous im-mune globulin in pregnant women with common variable hypogammaglobulinemia. Am J Med 1984; 76:73–77.

38. Morell A, Sidiropoulos D, Herrmann U, et al. IgG subclasses and antibodies to group B streptococci in preterm neonates after intravenous infusion of immunoglobulin to the moth-ers. Pediatr Infect Dis J 1986; 5:S195–S197.

39. Sidiropoulos D, Herrmann U, Morell A, Muralt Gv, Barandun S. Transplacental passage of intravenous immunoglobulin in the last trimester of pregnancy. J Pediatr 1986; 109:505–508.

40. Williams PE, Leen CL, Heppleston AD, Yap PL. IgG replacement therapy for primary hypogammaglobulinemia during pregnancy: report of 9 pregnancies in 4 patients. Blut 1990; 60:198–201.

41. Madsen DL, Catanzarite VA, Valela-Gittings F. Common variable hypogammaglobulinemia in pregnancy: treatment with high-dose immunoglobulin infusions. Am J Hematol 1986; 21:327–329.

42. Kaaja R, Julkunen H, Ammala P, Palosuo T, Kurki P. Intravenous immunoglobulin treat-ment of pregnant patients with recurrent pregnancy losses associated with antiphospholipid antibodies. Acta Obstet Gynecol Scand 1993; 72:63–66.

43. Valenise H, Vaquero E, De Carolis C. Normal fetal growth in women with antiphospholipid syndrome treated with high-dose intravenous immunoglobulin. Prenat Diagn 1995; 15:509–517.

44. Leen CLS, Yap PL, McClelland DBL. Increase of serum immunoglobulin level into the normal range in primary hypogammaglobulinaemia by dosage individualisation of intrave-nous immunoglobulin. Vox Sang 1986; 51:278–286.

45. Wilfert CM, Buckley RH, Mohanakumar T, et al. Persistent and fatal central nervous sys-tem echovirus infections in patients with agammaglobulinemia. N Engl J Med 1977; 296:1485–1489.

46. Bardelas JA, Winkelstein JA, Seta DSY. Fatal ECHO 24 infection in a patient with hypogammaglobulinemia: relationship to dermatomyositis-like syndrome. J Pediatr 1977; 90:396–399.

47. Weiner LS, Howell JT, Langford MP. Effect of specific antibodies on chronic echovirus type 5 encephalitis in a patient with hypogammaglobulinemia. J Infect Dis 1979; 140:858–863.

48. Mease PJ, Ochs HD, Wedgwood RJ. Successful treatment of ECHO virus meningoencephalitis and myositis-fasciitis with intravenous immune globulin therapy in a patient with X-linked agammaglobulinemia. N Engl J Med 1981; 304:1278–1281.

49. Dwyer JM, Erlendsson K. Intraventricular gamma-globulin for the management of enterovirus encephalitis. Pediatr Infect Dis J 1988; 7:S30–S33.

50. McKinney RE, Katz SL, Wilfert CM. Chronic enteroviral meningoencephalitis in agammaglobulinemic patients. Rev Infect Dis 1987; 9:334–356.

51. Duhem C, Dicato MA, Ries R. Side-effects of intravenous immune globulins. Clin Exp Immunol 1994; 97(suppl 1):79–83.

52. Schiff RI. Intravenous gammaglobulin, 2: pharmacology, clinical uses and mechanisms of action. Pediatr Allergy Immunol 1994; 5:127–156.

53. Roberton DM, Hosking CS. Use of methylprednisolone as prophylaxis for immediate adverse infusion reactions in hypogammaglobulinemic patients receiving intravenous immunoglobulin: a controlled trial. Aust Ped J 1988; 24:174–177.

54. Lederman HM, Roifman TM, Lavi S, Gelfand EW. Corticosteroids for prevention of adverse reactions to intravenous immune serum globulin infusions in hypogammaglobulinemic patients. Am J Med 1986; 81:443–446.

55. Vyas GN, Perkins HA, Fudenberg HH. Anaphylactoid tranfusion reactions associated with anti-IgA. Lancet 1968; 2:312–315.

56. Schmidt AP, Taswell HF, Gleich GJ. Anaphylactic transfusion reactions associated with anti-IgA antibody. N Engl J Med 1969; 280:188–193.

57. Burks AW, Sampson HA, Buckley RH. Anaphylactic reactions after gamma globulin administration in patients with hypogammaglobulinemia. N Engl J Med 1986; 314:560–564.

58. Björkander J, Hammarström L, Smith CIE, Buckley RH, Cunningham-Rundles C, Hanson LÅ. Immunoglobulin prophylaxis in patients with antibody deficiency syndromes and anti-IgA antibodies. J Clin Immunol 1987; 7:8–15.

59. Ferreira A, Garcia Rodriguez MC, Fonta G. Follow-up of anti-IgA antibodies in primary immunodeficient patients treated with gammaglobulin. Vox Sang 1989; 56:218–222.

60. Ropars C, Caldera LH, Griscelli C, Homberg JC, Salmon C. Anti-immunoglobulin antibodies in immunodeficiencies: their influence on intolerance reactions to γ-globulin administration. Vox Sang 1974; 27:294–301.

61. Björkander J, Cunningham-Rundles C, Lundin P, Olsson R, Söderström R, Hanson LÅ. Intravenous immunoglobulin prophylaxis causing liver damage in 16 of 77 patients with hypogammaglobulinemia or IgG subclass deficiency. Am J Med 1988; 84:107–111.

62. Bjøro K, Froland SS, Yun Z, Samdal HH, Haaland T. Hepatitic C infection in patients with primary hypogammaglobulinemia after treatment with contaminated immune globulin. N Engl J Med 1994; 331:1607–1611.

63. Lane RS. Non-A, non-B hepatitis from intravenous immunoglobulin. Lancet 1983; 2:974–975.

64. Lever AML, Webster ADB, Brown D, Thomas HC. Non-A, non-B hepatitis occurring in agammaglobulinaemic patients after intravenous immunoglobulin. Lancet 1984; 2:1062–1064.

65. Webster ADB, Lever AML. Non-A, non-B hepatitis after intravenous gammaglobulin. Lancet 1986; 1:322–323.

66. Ochs HD, Fischer SH, Virant FS, Lee ML, Kingdon HS, Wedgwood RJ. Non-A, non-B hepatitis and intravenous immunoglobulin. Lancet 1985; 1:404–405.

67. Ochs HD, Fischer SH, Virant FS, et al. Non-A, non-B hepatitis after intravenous gammaglobulin. Lancet 1986; 1:322–323.

68. Weiland O, Mattsson L, Glaumann H. Non-A, non-B hepatitis after intravenous gammaglobulin. Lancet 1986; 1:976–977.

69. Williams PE, Yap PL, Gillon J, Crawford RJ, Urbaniak SJ, Galea G. Transmission of non-A, non-B hepatitis by pH4-treated intravenous immunoglobulin. Vox Sang 1989; 57:15–18.

70. Leen CLS, Yap PL, Neill G, McClelland DBL, Westwood A. Serum ALT levels in patients with primary hypogammaglobulinaemia receiving replacement with intravenous immunoglobulin or fresh frozen plasma. Vox Sang 1986; 50:26–32.

71. CDC. Outbreak of hepatitis C associated with intravenous immunoglobulin administration—United States, October 1993–June 1994. MMWR 1994; 43:505–509.

72. Rousell RH, Good RA, Pirofsky B, Schiff RI. Non-A non-B hepatitis and the safety of intravenous immune globulin, pH 4.2: a retrospective survey. Vox Sang 1988; 54:6–13.

73. Lee ML, Courter SG, Tait D, Kingdon HS. Long-term evaluation of intravenous immune

globulin preparation with regard to non-A, non-B hepatitis safety. Viral Hepatitis Liver Dis 1988; 596–599.

74. Rousell RH, Budinger MD, Pirofsky B, Schiff RI. Prospective study on the hepatitis safety of intravenous immunoglobulin, pH 4.25. Vox Sang 1991; 60:65–68.

75. Buckley RH. Plasma therapy in immunodeficiency diseases. Am J Dis Child 1972; 124:376–381.

76. Berger M, Cupps TR, Fauci AS. Immunoglobulin replacement therapy by slow subcutaneous infusion. Ann Intern Med 1980; 93:55–56.

77. Ugazio AG, Duse M, Plebani A, Notarangelo LD, Burgio GR. Subcutaneous infusion of gamma globulins in the management of agammaglobulinemic patients. Birth Defects: Original Article Series 1983; 19:213–215.

78. Schiff RI, Sedlak D, Buckley RH. Rapid infusion of Sandoglobulin in patients with primary humoral immunodeficiency. J Allergy Clin Immunol 1991; 88:61–67.

79. Polmar SH, Smith TF, Pirofsky B, Cox DG, Rechtman D. Rapid infusion of intravenous immunoglobulin in patients with primary immunodeficiency diease. J Allergy Clin Immunol 1992; 89:166A.

80. Ashida ER, Saxon A. Home intravenous immunoglobulin therapy by self-administration. J Clin Immunol 1986; 6:306–309.

81. Ochs HD, Lee ML, Fischer SH, Delson ES, Chang BS, Wedgwood RJ. Self-infusion of intravenous immunoglobulin by immunodeficient patients at home. J Infect Dis 1987; 156:652–654.

82. Sorensen RU, Kallick MD, Berger M. Home treatment of antibody-deficiency syndromes with intravenous immune globulin. J Allergy Clin Immunol 1987; 80:810–815.

83. Kobayashi RH, Kobayashi AD, Lee N, Fischer S, Ochs HD. Home self-administration of intravenous immunogloublin therapy in children. Pediatrics 1990; 85:705–709.

84. Daly PB, Evans JH, Kobayashi RH, et al. Home-based immunoglobulin infusion therapy: quality of life and patient health perceptions. Ann Allergy 1991; 67:504–510.

15

Intravenous Immunoglobulin Treatment for IgG Subclass Deficiency

Thomas F. Smith

Washington University School of Medicine, St. Louis Children's Hospital, St. Louis, Missouri

INTRODUCTION

Antibody replacement using human gammaglobulin is essential in the treatment of patients with profound deficiency of immunoglobulin (1). Deficiency of IgG subclasses has been associated with a number of immunodeficiency syndromes; the discussion below addresses IgG subclass deficiency as a distinct entity. Assessing efficacy of intravenous immunoglobulin (IVIG) (or any form of therapy) for patients who have selective deficiency of IgG subclasses will be difficult until confusion about this syndrome has been resolved.

HOST DEFENSE AGAINST INFECTIONS

The main source of confusion about IgG subclass deficiency (IgGSD) is disagreement about the role of a given subclass of IgG in host defense against infection. Specifically, although it is clear that there is a relationship between decreased serum levels of IgG subclasses and increased susceptibility to infection (2–17), it is unlikely that there is a direct cause-and-effect relationship (18,19). Previous consideration was given to the possibility that certain antibody responses were restricted to one IgG subclass. In particular, early reports of a correlation between serum IgG2 concentrations and the antibody response to bacterial polysaccharide antigens (20) suggested that patients who were IgG2-deficient experienced recurrent respiratory infections with encapsulated pathogens such as *Haemophilus influenzae* and *Streptococcus pneumoniae* because of their decreased ability to make IgG2. In truth, distribution of antibody responses to carbohydrate antigens appears to depend on both the antigen (21) and the age of the subject (22), and there is not a direct relationship between antigen type and selective IgG subclass expression. Furthermore, healthy individuals who have no IgG2 have been reported (23–26); in most cases, this absence was shown to be the result of deletions of the gamma-2 heavy-chain constant region gene. Not unexpectedly, these patients have a skewed pattern of antipolysaccharide antibodies, with a shift to IgG1 and IgG3 (26-28). Their well-being argues that IgG2 is not essential for host defense.

There has also been discussion that protection against infection might be mediated more effectively by antibodies in one subclass than another. For example, Swedish investigators found that the serum of otitis-prone children contained less IgG2 antibody to pneumococcal polysaccharides than did the serum of normal children (29,30). Differences between subclasses in affinity, avidity, neutralization capacity, and antibody-dependent cell-mediated cytotoxicity have been demonstrated in vitro by Persson and co-workers (31,32). On the other hand, several studies have demonstrated that IgG1 and IgG2 are equally protective in complement-mediated bacteriolysis or rat protection activity in vivo against *H. influenzae* (33,34).

Although it does not appear that an inability to produce an adequate level of an IgG subclass directly causes deficiency of antibody, it seems likely that the patients with deficiency of a subclass who experience recurrent infections do so because of poor antibody responses that result from underlyng aberrations in T-cell and B-cell interaction and function (18). Oxelius's report in 1974 documented that her patients with IgGSD had absent antibody responses to bacterial polysaccharide antigens (3), and this association has been found in subsequent studies in which both IgG subclass levels and antibody levels or responses have been measured in the same patients (9,17,22,35–37). It should be noted that patients with recurrent infections who have low levels of a subclass often are unable to make antibodies in other subclasses (17,38). It seems an omission that many reports of patients with IgG subclass deficiencies have not included any assessment of antibody-forming capacity.

The inability to produce specific antibodies has also been well documented in patients with normal serum total IgG as well as normal serum levels of IgG subclasses (39–44); this is often termed "selective antibody deficiency." The classic example of this is Wiskott-Aldrich syndrome, in which patients are unable to make antipolysaccharide antibodies but have normal levels of all IgG subclasses (including IgG2) (45). It is unfortunate that reports that have found patients with antibody deficiency with or without abnormal levels of IgG subclasses often seem to emphasize the IgG subclass levels rather than the antibody deficiency.

IVIG THERAPY IN PATIENTS WITH IgGSD

No one would argue that inability to produce specific antibodies is an acceptable reason to consider antibody replacement therapy. In light of the discussion in the previous section, it would seem reasonable to request measurement of antibody responses as part of the assessment of patients with recurrent infections who are not hypo- or agammaglobulinemic before instituting such therapy. The presence or absence of this information should be kept in mind in addressing studies of the use of IVIG in patients with IgGSD.

There have been three prospective studies that address the diagnosis of subsequent treatment of patients with IgGSD. My colleagues and I studied the effect of IVIG in a prospective, double-blind, placebo-controlled trial in 50 children with chronic chest symptoms (46). We measured serum immunoglobulin levels, IgG subclass levels, and antibody levels to diphtheria, tetanus, and 12 pneumococcal serotypes before and after immunization, before treatment. During the study, children in both IVIG and placebo groups were remarkably well compared with how they had been prior to the study. Children who received IVIG experienced a decrease in both upper and lower respiratory tract symptoms compared with those who received placebo. We found no relationship between immunoglobulin or antibody measurements and clinical symptoms, medicine use, or improvement in either treatment group. We suggested that IVIG might benefit host defense specifically or nonspecifically, apart from provision of antibodies against infectious agents, because we did not detect a difference between our treatment groups in number of infections. This may have been the result of the low frequency of infections in both groups.

Söderström et al. studied the effect of IVIG in 43 adults with IgGSD using a prospective blind crossover protocol; 19 were later included in an open study using a higher dose of IVIG (18). No measurements of antibody levels or responses were made. The authors reported at a symposium that the patients receiving IVIG experienced a significant reduction in days with infections. Results for individual subjects were not included in the published report, and it is not possible to determine if all or only a subset of their subjects actually achieved benefit. It is not clear whether the outcome of the open study was included.

Bernatowska-Matuszkiewicz and co-workers conducted a prospective open trial in which they administered IVIG for 1 year to 20 children with "severe chest disease," including recurrent sinopulmonary infections (11 children) or steroid-dependent asthma (19 children) (47). Twenty of the 30 subjects had low serum levels of one or more IgG subclasses, including nine with deficiency only of IgG3 $\pm$ IgG4. The authors reported that mean IgG and IgM antibody titers to pneumococcal polysaccharides in these children were comparable to those obtained in 10 healthy children within the same age range, although what is meant by mean antibody titers and the details of the assay(s) used was not specified. Clinical improvement as documented by days in hospital, use of antibiotics, and use of steroids was seen in the study group as a whole and in the nine subjects with IgG3 deficiency. Results for individual subjects were not included in this report either, and again it is not possible to determine if all or only a subset of their subjects actually achieved benefit. Because the IgG3-deficient patients benefited from an IVIG preparation that contained only trace amounts of IgG3, the authors concluded that the mode of action of IVIG was not from replacement of a deficient isotype. They speculated that the benefit might come from preventing repeated viral infections.

Knutson reported the initiation of a multicenter, double-blind, placebo-controlled trial of IVIG in children with selective IgG2 deficiency and/or impaired antibody responses to bacterial capsular polysaccharide antigens (48), but the study could not be completed because of insufficient enrollment. Apparently this was in part because the investigators chose poor antibody response to pneumococcal serotype 3 as an inclusion criterion, when virtually everyone responds to type 3 antigen (49). Furthermore, it has been suggested that potential subjects and their parents were unwilling to risk being assigned to the placebo arm of the study.

There also are a number of anecdotal testimonials or reports of limited numbers of subjects concerning the use of IVIG in patients with IgGSD (14,36,50–54) (see Table 1), all of which are provocative but should be viewed as preliminary. The authors of these studies have all suggested that prospective studies would be warranted.

For example, Page et al. reported improvement during IVIG therapy in clinical outcome and pulmonary function tests in four of five children with asthma who also had IgGSD (14). Two of the five were said to have normal functional antibody titers,

Table 1 Reports of the Effect of IVIG in Patients with IgGSD

Reference No.	46	18	47	14	36	50	51	52	53	54
No. of subjects (adults or children)	50 child	43[a] adult	30 child	5 child	9 child	10 adult	NG[b]	3 child	1 adult, 3 child	1 adult
IgGSD[c]	S (mixed)	A (mixed)	S (mixed)	A (mixed)	S (IgG2)	A (mixed)	A (IgG4)	A (mixed)	A (mixed)	A (IgG3)
Antibody responses	Y	N	N	Y	Y	N	N	Y	Y	N
Double-blind	Y	Y	N	N	N	N	N	N	N	N
Placebo-controlled	Y	Y	N	N	N	N	N	N	N	N
Dose of IVIG (mg/kg)	200 q3wk	25 mg/wk	400 q4wk	1–300 q4wk	3–400 q3–4wk	NG	NG	NG	1–300 q4wk	400 q4wk
Duration	7 doses	1 yr/ arm	1 yr	10–30 mos	1 yr	NG	NG	NG	6 mo–2 yr	NG
Benefit	Y	Y	Y	4/5	Y	Y	Y	Y	Y	Y
Benefit by IgG subclass?[d]	N	N	N	N	Y	?	?	?	?	N

[a]19 subjects received 59 mg/kg/wk for an additional 6 months in an open trial.
[b]NG = not given in the report.
[c]Denotes whether all (A) or only some (S) patients had IgGSD and which IgG subclasses were deficient.
[d]Y = IgGSD predicted benefit; N = IgGSD did not predict benefit or IVIG did not contain significant amounts of deficient IgG subclass (IgG3).

although it is difficult to determine this from the results presented. The one subject whose symptoms were unchanged by IVIG had low pneumococcal antibodies before and after immunization. The authors suggested a number of possible explanations for the improvement seen in the other four children, primarily relating to provision of passive immunity.

Another such report was from Silk and co-workers, who studied the effect of open treatment with IVIG in nine children who were experiencing recurrent sinopulmonary infections and had a poor response to immunization with the unconjugated *H. influenzae* type b (Hib) vaccine (36). Five of the children had IgGSD (specifically, deficiency of IgG2), and four had normal IgG subclass levels. All patients had fewer episodes of sinusitis and otitis media while receiving IVIG. All also had a significant increase in total serum IgG, IgG2, and IgG anti-Hib antibodies. It should be noted that in this study the five children with IgG2 deficiency could not be distinguished clinically from those with normal IgG2.

The prospective studies cited above argue strongly against using IgG subclass levels as criteria for treatment with IVIG. On the other hand, it is reasonable to consider treatment of patients who have selective antibody deficiency with IVIG as antibody replacement therapy. Selective antibody deficiency cannot be detected reliably by measuring levels of IgG subclasses. As noted above, patients with normal levels of IgG subclasses may have deficiencies of specific antibodies, and patients with deficiencies of IgG subclasses may have normal specific antibody levels and be healthy. Nonetheless, selective antibody deficiency can be approached successfully through the combination of past medical history and measurement of specific antibody responses.

SELECTIVE ANTIBODY DEFICIENCY

Although ongoing research may expand its role in the future, at present the decision to treat a patient with IVIG should be based on documentation of the inability to make appropriate amounts of antibodies in response to appropriate challenges in the context of significant clinical symptoms. The use of multiple protein and polysaccharide antigens for challenge of the immune system makes overestimating antibody-forming capacity unlikely; therefore, empirical trials of antibody replacement therapy for the most part are unwarranted.

The optimum dose and frequency of administration of IVIG for a given patient are those which produce optimum clinical improvement. In the case of hypogammaglobulinemia, this usually occurs when serum IgG levels are maintained at about the mean concentration found in healthy individuals. Obviously, serum level of IgG is not a useful measurement in adjusting dosing of IVIG for children who have IgG subclass or selective antibody deficiencies but normal levels of IgG. Although levels of specific antibodies may be measured after IVIG is administered (55,56), they have not been used to adjust dosing of IVIG in antibody-deficient patients. Roifman et al. demonstrated that patients with hypogammaglobulinemia and chronic lung disease experienced a decrease in the frequency of infections and improvement in pulmonary function when treated with high-dose (600 mg/kg) IVIG compared to low-dose IVIG (300 mg/kg) (57). The dose and frequency of IVIG for a given patient should be adjusted according to clinical response. Although the dose of IVIG often needs to be increased above that used initially, the frequency of dosage can often be decreased after a satisfactory clinical state has been achieved. It should be noted that dosages needed cannot be realistically achieved using intramuscular replacement therapy. They can apparently be achieved when IVIG is given subcutaneously in immunodeficient patients (58–60). Multiple suitable IVIG preparations are available in the United States. Although these are not identical products (61), there is little to suggest that any one is more effective than another in the treatment of patients with antibody deficiency diseases.

It has been asserted that children whose deficiency of antibody or IgG might resolve eventually should not receive IVIG because of worries about (1) cost and efficacy of therapy; (2) negative effect of exogenous immunoglobulin on endogenous antibody production, especially on acquisition of future antibody responses; and (3) risk of production of antiallotype antibodies that might be harmful (e.g., immunizing girls against allotypes that might appear in future pregnancies). In our prospective study of the use of IVIG in children with chronic chest symptoms (46), we could not substantiate that the latter occurs, and we detected no effect of IVIG on IgG levels after treatment with IVIG was discontinued. No data support the hypothesis that a course of IVIG will alter immunological responsiveness after treatment is stopped. The beneficial effect of IVIG in treating patients with hypogammaglobulinemia is clear, and there is sufficient evidence to support its use in patients with selective antibody deficiencies. However, IVIG is expensive, and this alone would argue against its use in a patient who is well while receiving less expensive therapies such as prophylactic antibiotics.

It is unlikely that patients with congenital immunoglobulin deficiency disorders will begin producing antibodies; they generally require lifelong treatment with antibody replacement therapy. Those with common variable immunodeficiency also are likely to require lifelong treatment, although recovery of antibody function can occur. At present, however, the future immunological status of any single patient with selective antibody deficiency cannot be predicted with confidence. While adolescents and adults with selective antibody deficiency are likely to have a permanent defect, children with these syndromes may experience resolution of their clinical symptoms and immunological abnormalities over time (17). It should be noted that expansion of immunodeficiency over time is also possible (62). Routine reevaluation of children (and adolescents) not clearly shown to have a permanent immunological defect seems warranted.

CONCLUSION

The observation that there is a clinical association between IgG2 deficiency and recurrent respiratory tract infections has maintained interest in IgG subclasses. At present, however, there is little to support this or any subclass having an indispensable (if not unique) role in host defense. It is possible that there is a preferential relationship between a particular subclass and a set of V genes that results in special antibodies (or a certain specificity or affinity) in that subclass. Selective IgG subclass expression is certainly not absolute; antibody responses to most antigens may occur in multiple subclasses in various clinical situations. The presence of a low level of an IgG subclass suggests the possibility of a selective deficiency of antibody that is the result of underlying aberrations in T-cell and B-cell interaction and function. It is reasonable to consider treatment of patients who have selective antibody deficiency, with or without concomitant IgGSD, with IVIG as antibody replacement therapy.

REFERENCES

1. Huston DP, Kavanaugh AF, Rohane PW, Huston MM. Immunoglobulin deficiency syndromes and therapy. J Allergy Clin Immunol 1991; 87 (1 Pt 1):1–17.
2. Schur PH, Borel H, Gelfand EW, Alper CA, Rosen FS. Selective gamma-g globulin deficiencies in patients with recurrent pyogenic infections. N Engl J Med 1970; 284:631–634.
3. Oxelius V-A. Chronic infections in a family with hereditary deficiency of IgG2 and IgG4. Clin Exp Immunol 1974; 17:19–27.
4. Oxelius V-A. Quantitative and qualitative investigations of serum IgG subclasses in immunodeficiency diseases. Clin Exp Immunol 1979; 36(1):112–116.
5. Oxelius V-A, Laurell AB, Lindquist B, et al. IgG subclasses in selective IgA deficiency: importance of IgG2-IgA deficiency. N Engl J Med 1981; 304(24):1476–1477.
6. Smith TF, Morris EC, Bain R. IgG subclasses in non-allergic children with chronic chest symptoms. J Pediatr 1984; 105:896–900.
7. Braconier JH, Nilsson B, Oxelius VA, Karup-Pedersen F. Recurrent pneumococcal infections in a patient with lack of specific IgG and IgM pneumococcal antibodies and deficiency of serum IgA, IgG2 and IgG4. Scand J Infect Dis 1984; 16(4):407–410.
8. Björkander J, Bake B, Oxelius VA, Hanson LÄ. Impaired lung function in patients with IgA deficiency and low levels of IgG2 or IgG3. N Engl J Med 1985; 313(12):720–724.
9. Umetsu DT, Ambrosino DM, Quinti I, Siber GR, Geha RS. Recurrent sinopulmonary infection and impaired antibody response to antibacterial capsular polysaccharide antigen in children with selective IgG-subclass deficiency. N Engl J Med 1985; 313(20):1247–1251.
10. Beard LJ, Ferrante A, Oxelius VA, Maxwell GM. IgG subclass deficiency in children with IgA deficiency presenting with recurrent or severe respiratory infections. Pediatr Res 1986; 20(10):937–942.
11. Lane PJ, MacLennan IC. Impaired lung function in patients with IgA deficiency and low levels of IgG2 or IgG3. N Engl J Med 1986; 314:924–926.
12. Shackelford PG, Polmar SH, Mayus JL, Johnson WL, Corry JM, Nahm MH. Spectrum of IgG2 subclass deficiency in children with recurrent infections: prospective study. J Pediatr 1986; 108(5 Pt 1):647–653.
13. Umetsu DT, Ambrosino DM, Geha RS. Children with selective IgG subclass deficiency and recurrent sinopulmonary infection: impaired response to bacterial capsular polysaccharide antigens. Monogr Allergy 1986; 20:57–61.
14. Page R, Friday G, Stillwagon P, Skoner D, Caliguiri L, Fireman P. Asthma and selective immunoglobulin subclass deficiency: improvement of asthma after immunoglobulin replacement therapy. J Pediatr 1988; 112(1):127–131.
15. Söderström T, Söderström R, Avanzini A, Brandtzaeg P, Karlsson G, Hanson LA. Immunoglobulin G subclass deficiencies. Int Arch Allergy Appl Immunol 1987; 82(3–4):476–480.
16. Wong KS, Huang SC. IgG subclass deficiency in children with recurrent infections. Acta Paediatr Sin 1989; 30(3):165–171.
17. Shackelford PG, Granoff DM, Polmar SH, et al. Subnormal serum concentrations of IgG2 in children with frequent infections associated with varied patterns of immunologic dysfunction. J Pediatr 1990; 116(4):529–538.
18. Söderström T, Söderström R, Enskog A. Immunoglobulin subclasses and prophylactic use of immunoglobulin in immunoglobulin G subclass deficiency. Cancer 1991; 68(6 Suppl):1426–1429.
19. Shackelford PG. IgG subclasses: importance in pediatric practice. Pediatr Rev 1993; 14(8):291–296.
20. Siber GR, Schur PH, Aisenberg AC, Weitzman SA, Schiffman G. Correlation between serum IgG2 concentrations and the antibody response to bacterial polysaccharide antigens. N Engl J Med 1980; 303:178–182.

21. Scott MG, Briles DE, Nahm MH. Selective IgG subclass expression: biologic, clinical and functional aspects. In: Shakib F, ed. The Human IgG Subclasses: Molecular Analysis of Structure, Function, and Regulation. New York: Pergamon Press, 1990:161–183.

22. Smith TF, Bain RP, Schiffman G. Relationship between serum IgG2 concentrations and antibody responses to pneumococcal polysaccharides in children with chronic chest symtpoms. Clin Exp Immunol 1990; 80:339–343.

23. Hammarström L, Smith CIE. IgG2 deficiency in a healthy blood donor. Concomitant lack of IgG2, IgA, an IgE immunoglobulins and specific anti-carbohydrate antibodies. Clin Exp Immunol 1983; 51:600–604.

24. Lefranc MP, Lefranc G, Rabbitts TH. Inherited deletion of immunoglobulin heavy chain constant region genes in normal individuals. Nature 1982; 300:760–762.

25. Migone N, Oliviero S, de Lange G, et al. Multiple gene deletions within the human immunoglobulin heavy-chain cluster. Proc Natl Acad Sci USA 1984; 81:5811–5815.

26. Plebani A, Ugazi AG, Meini A, et al. Extensive deletion of immunoglobulin heavy chain constant region genes in the absence of recurrent infections: when is IgG subclass deficiency clinically relevant? Clin Immunol Immunopathol 1993; 68(1):46–50.

27. Hammarström L, Carbonara AO, DeMarchi M, Lefranc G, Lefranc MP, Smith CI. Generation of the antibody repertoire in individuals with multiple immunoglobulin heavy chain constant region gene deletions. Scand J Immunol 1987; 25:189–194.

28. Hammarström L, Carbonara AO, DeMarchi M, et al. Sublass restriction pattern of antigen-specific antibodies in donors with defective expression of IgG or IgA subclass heavy chain constant region genes. Clin Immunol Immunopathol 1987; 45:461–70.

29. Freijd A, Hammarström L, Persson MAA, Smith CIE. Plasma anti-pneumococcal antibody activity of the IgG class and subclass in otitis prone children. Clin Exp Immunol 1984; 56:233–238.

30. Freijd A, Oxelius V-A, Rynnel-Dagöö B. A prospective study demonstrating an association between plasma IgG2 concentrations and susceptibility to otitis media in children. Scand J Infect Dis 1985; 17:115–120.

31. Persson MA, Brown SE, Steward MW, et al. IgG subclass-associated affinity differences of specific antibodies in humans. J Immunol 1988; 140(11):3875–3879.

32. Mathiesen T, Persson MA, Sundqvist VA, Wahren B. Neutralization capacity and antibody dependent cell-mediated cytotoxicity of separated IgG subclasses 1, 3 and 4 against herpes simplex virus. Clin Exp Immunol 1988; 72(2):211–215.

33. Weinberg GA, Granoff DM, Nahm MH, Shackelford PG. Functional activity of different IgG subclass antibodies against type b capsular polysaccharide of *Hæmophilus influenzae*. J Immunol 1986; 136(11):4232–4236.

34. Amir J, Scott MG, Nahm MH, Granoff DM. Bactericidal and opsonic activity of IgG1 and IgG2 anticapsular antibodies to *Hæmophilus influenzae* type b. J Infect Dis 1990; 162(1):163–171.

35. Insel RA, Anderson PW. Response to oligosaccharide-protein conjugate vaccine against *Hæmophilus influenzae* B in two patients with IgG2 deficiency unresponsive to capsular polysaccharide vaccine. N Engl J Med 1986; 315:1584–1590.

36. Silk HJ, Ambrosino D, Geha RS. Effect of intravenous gammaglobulin therapy in IgG2 deficient and IgG2 sufficient children with recurrent infections and poor response to immunization with *Haemophilus influenzae* type b capsular polysaccharide antigen. Ann Allergy 1990; 64(1):21–25.

37. De Gracia J, Rodrigo MJ, Morell F, et al. IgG subclass deficiencies associated with bronchiectasis. Am J Respir Crit Care Med 1996; 153(2):650–655.

38. Hammarström L, Lefranc G, Lefranc MP, Persson MAA, Smith CIE. Aberrant pattern of anti-carbohydrate antibodies in immunoglobulin class or subclass-deficient donors. Monogr Allergy 1986; 20:50–56.

39. Rothbach C, Nagel J, Rabin B, Fireman P. Antibody deficiency with normal immunoglobulins. J Pediatr 1979; 94(2):250–253.

40. French MA, Harrison G. Systemic antibody deficiency in patients without serum immunoglobulin deficiency or with selective IgA deficiency. Clin Exp Immunol 1984; 56(1):18–22.

41. Knutsen AP, O'Connor DM. Antibody deficiency with normal immunoglobulins in a child with hypoplastic anemia. Clin Immunol Immunopathol 1985; 36(3):330–337.

42. Ambrosino DM, Umetsu DT, Siber GR, et al. Selective defect in the antibody response to *Haemophilus influenzae* type b in children with recurrent infections and normal serum IgG subclass levels. J Allergy Clin Immunol 1988; 81(6):1175–1179.

43. Herrod HG, Gross S, Insel R. Selective antibody deficiency to *Haemophilus influenzae* type B capsular polysaccharide vaccination in children with recurrent respiratory tract infection. J Clin Immunol 1989; 9(5):429–434.

44. Epstein MM, Gruskay F. Selective deficiency in pneumococcal antibody response in children with recurrent infections. Ann Allergy Asthma Immunol 1995; 75(2):125–131.

45. Nahm MH, Blaese RM, Crain MJ, Briles DE. Patients with Wiskott-Aldrich syndrome have normal IgG2 levels. J Immunol 1986; 137(11):3484–3487.

46. Smith TF, Muldoon MF, Bain RP, et al. Clinical results of a prospective, double-blind, placebo controlled trial of intravenous γ-globulin in children with chronic chest symptoms. Monogr Allergy 1988; 23:168–176.

47. Bernatowska-Matuszkiewicz E, Pac M, Skopcynska H, Pum M, Eibl MM. Clinical efficacy of intravenous immunoglobulin in patients with severe inflammatory chest disease and IgG3 subclass deficiency. Clin Exp Immunol 1991; 85(2):193–197.

48. Knutsen AP. Patients with IgG subclass and/or selective antibody deficiency to polysaccharide antigens: initiation of a controlled clinical trial of intravenous immune globulin. J Allergy Clin Immunol 1989; 84(4 Pt 2):640–645.

49. Herrod HG. Management of the patient with IgG subclass deficiency and/or selective antibody deficiency. Ann Allergy 1993; 70(1):3–8.

50. Björkander J, Oxelius V-A, Söderström R, Hanson LÅ. Immunoglobulin treatment of patients with selective IgG subclass and IgA deficiency states. Monogr Allergy 1988; 23:160–167.

51. Heiner DC, Lee SI, Kim K, Schoettler J. Replacement therapy in IgG4-deficient patients. Monogr Allergy 1988; 23:187–193.

52. Beard LJ, Ferrante A. IgG replacement therapy in IgG subclass-deficient children. Monogr Allergy 1988; 23:194–203.

53. Beard LJ, Ferrante A. Aspects of immunoglobulin replacement therapy. Pediatr Infect Dis J 1990; 9(8 suppl):S54–S61.

54. Snowden JA, Milford-Ward A, Reilly JT. Symptomatic IgG3 deficiency successfully treated with intravenous immunoglobulin therapy. Postgrad Med J 1994; 70(830):924–926.

55. Mankarious S, Lee M, Fischer S, et al. The half-lives of IgG subclasses and specific antibodies in patients with primary immunodeficiency who are receiving intravenously administered immunoglobulin. J Lab Clin Med 1988; 112(5):634–640.

56. Fischer SH, Ochs HD, Wedgwood RJ, et al. Survival of antigen-specific antibody following administration of intravenous immunoglobulin in patients with primary immunodeficiency diseases. Monogr Allergy 1988; 23:225–235.

57. Roifman CM, Levison H, Gelfand EW. High-dose versus low-dose intravenous immunoglobulin in hypogammaglobulinaemia and chronic lung disease. Lancet 1987; 1(8541):1075–1077.

58. Gardulf A, Björvell H, Gustafson R, Hammarström L, Smith CI. Safety of rapid subcutaneous gammaglobulin infusions in patients with primary antibody deficiency. Immunodeficiency 1993; 4(1–4):81–84.

59. Waniewski J, Gardulf A, Hammarström L. Bioavailability of gamma-globulin after subcu-

taneous infusions in patients with common variable immunodeficiency. J Clin Immunol 1994; 14(2):90–97.

60. Gardulf A, Andersen V, Björkander J, et al. Subcutaneous immunoglobulin replacement in patients with primary antibody deficiencies: safety and costs. Lancet 1995; 345(8946):365–369.

61. Greenbaum BH. Differences in immunoglobulin preparations for intravenous use: a comparison of six products. Am J Pediatr Hematol-Oncol 1990; 12(4):490–496.

62. Söderström T, Söderström R, Andersson R, Lindberg J, Hanson LÅ. Factors influencing IgG subclass levels in serum and mucosal secretions. Monogr Allergy 1988; 23:236–243.

16

Prevention of Infections in B-Cell Lymphoproliferative Diseases

Helen Griffiths and Helen Chapel
Oxford Radcliffe Hospital, Oxford, England

INTRODUCTION

Recurrent infections are a common clinical problem in patients with B-cell lympho-proliferative diseases such as chronic lymphocytic leukemia (CLL) and multiple my-eloma. Many of these patients are elderly, and infectious diseases are a major cause of morbidity and mortality in such a population; however, there is a higher rate of infection in such patients when compared with age-matched controls. Twomey followed 45 patients with CLL, 50 patients with multiple myeloma, and a control group of 50 patients of a similar age range who had survived myocardial infarction. The annual infection rate was five times higher in patients with CLL and 15 times higher in patients with multiple myeloma compared with the age-matched control group (Fig. 1). Infections contributed to the higher mortality in patients with CLL and multiple myeloma (1). The increased infection rate seen in patients with multiple myeloma is not reflected in other plasma cell disorders, such as Waldenstrom's macroglobulinemia or monoclonal gammopathy of uncertain significance (2) (Table 1). Prevention of infection in patients with CLL and multiple myeloma should considerably reduce morbidity and mortality in this group of patients, with subsequent improvement in quality of life (3).

CHRONIC LYMPHOCYTIC LEUKEMIA

Chronic lymphocytic leukemia is a clonal proliferation of B lymphocytes whose maturation is arrested. It is the most common leukemia in Europe and North America. Cases of T CLL are uncommon.

Incidence of Infection

The occurrence of infection in patients with CLL is not a new observation. In the 1930s infections were described as a complication of this disease, but the first large series in which considerable morbidity and mortality became apparent appeared in the 1950s

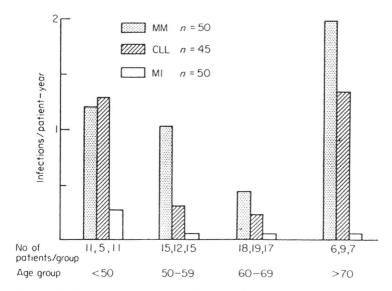

Figure 1 A comparison of rates of infection in patients with multiple myeloma, chronic lymphocytic leukemia, and age-matched controls (from Ref. 1). MM = multiple myeloma; CLL = chronic lymphocytic leukemia; MI - myocardial infarction.

(4,5). A more recent review of the literature suggests that infection will be a problem at some time in up to half of all patients with CLL (6).

Timing of Infections

Patients with advanced stages of disease tend to have an increased risk of infection whereas patients with early disease have fewer infections. In one large series, 159 infections were documented in 60 patients, with over half the infections occurring in those patients with advanced disease (7). This was confirmed more recently in a study of 59 unselected patients with CLL; patients with lower stages of disease tended to have fewer infections (Table 2) (8). The use of intensive chemotherapy regimens in those patients with progressive disease may further increase the risk of infection.

Table 1 Serious Infection Rates in Patients with Multiple Myeloma (MM), Waldenström's Macroglobulinemia (WM), or Monoclonal Gammopathy of Uncertain Significance (MGU)

	MM	WM	MGUS
Total number of patients	86	14	19
Observation period (months)	921	239	203
Mean observation period per patient (months)	11	17	11
Total number of deaths	26	4	1
Number of deaths due to infection	12	1	0
Serious infections	77	2	4
Serious infection rate (per patient per year)	1.0[a]	0.1	0.2

Source: Ref. 2.

[a]$P < .01$ (significant increase in infection rate in myeloma; cf. both other groups).

Table 2 Number of CLL Patients Divided According to Stage of Disease and Infection History

Stage of disease	Infection history			
	Minimal	Recurrent	Severe/multiple	Total
0	10	0	0	10
I	3	2	2	7
II	8	3	0	11
III	2	3	5	10
IV	7	3	11	21
Total	30	11	18	59

Source: Ref. 8.

Types of Infections

The type of infection seen in patients with CLL is predominantly bacterial. The organisms responsible are mainly encapsulated bacteria such as *Streptococcus pneumoniae* and *Haemophilus influenzae*. The majority of infections affect the upper and lower respiratory tracts, skin, and urinary tract with a significant incidence of septicemia (9). Viral infections, including herpes simplex and herpes zoster, have been noted in several published series though these are not common. Nineteen (19) out of 159 infections occurring in 60 patients in one series were of viral etiology, and 15 were due to herpes virus (7); however, over half of these infections were in patients with advanced disease, suggesting some impairment of cell-mediated immunity possibly as a result of chemotherapy.

Severity of Infections

Several studies over the past 40 years have shown that infection is a major cause of mortality in patients with CLL. In one large series, infection contributed to death in 85% of patients (10). However, many infections are probably not life-threatening provided they are diagnosed and treated effectively.

Mechanisms of Susceptibility to Infection

General

The preponderance of bacterial infections in patients with CLL suggests that the underlying defect is related to a functional abnormality of B lymphocytes, resulting in impaired antibody production in response to various antigens. Antigens are conventionally divided into thymus-dependent antigens such as proteins, which require T-cell help for the production of antibodies; and thymus-independent antigens such as bacterial polysaccharides, which directly stimulate specific B lymphocytes to induce antibody production. Thymus-independent responses are short-lived and induce poor immunological memory. The production of antibody in response to a variety of bacterial pathogens therefore requires the presence of functionally intact antigen presenting cells, B lymphocytes, and T lymphocytes. Impaired antibody production is likely to be due to defects in one or more of these components of the immune system.

Hypogammaglobulinemia

The first report of hypogammaglobulinemia secondary to CLL which resulted in infection was a case report by Jim and Reinhard in 1956 (11), although low levels of gammaglobulin had been reported in two patients with longstanding CLL as long ago as 1948 (12). With the introduction of better techniques for measuring gammaglobulin levels, Fairley and Scott (13) found in 1961 that 74 out of 110 patients had gammaglobulin levels below the lower limit of normal for their laboratory. Hypogammaglobulinemia may occur early in the disease but is often a late manifestation; several authors have reported a correlation between disease duration and low immunoglobulin levels (14) (Fig. 2). The prognostic significance of hypogammaglobulinemia has been addressed by a series of sequential studies on untreated patients with CLL. The presence of hypogammaglobulinemia significantly affected the probability of survival in this group of patients (15). More recent studies, using modern methods for the detection of isotype-specific immunoglobulins, have confirmed the finding of hypogammaglobulinemia in patients with CLL. Serum IgG levels were compared in a group of 59 randomly selected CLL patients attending outpatient clinics in Oxford with IgG levels in a group of 58 healthy individuals of similar ages (8). Over half the patients had serum IgG levels below the institutional lower limit of normal compared with none of the control group ($P = 8.8 \times 10^{-11}$). When patients were divided according to their infection history, there was a significant correlation between low IgG levels and severe or multiple infections ($P < .001$) (Fig. 3). There was a tendency for a long duration of the disease to be associated with low serum IgG levels, confirming the ear-

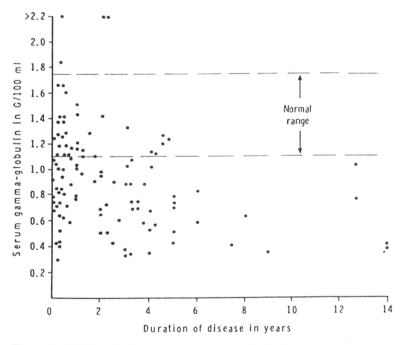

Figure 2 Relationship between serum gammaglobulin levels and duration of CLL. (From Ref. 13.)

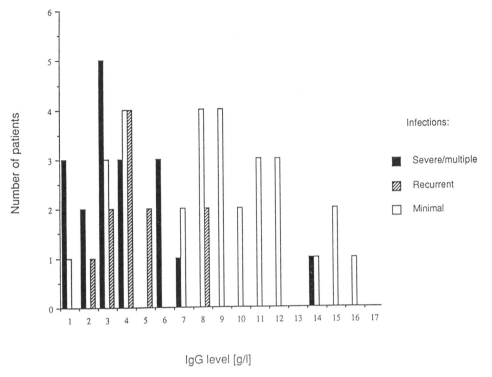

Figure 3   Infection history related to serum IgG level in patients with CLL. The lower limit of normal for IgG levels is 6.0 g/L.

lier findings of Fairley and Scott (13). In this study, low IgG levels tended to be associated with advanced stage of disease, but this did not reach significance (P = .08). Hypogammaglobulinemia appears to develop spontaneously during the course of the disease and is not related to chemotherapy. Forty-eight percent of patients with hypogammaglobulinemia in one study were untreated (9).

Specific Antibody Deficiency

Although hypogammaglobulinemia is associated with infections in many patients with CLL, there are patients with low IgG levels who do not suffer from recurrent infections. Levels of specific antibodies may be a better indicator of infection risk. In the Oxford study, lower pneumococcal IgG antibody levels were found in patients with CLL than in an elderly normal control group, and there was a clear correlation between low pneumococcal antibody levels and severe, multiple, or recurrent infections (P < .00001) (Fig. 4). Although low pneumococcal antibody levels showed a strong correlation with the presence of hypogammaglobulinemia in the CLL patients (P < .001), there were 12 patients (20%) with low serum IgG levels but normal pneumococcal antibody levels. Only two of these patients suffered from severe or multiple infections. In contrast, low pneumoccocal antibody levels in the presence of a normal total IgG were found in only three of the 59 patients studied.

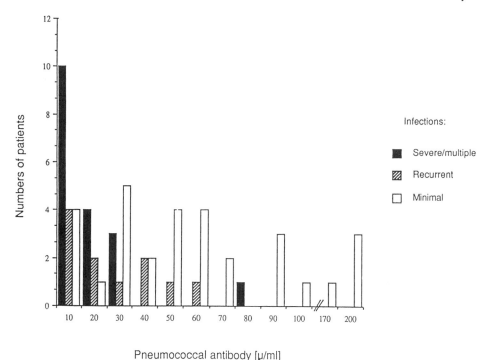

Figure 4   Infection history related to pneumococcal antibody levels in patients with CLL. The lower limit of normal for pneumococcal antibody levels is 20 U/ml.

Immunization Responses

Impaired production of antibodies to the pneumococcal capsular polysaccharide may reflect a more widespread impairment of response to other encapsulated organisms such as *Haemophilus influenzae*. Poor response to Pneumovax II, a pneumococcal vaccine, has been demonstrated in a group of patients with CLL when compared to an age-matched healthy control population. Only one of 13 CLL patients showed at least a twofold increase in IgG pneumococcal antibody levels following vaccination, compared with 13 of 13 controls, demonstrating impairment of the T-independent antibody response (A. M. O'Hay, personal communication). In this study, there was no attempt to correlate immunization responses with infection history. Immunization responses to diphtheria, typhoid, influenza, and mumps vaccines have also been studied in selected

Table 3   Relationship Between IgG and Pneumococcal Antibody Levels with Infection in Patients with CLL

Infection history	IgG normal; pneumococcal antibody normal	IgG normal; pneumococcal antibody low	IgG low; pneumococcal antibody low	IgG low; pneumococcal antibody normal
Minimal (N = 30)	21	1	3	5
Recurrent (N = 11)	1	1	4	5
Severe/multiple (N = 18)	2	1	13	2

patients with CLL, none of whom had been treated with steroids or cytotoxic therapy (9). All four antigens gave poor responses when compared with a normal control group. Similarly, Cone and Uhr (16) demonstrated impaired secondary antibody responses to diphtheria toxoid, presumed to have been encountered previously, in 10 untreated patients with CLL, all of whom were hypogammaglobulinemic. In addition, none of these patients responded to primary immunization with the bacteriophage øx 174. These studies demonstrate impaired responses to both T-dependent and T-independent antigens.

Cell-Mediated Immunity

Other factors affecting response to infection have been studied in patients with CLL. Miller and Karnofsy (17) showed poor skin recall antigen tests to tuberculin, mumps, and *Candida* antigens in 11 patients with CLL selected for recurrent infections when compared with 11 patients with no infection history. Cone and Uhr (16) studied eight untreated CLL patients for delayed-type hypersensitivity reactions to eight commonly encountered antigens and found that 50% of patients gave a positive response to only one antigen. We have recently looked at recall skin tests in 23 unselected CLL patients and found 48% of them to be anergic (J. North, unpublished data). There was no correlation between frequency of infection and anergy or between infection and treatment. In this study, chemotherapy was associated with poor recall skin testing and reduced numbers of circulating T lymphocytes, suggesting that some of the defective cell-mediated immunity in this group of patients follows chemotherapy.

Other Immune Defects

Other factors may be involved in susceptibility to infection. Neutropenia secondary to chemotherapy and defective complement activity have been suggested as additional reasons for infection risk. Neutrophils have been shown to be functionally normal in inflammatory exudates in patients with CLL (18), and complement abnormalities do not correlate with infection history (17).

Summary

The major immune defect contributing to the increased susceptibility to bacterial infection in patients with CLL is failure of polyclonal antibody production and the inability to respond to both T-dependent and T-independent antigens. Neutropenia may contribute to an increased risk of infection at some point in patients undergoing intensive chemotherapy.

MULTIPLE MYELOMA

Multiple myeloma is a progressive neoplastic proliferation of a single clone of plasma cells, resulting in the production of a monoclonal immunoglobulin. The rate of tumor growth is initially rapid in the preclinical phase, but as it becomes larger, the growth rate slows until at the time of presentation it has reached a plateau. Following successful chemotherapy, a stable plateau phase is attained.

Incidence of Infection

Several studies over the past 40 years have all demonstrated a high incidence of infection in patients with multiple myeloma. The exact incidence varies considerably with different studies due to varying methods of definition and classification of infection, the number of patients studied, and the period of study, In a retrospective study carried out from 1960 to 1980 involving 144 patients, 106 infections were recorded in 81 patients, a per-patient incidence of 56% (19). A more recent prospective study of 102 patients with multiple myeloma, monitored carefully over a 12-month period, confirmed the high incidence and high recurrent rates of infection (20). One hundred seventy-two episodes of infection were recorded in 84.8 patient years. Only 24 patients (23.5%) were infection-free during the study period; 56 patients (54.9%) suffered one infection, and 22 patients (21.6%) suffered more than one infection.

Timing of Infections

The risk of serious infection in patients with multiple myeloma varies with time after diagnosis. A small proportion of patients (5–14%) present with serious infection at the time of diagnosis (21). In the remaining patients, there appear to be three phases of susceptibility: the first three monthly immediately after diagnosis; the stable plateau disease phase; and the relapse phase. Infections are most frequent in periods of disease in which chemotherapy is used, especially in the initial treatment period and in relapse. In our study of 102 patients with myeloma, the infection rate during induction chemotherapy was 1.58 serious infections per patient-year (21 infections in 13.3 years of observation) compared with 0.49 in plateau phase (27 infections in 55.7 years) and 1.90 during relapse/progressive phase (30 infections during 15.8 years) (20). The increased rate of infection in the early period confirms the findings of Savage et al. (19), who also found an increased incidence of infection during periods of chemotherapy.

Type of Infection

Infections associated with the initial phase of the disease and relapse are of viral, fungal, and bacterial etiology, reflecting multiple defects in the immune response. During the stable plateau phase, infections are predominantly bacterial, with viral and fungal infections less frequent. The commonest sites of infection are the respiratory tract, urinary tract, and skin. Septicemia, though less frequent, is important because of its life-threatening nature. The organisms responsible are predominantly encapsulated bacteria such as *Streptococcus pyogenes* and *H. influenzae*. Gram-negative organisms such as *Escherichia coli*, *Klebsiella*, and *Proteus* species are commonly found in urinary tract infections and gram-negative septicemia. *Staphylococcus aureus* is the most common isolate from skin (1). Savage et al. (19) showed that the organisms responsible for infections in patients with myeloma were different at different stages of the disease, with Gram-negative organisms accounting for infections at times of neutropenia and encapsulated bacteria such as *S. pneumoniae* and *H. influenzae* at other times. Gram-negative bacilli and *S. aureus* accounted for 92% of infection-related deaths in this study.

Severity of Infections

The clinical severity of infections in patients with multiple myeloma is well described. Both Twomey (1) and Savage (19) have shown that infection is a major cause of death in up to one-third of patients. We found 78 episodes of serious infection in 49 patients during the study period (20). Thirty-three of these episodes were major infections, including pneumonia and septicemia. A third of these major infections were fatal (Table 4). Twenty-two patients suffered two or more serious infections during this period.

Mechanisms of Susceptibility to Infection

General

The type of infection seen in multiple myeloma patients with stable or plateau phase disease are typical of a depressed humoral immunity state and similar to that seen in patients with CLL, and primary antibody deficiency diseases. The contribution of chemotherapy and subsequent neutropenia to susceptibility to infection may be an important factor at other stages of the disease (Fig. 5).

Hypogammaglobulinemia

Polyclonal humoral immunosuppression is a major factor in susceptibility to infection in patients with myeloma. Some degree of nonparaprotein immunosuppression has been described in up to 90% of patients (19). The degree of immunosuppression has been shown to be related to the stage of disease at presentation (22). Nonparaprotein immunoglobulin levels have been shown to return to normal following intensive chemotherapy regimes (23).

A recent study to identify potential immunological risk factors predisposing to serious infection showed that 75% of patients studied demonstrated suppression of at least one nonparaprotein immunoglobulin class. Nonparaprotein serum IgG and IgA levels were both significantly reduced in patients with serious infections ($P < .001$)

Table 4 Types and Severity of Infection in Patients with Multiple Myeloma

Infection class	No. of infections
Minor	94
Moderate	45
Respiratory tract (B)[a]	19
Urinary tract (B)	10
PUO (U)	2
Skin (B)	2
Herpes zoster (V)	6
Other (U)	6
Major	22
Septicemia (B)	5
PUO/other (U)	3
Meningitis (B)	0
Pneumonia (B)	14
Resulting in death	11
Septicemia (b)	5
Pneumonia (b)	6
Total serious infection rate[b]	0.92

Source: Ref. 20.
[a]Infection type: B = bacterial; U = unknown; V = viral; PUO = pyrexia of unknown origin.
[b]Major and moderate infections per patient-year.

Infection in Myeloma

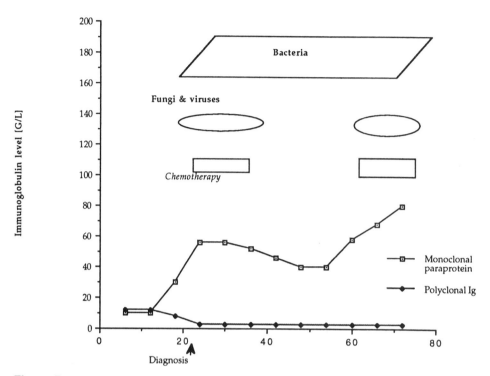

Figure 5   Types of infection during different stages of disease in multiple myeloma.

(20). Almost half of the patients with both low IgA and IgG2 levels (8/21) suffered from pneumonia compared with only a few of those patients (2/13) with normal serum levels for those two isotypes ($P = .16$). In this study there was no correlation between humoral immunosuppression and tumor load as assessed by clinical staging.

Specific Antibodies

Specific antibody levels have been suggested to be more sensitive markers of immunosuppression in myeloma. Low levels of antilipopolysaccharide antibodies have been reported in multiple myeloma in association with an increased risk of Gram-negative sepsis (24). We have found significantly low IgG antibody levels to both protein (diphtheria toxoid and tetanus toxoid) and carbohydrate (pneumococcal capsular polysaccharide) antigens when compared with an age-matched control population (20). Anti-*E. coli* lipopolysaccharide antibodies were also lower in the patient group, but the difference was not significant. Fifteen out of the group of 102 patients had low levels of both pneumococcal antibodies and *E. coli* antibodies and at least one serious infection since diagnosis compared with only two patients in this group with such low levels and no serious infections ($P = .035$). Patients with an IgG paraprotein showed significantly lower IgG pneumococcal antibody levels compared with patients with an IgA or light chain paraprotein ($P = .006$).

Immunization Responses

Impaired response to pneumococcal vaccine has been demonstrated in several studies of patients with multiple myeloma (25,26). Both of these studies showed suboptimal responses compared to healthy controls. More recently reported studies failed to demonstrate an association between immunization response and polyclonal immunosuppression and did not correlate response with susceptibility to infection (27,28). We have demonstrated impaired responses to immunization with both protein and carbohydrate antigens in patients with predominantly plateau phase myeloma (20). Thirty-eight percent of patients failed to respond to Pneumovax II, 35% failed to respond to tetanus toxoid, and 60% to diphtheria toxoid, suggesting impairment of both the T-independent and T-dependent pathways. There was a significant association between a poor IgG antibody, response to Pneumovax II, and the occurrence of septicemia. Five of 22 patients with poor or intermediate immunization responses had septicemia compared with none of the 18 good responders ($P = .03$). Poor response to Pneumovax II was not significantly associated with a poor response to tetanus or diphtheria toxoids, nor with disease stage.

Cell-Mediated Immunity

Both normal and impaired skin test response to commonly encountered antigens have been described in some patients with multiple myeloma (16,29). However, recurrent viral and fungal infections, characteristic of defects in cell-mediated immunity, do not occur with increased frequency in patients with plateau phase multiple myeloma.

Other Immune Defects

Specific complement component defects have been described in individual patients with multiple myeloma in addition to functional defects of the alternative pathway (30–32); however, no consistent pattern has emerged. Neutropenia is an important factor during periods of intensive chemotherapy.

Summary

Polyclonal humoral immunosuppression and inability to respond to immunization are the major factors resulting in increased susceptibility to bacterial infection in patients with multiple myeloma in the plateau or stable phase. The mechanisms responsible for this immunosuppression are not clear but are likely to be associated with defective regulatory mechanisms during cell proliferation or during synthesis and secretion of antibody. Antigen recognition processes have been shown to be intact (33).

OVERVIEW

The clinical features of infections in patients with CLL and myeloma resemble those in patients with primary antibody deficiency—namely, involvement of the upper and lower respiratory tract and skin with a similar range of bacterial pathogens. In all these conditions, the major immune defect is hypogammaglobulinemia and an inability to produce specific antibodies in response to bacterial pathogens. In patients with CLL and multiple myeloma, the hypogammaglobulinemia is likely to have developed much more rapidly than in patients with primary antibody deficiency disease and is unlikely to have preceded the onset of clinical disease. Patients rarely survive long enough to develop the chronic consequences of recurrent bacterial infection, especially of the respiratory tract since the diagnosis of polyclonal hypogammaglobulinemia is made earlier than with primary antibody deficiency disorders.

It is well established that patients with primary antibody deficiency benefit from regular parenteral immunoglobulin replacement with a reduction in bacterial infections, antibiotic requirements, and improved quality of life (34,35). Patients with hypogammaglobulinemia secondary to CLL and multiple myeloma should logically respond in a similar fashion.

IMMUNOGLOBULIN REPLACEMENT

Immunoglobulin replacement therapy for the secondary antibody deficiency disorders was initially tried in the 1960s in patients with CLL and multiple myeloma with intramuscular injections (36). However, results were poor due both to the low dose that can be given by this route and the lack of compliance with these painful, weekly injections, which were not well tolerated. The method of choice for replacement therapy in most cases of primary antibody deficiency disorders is with intravenous immunoglobulin (IVIG) (37), which can be given safely and in much larger doses than by the intramuscular route. This raised the possibility of IVIG replacement therapy in patients with secondary antibody deficiency disorders. Besa (38) published anecdotal reports on the beneficial effect of intravenous immunoglobulin in three patients with CLL; no new infections were reported during their period of treatment with IVIG at a dose of 300 mg/kg every 3–4 weeks. However, no infection data were presented on these patients. Similarly, Schedel (39) reported a reduction in the number of infections in patients with multiple myeloma and CLL treated with IVIG, though the crossover design of this study is questionable. Subsequent studies were undertaken formally to answer the question of whether IVIG would work in secondary antibody deficiency disorders.

Intravenous Immunoglobulin Replacement Therapy in CLL

Multicenter Study

A multicenter double-blind placebo-controlled study was designed to assess the effect of regular intravenous immunoglobulin replacement on the incidence of infections in patients with CLL. Eighty-one patients who were considered to be at risk of infection because of hypogammaglobulinemia, a history of infection, or both were randomized to receive either IVIG 400 mg/kg or an equivalent volume of normal saline every 3 weeks for 1 year. The patients were carefully monitored throughout the study year for type, severity, and frequency of infections. Patients in the two treatment arms were well matched for age, sex, disease duration, stage of disease at diagnosis and entry, previous chemotherapy, infection history, hematological parameters, and serum IgG levels. (40). Bacterial infections were significantly less frequent in the group receiving IVIG ($P = .01$). There were 23 bacterial infections in the immunoglobulin-treated group and 42 in the placebo group. The incidence of viral and fungal infections was similar in the two groups, as was the proportion of patients who remained free from infection during the study period (Table 5). The sites of infection (Table 6) and the organisms isolated were typical of other studies of infection in patients with CLL (1).

Table 5 Types and Severity of Infection During Treatment and Placebo Periods

	Immunoglobulin	Placebo	P value
Bacterial infections			
Total	23	42	0.01
Major	8	11	0.25[a]
Moderate	10	21	0.026
Trivial	5	10	0.10
Viral infections			
Total	40	37	0.65
Major	2	3	
Moderate	6	7	
Trivial	32	27	
Fungal or candidal infections	3	2	
Patients free of any infection	13	11	0.68

Source: Ref. 40.
[a]For major and moderate bacterial infections combined, $P = .026$.

The reduction in bacterial infections was most marked in the 57 patients who completed the full year of study; 14 in 28 IVIG patients versus 36 in 29 controls ($P = .001$). The recurrence rate in individual patients was also reduced by IVIG. There was a reduction in the number of bacterial infections in patients with all stages of disease, the reduction being most marked in stage C patients. Patients who received IVIG remained free of serious bacterial infections for a longer period of time after entering the study than those receiving placebo ($P < .05$).

Crossover Study

A crossover study was subsequently performed using the same treatment regime in Oxford (41). After completion of the year of the multicenter study, seven patients went on to receive the alternative product every 3 weeks for a further 12 months. In addi-

Table 6 Sites of Infection During Treatment and Placebo Periods

	Number of bacterial infections	
Type of infection	IVIG group	Placebo group
Septicemia	5	3
Pneumonia	3	12
Other respiratory infections	4	7
Otitis media	1	1
Conjunctivitis	1	0
Dental abscess	1	4
Pericarditis	0	1
Skin or wound infection	5	8
Urinary tract	1	3
Pyrexia of unknown origin	2	3
Total	23	42

tion, four patients with low-grade non-Hodgkin's lymphoma with low serum immuno-globulin levels (originally entered into the multicenter study but not included in the analysis) also crossed over to the alternative product for a further year. A similar reduction in the number of bacterial infections was seen in the crossover study using the same dose of IVIG and the same infusion schedule.

There was a major reduction in life-threatening bacterial infections in the patients who received IVIG: nine episodes of 162 placebo treatment periods compared with none in 191 IVIG treatment periods ($P = .001$). Similarly, non-life-threatening bacterial infections were also reduced: 11 episodes in the saline period versus three during the IVIG period ($P = .033$) (Table 7). All serious infections tended to occur in periods when the serum IgG level was less than 6.4 g/L ($P = 0.046$).

Half-Life of IVIG in CLL

The half-life of IgG has been shown to be normal in patients with CLL (42), suggesting that the interval between infusions could be longer than 3 weeks. Furthermore, the data suggest that the catabolic rate of IgG is normal in patients with low-grade B-cell tumors. Serum samples taken at 3-month intervals from CLL patients on regular IVIG replacement therapy showed that the rate of postinfusion fall in IgG concentrations did not change over a year (42). This is reassuring evidence that, once a protective serum IgG level has been reached, a steady state is obtained. The level at which this is obtained, however, may vary in individual patients.

Treatment Schedule and Dose of IVIG

The optimal dose and treatment schedule for IVIG in patients with CLL has been further analyzed in subsequent studies (43). A prospective double-blind multicenter comparative study of two doses of IVIG, one equivalent to the dose used in the multicenter study (500 mg/kg every 4 weeks) and the other equivalent to half that amount (250 mg/

Table 7 Number and Infections According to Etiology and Severity During Placebo and Treatment Periods

	IVIG	Saline
Patients free of serious infections	6	1
Major		
Bacterial	0	9
Viral	1	1
Fungal	1	0
Total	2	10
Moderate		
Bacterial	3	11
Viral	3	0
Fungal	0	1
Unknown	1	1
Total	7	13
Trivial		
Total	23	22
Total cycles of therapy		
(3 weekly periods)	191	162

Source: Ref. 41.

kg every 4 weeks) was carried out over the course of a year in 34 patients with CLL. Eighteen patients were randomized to the low-dose group, and 16 to the high-dose group. Both groups were comparable with regard to age, sex, stage of disease, chemotherapy, and serum IgG level. The rate of infection was similar to that observed in IVIG-treated patients in previous studies.

There was no significant difference between the number of bacterial infections in the two groups. Eleven patients remained free from serious infection in the high-dose group, and 10 patients in the low-dose group ($P = .41$). There were five serious bacterial infections in the high-dose group and seven in the low-dose group ($P = .68$). Both dosage regimens in this study achieved trough serum IgG levels greater than 6 g/ L.

The effect of lower-dose immunoglobulin replacement therapy has been further studied in a group of patients with CLL who had a history of recurrent infections and hypogammaglobulinemia (44). Fifteen patients received 10 g gammaglobulin intravenously every 3 weeks. There was a significant reduction in the number of admissions to hospital ($P = .05$) and in the number of febrile episodes ($P = .004$) in the 169 patient-months of therapy compared with the 168 patient-months prior to therapy. There was also a reduction in the number of prescriptions for antibiotics from 78 to 56, but this reduction was not significant. These results suggest that the dose and/or frequency of IVIG may be reduced without compromising effectiveness.

Subcutaneous Immunoglobulin

Rapid subcutaneous infusions of preservative-free intramuscular immunoglobulin are currently being used in the treatment of selected patients with primary antibody deficiency disorders. This has been recommended as the preferred form of treatment in some patients because of the ease of administration, the low incidence of adverse reactions, and the lower cost (45,46). This method of administration has been assessed in a group of patients with secondary hypogammaglobulinemia (47). Seventeen patients (14 with CLL, one with lymphoma, and two with Waldenström's macroglobulinemia) were treated with subcutaneous immunoglobulin at a dose of 50 mg/kg weekly for a period of 6–43 months. There was a significant reduction in the number of hospital admissions due to infection ($P < .05$) and in the number of courses of antibiotics ($P < .05$) in the group as a whole while on treatment. Eleven of the 17 patients who benefited from this treatment showed a reduction in the time hospitalized due to infection from 272 days to 112 days. The remaining six patients experienced no beneficial effects; however, most of these patients were neutropenic at the time of infection. Although this method of administration of immunoglobulin caused an increase in baseline serum IgG levels after 6 months of therapy, the levels remained below normal. Higher doses of subcutaneous immunoglobulin may be required.

Intravenous Immunoglobulin Replacement Therapy in Multiple Myeloma

Multicenter Double-Blind, Placebo-Controlled Study

A randomized double-blind, placebo-controlled trial of IVIG was undertaken in a group of 82 selected patients with stable myeloma to determine whether IVIG was effective in the prevention of infection (48). To be eligible, patients had to be considered fit to travel to the hospital regularly for infusions and were expected to complete at least 6

Table 8 Number of Sites of Serious Infections Occurring in Patients with Multiple Myeloma on IVIG and Placebo

	IVIG	Placebo	P (two-tailed value)[a]
Septicemia	0	3	.045
Pneumonia	0	7	.005
Chest infections (other than pneumonia)	6	18	.0097
Urinary tract infections	8	5	NS
Skin sepsis/abscess/cellulitis	2	0	NS
PUO	2	0	NS
Other	1	5	NS
Total	19	38	

Source: Ref. 48.
[a]NS = not significant.

months of the study. Forty-one patients received intravenous infusions of IVIG, 400 mg/kg body weight, and 41 an equivalent volume of placebo (0.4% albumin) every 4 weeks on an outpatient basis. Sixty patients completed a full year on study. There were no differences between the treatment arms at entry or during the study period with respect to clinical or laboratory variables. The patients were closely monitored for infections, which were classified according to type, severity, and frequency. There was a significant reduction in the incidence of serious infections in the group receiving IVIG (Table 8). There were no episodes of life-threatening infections (septicemia or pneumonia) in the patients receiving IVIG, compared with 10 such episodes in the placebo group ($P = .002$). There were a total of 138 infective episodes in the study, of which 57 were serious; 19 serious infections occurred in 449 patient-months in the immunoglobulin arm compared with 38 in 470 patient-months in the placebo arm ($P = .019$). Forty-four of the 57 serious infections were bacterial. There were 15 serious bacterial infections in patients receiving IVIG compared with 29 in patients receiving placebo ($P = .05$). There was a reduction in the number of chest infections other than pneumonia; however, there was no reduction in the number of minor infections or skin infections, but these are not usually life-threatening. There was also a significant reduction in the recurrence rate of infections in individual patients receiving IVIG ($P = .021$) (Table 9). Although most of the patients suffered an infection by the end of the study, IVIG delayed the time to the first infection ($P = .008$). Fifty-four of the 82 patients had been immunized with Pneumovax II 1 month before the start of the infusions.

Table 9 Frequency of Infection in Patients with Multiple Myeloma on IVIG and Placebo

No. of infections	IVIG group	Placebo group
1	12	4
2	4	11
3	4	7
4 or more	4	4

Patients who had less than a twofold increase in IgG pneumococcal antibody level (i.e., poor responders) had maximum benefit from IVIG. There were six episodes of serious infection in 128 patient-months on IVIG compared with 16 episodes in 128 patient-months on placebo ($P = .033$) in the poor Pneumovax responders. There was no significant protection in those patients who had demonstrated a good IgG antibody response to Pneumovax.

SAFETY OF INTRAVENOUS IMMUNOGLOBULIN IN CLL AND MULTIPLE MYELOMA

Infusion-related effects of IVIG range in severity from mild adverse reactions such as headache, backache, and nausea to extremely rare anaphylactoid reactions. The frequency of nonanaphylactoid reactions in patients with primary antibody deficiency disorders having regular IVIG replacement therapy is reported to range from 1% to 15% of infusions (49). In the group of elderly patients with secondary antibody deficiency due to underlying lymphoid malignancy, there is a small but significant incidence of infusion-related reactions, particularly in patients with multiple myeloma. Reactions have been observed in the double-blind studies in patients receiving both immunoglobulin and placebo, perhaps reflecting underlying pathology of the primary disease.

In the multicenter CLL study, minor adverse reactions were noted in less than 2% of infusions given: 16 reactions occurred in the immunoglobulin-treated group, and seven in the control group. Mild chills, fever, and sleepiness were the most frequent effects seen in the immunoglobulin-treated group. Chills, flushing, transient weakness, anxiety, and sleepiness were reported in the control group. In the study of IVIG in patients with multiple myeloma, adverse effects were more frequent but again minor, and occurred in both the control and treatment groups. Reactions occurred with 12% of immunoglobulin infusions and 5% of placebo infusions (Table 10). Three moderate reactions of rigors, vomiting, and hypotension responded to reduction in the rate of infusion and intravenous hydrocortisone. In this study, two patients developed renal failure while receiving IVIG. In retrospect, deterioration in renal function was present before their first infusion. No patient's serum creatinine rose more than 20 µmol/L during the study. A subsequent study of IVIG in patients with nephrotic syndrome has found transient rises in serum creatinine related to IVIG infusions, but no long-term sequelae (50). The administration of high-dose IVIG causes slight increases in plasma and whole blood viscosity (51), and could favor thrombosis in patients already at risk of thromboembolic events. However, such complications have not occurred in patients to whom replacement doses of IVIG have been given.

PATIENT SELECTION FOR PROPHYLACTIC INTRAVENOUS IMMUNOGLOBULIN REPLACEMENT THERAPY

These studies clearly demonstrate the efficacy of IVIG in the prevention of bacterial infections in patients with CLL and multiple myeloma; however, an appropriate selection of patients for IVIG replacement therapy needs to be addressed before recommend-

Table 10 Adverse Reactions in Multiple Myeloma Patients Receiving Either IVIG or Placebo

Adverse Reactions	IVIG	Placebo
Mild		
Lethargy/malaise	14	7
Shivers	7	6
Headaches	6	1
Felt cold	9	5
Nausea/vomiting/diarrhea	3	1
Epigastric pain	5	0
Drowsy	3	0
Fever	1	0
Blurred vision	1	0
Tingling tongue	1	0
Joint pain	0	1
Moderate		
Rigors and vomiting	2[a]	1
Hypotension	1	0
Total	53	23
	12% of infusions	5% of infusions

Source: Ref. 48.
[a]Same patient on two occasions.

ing its widespread use. The careful selection of patients with low levels of antibodies to pneumococcal capsular polysaccharide and impaired IgG antibody response to immunization are useful indicators of patients most at risk of infection.

COST-EFFECTIVENESS OF IVIG IN CLL AND MULTIPLE MYELOMA

The question of cost-effectiveness of prophylactic IVIG in patients with CLL has been raised by Weeks and colleagues (52) following independent analysis of the multicenter study of IVIG in patients with CLL using the views of oncologists rather than those of patients. It was suggested that this type of treatment is extremely expensive when compared with other treatments that are accepted as cost-effective. The clinical efficacy of IVIG was not questioned but was dismissed on theoretical and cost-effective grounds. To counter this analysis, a recalculation of the cost-effectiveness of IVIG was carried out by obtaining information directly from affected individuals, as recommended by Gill and Feinstein (53), on the use of IVIG and its impact on their quality of life. A vastly different response was obtained using this information, compared with that reported by expert physicians (3). Treatment with IVIG is costly, and an attempt has been made to reduce these costs by modifying the interval between infusions and the dose administered. The precise dose can be tailored to the clinical state of the patient and the incidence of breakthrough infections, as in primary antibody deficiency diseases (54).

CONCLUSIONS

Intravenous immunoglobulin can be given safely to patients with B-cell lympho-proliferative disease. It protects against life-threatening infections and reduces the risk of recurrent bacterial infections. Furthermore, it can be shown by appropriate financial costing to be cost-effective and to improve the quality of life in a carefully selected group of patients.

REFERENCES

1. Twomey J. Infections complicating multiple myeloma and chronic lymphatic leukaemia. Arch Intern Med 1973; 132:562–565.
2. Chapel HM, Lee M. The use of intravenous immunoglobulin in multiple myeloma. Clin Exp Immunol 1994; 97(suppl 1):21–24.
3. Lee ML, Chapel H, Brennan V, Gamm H, Dicato M, Courter SG. Quality of life assessments and clinical outcome measures in patients with B-cell lymphoproliferative disease receiving intravenous immune globulin. Proceedings of the 4th Conference on Biological Agents in Autimmune Disease, 1995. in press.
4. Osgood EE, Seaman AJ. Treatment of chronic leukaemias. Results of therapy by titrated, regularly spaced total body radioactive phosphorus, or roentgen irradiation. JAMA 1952; 150:1372–1379.
5. Scott RB. Chronic lymphatic leukaemia. Lancet 1957; 1:1162–1167.
6. Bunch C. Management of infection in chronic lymphocytic leukaemia. In: Gale RP, Rai K, eds. Chronic Lymphocytic Leukaemia: Recent progress, Future Directions. New York. Liss, 1987:373–381.
7. Travade P, Dusart JD, Cavaroc M, Beytout J, Rey M. Les infections graves associees a la leucemie lymphoide chronique: 159 episodes infectieux observes chez 60 malades. Presse Med 1986; 15:1715–1718.
8. Griffiths H, Lea J, Bunch C, Lee M, Chapel HM. Predictors of infections in CLL. Clin Exp Immunol 1992; 89:374–377.
9. Shaw RK, Szwed C, Boggs DR, et al. Infection and immunity in chronic lymphocytic leukaemia. Arch Intern Med 1960; 106:467–478.
10. Hansen MM. Chronic lymphocytic leukaemia. Clinical studies based on 189 cases followed for a long time. Scand J Haematol 1973; 18:(suppl)1–282.
11. Jim RTS, Reinhard EH. Agammaglobulinemia and chronic lymphatic leukaemia. Ann Intern Med 1956; 44:790–796.
12. Brown RK, Read JT, Wiseman BK, France WG. Electrophoretic analysis of serum proteins of blood dyscrasias. J Lab Clin Med 1948; 33:1523–1533.
13. Fairley HG, Scott BG. Hypogammaglobulinemia in CLL. BMJ 1961; 4:920–924.
14. Hudson RP, Wilson SJ. Hypogammaglobulinemia and chronic lymphatic leukaemia. Cancer 1960; 13:200–204.
15. Rozman C, Montserrat E, Viñolas N. Immunoglobulins in B-chronic lymphocytic leukaemia. Natural history and prognostic significance. Cancer 1988; 279–283.
16. Cone L, Uhr JW. Immunological deficiency disorders associated with chronic lymphocytic leukaemia and multiple myeloma. J Clin Invest 1964; 43:2241–2248.
17. Miller D, Karnofsky DA. Immunologic factors and resistance to infection in chronic lymphatic leukaemia. Am J Med 1961; 747–757.
18. Boggs DR. Cellular composition of inflammatory exudates in human leukaemia. Blood 1960; 15:466–475.

19. Savage D, Lindenbaum J, Garret T. Biphasic pattern of bacterial infection in multiple myeloma. Ann Intern Med 1982; 96:47–50.
20. Hargreaves RM, Lea JR, Griffiths H, et al. Immunological factors and risk of infection in plateau phase myeloma. J Clin Pathol 1995; 48:260–266.
21. Kyle R. Multiple myeloma: review of 869 cases. Mayo Clin Proc 1975; 50(1):29–40.
22. Pruzanski W, Gidon MS, Roy A. Suppression of polyclonal immunoglobulins in multiple myeloma: relationship to staging and other manifestations at diagnosis. Clin Immunol Immunopathol 1980; 17:280–286.
23. Gore ME, Selby PJ, Viner C, et al. Intensive treatment of multiple myeloma and criteria for complete remission. Lancet 1989; 332:879–882.
24. Stoll C, Schedel I, Peest D. Serum antibodies against common antigens of bacterial lipopolysaccharides in healthy adults and in patients with multiple myeloma. Infection 1985; 13:115–119.
25. Larson DL, Tomlinson LJ. Quantitative antibody studies in man: 11. The relation of the level of serum proteins to antibody production. J Lab Clin Med 1952; 39:129–134.
26. Zinneman HH, Hall WH. Recurrent pneumonia in multiple myeloma and some observations on immunologic response. Ann Intern Med 1954; 41:1152–1163.
27. Birgens HS, Esperson F, Hertz JB, Pederson FK, Drivsholm A. Antibody response to pneumococcal vaccination in patients with myelomatosis. Scand J Haematol 1983; 30:324–330.
28. Lazarus HM, Lederman M, Lubin A, et al. Pneumococcal vaccination: the response of patients with multiple myeloma. Am J Med 1980; 69:419–423.
29. Glenchur H, Zinneman H, Wendell H. A review of 51 cases of multiple myeloma. Arch Intern Med 1982; 103:173–183.
30. Cheson BD, Walker HS, Heath ME, Gobel RJ, Janatova J. Defective adherence of the third component of complement (C3) to *Streptococcus pneumoniae* in multiple myeloma. Blood 1984; 63:949–957.
31. Zurlo JJ, Schecter GP, Fries LF. Complement abnormalities in multiple myeloma. Am J Med 1989; 87:411–420.
32. Kraut EH, Sagone AL. Alternative pathway of complement in multiple myeloma. Am J Hematol 1981; 11:335–345.
33. Paglieroni T. MacKenzie MR. Studies on the pathogenesis of an immune defect in multiple myeloma. J Clin Invest 1977; 59:1120–1133.
34. Buckley RH. Long term use of intravenous immunoglobulin in patients with primary immunodeficiency diseases. Inadequacy of current dosage practices and approaches to the problem. J Clin Immunol 1982; 2 (April suppl):15–21.
35. Cunningham-Rundles C, Siegal FP, Smithwick EM, et al. Efficacy of intravenous immunoglobulin in primary humoral immunodeficiency disease. Arch Intern Med 1984; 101:435–439.
36. Fahey J, Scoggin R, Utz J, Swed C. Infection antibody response and gammaglobulin components in multiple myeloma and macroglobulinemia. Arch J Med 1963; 35:698–707.
37. Spickett GP, Misbah SA, Chapel HM. Primary antibody deficiency in adults. Lancet 1999; 337:281–284.
38. Besa EC. Use of intravenous immunoglobulin in chronic lymphocytis leukaemia. Am J Med 1984; 76:209–218.
39. Schedel I. Application of immunoglobulin preparations in multiple myeloma. In: Morell A, Nydegger U, eds. Clinical Uses of Intravenous Immunoglobulins. London: Academic Press, 1986:123–130.
40. Co-operative Group for the Study of Immunoglobulin in Chronic Lymphocytic Leukaemia. Intravenous immunoglobulin for the prevention of infection in chronic lymphocytic leukaemia, a randomised controlled clinical trial. N Engl J Med 1988; 319:902–907.
41. Griffiths H, Brennan V, Lea J, Bunch C, Lee M, Chapel H. Crossover study of immuno-

globulin replacement therapy in patients with low grade B-cell tumours. Blood 1989; 73:366–368.

42. Chapel HM, Lee M. Immunoglobulin replacement in patients with chronic lymphocytic leukaemia (CLL); kinetics of immunoglobulin metabolism. J Clin Immunol 1992; 12:17–20.

43. Chapel H, Dicato M, Gamm H, et al. Immunoglobulin replacement in patients with chronic lymphocytic leukaemia: a comparison of two dose regimes. Br J Haematol 1994; 88:209–212.

44. Jurlander J, Geisler CH, Hansen MM. Treatment of hypogammaglobulinemia in chronic lymphocytic leukaemia by low dose intravenous gammaglobulin. Eur J Haematol 1994; 53:114–118.

45. Gardulf A, Hammarstrom L, Smith CIE. Home treatment of hypogammaglobulinemia with subcutaneous gammaglobulin by rapid infusion. Lancet 1991; 338:162–166.

46. Thomas MJ, Brennan VM, Chapel HM. Rapid subcutaneous immunoglobulin infusions in children. Lancet 1993; 342:1432–1433.

47. Hammarström L, Samuelson J, Grimfors G. Subcutaneous gammaglobulin for patients with secondary hypogammaglobulinemia. Lancet 1995; 345:382–383.

48. Chapel HM, Lee M, Hargreaves R, Pamphilon DH, Prentice AG. Randomized trial of intravenous immunoglobulin as prophylaxis against infection in plateau-phase multiple myeloma. Lancet 1994; 343:1059–1063.

49. Duhem C, Dicato MA, Ries F. Side effects of intravenous immune globulins. Clin Exp Immunol 1994; 97(suppl 1):79–83.

50. Schifferli J, Leski M, Favre H, Imbach P, Nydeggar U, Davies K. High dose intravenous IgG treatment and renal function. Lancet 1991; 337:457–458.

51. Reinhart WH, Berchtold PE. Effect of high dose intravenous immunoglobulin therapy on blood rheology. Lancet 1992; 339:662–664.

52. Weeks JC, Tierney MR, Weinstein MC. Cost effectiveness of prophylactic administration of intravenous immune globulin in chronic lymphocytic leukaemia. N Engl J Med 1991; 324:81–86.

53. Gill TM, Feinstein AR. A critical appraisal of the quality of quality-of-life measurements. JAMA 1994; 272:619–626.

54. Chapel HM for the Consensus Panel for the Diagnosis and Management of Primary Antibody Deficiencies. Consensus on diagnosis and management of primary antibody deficiencies. Br Med J 1994; 308:581–585.

17

Etiology and Prevention of Infection Following Thermal Injury

Khan Z. Shirani, George M. Vaughan, Albert T. McManus, and Arthur D. Mason, Jr.,
U.S. Army Institute of Surgical Research, Fort Sam Houston, Texas

Basil A. Pruitt, Jr.
University of Texas Health Science Center, San Antonio, Texas

INTRODUCTION

The risk of nosocomial infection in the burned patient is proportional to the extent of injury. Local and systemic factors may promote such a relationship. Loss of the protective skin barrier and the need for invasive monitoring provide endogenous bacteria opportune access to the vulnerable tissues of the body and predispose the burned host to systemic infection. Though laboratory results suggest global immunosuppression in the immediate postburn period, infectious complications are usually delayed to the second week postburn or beyond in patients treated with current techniques. Progressive improvements in general patient care, fluid therapy of shock, wound management, patient isolation techniques, and effective management of pulmonary and other septic complications have significantly improved burn patient survival in recent decades (1). However, despite the recent improvements in burn patient management, infection remains the major cause of morbidity and mortality following extensive injury. In this chapter we review some of the pertinent causes of increased susceptibility of a burn

The opinions or assertions contained herein are the private views of the authors and are not to be construed as official or as reflecting the views of the Department of the Army or the Department of Defense.

Citations of commercial organizations and trade names in this report do not constitute an official Department of the Army endorsement or approval of the products or services of these organizations.

Human subjects participated in these studies after giving their free and informed voluntary consent. Investigators adhered to AR 70-25 and USAMRDC Reg 70-25 on Use of Volunteers in Research.

Research was conducted in compliance with the Animal Welfare Act and other Federal statutes and regulations relating to animals and experiments involving animals and in adherence with the Guide for the Care and Use of Laboratory Animals, NIH publication 80-23, 1985 edition.

patient to infection. In addition, we outline available measures that help reduce the risk of infection in patients with burn injury.

LOCAL HOST DEFENSES

Thermal injury destroys the protective skin barrier which ordinarily prevents bacterial entry to the underlying vital tissues of the body. Moreover, in the extensively burned patient the risk of infection is further amplified by the use of invasive therapeutic measures and monitoring devices that transgress normal anatomical barriers, function as foreign bodies, and may serve additionally as portals of bacterial entry. Further, prolonged hospitalization in an intensive care unit in which the patient may be exposed to multiple drug-resistant bacteria and may receive repetitive courses of perioperative antibiotics allows infection with organisms that are difficult to control.

Skin Defenses

Through a variety of mechanisms, normal skin offers a hostile environment to pathogenic bacteria. The low skin surface pH (5–6) retards bacterial growth, and its commensal flora helps quell the growth of several pathogens, including fungi, through competitive inhibition. Intact skin is impermeable to most pathogens, except *Staphylococcus aureus*, which may infect normal viable hair follicles or sweat glands. The anaerobic flora of skin is comprised of mostly *Propionibacterium* species that hydrolyze sebum triglycerides into fatty acids which exhibit antifungal and antibacterial properties (2). Most aerobic gram-negative bacilli, *Streptococcus pyogenes*, and *Staphylococcus* species are sensitive to these sebum-derived fatty acids. Through destruction of the normal chemical environment of the skin, burn injury facilitates microbial proliferation at the wound surface and thus increases the risk of burn wound infection. Use of systemic antibiotics for the treatment or prophylaxis of infection can alter the composition of normal body flora and render a burn patient vulnerable to superinfection with opportunistic organisms, including fungi and drug-resistant bacteria.

Airway Defenses

A unique combination of physical, cellular, and immunological attributes defends the respiratory tract against inhaled pathogens (3). The nasal hair, turbinates, and convolutions of the upper airways render inspired air turbulent. As a result, the inhaled particles striking against these anatomic barriers are deposited in the posterior nasopharynx for easy removal. The moist mucosal lining of the respiratory tract, covered with a thick mucous blanket, captures the inhaled organisms which are then propelled toward the nasopharynx by the mucociliary action of the epithelium, aided by the cough reflex (4). In the burn patient a defective cough mechanism, due for instance to smoke inhalation injury or an indwelling endotracheal or nasogastric tube, seriously impairs the ability of the airway to protect against inhaled pathogens, predisposing the patient to bronchopulmonary infection. Further, breathing of warm dry room air interferes with the removal of inspissated secretions, and should be avoided in patients with inhalation injury.

The removal of inhaled particles beyond the level of the terminal bronchioles, where the ciliated epithelium ends, is performed by alveolar macrophages (4) that first ingest the deposited material and then migrate either to the mucociliary area or traverse the pulmonary interstitium to arrive at terminal bronchioles for excretion in the airways (5). Less frequently, when the other two routes of disposal are overburdened, macrophages migrate via lymphatic channels. A disruption of the airway protective mechanisms due to inhalation injury, and the resultant tracheobronchitis and pneumonitis, increase the risk of pulmonary complications.

Microorganisms that evade the mechanical and biological barriers of the lung are handled through immunological mechanisms. Compared to systemic immunity, local airway immunity appears to provide better protection against previously encountered antigens (6). The upper respiratory tract is protected by IgA, IgE, and low-molecular-weight mediators; the lower respiratory tract is protected by IgG, IgM, and high-molecular-weight mediators. The most important respiratory tract defense against bacteria, however, is IgA, a product of plasma cells underlying the respiratory epithelium. IgA inhibits bacterial adherence to the respiratory mucosa and prevents microorganisms from establishing a nidus of infection in the nasopharynx and tracheobronchial tree (7).

Mucosal damage from inhalation injury compromises the mechanical barrier of the respiratory tract, attenuates the immunological responses of the lung, and predisposes the burn patient to pulmonary infection. In one study of 1058 burn patients admitted to this institute between 1980 and 1984, the incidence of pneumonia in patients with inhalation injury was 38%, as opposed to 9% in patients without inhalation injury (8).

SYSTEMIC HOST DEFENSES

Immunity Changes

Burns alter immunity depending on the extent of injury. Alone or conjoined, the humoral system, phagocytic function, and cell-mediated immunity mount a systemic response to infection. Polymorphonuclear leukocytes (PMNs; neutrophils), together with the humoral opsonic component of immunity, composed of complement and immunoglobulins, provide the first line of defense against invading bacteria. Complement aids immune adherence, PMN chemotaxis and phagocytosis, and the lysis of organisms. Complement, IgG, and IgM opsonize (coat) the bacteria and enhance phagocytosis and intracellular killing by the PMNs. Monocytes, T and B lymphocytes, and macrophages form the second line of defense against bacteria. Similar to those of PMNs, the chemotactic and phagocytic activities of monocytes are enhanced by complement and immunoglobulins. Macrophages process the microbial antigens and migrate to local and regional lymph nodes via lymphatics to initiate the production of specific antibodies. Separate from the effect of local barrier disruption at the sites of injury, severe thermal injury appears to evoke systemic inhibition of resistance to microbial invasion.

PMN Changes

Inflammation is the first and basic response to infection and constitutes a common pathway of immunological injury. Burn injury triggers a multitude of cellular and humoral responses that induce production and release of vasoactive mediators and cytokines. In the initial 24 h postburn, the cellular portion of the inflammatory exudate consists mainly of PMNs, which are later supplanted by peripheral blood mononuclear cells (lymphocytes and monocytes). The fluid portion of the exudate consists of IgG, IgM, and complement, which opsonize the offending organisms and facilitate their phagocytosis.

The predilection of a burn patient to infection depends in part on PMN dysfunction from thermal injury. In direct proportion to the extent of injury, burns suppress neutrophil chemotactic and phagocytic activities, both of which are restored by incubating PMNs in normal serum (9). Burns are reported to downregulate C5a receptor expression by the PMN and increase formyl-methionyl-leucyl-phenylalanine (FMLP) receptor expression, but reduce PMN responsiveness to FMLP stimulation, enhance CR1 and CR3 receptor expression, and increase the oxidative activity of resting PMNs. These findings are consistent with the notion of early activation of PMNs that may explain PMN hyporesponsiveness to subsequent infectious challenges in the burn patient.

Phagocytic cells kill bacteria through oxidative damage. Granulocyte oxidative activity is depressed early in the course of burn injury, but following resuscitation it depends on the clinical condition of the patient. In burn patients with infection, granulocyte peroxidase activity is elevated and often associated with toxic granulation of the neutrophils. In preterminal patients, however, the membrane-associated granulocyte oxidase activity progressively declines, indicating bone marrow exhaustion. Reduced serum opsonic activity and deficient leukocyte oxygenation capacity have been temporally correlated with the development of sepsis in burn patients (10).

Lymphocyte Changes

That burns suppress cell-mediated immunity has long been recognized. Prolonged skin allograft survival, suppressed delayed hypersensitivity, and impaired in vitro lymphoproliferative responses have been observed in experimental animals and humans with burns of 20% or more of the total body surface area (TBSA) (11–13).

Postburn cellular changes typically involve the lymphocyte phenotype and numbers. The first postburn week is marked by peripheral blood leukocytosis, relative lymphocytopenia, and a reduction in the number of CD3 + (T) and CD4 + (helper/inducer T) cells (11–14). Most of these cellular abnormalities, however, resolve in the second to third postburn week, particularly in patients making a satisfactory recovery. Though an abnormal CD4/CD8 ratio beyond the second postburn week has been implicated in the development of clinical sepsis, experimental work from this institute suggests that the reversal of CD4+/CD8+ ratio is a consequence rather than the cause of infection after burn injury (15). Despite a reduction in absolute numbers of CD3+, CD4+, and CD8+ cells in the circulation 48 h postburn, studies based on cell analysis by flow cytometry indicate that the expression of cell surface markers of lymphocyte activation, such as CD25, CD69, and CD71, and integrin adhesion molecules (CD11c, CD49a, CD54), is increased. These findings suggest the redistribution of activated lymphocytes from circulation to the tissues as a cause of peripheral lymphocytopenia that may contribute to the immunosuppression of burn injury (16).

In burn patients elevated serum interleukin-2 (IL-2) and IL-2 receptor levels (17) and increased spontaneous and IL-2-induced expression of CD25 by the peripheral blood lymphocytes (14,18) suggest that the T cells are activated early in the course. This perhaps renders the T cells unable to mount specific immunological responses later.

However, other investigators using in vitro mitogen stimulation and two-color flow cytometry observed a decreased expression of CD25 and transferrin receptors by the peripheral blood CD4+ and CD8+ T cells (19) following burns. Some findings appear to challenge the notion of burn-induced immunosuppression, and the clinical significance of these disparate laboratory findings remains unclear.

Serial measurements in burn patients indicate that time postburn and the presence of infection influence the expression of CD4+ and CD8+ receptors. In one study, burn patients who developed infection exhibited proportionately greater CD4+ and CD8+ cells, 50% fewer natural killer cells, markedly reduced β-integrin-bearing CD11b cells, and slightly decreased CD45RO+ memory cells, compared to uncomplicated patients. The percentage of cells that expressed early activation antigens, IL-2 and CD69, was significantly increased in the patients who developed infection (20). The application of a classification function based on patient age, burn size, and the percentage of CD4+ cells that expressed CD69 and HLA-DR permitted investigators at this institute to identify with 87% accuracy the samples of infected patients (21). A prospective confirmation of these findings would aid in the early identification of patients at greater risk of infection and thus in need of more intense monitoring and possible prophylactic therapy.

Studies suggest that the postburn in vitro lymphocyte suppression may not result from inherent T-cell defects, but from experimental conditions under which the T cells are cocultured with nonlymphoid cells. The prior removal of contaminating nonlymphoid cells from the peripheral blood mononuclear cells (PBM) of burned subjects normalized T-cell responses to mitogens and alloantigens (21,22). In one study in burn patients increased prostaglandin-E2 synthesis (PGE-2) by the burn/infection-activated monocytes and macrophages reduced T-cell IL-2 production and mitogen-induced T-cell responses. The addition of PGE-2 inhibitor, indomethacin, to the PBL restored both IL-2 production and mitogen responses, suggesting a possible therapeutic value of cyclooxygenase inhibitors in immune modulation of burn injury (23). In a murine model of burn injury, concanavalin-A stimulated splenocyte proliferation was suppressed compared to unburned controls. The removal of macrophages from the cell culture of burned animals improved lymphoproliferation, while addition of burned mouse macrophages to the unburned mouse lymphocyte culture inhibited lymphoproliferation (24). These findings suggested the possibility that burn injury may lead to the production of immunosuppressive macrophages.

HLA-DR expression by the PBMs is reduced on the first postburn day and remains subnormal during the initial 3 weeks of injury. Such a reduction in the expression of class II MHC antigens possibly interferes with the PBM ability to present antigens to CD4+ T cells and may explain, in part, the immune suppression of burn injury (14).

At a more general level, prolonged sympathoadrenal and pituitary-adrenocortical activation after burn injury (25,26) probably exerts an overall suppression of cellular inflammatory and immune responses, and the neuroendocrine surge itself may be stimulated by the cellular mediators activated by injury or infection.

Cytokine Changes

IL-1

Altered synthesis and release of cytokines may play a role in burn-induced immunosuppression. In one study, PBM harvested from patients whose burns averaged 70%

TBSA and who developed multiple organ failure showed reduced in vitro IL-2 production, interpreted to be a consequence of prior hyperstimulation of those cells at the time of injury. In addition, those patients had elevated serum C-reactive protein levels, suggesting that in vivo IL-1 release stimulated the production of acute phase protein by the hepatocytes (27). Studies from this institute indicated that plasma IL-1β is elevated roughly in proportion to burn size during the first week postburn and that TNF and IL-6 did not seen to correlate with the extent of burns (28). However, some cytokine measurements in the circulation typically have limited precision and accuracy at the levels present.

Consequently, the influence of infection on plasma IL-1 levels in burn patients is as yet uncertain. Moreover, increased levels of plasma IL-1 receptor antagonist (IL-1Ra), a macrophage product that blocks IL-1 actions, have been observed in burn patients (29). The clinical relevance of these findings remains uncertain since the IL-1Ra levels rose further with burn wound excision and grafting and, in addition, remained elevated in patients with lethal injury, suggesting that IL-1Ra may be a nonspecific marker of a variety of stimuli.

IL-2

Systemic infection in the burn patient with impaired cellular immune function remains a constant threat (14) and may be related to changes in IL-2 synthesis. IL-2 production by the PBMs of burned humans is suppressed, proportional to the extent of injury, and is further reduced during episodes of sepsis (30). Following burns, human PBM and murine splenocytes exhibit reduced IL-2 mRNA (31) levels, diminished IL-2 (31,32) production, and impaired proliferative responses that are normalized by the addition of recombinant IL-2 to the culture medium. Burn patients are reported to have elevated levels of soluble serum IL-2 receptor (IL-2R) (33,34) capable of competitively inhibiting the IL-2-dependent immune responses. IL-2 changes may partly explain the immune dysfunction of burn injury. Similarly, IL-2 gene transcription by the PBMs of patients with mechanical trauma is also reduced. This is thought to result from a defective transmembrane signaling mechanism since addition of phorbol myristate acetate, a surrogate "second messenger" to the PBM, increased both IL-2 levels and IL-2 production (35).

IL-2 administration improved survival in burned mice challenged with cecal ligation and puncture (32), suggesting a possible role of IL-2 therapy to enhance immune competence. In contrast, however, though addition of exogenous IL-2 to PBMs isolated from burn patients enhanced IL-2R expression, PBM proliferative responses did not improve, suggesting that the IL-2R present on PBMs of burn patients may be either nonfunctional or of low affinity (36).

IL-6

Proinflammatory cytokines appear to play a role in postburn immune defects. Burn-activated monocytes secrete IL-6 (37), the serum levels of which rise within hours of injury and remain elevated in patients for several weeks postburn (38). Both IL-1 and tumor necrosis factor-α (TNF-α) induce monocyte production of IL-6, which can cause fever and stimulate the synthesis of acute-phase liver proteins such as fibrinogen, C-reactive protein, α-1-antitrypsin, and immunoglobulins, all of which increase to a varying extent after burn injury. Compared to unburned mice, IL-6 secretion was increased in the splenocytes of burned mice in response to LPS challenge (37), suggesting that bacterial infection may potentiate IL-6 synthesis in the postburn period. The addition of IL-6 to cultured murine splenocytes suppresses mitogen responses (39), suggesting that such in vitro T-cell unresponsiveness may contribute to in vivo immunosuppression. A 2-week LPS pretreatment in mice subjected to 30% full thickness burns and immediately seeded with *Pseudomonas aeruginosa* resulted in significantly less weight loss, improved survival, and diminished C-reactive protein, IL-6, and TNF production (40). From those data, one is tempted to surmise that LPS pretreatment would induce tolerance and protect burned animals or humans from infection. Though manipulation of cytokine production or action of other defense responses to bacterial components may hold theoretical promise, interpretation of relevant observations warrants caution.

TNF and Other Cytokines

Stimulation of reticuloendothelial or other host defense cells and the resultant increased synthesis of tumor necrosis factor (TNF) could be detrimental to the host. In vitro PGE-2 treatment of Kupffer cells harvested from the burned rat abrogates increased TNF-α synthesis, suggesting the possibility that a PGE-2 deficiency may promote increased TNF-α production following burns (41). TNF-α production by the LPS-stimulated alveolar macrophages harvested from rats with a 40% burn is increased without a rise in TNF-α mRNA levels, indicating that posttranscriptional mechanisms control TNF-α release (42).

Thermal injury in a murine model reduced mitogen-stimulated lymphocyte responses and, in addition, impaired the splenocytes ability to produce IFN-γ and IL-10, a cytokine that downregulates macrophage synthesis of cytokines and inhibits nitric oxide production by the activated macrophages. In vitro pharmacological inhibition of nitric oxide normalized IL-10 production, improved splenocyte proliferative responses, but had no effect on IFN-γ production (43).

It is not yet possible to define the net role of changes of individual mediators in the overall immune response to burn or in postburn resistance to microbial invasion, though the latter appears inhibited.

Immune Cells

While on the first postburn day circulating granulocytes and monocytes begin to rise (12), serum immunoglobulin G (IgG) levels decrease and remain depressed for 2–4 weeks postburn. During the second to fifth postburn week, a decreased expression of a B-cell activation marker CD23 on both unstimulated and IL-4-stimulated cells (17) suggests B-cell downregulation and inability to respond normally. Active immunization with tetanus toxoid in a murine model, either prior to or at the time of thermal injury, resulted in an increased number of antigen-specific B cells without concomitant rise in the tetanus-specific IgG, suggesting an injury-induced inability of B cells to propagate normal IgG responses (44). In burned humans, the primary serum antibody response to injected alligator red cells was suppressed and allograft rejection appeared delayed. However, the anamnestic serum antitoxin response to tetanus toxoid (in individuals previously immunized) was enhanced and advanced in burn patients compared to controls (45). Following burns, IgM expression on murine mesenteric and spleen cells is increased without a corresponding rise in IgM production (46), again indicating reduced

B-cell immunoglobulin secretion following burn injury. In contrast, however, spontaneous in vitro IgG production by burn patient lymphocytes is increased, and exogenous administration of IgG in burn patients restores the depressed in vivo IgG levels to normal, but without improving patient mortality (47). The activity of peripheral blood natural killer (CD16+) cells in burn patients is reduced without concomitant reduction in the number of T cells (14).

As is the case with most other elements of overall host defense, it is difficult to tell whether postinjury changes in immune cells and immunoglobulin functions are beneficially adaptive or adversely affect the course of burn disease.

Serum Factors

Several studies support the notion that burn patient serum contains factors that suppress immunity. A multitude of immunosuppressive agents including complement degradation products, which suppress phagocytosis (10), immunoglobulin fragments, intermediate products of fibrinolysis and coagulation systems (48), endotoxin and prostaglandins (49) have been isolated from the sera of burn patients. Burn patient serum is known to suppress neutrophil function, inhibit neutrophil chemotaxis, and impair neutrophil chemiluminescence (9). Burn serum reportedly contains a 10-kD-molecular-weight polypeptide that inhibits mitogen-induced lymphoproliferation (50). Similarly, subeschar tissue fluid contains factors that suppress in vitro cell-mediated immunity and thus perhaps facilitate bacterial invasion of the burn wound (51).

The interpretation of observed suppressive (or stimulatory) elements within the complicated postinjury response, however, must be tempered with the realization that inflammatory and immune responses can damage uninjured tissue. The various response elements may seek a balance between preventing their own damaging potential and destroying microbes. Therapies directed at promoting or blocking inflammation or immunity may thus be inherently fraught with difficulties arising from a balance (between stimulation and suppression), the optimal setting of which is so far only cryptic. What is expressed as a compromise in host defense might also be a restriction of processes that would otherwise damage organs and magnify mortality.

SITE-SPECIFIC INFECTIONS

Burn Wound Infection

The avascular burn wound impedes diffusion of humoral antibodies, immune cells, and infused antibiotics, and thus permits uninhibited bacterial growth at the wound surface. In addition, the nonviable burn eschar forms an excellent culture medium that promotes bacterial proliferation. As a result, rapidly proliferating pathogens on the wound surface may invade underlying viable tissues and disseminate to distant sites in the immunocompromised host.

Certain bacterial characteristics such as virulence, toxin production, and drug resistance influence the development and course of infection. Members of the endogenous microbial flora, usually gram-positive organisms, chiefly *Staphylococcus aureus*, a commensal present on moist skin surfaces and the anterior nares of about 40% of the normal population (52), are the initial colonizers of wounds. The density and species-specific characteristics, such as virulence and drug resistance, of the colonizing microorganisms influence the course of infection. For instance, to produce a pustule in volunteers, an intradermal or subcutaneous injection of about 7.5×10^6 *Staphylococcus aureus* is required (53,54). Cell walls of several strains of *S. aureus* contain peptidoglycan, a mucopeptide that mimics endotoxin, can activate both the classic and alternate complement pathways, and elicit cell-mediated immunity (55). An intradermal injection of staphylococcal peptidoglycan in experimental animals inhibits leukocyte migration and edema accumulation at the injection site, and thus facilitates localized abscess formation (56). Surface-associated exopolysaccharide, or slime (57), is a virulence factor associated with some staphylococci and many gram-negative organisms, which impairs phagocytosis and inhibits neutrophil (58) catalase activity and thus protects the bacteria against PMN-induced lethal oxidant injury.

Gram-negative bacteria and fungi usually colonize the burn wound later in the course of the disease. The cell wall of gram-negative organisms contains endotoxin, a heat-stable antigen that elicits in dose-related fashion fever, initial leukopenia followed by leukocytosis, progressive hemodynamic instability, and even death. Particularly aggressive pathogens, among the gram-negative aerobic rods that infect the burn patient, belong to the *Pseudomonas* species, which was once considered nonpathogenic. *Pseudomonas aeruginosa* excretes pyocyanin and fluorescent pigments which impart a bluish-green hue to the infected wound. *Pseudomonas aeruginosa* was the most common cause of life-threatening infection in burn patients in the late 1950s and early 1960s at this institute. Since the introduction of effective topical chemotherapy in 1964, infections caused by that organism have progressively decreased in number, and over the past two decades (since 1977) the recovery of *Pseudomonas* from the wound and blood of patients treated at this burn center has precipitously declined. Even so, the burn patient remains susceptible to opportunistic infections and *Providencia stuartii*, *Enterobacter cloacae*, and *Klebsiella* species have caused successive miniepidemics of infection in our patients. In recent years a striking reduction in infection has coincided with the effective control of microbial density of the burn wound with routine use of topical agents, "early" excision of heavily colonized wounds, and patient isolation that prevents cross-contamination with drug-resistant organisms.

Burn Wound Management

Limitation of bacterial proliferation in the wound is essential for prevention and control of burn wound infection. This imperative can be achieved through wound care with topical antimicrobial agents along with timely excision and grafting of the wound. As soon as the condition of a burn patient permits, topical wound therapy should be initiated to maintain bacterial density at low levels and to prevent invasive wound infection. The burn wound should be debrided to remove loose necrotic tissue, including bullae, and the patient should be bathed with a nonirritating detergent disinfectant, such as chlorhexadine, followed by copious warm water irrigation. The burn wound should then be treated with a topical antimicrobial agent. The goal of topical wound therapy is to prevent infection until spontaneous wound healing or surgical closure of the wound occurs.

The risk of bacterial colonization and subsequent invasion of the underlying viable tissues rises with increasing burn size (59). If untreated, the microbial density of the wound increases with time, and the proliferating bacteria penetrate burn eschar, migrate along the viable sweat glands and hair follicles, and gain access to the underlying viable tissues. A bacterial density of 10^5 or more bacteria per gram of tissue at the viable/nonviable tissue interface may herald in imminent wound invasion but cannot be used to differentiate wound colonization from invasion (60).

Of documented clinical efficacy are three antimicrobial agents—11.1% mafenide acetate cream, 1% silver sulfadizine cream, and 0.5% silver nitrate solution—widely used to prevent burn wound infection. Topical mafenide acetate provides a wide antimicrobial spectrum that encompasses most gram-negative organisms, including *Pseudomonas*. This agent readily penetrates the burn eschar and reaches an effective antibacterial concentration at the viable/nonviable tissue interface, where the wound invasion begins. Both silver-containing agents exhibit a broad spectrum of antibacterial activity, except for a few gram-negative organisms. All three agents effectively prevent burn wound invasion and sepsis. However, because of minimal eschar penetration, the silver-containing agents are most effective when application can be started immediately after the burn injury to less contaminated wounds to function as a surface barrier to organisms that are not yet beneath the surface.

After the daily cleansing and prior to the application of antimicrobial agents, the burn wound should be inspected at least once each day to detect subeschar purulence or presence of tinctorial changes indicative of wound infection. All skin lesions that appear to be infection-related should be biopsied under local anesthesia. One-half of the biopsy specimen should be submitted for a rapid histological examination, and the other half for quantitative bacterial cultures. Burn wounds with increasing bacterial density in surveillance specimens even without evidence of wound invasion should be treated with mafenide acetate (Sulfamylon) cream, and other topical agents should be discontinued. To prevent the systemic dissemination of infection in patients with histologically confirmed microbial invasion of the viable tissues, the infected burn wound should undergo subeschar clysis with antibiotics, usually with a broad-spectrum penicillin, followed by prompt excision.

Surgical Therapy of the Burn Wound

Most partial-thickness burns managed under the protective umbrella of antimicrobial topical therapy heal spontaneously in 2–3 weeks. Partial-thickness burns assessed as unlikely to heal within 2–3 weeks and full-thickness burns require excision and grafting. Following resuscitation, usually between the third and fifth postburn day, surgical excision of the burn wound should be carried out as a single or staged procedure, depending on donor site availability and the location and extent of injury. Patients with 15–20% body surface area burns can be safely excised and simultaneously autografted. Burn wound excision in excess of 20% body surface area at a single sitting, however, may cause undue hemodynamic instability in the patient and should be avoided. Timely excision and definitive wound closure, which remain the central themes of burn wound therapy, minimize the risk of bacterial infection of the wound and the occurrence of invasive burn wound sepsis.

Three pertinent variables—severity (extent and depth) of burn, microbial density of the wound, and specific traits of infecting bacteria—determine the risk of infection. The use of topical wound therapy achieves effective control of bacterial density; timely excision and definitive wound closure reduce the extent of burn wound at risk of infection; and the control of the patient's environment reduces the risk of patient cross-contamination with multiple drug-resistant organisms.

Pulmonary Infection

Effective control of invasive burn wound infection has been associated with the emergence of pulmonary sepsis as the leading cause of death in burn patients. Prior to the routine use of topical antimicrobial chemotherapy in burn wound management, hematogenous pneumonia was a common pulmonary infection that most often resulted from bacterial dissemination from an infected wound to the lung. In addition to the burn wound, infection at other sites such as heart valves, previously cannulated veins, soft tissues, and the abdominal or other body cavities may also metastasize to the lung.

Today, however, the most frequent pulmonary infection in the burn patient is bronchopneumonia that begins as bronchiolitis and spreads to adjacent alveoli. Burn patients with an underlying inhalation injury (8) and those requiring mechanical support of ventilation (61) are at an increased risk of developing pneumonia. Pulmonary infection in the critically ill patient is of multifactorial origin. The endotracheal tube in intubated patients becomes heavily colonized with endogenous bacteria, which, upon routine suctioning, may be dislodged and inoculate the lung and cause pneumonia (62). In acutely ill patients, undetected aspiration of contaminated oropharyngeal secretions has been implicated as the cause of pneumonia. Gut decontamination to control that potential pathogenetic factor has been reported to decrease the occurrence of gram-negative pneumonia but has exerted no effect on mortality (63).

Bacterial colonization of the upper gastrointestinal tract in critically ill patients receiving antacid therapy for the prevention of Curling's ulcers has been invoked as a cause of pneumonia. In a prospective trial at this institute (64), burn patients were randomized to receive antacids and H_2 blockers or a nonantacid agent sucralfate. Both regimens provided stress ulcer control, and, in addition, in both groups the frequency and time of gram-negative colonization of the airway were comparable. The incidence of pneumonia in the sucralfate-treated, mechanically ventilated patients was higher, indicating that the reduction of gastric acidity appears to play no role in susceptibility to nosocomial pneumonia.

Bacterial translocation from increased intestinal permeability, thought to follow postischemic reperfusion of the gut, has been proposed as a cause of nosocomial pneumonia in critical patients (65). Intestinal permeability was estimated by determining the clearance ratios of orally administered lactulose and mannitol in burn patients at this institute (66). The patients who subsequently developed an infection had an elevated lactulose to mannitol clearance ratio, indicating increased intestinal permeability and suggesting the possibility of increased infection with enteric flora in these patients. The pneumonia in patients with increased intestinal permeability was, however, due predominatly to gram-positive and not gram-negative organisms, as would be anticipated on the basis of bacterial translocation from the gut.

The recent change in the predominant form of pneumonia from bloodborne to airborne reflects the decreased incidence of burn wound infection and the improved survival of patients with inhalation injury and those receiving mechanical ventilation. Bronchopneumonia in the burn patient is commonly caused by *Staphylococcus* and to a lesser extent by other opportunistic organisms including gram-negative bacteria.

High-Frequency Ventilation

High-frequency percussive ventilation, which permits use of lower airway pressures and lower concentrations of inspired oxygen, helps maintain airway patency and facilitates clearance of tracheobronchial secretions (67). Prophylactic use of high-frequency interrupted flow-positive pressure ventilation (HFIFPPV) has been reported to decrease the incidence of pneumonia and increase the survival of burn patients with inhalation injury (67). Over the past 6–8 years, prophylactic use of HFIFPPV in burn patients with inhalation injury has been associated wtih a significant reduction in mortality overall, and the comorbid effect of mild inhalation injury has been abrogated—i.e., observed mortality in those patients corresponded to that predicted on the basis of age and burn size alone (68).

GENERAL PROPHYLACTIC MEASURES

Immune Therapy

The apparent association of cellular and humoral defects with an increased risk of infection in the burn patient forms the basis for immunomodulatory therapy to augment host defenses and thereby prevent systemic infection.

GM-CSF Therapy

Granulocyte-macrophage colony-stimulating factor (GM-CSF) has been studied as a means of correcting burn-induced impairment of cellular immunity. GM-CSF prolongs the life-span of neutrophils and macrophages; enhances the expression of cell surface HLA class II, CD11b, and CR1 and CR3 receptors; and increases the PMN responsiveness to chemotactic agents. The agent, in addition, augments PMN phagocytic and bactericidal activities. Compared to controls, GM-CSF pretreatment improved survival and diminished bacterial translocation to the mesenteric nodes, spleen, and liver of burned mice subjected to blood transfusion and cecal ligation and puncture (69). These findings suggested that intact neutrophil and macrophage function were necessary to combat infection; however, the clinical relevance for these findings in critically ill patients is not clear. In addition, further activation of neutrophils prestimulated by burn injury could be detrimental to circulation-rich organs such as the lung, where PMN sequestration is thought to contribute to the development of adult respiratory distress syndrome.

In a group of 10 burn patients (extent of burn 20–54% TBSA), GM-CSF administration for the first 3 weeks after the burn injury augmented the postburn elevation of total white cell count during the second week without changing the granulocyte fraction. However, during and after administration, it did not change the elevated unstimulated granulocyte cytosolic peroxidase activity, and it reduced the phorbol myristate acetate-stimulated activity of this enzyme compared to that in matched untreated control burn patients. It appeared to reduce the elevated neutrophil myeloperoxidase activity during the second week of treatment. A biacridinium probe was used to assess the chemiluminogenic activity of superoxide and other oxidative species. A fall in this activity below normal was seen in the untreated patients after 3 weeks postburn, though such a fall at this time was prevented in burn patients receiving GM-CSF for the first 3 weeks after injury. Fever, pruritis, and possibly other adverse effects were reported, and it is not yet possible to determine whether the noted effects on granulocytes would produce any net benefit for burn patients (70).

IVIG Therapy

The influence of serum IgG augmentation on the incidence of infection was studied in a randomized trial of 69 adult burn patients (34 controls, 35 IgG therapy) admitted to this institute within 5 days of injury (71). Patients in the two groups were comparable in age, burn size, and the presence of inhalation injury. IgG (Cutter Biological-Miles, 500 mg/kg) was infused twice weekly for a minimum of 2 weeks. Patients with large open wounds received IgG beyond 2 weeks until complete wound closure.

Though IgG replacement resulted in a more swift and sustained augmentation of serum IgG levels, the serum IgG normalized in both groups within 2 weeks postburn. Pneumonia developed in 20 IgG-treated and in 21 control patients, and 11 patients in each group developed bacteremia. Other infections observed in the IgG-treated versus control patients were: burn wound invasion (1/3), urinary tract infection (4/4), and cellulitis (3/4). About one-half of all infections in patients in both groups were due to gram-positive bacteria, and the rest due to gram-negative organisms and *Candida* species. Overall patient mortality and number of intensive care days in the survivors were similar in both groups. From these data we concluded that early augmentation of serum IgG with exogenous IgG infusions is unwarranted.

Despite demonstrable abnormalities in humoral and cellular elements of immunity, the exact relationship between burn-induced immune defects and susceptibility of a burn patient to infection remains unclear. The limited use of various vaccines and immunomodulating agents and their uncertain success in preventing infection or improving burn patients' survival precludes the routine use of such agents in burn patient care.

Bacterial Surveillance

Because of the loss of both physical and immunological barriers and the intensity and duration of necessary care, burn patients represent one of the most infection-susceptible hospital populations. The high probability of nosocomial infection in the intensive burn care environment justifies both intense surveillance of infections and prompt identification of the origin of offending pathogens. The added risk of acquiring and perpetuating virulent, possibly multiple antibiotic-resistant endemic strains of microorganisms in a specialized care facility must be minimized. Patient care policies, including isolation procedures and the work assignments of burn care providers, should be designed to minimize traffic between patients to prevent cross-contamination. A protocol-based microbial surveillance system of scheduled cultures of wound, sputum, and urine from the time of admission and throughout care ensures documentation of the introduction and spread of antibiotic-resistant hospital-associated strains. These organisms are uncommon in the community and are most often introduced on transferred patients. The absence of such organisms should not be used as a transfer criterion, but the presence of such organisms must be considered in patient care planning.

The information gained by a microbial surveillance system may be used as a quality improvement mechanism for burn care and may also be used as documentation of cost control efforts. Identification of potential pathogens at the colonization phase allows a rational basis for selection of antimicrobial therapy should infection occur. Documentation of sensitivity of an infecting organism to older (perhaps generic) antimicrobial agents will justify their use as less expensive, first-line therapy. The savings that result from the lesser use of newer expensive antimicrobial agents amply justifies the expense of microbial surveillance and other infection control programs.

Patient Isolation

Organization of patient care should be based on patient acuity and available staffing. Assignment of individual patient care teams (team nursing) may be used to minimize between-patient contacts. Each team should be assigned to specified patients, and team members should not participate in the care of patients assigned to other teams. The identification of an organism known to present an exceptional risk, such as a multiply resistant *Psuedomonas aeruginosa*, may require assignment of patient-specific nurses or team (cohort nursing). To curtail interpatient bacterial transfer, strict environmental control measures should be enforced, including the use of protective gowns, gloves, masks, and caps while attending patients; use of impervious aprons during wound care; hand washing between patient contacts; and physical isolation of patients in single rooms.

Such practices have been found to be effective in reducing the incidence of burn ward–associated infections (72,73). When such measures are strictly enforced, the occurrence of infection by multiply resistant organisms is a rare event, underscoring the role of lax environmental control (rather than aggressive antibiotic therapy) in the development of nosocomial infections by such organisms. Multiply resistant organisms may occasionally be introduced by a given patient, but their spread in the unit can be prevented by enviromental control, and their progression from colonizers to invaders can be minimized by proper wound care and present-day techniques of organ system support.

REFERENCES

1. Pruitt BA Jr, Mason AD Jr. Epidemiological, demographic and outcome characteristics of burn injury. In: Herndon DN, ed. Total Burn Care. London: W. B. Saunders, 1995:5–15.
2. McGinley KJ, Webster GF, Leyden JJ. Regional variations of cutaneous propionibacteria. Appl Environ Microbiol 1978;35:62.
3. Proctor DF, Anderson I, Lundgvist G. Clearance of inhaled particles from the human nose. Arch Intern Med 1973;131:132.
4. Rhodin JAG. Ultrastructure and function of the human tracheal mucosa. Annu Rev Respir Dis 1966;93:1.
5. Hocking WG, Golde DW. The pulmonary-alveolar macrophage. N Engl J Med 1979;301:580.
6. Ganguly C, Waldman RH. Local immunity and local immune defenses. Prog Allergy 1980;27:1.
7. Cohan AB, Gold WM. Defense mechanisms of the lungs. Annu Rev Physiol 1975;37:325.
8. Shirani KZ, Pruitt BA Jr, Mason AD Jr. The influence of inhalation injury and pneumonia on burn mortality. Ann Surg 1987;205:82.
9. Allen RC, Pruitt BA Jr. Humoral-phagocyte axis of immune defense in burn patients. Chemiluminigenic probing. Arch Surg 1982;117:133.
10. Alexander J. Alteration of opsonic activity after burn injury. Proceedings of the 40th Anniversary Symposium, U.S. Army Institute of Surgical Research, Fort Sam Houston, TX, 1989;126–130.
11. McIrvine AJ, O Mahony JB, Saprorschetz I, et al. Depressed immune response in burn patints: use of monoclonal antibodies and funcctional assays to define the role of suppressor cells. Ann Surg 1982;196:297.

12. Calvano SE, DeRiesthal HF, Marano MA, et al. The decrease in peripheral blood CD4+ and T cells following thermal injury in humans can be accounted for by a concomitant decrease in suppressor-inducer CD4+ and T cells as assessed using anti-CD45R. Clin Immunol Immunopathol 1988;47:164.

13. Sakai H, Daniels JC, Beathard GA, et al. Mixed lymphocyte culture reaction in patients with acute thermal burns. J Trauma 1974;14:53.

14. Schluter B, Konig W, Koller M, et al. Differential regulation of T- and B-lymphocyte activation in severely burned patients. J Trauma 1991;31:239.

15. Burleson DG, Vaughn GK, Mason AD Jr, et al. Flow cytometric measurement of rat lymphocyte subpopulations after burn injury and burn injury with infection. Arch Surg 1987; 122:216.

16. Maldonado MD, Venturoli A, Franco A, Nunez-Roldan A. Specific changes in peripheral blood lymphocyte phenotype from burn patients. Probable origin of the thermal injury-related lymphocytopenia. Burns 1991;17:188.

17. Teodorczyk-Injeyan JA, Sparkes BG, Mills GB, Peters WJ. Immunosuppression follows systemic T lymphocyte activation in the burn patient. Clin Exp Immunol 1991;85:515.

18. Deitch EA, Landry KN, McDonald JC. Postburn impaired cell-mediated immunity may not be due to lazy lymphocytes but to overwork. Ann Surg 1985;201:793.

19. Zapata-Sirvent RL, Hansbrough JF. Temporal analysis of human leukocyte surface antigen expression and neutrophil respiratory burst activity after thermal injury. Burns 1993;19:5.

20. Burleson DG, Cioffi WG Jr, Wolcott KM, Mason AD Jr, Pruitt BA Jr. Lymphocyte surface antigen expression after infection in burned patients. In: Faist E et al., eds. The Immune Consequences of Trauma, Shock, and Sepsis, Vol. 1. Lengerich, Germany: Pabst Science Publishers, 1996:295–299.

21. Burleson DG, Mason AD Jr, Pruitt BA Jr. Changes in lymphocyte surface antigen that precede infection in burned patients. FASEB J 1995;9(3):A520.

22. Xu DZ, Deitch EA, Sitting K, et al. In vitro cell-mediated immunity after thermal injury is not impaired. Density gradient purification of mononuclear cells is associated with spurious (artifactual) immunosuppression. Ann Surg 1988;208:768.

23. Grbic JT, Mannick JA, Gough DB, Rodrick ML. The role of prostaglandin E2 in immune suppression following injury. Ann Surg 1991;214:253.

24. Yang L, Hsu B. The roles of macrophage (M0) and PGE-2 in postburn immunosuppression. Burns 1992;18:132.

25. Vaughan GM. Neuroendocrine and sympathoadrenal response to thermal trauma. In: Dolecek R, Brizio-Molteni L, Molteni A, Traber D, eds. Endocrine Response to Thermal Trauma. Philadelphia: Lea & Febiger, 1990;267–306.

26. Vaghan GM, Pruitt BA Jr, Mason AD Jr. Burn trauma as a model of severe non-thyroidal illness. In: Dolecek R, Brizio-Molteni L, Molteni A, Traber D, eds. Endocrine Response to Thermal Trauma. Philadelphia: Lea & Febiger, 1990;307–349.

27. Liu XS, Yang ZC, Luo ZH, Li A. Clinical significance of the change of blood monocytic interleukin-1 production in vitro in severely burned patients. Burns 1994;20:302.

28. Drost AC, Burleson DG, Cioffi WG Jr, Jordan BS, Mason AD Jr, Pruitt BA Jr. Plasma cytokines following thermal injury and their relationship with patient mortality, burn size, and time postburn. J Trauma 1993;35:335–339.

29. Mandrup-Poulsen T, Wogensen LD, Jensen M, et al. Circulating interleukin-1 antagonist concentration are increased in adult patients with thermal injury. Crit Care Med 1995;23:26.

30. Wood JJ, Rodrick ML, O'Mahony JB, et al. Inadequate interleukin 2 production. A fundamental immunological deficiency in patients with major burns. Ann Surg 1984;200:311.

31. Horgan AF, Mendez MV, O Riordan DD, et al. Altered gene transcription after burn results in depressed T-lymphocyte activation. Ann Surg 1994;220:342.

32. Gough DB, Moss NM, Jordan A, et al. Recombinant interleukin-2 (rIL-2) improves immune response and host resistance to septic challenge in thermally injured mice. Surgery 1988;104:292.

33. Teodorczyk-Injeyan JA, Sparkes BG, Mills GB, et al. Increase of serum interleukin 2 receptor level in thermally injured patients. Clin Immunol Immunopathol 1989;51:205.

34. Xiao GX, Chopra RK, Adler WH, et al. Altered expression of lymphocyte IL-2 receptors in burned patients. J Trauma 1988;28:1669.

35. Faist E, Schinkel C, Zimmer S, et al. Inadequate interleukin-2 synthesis and interleukin-2 messenger expression following thermal and mechanical trauma in humans is caused by defective transmembrane signaling. J Trauma 1993;34:386.

36. Tedorczyk-Injeyan JA, Sparkes BG, Mills GB, et al. Impaired expression of interleukin-2 receptor (IL-2R) in the immunosuppressed burn patient: reversal by exogenous IL-2. J Trauma 1987;27:180.

37. O Riordan MG, Collins KH, Pilz M, et al. Modulation of macrophage hyperactivity improves survival in a burn-sepsis model. Arch Surg 1992;127:152.

38. Nijsten MWN, Hack CE, Helle M, ten Duis HJ, Klasen HJ, Aarden LA. Interleukin-6 and its relation to the humoral immune response and clinical parameters in burned patients. Surgery 1991;109:761–767.

39. Zhou D, Munster AM, Winchurch RA. Inhibitory effects of interleukin 6 on immunity: possible implications in burn patients. Arch Surg 1995;127:65.

40. He W, Fong Y, Marano MA, et al. Tolerance to endotoxin prevents mortality in infected thermal injury: association with attenuated cytokine responses. J Infect Dis 1992;165:859.

41. Dong Y-L, Ko F, Huang H-Q, et al. Evidence for Kupffer cell activation by burn injury and *Pseudomonas* exotoxin A. Burns 1993;19:12.

42. Minei JP, Williams JG, Hills SJ. Augmented tumor necrosis factor response to lipopolysaccharide after thermal injury is regulated post-transcriptionally. Arch Surg 1994;129:1198.

43. Napolitano LM, Campbell C. Nitric oxide inhibition normalizes splenocyte interleukin-10 synthesis in murine thermal injury. Arch Surg 1994;129:1276.

44. Malloy RG, Nestor M, Collins KH, et al. The humoral immune response after thermal injury: an experimental model. Surgery 1994;115:431.

45. Alexander WJ, Moncrief JA. Alterations of the immune response following severe thermal injury. Arch Surg 1966;93:75–83.

46. Tabata T, Meyer AA, Effects of burn injury class-specific B-cell population and immunoglobulin synthesis in mice. J Trauma 1993;35:750.

47. Burleson DG, Mason AD Jr, McManus AT, Pruitt BA Jr. Lymphocyte phenotype and function changes in burn patients after intravenous IgG therapy. Arch Surg 1988;123:1379–1382.

48. Ozkan AN, Hoyt DB, Ninnemann JL. Generation and activity of suppressor peptides following traumatic injury. J Burn Care Rehabil 1987;8:527.

49. Warden GD. Burn-related humoral immunosuppressants. Proceedings of the 40th Anniversary Symposium, U.S. Army Institute of Surgical Research, Fort Sam Houston, TX, 1989;134.

50. Constantian MB. Association of sepsis with an immuno suppressive polypeptide in the serum of burn patients. Ann Surg 1978;188:209.

51. Ferrara JJ, Dyess DL, Luterman A, et al. The suppressive effect of subeschar tissue fluid upon in vitro cell-mediated immunologic function. J Burn Care Rehabil 1988;9:584.

52. William REO, Blowers R, Garrod LP, Shooter RA. Hospital Infections, 2nd ed. London: Lloyd-Luke, 1966.

53. Levenson SM, Kan-Gruber D, Gruber C, et al. Wound healing accelerated by *Staphylococcus aureus*. Arch Surg 1983;118:310.

54. Elek SD, Concen PE: The virulence of *Staphylococcus pyogenes* for man: a study of wound infection. Br J Exp Pathol 1957;38:573.

55. Rotta J. Endotoxin-like properties of the peptidoglycan. Z Immunitaetsforsch 1975;149:230.

56. Van der Vijver JCM, Van Es-Boon MM, Michel MF. A study of virulence factors with induced mutants of *Staphylococcus aureus*. J Med Microbiol 1975;8:279.

57. Gristina AG, Oga M, Webb LX, Hobgood DC. Adherent bacterial colonization in the pathogenesis of osteomyelitis. Science 1985;228:990.

58. Mandell GL. Catalase, superoxide dismutase, and virulence of *Staphylococcus aureus*. In vitro and in vivo studies with emphasis on staphylococcal-leukocyte interaction. J Clin Invest 1975;55:561.

59. Pruitt BA Jr, Goodwin CW, Cioffi WG Jr. Thermal injuries. In: Davis JH, Sheldon GF, eds. Surgery: A Problem-Solving Approach, 2nd ed. New York: Mosby, 1995:222.

60. Pruitt BA Jr, Goodwin CW, Cioffi WG Jr. Thermal injuries. In: Davis JH, Sheldon GF, eds. Surgery: A Problem-Solving Approach, 2nd ed. New York: Mosby, 1995:185.

61. Rue LW III, Cioffi WG, Mason AD Jr, et al. The risk of pneumonia in thermally injured patients requiring ventilatory support. J Burn Care Rehab 1995;16(Pt 1):262–268.

62. Sottile FD, Marrie TJ, Prough DS, et al. Nosocomial pulmonary infection: possible etiologic significance of bacterial adhesion to endotracheal tubes. Crit Care Med 1986;14:265–270.

63. Stoutenbeek DP, van Saene KF, Miranda DR, et al. The effect of oropharyngeal decontamination using topical nonabsorbable antibiotics on the indicence of nosocomimal respiratory tract infections in multiple trauma patients. J Trauma 1987;27:357–1364.

64. Cioffi WG, McManus AT, Rule LW III, Mason AD, McManus WF, Pruitt BA Jr. Comparison of acid neutralizing and non-acid neutralizing stress ulcer prophylaxis in thermally injured patients. J Trauma 1994;36:544–547.

65. Fiddian-Green RG, Baker S. Nosocomial pneumonia in the critically ill: product of aspiration or translocation? Crit Care Med 1991;19:763–769.

66. LeVoyer T, Cioffi WG Jr, Pratt L, et al. Alterations in intestinal permeability after thermal injury. Arch Surg 1992;127:26–30.

67. Cioffi WG Jr, Rue LW III, Graves TA, McManus WF, Mason AD Jr, Pruitt BA Jr. High-frequency percussive ventilation in patients with inhalation injury. Ann Surg 1991: 213:575–582.

68. Rue LW III, Cioffi WG, Mason AD, McManus WF, Pruitt BA Jr. Improved survival of burned patients with inhalation injury. Arch Surg 1993;128:778–780.

69. Gennari R, Alexander JW, Gianotti L, et al. Granulocyte macrophage colony-stimulating factor improves survival in two models of gut-derived sepsis by improving gut barrier function and modulating bacterial clearance. Ann Surg 1994;220:68.

70. Cioffi WG Jr, Burleson DG, Jordon BS, et al. Effects of granulocyte-macrophage colony-stimulating factor in burn patients. Arch Surg 1991;126:74–79.

71. Shirani KZ, Vaughan GM, McManus AT, et al. Replacement therapy with modified immunoglobulin G (IgG) in burn patients: preliminary kinetic studies. Proceedings of a Symposium on Intravenous Immune Globulin and the Compromised Host. Am J Med 1984;76:175–180.

72. McManus AT, Mason AD Jr., McManus WF, Pruitt BA Jr. A decade of reduced gram-negative infections and mortality associatd with improved isolation of burned patients. Arch Surg 1994;129:1306–1309.

73. Shirani KZ, McManus AT, Vaughan GM, McManus WF, Pruitt BA Jr, Mason AD Jr. Effects of environment on infection in burn patients. Arch Surg 1986;121:31–36.

18

Prevention and Treatment of Viral Infection

Martha M. Eibl and Hermann M. Wolf

Institute of Immunology, University of Vienna, Vienna, Austria

INTRODUCTION

Most viruses are strong antigens and stimulate a considerable antibody response. Viruses contain a large number of antigenic epitopes on viral proteins, and there is amplification in the quantity of antigenic material due to viral replication. Only a few of the antibodies induced, however, play a significant role in protecting the host against infection and/or disease. It might be that these antibodies do not in all instances prevent infection, but are rather involved in controlling infection and thereby preventing disease. However, in some viral infections antibodies themselves may be implicated in disease pathogenesis (e.g., dengue virus infection) (1,2).

Antibodies that inhibit the infectivity of viral particles are referred to as neutralizing antibodies. Viral infectivity may be reduced because neutralizing antibodies inhibit attachment, penetration, or uncoating of virus; produce aggregation of virions; accelerate viral degradation; enhance viral opsonization and subsequent phagocytosis; or mediate antibody-dependent cellular cytotoxicity of virus-infected cells.

Standard immunoglobulin products are prepared from more than 5000 plasma donations, and antibody concentrations to certain common pathogens are normally present in sufficient amounts to be protective against infections with these pathogens in antibody-deficient individuals (3). Intravenous immunoglobulin preparations will provide protection against most common infectious diseases usually occurring in the population if the mode of preparation is such that the function and the half-life of 7 S antibodies is unimpaired. It has to be recognized, however, that lot-to-lot differences in certain antibody activities do exist even within products of the same manufacturer and even more so among different manufacturers. Especially, antibody titers to specific viruses vary over a 10-fold range in different pooled lots of gammaglobulin, and the fairly large doses of intravenous immunoglobulin given in order to obtain significant antiviral antibody titers in the patient may have additional wanted or unwanted immune modulatory effects already known or as yet unrecognized.

Thus, it is important to emphasize that immunoglobulin concentrations and titers of specific antibodies against certain viral pathogens (antibodies binding to the pathogen vs. functional antibodies vs. protective antibodies) have to be looked upon individually in different preparations, and that immunoglobulin products similar in immunoglobulin concentrations, especially IVIG preparations, may show some variation in titers of antibodies binding to certain antigens as well as in functional and/or protective antibody activity (4). One of the reasons for the variability in titers of functional and protective antibodies may be that standardization of functional assays is much more difficult and variability is even more pronounced in experimental animals than in in vitro test systems.

As only certain antiviral antibodies are present in sufficient quantities in standard immunoglobulin preparations, hyperimmunoglobulin preparations are needed in the prevention and treatment of a number of viral diseases (4). Such hyperimmunoglobulins are prepared from selected high-titer plasma donations or obtained by donor immunization. While selection of high-titer plasma donations is usually based on the demonstration of high titers of virus antigen-binding antibodies, the importance of the presence of high titers of specific functional and/or protective antibodies in the hyperimmunoglobulin preparation, in addition to a high level of antigen-binding antibodies, cannot be overemphasized.

INDICATIONS FOR HUMAN IG IN THE PREVENTION OF VIRAL DISEASES

The primary use of immunoglobulins is in the substitution therapy of patients with primary antibody deficiency. Even though the most common infections in these patients are bacterial infections, recurrent or severe viral infections are also known to occur, and it is well established that regular immunoglobulin replacement therapy will be effective in preventing these infections. A rare but previously fatal complication seen in patients with severe antibody deficiency was a progressive encephalitis combined with symptoms of dermatomyositis, caused by different members of the echovirus family. High-dose treatment with IVIG allows for the control of this severe viral disease over lengthy periods of time (5). However, while obviously suppressing viral replication, treatment will not lead to the elimination of the viral pathogen. In consequence, high-dose IVIG treatment (1–2 g/kg/month) has to be continued for prolonged periods of time, and reducing the dose will lead to exacerbation of disease. Furthermore, in some individuals high-dose IVIG treatment is not as effective as in others. Varying antibody titers in different products and especially varying concentrations of antibodies against individual echovirus strains have been discussed in this context.

Treatment with human gammaglobulin prior to or shortly after exposure to viral pathogens is well accepted in the prevention of several viral diseases such as hepatitis A, measles, varicella zoster virus infection, and, concomitantly with active immunization, rabies, and hepatitis B (Table 1) (4,6,7). Standard intramuscular gammaglobulin is indicated for the prevention of measles and hepatitis A (8). Minimal antibody titers have to be present against both viral pathogens. Hyperimmunoglobulins (i.e., immunoglobulin preparations made from plasma with high antibody titers against specific antigens) specific for cytomegalovirus, varicella zoster virus, hepatitis B, and rabies are available and indicated in certain well-defined situations (8). At times when vaccination against smallpox was ongoing, vaccinia hyperimmunoglobulin has been used both prophylactically and therapeutically to prevent or treat disease complications.

Table 1 Indications for Human Immunoglobulin Preparations in the Prevention of Viral Diseases

Immunoglobulin preparation	Indication(s)
Standard human immune globulin	Pre- and postexposure prophylaxis of hepatitis A and postexposure prophylaxis of measles in susceptible persons
Hepatitis B immune globulin	Postexposure prophylaxis of hepatitis B in susceptible persons in conjunction with active immunization
Rabies immune globulin	Postexposure prophylaxis of rabies in susceptible persons in conjunction with active immunization
Varicella zoster immune globulin	Postexposure prophylaxis of susceptible immunocompromised persons or pregnant women, perinatally exposed newborns, and hospitalized premature infants
Vaccinia immune globulin	Treatment of eczema vaccination, vaccinia necrosum, and ocular vaccinia
Cytomegalovirus immune globulin, intravenous	Prophylaxis of CMV disease in bone marrow and kidney transplant recipients

Source: Modified from CDC (88).

Standard human immunoglobulin can be given to prevent or modify measles in a susceptible person within 6 days of exposure (recommended dose: a single dose of 0.25 ml/kg of body weight given as soon after exposure as possible) (8).

Gammaglobulin is especially indicated in susceptible household or hospital contacts of measles patients if these household contacts are younger than 1 year of age or in pregnant women. If the risk of severe morbidity from the disease is extremely high, as in immunocompromised persons, a higher dose of immunoglobulin should be administered (0.5 ml/kg). For patients receiving regular IVIG substitution therapy, the usual dose (400 mg/kg every 3–4 weeks) should be sufficient for measles prophylaxis (8).

Standard gammaglobulin is also being used for prophylaxis of hepatitis A in travelers to foreign countries (recommended dose 0.02 ml/kg for a 3-month or shorter stay, 0.06 ml/kg for up to 6 months). Application of immunoglobulin is also recommended in hepatitis A outbreaks in child care facilities or hospitals (dose 0.02 ml/kg) (9). Protection against hepatits A is likely to last for several months after gammaglobulin administration. Fujiyama et al. (10) investigated in vivo recovery and pharmacokinetics of hepatitis A antibodies after application of gammaglobulin. Ten antibody-negative volunteers were injected with 7.5 mg/kg and 15 mg/kg, respectively, of serum immunoglobulin, and hepatitis A antibody titers were measured for 28 weeks. Positive serum-neutralizing antibody titers persisted for 14 weeks in individuals who received the low dose and for 18 weeks in the recipients of the higher dose.

Immunoglobulins are also known to be beneficial in postexposure prophylaxis of certain viral diseases where simultaneous passive/active immunization is recommended— i.e., where immunoglobulins and vaccines are applied at the same time. In postexposure prophylaxis of hepatitis B, simultaneous application of hepatitis B immune globulin and hepatitis B vaccine is recommended for newborn infants born to HBs antigen-positive mothers (recommended dose of hepatitis B immunoglobulin: 0.5 ml). A similar regime is indicated in household contacts of individuals with acute HBV infection if these household contacts are below 12 months of age (dose 0.5 ml) or are sexual partners of persons with acute HBV infection (recommended dose 0.06 ml/kg). Furthermore, susceptible individuals who have had an acute exposure to blood that might contain hepatitis B virus (e.g., needlestick injuries) should receive hepatitis B immune globulin concomitantly with active immunization (recommended dose 0.06 ml/kg) (11).

In suspected infection with rabies virus, rabies hyperimmunoglobulin and rabies vaccination are indicated to be applied simultaneously (12). Experimental evidence suggests that rabies virus will migrate into the central nervous system without prior local replication; antirabies antibodies were shown to be effective in this experimental model as long as the infection of the central nervous system did not take place.

Prevention of Viral Disease in Immunocompromised Populations

An increasing segment of the population has to be considered immunocompromised. Premature infants, neonates, patients with genetic immunodeficiencies, patients with hematological and other malignancies, patients with chronic disease like renal failure and chronic liver disease, patients on chemotherapy or those receiving radiation, patients with certain viral infections like HIV, and patients receiving organ or bone marrow transplants are unduly susceptible to infection. They may also be overexposed to viral pathogens—e.g., a CMV-seronegative individual receiving an organ transplant from a CMV-positive donor. At the same time, their ability to mount an effective immune response may be impaired. A viral infection that might be relatively harmless in the healthy population may cause substantial morbidity and mortality in these individuals, and immunoglobulins, either standard or enriched for certain antibody specificities, may be life-saving by preventing and/or attenuating viral disease. Vaccination with live attenuated vaccines is often contraindicated, and killed vaccines may not be effective in inducing an immune response. In these populations, the use of immunoglobulins for the prevention of certain infectious diseases has been described to be greatly advantageous (13).

IVIG Substitution Therapy in Patient Populations with Secondary Immune Deficiency

The regular long-term application of intravenous immunoglobulins in patient populations with antibody deficiency should be mentioned only briefly in this context, as it will be treated in more detail in other chapters of this book. Provision of polyclonal antibodies will prevent and modify upper and lower respiratory tract infections (mostly of viral origin) including viral and bacterial pneumonia in patients with hematological malignancies (e.g., lymphocytic leukemia and antibody deficiency) in patients with multiple myeloma, in children with ALL, and in patients with small cell carcinoma of the lung (14).

Prophylaxis of CMV-Associated Disease in Transplant Recipients

Cytomegalovirus (CMV) immunoglobulin has been developed for prophylaxis of CMV-associated disease in seronegative transplant recipients. However, the results of its use in prevention of CMV transmission in other susceptible populations, e.g., newborn infants, are inconclusive. Titers of functional CMV antibodies show great variation in different immunoglobulin products (15), and, as correlations of antibody assays with efficacy in clinical use are unknown, CMV antibodies will have to be looked upon as markers for lot-to-lot consistency rather than as indicators of therapeutic efficacy. Several controlled studies examined possible efficacy of CMV hyperimmunoglobulin in recipients of organ allografts and in bone marrow transplantation (4,16–25). In a large meta-analysis, Glowacki and Smaill (22) reviewed the evidence for the use of immunoglobulin in the prevention of CMV disease in transplant recipients. The time frame was 1980–1991, and 18 studies were analyzed. The results of this analysis combining trials of polyvalent immunoglobulin and hyperimmunoglobulin in solid organ as well as in bone marrow recipients revealed for the treated group as compared to the untreated group a common odds ratio of 0.58 (95% C.I. 0.42–0.77). The patient population who profited most were CMV antibody-negative recipients receiving transplants from CMV-positive donors.

Bone marrow transplantation. Bone marrow transplant recipients are severely immunocompromised in consequence of supralethal doses of chemotherapy and/or radio therapy prior to transplantation. The patients have multiple immunological deficiencies which persist for 6–12 months, and during this time they are at high risk of developing a variety of infections (26). T- and B-cell abnormalities may be seen for years, even in patients with normal numbers of lymphocytes and despite normal levels of immunoglobulins. A subset of patients with chronic graft-versus-host disease (GvHD) is especially at risk for acquiring recurrent infections. IVIG treatment has been beneficial in reducing GvHD and transplant-related mortality in adult recipients of related bone marrow transplants as well as in reducing interstitial pneumonia, fatal CMV disease, and septicemia (16–19,27).

Kidney transplantation. In renal transplant recipients Snydman and co-workers conducted an open-label trial of CMV IVIG (28). The transplant recipients were CMV-negative and received kidneys from CMV-positive donors. The results of this study were difficult to evaluate because the patients treated had more immune suppressive treatment due to a higher rejection rate. In a controlled trial by the same group, a significant reduction in virologically confirmed CMV-associated syndromes could be observed, and graft loss was less frequent in the immunoglobulin recipients (29). Furthermore, superinfection (especially fungal infection) was less frequent in the treated group. Similar results were obtained by Steinmuller et al. (20) and by Metselaar et al. (30) in kidney transplant recipients. Other studies, smaller in size, did not show significant protection (31,32). In addition, prophylaxis of primary CMV disease in renal transplantation has been studied in 51 consecutive CMV serum-negative patients who received renal allografts from serum-positive donors from 1990 to 1992 and were randomized to receive CMV prophylaxis with seven doses of IVIG for 6 weeks or low-dose IV ganciclovir for 3 weeks (23). Results were compared to historical controls who did not receive prophylaxis. Both regimens significantly reduced the incidence of invasive CMV infection ($P < .05$). The cost of ganciclovir was substantially lower. It appears likely that high-titer IgG antibodies against CMV have a certain beneficial effect in organ recipients. However, this effect seems to be limited and is found only if all severe CMV-related symptoms are evaluated as a single entity. On the basis of several studies, CMV immunoglobulin appears to be moderately effective in kidney transplant recipients who receive 150 mg/kg every other week.

CMV immunoglobulin therapy might also be beneficial in other organ transplant recipients. In the evaluation of patients with CMV pneumonitis after lung transplantation in a large single center between 1987 and 1992, 74 lung transplantations were performed, and when the organ from a positive donor was transplanted into a negative recipient, a course of hyperimmune CMV globulin was given. Both ganciclovir and hyperimmunoglobulin have been given, and this treatment appeared to be beneficial when results were compared to results in historical controls (33).

RECENT ATTEMPTS FOR PREVENTION OF VIRAL DISEASE BY HUMAN IMMUNOGLOBULIN PREPARATIONS

Prevention of Viral Disease in Endemic (Hospital) Settings

Enteroviruses

Enteric infections are important causes of morbidity in children in Western countries and contribute to mortality of infants and children in developing countries (34). Enteric infections are also an important threat for immunocompromised populations—e.g., patients with cancer chemotherapy, malnutrition, HIV infection, etc. A subset of these infections is caused by viral pathogens, some of which, even though they mainly replicate in the gastrointestinal tract, may also cause other clinical symptoms—e.g., meningitis, neurological disease, or respiratory infections. Anecdotal studies of gammaglobulin application in enterovirus disease (35) in the first 2 weeks of life showed some advantage of gammaglobulin application in infants with early-onset illness, multisystem disease, and/or viremia, but other studies failed to confirm these results (36).

The agent most frequently encountered in viral gastroenteritis in young children is rotavirus, a double-stranded RNA virus. The acute infection leading to epithelial cell destruction is often associated with vomiting followed by acute diarrhea. As the newly regenerated epithelium may lack certain digestive enzymes, a prolonged intolerance to lactose and other disaccharides may lead to a vicious circle. Rotavirus infection is often accompanied by fever and may be associated with respiratory disease, hepatitis, and neurological abnormalities (37,38). Patients with impaired T-cell function are more likely to develop prolonged infection and may shed virus for several months (39–41).

As rotavirus infection is highly prevalent in the adult population, antibodies to rotavirus are present in varying concentrations in immunoglobulin products. The question also arises, will intravenously administered immunoglobulin be transported to the gut? Yolken et al. (42) investigated the pharmacokinetics of IgG following administration of IVIG by measuring maximal intestinal IgG levels. These authors observed that the highest levels could be detected in intestinal fluids of children with ileostomies and colostomies, but IgG could also be detected in the stools of the babies, even though in smaller quantities. An earlier report by the same group (43) examined the pharmacokinetics of human serum immunoglobulin possessing antirotavirus activity when administered orally to children with primary immunodeficiency syndromes. They used biotin or ^{125}I for labeling. About half of the excreted activity in the stool was in a macromolecular fraction; the remainder was excreted in the urine as low-molecular-weight fragments. Immune complexes composed of rotavirus and specific immunoglobulin could also be identified. These studies indicated that orally administered IgG can survive passage in the gut in an immunologically active form.

Several studies, both controlled and anecdotal, indicated that rotavirus antibodies may be effective in the prevention and treatment of acute rotavirus infection. The antibodies applied were homologous human IgG as available in immunoglobulin products for intramuscular use, as well as bovine antibodies, obtained from the colostrum or milk. Barnes et al. (35) reported results of a randomized trial of oral gammaglobulin in low-birth-weight infants infected with rotavirus. By feeding human immunoglobulins they concluded that gammaglobulin administration was associated with delayed excretion of rotavirus and milder symptoms of infection. Guarini et al. (44) described similar results and also showed a reduction in the time for viral shedding in two patients. Several other investigations (45–47) demonstrated the beneficial effect of bovine antibodies, using milk or colostrum, by documenting a significant reduction in clinical symptoms—e.g., in the number of days with diarrhea and/or a reduction of time of viral shedding. Furthermore, according to an Australian study, bovine antibodies were also effective prophylactically in protecting against rotavirus infection (46).

Respiratory Syncytial Virus

Respiratory syncytial virus (RSV) is the single most important respiratory pathogen in infancy and early childhood. Predictable yearly outbreaks of RSV disease last from the late fall into the spring months and are frequently occurring in hospital units. Primary RSV infection results in bronchiolitis and pneumonia in ca. 40% of the cases in children less than 6 months of age, and preterm infants and infants with underlying pulmonary or cardiac disease are unduly susceptible. Epidemiological studies demonstrated protection against RSV in babies born to mothers with high levels of RSV antibodies. Specificity against fusion or F protein appeared important in protection against disease (48). Different studies in full-term infants (49–54) indicate that high serum titers of RSV-neutralizing antibody (between 1:200 and 1:400) prevent RSV infection in the lower respiratory tract. Studies performed in experimental animals (55–60) clearly indicated that serum titers of RSV-neutralizing antibodies are associated with prevention of RSV infection of the lower respiratory tract, and that protection against nasal challenge can be achieved by moderate titer immunoglobulin in cotton rats (61).

Despite the recognition of humoral immunity against RSV as a protective principle, active immunization is problematic because augmentation of the immune response may also result in more severe pulmonary complications. Antibody titers to respiratory viruses were shown to vary greatly in immunoglobulin products (62). Antibodies quantified by ELISA were poor predictors of in vivo protection in a mouse model for RSV infection (63); neutralization assays are better correlates of protection. As levels of functional antibody against respiratory viruses and especially against RSV are low and vary greatly, regular gammaglobulin products are not suited in prophylactic attempts for this disease. As lung damage in babies may occur very early following the infection, prevention of RSV would be preferable to treatment. Evidence indicating that active immunization of the mother could be protective for the baby in the first month of life suggests that antibodies could be effective in preventing or attenuating the disease in high-risk children (48). The question of prophylactic administration of RSV immunoglobulin has been addressed in several studies. However, a licensed product is not available at present.

A large multicenter clinical trial has been conducted in 249 infants who had bronchopulmonary dysplasia, congenital heart disease, or prematurity alone, and who received high-dose (750 mg/kg) or low-dose (150 mg/kg) hyperimmunoglobulin or no immunoglobulin (64). There were significantly fewer lower respiratory tract infections, fewer hospitalizations, fewer hospital days, fewer days in the intensive care unit, and less use of ribavirin in the group with high-dose hyper-Ig treatment, and the authors concluded that administration of high-dose RSV immunoglobulin is a safe and effective means of preventing lower respiratory tract infection in infants and young children at high risk for this disease.

An accompanying editorial shared the view of the authors (65). In a letter to the editor, however, members of the FDA expressed serious criticism on the quality of the study, especially with regard to randomization and a possible bias due to a large number of dropouts not evenly distributed between the treatment and control arms (66). In addition, a higher mortality in the treated children who had a congenital heart disease could be observed. Even though the difference was not significant, it is a serious concern.

In conclusion, even though epidemiological and experimental studies indicate a protective role of RSV antibodies against disease, results of controlled clinical trials will still have to prove whether RSV hyperimmunoglobulin is safe and efficacious in preventing and/or treating RSV-associated disease.

Herpes Viruses

In spite of the availability of antiviral treatment, neonatal herpes simplex virus infections are still the cause of significant morbidity and mortality. These infections may involve the skin, the eye, and the mouth and may cause encephalitis or disseminated infection. Dangerous, life-threatening complications lead to a mortality of 50% in the babies, and severe sequelae may occur in children who survive. Treatment with high-titer antibodies, e.g., monoclonal antibodies or hyperimmunoglobulins, are considered additional tools in the therapy of babies with disseminated or cerebral disease (67). However, envisaging the theoretical possibility of enhancement of viral replication, results on the safety of IVIG in this setting would be desirable.

The question of possible efficacy of antibodies in herpesvirus infection has been addressed in several experimental studies. McDermott et al. (68) demonstrated that intravenous transfer of antiviral monoclonal antibodies protected against systemic HSV-2 infection but was ineffective against vaginal infection. The antibodies failed to protect against mucosal challenge because of insufficient transport into the secretions. In other studies (69,70), pooled human IVIG was evaluated in the prophylaxis and treatment of herpes simplex encephalitis in a mouse model after intranasal challenge. IVIG was protective against death in a dose-dependent fashion. Interestingly, the antibody-mediated protection was dependent on the Fc part of the immunoglobulin molecule but did not require virus-neutralizing activity. The protective effect of immunoglobulin could be observed when Ig was given up to 4 h postinfection, and a delay in the course of disease without true effect on survival could be observed with treatment up to 3 days postchallenge.

Topical treatment with immunoglobulin in epithelial herpes simplex keratitis has been attempted in humans in a phase I/II study in combination with the antiviral drug trifluorothymidine (71). This anecdotal treatment proved to be safe, but the question of efficacy has still to be answered. Anecdotal use of IVIG in disseminated herpesvirus infection in babies as well as in immunocompromised individuals has been attempted, and there are no reports indicating severe adverse effects.

Another member of the herpesvirus family, Epstein-Barr virus, has been associated with severe virus-induced immune thrombocytopenia in rare instances. Anecdotal experience indicates the effectivity of IVIG in this disease, even in patients in whom steroid therapy failed (72,73).

Human Parvovirus B19

Human parvovirus B19 (B19) is a single-stranded DNA virus of the genus *Parvovirus*, and is the only human parvovirus that causes clinical illness (74). The diseases associated with B19 infection are mostly benign and self-limiting, and include erythema infectiosum, a common childhood exanthematous disease; and transient arthritis and rheumatic symptoms in adults. However, in certain individuals, such as pregnant women, patients with increased erythrocyte production, and patients with immunodeficiency, B19 infection can cause severe disease such as hydrops fetalis and anemia (acute aplastic and hypoplastic or chronic anemia). These disorders result from the capacity of B19 to infect fetal cells such as myocardial cells (75,76) and proliferating cells, especially late erythroid progenitor cells.

Human parvovirus B19 has worldwide distribution, and epidemics of B19 infection or sporadic cases may occur. The incidence of B19 IgG seropositivity is 40–60% in adults more than 20 years old (77). Standard IVIG preparations contain high titers of antibodies against parvovirus B19 (78), and antibodies in IVIG preparations have been shown to neutralize the virus (79). Anecdotal experience suggests that IVIG could be useful in the therapy of chronic or severe B19 infection (78–86). IVIG has been used successfully in the therapy of B19 infection in a hypogammaglobulinemic infant with neurological disorders and anemia (81). Passive administration of B19 antibodies present in the IVIG preparation appeared to clear viral infection in this patient, and clinical manifestations of the disease disappeared as well. Anecdotal results also indicate potential effectivity in other rare cases of red cell aplasia associated with parvovirus infection. Treatment attempts have been reported on single patients with this disease, with or without associated HIV infection. However, treatment results were inconsistent, ranging from dramatic improvement (78,80) to treatment failure (87).

FUTURE APPLICATIONS

Based on the experience that repeated high-dose IVIG treatment is advantageous in chronic echovirus infection, the question has been raised whether long-term treatment of other chronic viral diseases with immunoglobulin preparations containing high amounts of specific antibodies could be of benefit in other chronic viral infections as well. Controlled clinical trials will be necessary to prove this point, and the safety of the products used will be of crucial importance. HIV hyperimmunoglobulin is currently being studied in newborns of infected mothers, and this type of treatment has also been discussed in certain other HIV-infected populations.

REFERENCES

1. Porterfield JS. Antibody-dependent enhancement of viral infectivity. Adv Virus Res 1986; 31:335–355.

2. Mady BJ, Erbe DV, Kurane I, Fanger MW, Ennis FA. Antibody-dependent enhancement of dengue virus infection mediated by bispecific antibodies against cell surface molecules other than Fc gamma receptors. J Immunol 1991; 147:3139–3144.

3. Anonymous. Appropriate use of human immunoglobulin in clinical practice. Memorandum from an IUIS/WHO meeting. Bull World Health Organ 1982; 60:43–47.

4. Siber GR, Snydman DR. Use of mglobulins in the prevention and treatment of infections. Curr Clin Top Infect Dis 1992; 12:208–256.

5. Mease PJ, Ochs HD, Wedgwood RJ. Successful treatment of echovirus meningoencephalitis and myositis-fasciitis with intravenous immune globulin therapy in a patient with x-linked agammaglobulinemia. N Engl J Med 1981;304:1278–1281.

6. Stiehm ER. Standard and special human immune serum globulins as therapeutic agents. Pediatrics 1979; 63:301–319.

7. Janeway CA, Rosen FS. The gammaglobulins. Therapeutic uses of gamma globulin. N Engl J Med 1966; 275:826–831.

8. American Academy of Pediatrics. Passive immunization. In: Peter G, ed. 1994 Red Book Report of the Committee on Infectious Diseases. 23rd ed. Elk Grove Village, IL: American Academy of Pediatrics, 1994:40–43.

9. American Academy of Pediatrics. Hepatitis A. In: Peter G, ed. 1994 Red Book Report of the Committee on Infectious Diseases. 23rd ed. Elk Grove Village, IL: American Academy of Pediatrics, 1994:221–224.

10. Fujiyama S, Iino S, Odoh K, et al. Time course of hepatits A virus antibody titer after active and passive immunization. Hepatology 1992; 15:983–988.

11. American Academy of Pediatrics. Hepatitis B. In: Peter G. ed. 1994 Red Book Report of the Committee on Infectious Diseases. 23rd ed. Elk Grove Village, IL: American Academy of Pediatrics; 1994:224–238.

12. American Academy of Pediatrics. Rabies. In: Peter G, ed. 1994 Red Book Report of the Committee on Infectious Diseases. 23rd ed. Elk Grove Village, IL: American Academy of Pediatrics, 1994:221–224.

13. Centers for Disease Control and Prevention. Recommendations of the Advisory Committe on Immunization Practices (ACIP). Use of vaccines and immune globulins for persons with altered immunocompetence. MMWR 1993; 42(RR-5):1–18.

14. Morell A, Barandun S. Prophylactic and therapeutic use of immunoglobulin for intravenous administration in patients with secondary immunodeficiencies associated with malignancies. Pediatr Infect Dis J 1988; 7(5 Suppl):S87–S91.

15. Chemini J, Peppard J, Emanuel D. Selection of an intravenous immune globulin for the immunoprophylaxis of cytomegalovirus infections: an in vitro comparison of currently available and previously effective immune globulins. Bone Marrow Transplant 1987; 2:395–402.

16. Condie RM, O'Reilly RJ. Prevention of cytomegalovirus infection by prophylaxis with an intravenous, hyperimmune, native, unmodified cytomegalovirus globulin. Am J Med 1984; 76:134–141.

17. Winston DJ, Ho WG, Lin C-H, et al. Intravenous immune globulin for prevention of cytomegalovirus infection and interstitial pneumonia after bone marrow transplantation. Ann Intern Med 1987; 106:12–18.

18. Sullivan KM, Kopecky KJ, Jocom J, et al. Immunomodulatory and antimicrobial efficacy of intravenous immunoglobulin in bone marrow transplantation. N Engl J Med 1990; 323:705–712.

19. Bass EB, Powe NR, Goodman SN, et al. Efficacy of immune globulin in preventing complications of bone marrow transplantation: a meta analysis. Bone Marrow Transplant 1993; 12:273–282.

20. Steinmuller DR, Novick AC, Streem SB, Graneto D, Swift C. Intravenous immunoglobulin infusions for the prophylaxis of secondary cytomegalovirus infection. Transplantation 1990; 49:68–70.

21. Stratta RJ, Taylor RJ, Bynon JS, et al. Viral prophylaxis in combined pancreas-kidney transplant recipients. Transplantation 1994; 57:506–512.
22. Glowacki LS, Smaill FM. Use of immune globulin to prevent symptomatic cytomegalovirus disease in transplant recipients—a meta analysis. Clin Tranplantation 1994; 8:10–18.
23. Conti DJ, Freed BM, Gruber SA, Lempert N. Prophylaxis of primary cytomegalovirus disease in renal transplant recipients. A trial of gancyclovir vs immunoglobulin. Arch Surg 1994; 129:443–447.
24. Dunn DL, Gillingham KJ, Kramer MA, Schmidt WJ, Erice A. A prospective randomized study of acyclovir versus gancyclovir plus human immune globulin prophylaxis of cytomegalovirus infection after solid organ transplantation. Transplantation 1994; 57:876–884.
25. Mor E, Meyers BR, Yagmur O, et al. High-dose acyclovir and intravenous immune globulin reduce the incidence of CMV disease after liver transplantation. Transplant Int 1995; 8:152–156.
26. Lum LG. A review: the kinetics of immune reconstitution after human marrow transplantation. Blood 1987; 69:369–380.
27. Siadak MF, Kopecky K, Sullivan KM. Reduction in transplant-related complications in patients given intravenous immune globulin after allogeneic marrow transplantation. Clin Exp Immunol 1994; 97(suppl 1):53–57.
28. Snydman DR, Werner BG, Tilney NL, et al. A final analysis of primary cytomegalovirus disease prevention in renal transplant recipients with a cytomegalovirus immune globulin: interim comparison of a randomized and an open-label trial. Tranplant Proc 1988; 20:24–30.
29. Snydman DR, Werner BG, Heinze-Lacey B, et al. Use of cytomegalovirus immune globulin to prevent cytomegalovirus disease in renal transplant recipients. N Engl J Med 1987; 317:1049–1054.
30. Metselaar HJ, Rothbarth PH, Brouwer RML, et al. Prevention of cytomegalovirus-related death by passive immunization. Tranplantation 1989; 48:264–266.
31. Kasiske BL, Heim-Duthoy KL, Tortorice KL, et al. Polyvalent immune globulin and cytomegalovirus infection after renal transplantation. Arch Intern Med 1989; 149:2733–2736.
32. Khawand N, Light JA, Brems W, et al. Does intravenous immunoglobulin prevent primary cytomegalovirus disease in kidney transplant recipients? Transplant Proc 1989; 21:2072–2074.
33. Gould FK, Freeman R, Taylor CE, Ashcroft T, Dark JH, Corris PA. Prophylaxis and management of cytomegalovirus pneumonitis after lung transplantation: a review of experience in one center. J Heart Lung Transplant 1993; 12:695–699.
34. Maldonado Y, Yoken RH: Rotavirus. In: Farthing MJG, Keusch GT, eds. Enteric Infection: Mechanisms, Manifestations and Management. London: Chapman and Hall, 1989:365–376.
35. Barnes GL, Hewson PH, McLellan JA, et al. A randomized trial of oral gammaglobulin in low-birth-weight infants infected with rotavirus. Lancet 1982; 1:1371–1373.
36. Piedra PA, Kasel JA, Norton HJ, Gruber WC, Garcia-Prats JA, Baker CJ. Evaluation of an intravenous immunoglobulin preparation for the prevention of viral infections among hospitalized low birth weight infants. Pediatr Infect Dis J 1990; 9:470–475.
37. Santosham M, Yolken RH, Quiroz E, et al. Detection of rotavirus in respiratory secretions of children with pneumonia. J Pediatr 1983; 103:583–585.
38. Kinney JS, Eiden JJ. Enteric infectious disease in neonates. Epidemiology, pathogenesis, and a practical approach to evaluation and therapy. Clin Perinatol 1994; 21:317–333.
39. Townsend T, Yolken RH, Bishop CA, et al. Outbreak of Coxsackie A1 gastroenteritis: a complication of bone marrow transplantation. Lancet 1982; 1:820–823.
40. Saulsbury FT, Winkelstein JA, Yolken RH. Chronic rotavirus infection in immunodeficiency. J Pediatr 1980; 97:61–65.
41. Eiden J, Losonski GA, Johnson J, Yolken RH. Rotavirus RNA variation during chronic infection of immunocompromised children. Pediatr Infect Dis J 1985; 4:632–637.

42. Yolken R, Kinney J, Wilde J, Willoughby R, Eiden J. Immunoglobulins and other modalities for the prevention and treatment of enteric viral infection. J Clin Immunol 1990; 10(Nov. suppl):80S–87S.

43. Losonsky GA, Johnson JP, Winkelstein JA, Yolken RH. Oral administration of human serum immunoglobulin in immunodeficient patients with viral gastroenteritis. J Clin Invest 1985; 76:2362–2367.

44. Guarino A, Guandalini S, Albano F, Mascia A, de Ritis G, Rubino A. Enteral immunoglobulins for treatment of protracted rotaviral diarrhea. Pediatr Infect Dis J 1991; 10:612–614.

45. Turner RB, Kelsey DK. Passive immunization for prevention of rotavirus illness in healthy infants. Pediatr Infect Dis J 1993; 12:718–722.

46. Davidson GP, Daniels E, Nunan H, et al. Passive immunization of children with bovine colostrum containing antibodies to human rotavirus. Lancet 1989; 2:709–712.

47. Hilpert H, Brssow H, Mietens C, Sidoti C, Lerner L, Werchau H. Use of bovine milk concentrate containing antibody of rotavirus to treat rotavirus gastroenteritis in infants. J Infect Dis 1987; 156:158–166.

48. Englund JA. Passive protection against respiratory syncytial virus disease in infants: the role of maternal antibody. Pediatr Infect Dis J 1994; 13:449–453.

49. Parrott RH, Kim HW, Arrobio JO, et al. Epidemiology of respiratory syncytial virus infection in Washington, D.C. II. Infection and disease with respect to age, immunologic status, race and sex. Am J Epidemiol 1973; 98:289–300.

50. Glezen WP, Paredes A, Allison JE, Taber LH, Frank AL. Risk of respiratory syncytial virus infection for infants from low-income families in relationship to age, sex, ethnic group, and maternal antibody level. J Pediatr 1981; 98:708–715.

51. Bruhn FW, Yeager AS. Respiratory syncytial virus in early infancy: circulating antibody and the severity of infection. Am J Dis Child 1977; 131:145–148.

52. Lamprecht CL, Krause HE, Mufson MA. Role of maternal antibody in pneumonia and bronchiolitis due to respiratory syncytial virus. J Infect Dis 1976; 134:211–217.

53. Ogilvie MM, Vathenen AS, Radford M, Codd J, Key S. Maternal antibody and respiratory syncytial virus infection in infancy. J Med Virol 1981; 7:263–271.

54. Ward KA, Lambden PR, Ogilvie MM, Watt PJ. Antibodies to respiratory syncytial virus polypeptides and their significance in human infection. J Gen Virol 1983; 64:1867–1876.

55. Prince GA, Jenson AB, Horswood RL, Camargo E, Chanock RM. The pathogenesis of respiratory syncytial virus infection in cotton rats. Am J Pathol 1978; 93:771–791.

56. Prince GA, Horswood RL, Camargo E, Koenig D, Chanock RM. Mechanisms of immunity to respiratory syncytial virus in cotton rats. Infect Immun 1983; 42:81–87.

57. Prince GA, Jenson AB, Hemming VG, et al. Enhancement of respiratory syncytial virus pulmonary pathology in cotton rats by prior intramuscular inoculation of formalin-inactivated virus. J Virol 1986; 57:721–728. [Erratum: J Virol 1986; 59:193.]

58. Prince GA, Horswood RL, Chanock RM. Quantitative aspects of passive immunity to respiratory syncytial virus infection in infant cotton rats. J Virol 1985; 55:517–520.

59. Prince GA, Hemming VG, Horswood RL, Chanock RM. Immunoprophylaxis and immunotherapy of respiratory syncytial virus infection in the cotton rat. Virus Res 1985; 3:193–206.

60. Prince GA, Hemming VG, Horswood RL, Baron PA, Chanock RM. Effectiveness of topically administered neutralizing antibodies in experimental immunotherapy of respiratory syncytial virus infection in cotton rats. J Virol 1987; 61:1851–1854.

61. Sami IR, Piazza FM, Johnson SA, et al. Systemic immunoprophylaxis of nasal respiratory syncytial virus infection in cotton rats. J Infect Dis 1995; 171:440–443.

62. Hemming VG, Prince GA. Intravenous immunoglobulin G in viral respiratory infections for newborns and infants. Pediatr Infect Dis J 1986; 5:S204–S206.

63. Siber GR, Leszczynski J, Pena-Cruz V, et al. Protective activity of a human respiratory syncytial virus immune globulin prepared from donors with high antibody by microneutralization assay. J Infect Dis 1992; 165:456–463.

64. Groothuis JR, Simoes EAF, Levin MJ, et al. Prophylactic administration of respiratory syncytial virus immune globulin to high-risk infants and young children. N Engl J Med 1993; 329:1524–1530.
65. McIntosh K. Respiratory syncytial virus—successful immunoprophylaxis at last. N Engl J Med 1993; 329:1572–1573. Editorial.
66. Ellenberg SS, Epstein JS, Fratantoni JC, Scott D, Zoon KC. A trial of RSV immune globulin in infants and young children: the FDA's view. N Engl J Med 1994; 331:203–204. Letter.
67. Whitley RJ. Neonatal herpes simplex virus infections: is there a role for immunoglobulin in disease prevention and therapy? Pediatr Infect Dis J 1994; 13:432–438.
68. McDermott MR, Brais LJ, Evelegh MJ. Mucosal and systemic antiviral antibodies in mice inoculated intravaginally with herpes simplex virus type 2. J Gen Virol 1990; 71 (Pt 7):1497–1504.
69. Erlich KS, Dix RD, Mills J. Prevention and treatment of experimental herpes simplex virus encephalitis with human immune serum globulin. Antimicrob Agents Chemother 1987; 31:1006–1009.
70. Erlich KS, Mills J. Passive immunotherapy for encephalitis caused by herpes simplex virus. Rev Infect Dis 1986; 8(suppl 4):S439–S445.
71. Klager AJ, Buchi ER, Osusky R, Burek-Kozlowska A, Morel A. Topical immunoglobulins for epithelial herpes simplex keratitis. Ophthalmologica 1993; 207:78–81.
72. Hugo H, Linde A, Abom PE. Epstein-Barr virus induced thrombocytopenia treated with intravenous acyclovir and immunoglobulin. Scand J Infect Dis 1989; 21:103–105.
73. Duncombe AS, Amos RJ, Metcalfe P, Pearson TC. Intravenous immunoglobulin therapy in thrombocytopenic infectious mononucleosis. Clin Lab Haematol 1989; 11:11–15.
74. Luban NLC. Human parvoviruses: implications for transfusion medicine. Transfusion 1994; 34:821–827.
75. Porter HJ, Quantril AM, Kleming KA. B19 parvovirus infection of myocardial cells. Lancet 1988; 1:535–536. Letter.
76. Weiland HT, Vermey-Keers C, Salimans MM, Fleuren GJ, Verwey RA, Anderson MJ. Parvovirus B19 associated with fetal abnormality. Lancet 1987; 1:682–683. Letter.
77. Anderson LJ. Role of parvovirus B19 in human disease. Pediatr Infect Dis J 1987; 6:711–718.
78. Schwarz TF, Roggendorf M, Hottentrger B, Modrow S, Deinhardt F, Middeldorp J. Immunoglobulins in the prophylaxis of parvovirus B19 infection. J Infect Dis 1990; 162:1214. Letter.
79. Takahashi M, Koike T, Moriyama Y, Shibata A. Neutralizing activity of immunoglobulin preparation against erythropoietic suppression of human parvovirus. Am J Hematol 1991; 37:68. Letter.
80. Kurtzman G, Frickhofen N, Kimball J, et al. Pure red cell aplasia of 10 years' duration due to persistent parvovirus B19 infection and its cure with immunoglobulin therapy. N Engl J Med 1989; 321:519–523.
81. Nigro G, D'Eufemia P, Zerbini M, et al. Parvovirus B19 infection in a hypogammaglobulinemic infant with neurologic disorders and anemia: successful immunoglobulin therapy. Pediatr Infect Dis J 1994; 13:1019–1021.
82. Ramage JK, Hale A, Gane E, et al. Parvovirus B19-induced red cell aplasia treated with plasmapheresis and immunoglobulin. Lancet 1994; 343:667–668. Letter.
83. Finkel TH, Trk TJ, Ferguson PJ, et al. Chronic parvovirus B19 infection and systemic necrotising vasculitis: opportunistic infection or aetiological agent? Lancet 1994; 343:1255–1258.
84. Murray JC, Gresik MV, Leger F, McClain KL. B19 parvovirus-induced anemia in a normal child. Am J Pediatr Hematol Oncol 1993; 15:420–423.
85. Tang MLK, Kemp AS, Moaven LD. Parvovirus B19-associated red blood cell aplasia in

combined immunodeficiency with normal immunoglobulins. Pediatr Inf Dis J 1994; 13:539–542.

86. Nour B, Green M, Michaels M, et al. Parvovirus B19 infection in pediatric transplant patients. Transplantation 1993; 56:835–838.

87. Bowman CA, Cohen BJ, Norfolk DR, Lacey CJ. Red cell aplasia associated with human parvovirus B19 and HIV infection: failure to respond clinically to intravenous immunoglobulin. AIDS 1990; 4:1038–1039. Letter.

88. Centers for Disease Control. General recommendations on immunization. Recommendations of the Advisory Committee on Immunization Practices (ACIP). MMWR 1994; 43 (RR-1):1–38.

19

Intravenous Immunoglobulin Therapy of Neonates with Nonpolio Enteroviral Infections

Harry L. Keyserling
Emory University School of Medicine, Atlanta, Georgia

VIROLOGY

The enteroviruses are small, 24- to 30-nm particles with a single-stranded RNA genome. They are classified as Picornaviridae. In 1957, several groups of viruses (polio, Coxsackie, and echo) were combined into the enterovirus genus. Although polioviruses caused severe epidemics of paralytic disease in the first half of the 20th century, successful vaccine programs have eliminated polio from the Western hemisphere, and a multinational effort is under way to eradicate polio from the world. This leaves the nonpolio enteroviruses as the major neonatal viral infection during the summer months in the United States. Enteroviruses of human origin include the following:

1. Coxsackie viruses A: 23 types and several variants (Coxsackie viruses A1–A24 [Coxsackie virus type A 23 is the same virus as echovirus 9])
2. Coxsackie viruses B: types B1–B6
3. Echoviruses: 31 types (types 1-33 [echovirus 10 has been reclassified as reovirus type 1, and echovirus 28 as rhinovirus type 1A])
4. Enterovirus types 68–71

All enteroviruses contain four structural proteins: VP1, VP2, VP3, and VP4. The variability of these structural proteins accounts for the unique serotypes. Although minor mutations occur rapidly, the emergence of new serotypes is rare. Since the enteroviruses lack a lipid envelope, they resist inactivation by alcohol and ether.

EPIDEMIOLOGY

Humans are the only natural host for the identified human enteroviral serotypes. Enteroviruses are distributed worldwide. Infection is thought to provide lifelong protection against that particular serotype. Infections predominate during warm weather.

Therefore, infections occur year-round in tropical climates. The peak season in the United States is May through September. Transmission occurs by the fecal-oral or respiratory route. Most infections are subclinical. During the summer months, a significant proportion of children will be shedding enterovirus in their stools. The incubation period is 2–6 days. Nonpolio enteroviruses (Coxsackie A, B; echo) are common human pathogens that cause a diverse spectrum of clinical syndromes. Diseases include pharyngitis, upper respiratory infections, conjunctivitis, parotitis, myocarditis, hepatitis, pneumonia, pancreatitis, orchitis, pleurodynia, and meningitis. Although most infections are asymptomatic or self-limited, fulminant hepatitis and myocarditis may be fatal. Neurological sequelae may occur following meningitis.

Neonates are more susceptible to severe disease than older children and adults. Lake et al. (1) reported 27 symptomatic neonates in Denver, Colorado, between 1969 and 1975. All patients were hospitalized within the first 2 weeks of life. Only 19% had a gestational age of ≤37 weeks. Maternal illness compatible with enteroviral infection occurred in 59%. Symptoms included fever (93%), poor feeding (89%), diarrhea (81%), rash (41%), hepatomegaly (37%), jaundice (19%), and seizures (15%). Seventy-two percent were male. Four children had thrombocytopenia, and three were diagnosed with necrotizing enterocolitis. Three children died with Coxsackie B virus infections. All infants who died were symptomatic within 36 h of life, and their mothers had clinical illnesses that started less than 3 days before delivery.

Morens reviewed data from the Centers for Disease Control and Prevention (CDC) (2). During this time period, states and territories representing two-thirds of the population of the United States reported clinical data on enteroviral isolates. Of 338 isolates from infants less than 2 months of age during 1972–1975, 51% were echoviruses, 45% Coxsackie B viruses, and 4% Coxsackie A viruses. Sources of enteroviral isolates were stool (52%), throat or nasopharynx (20%), cerebrospinal fluid (CSF) (11%), blood (9%), tissue (5%), and urine (3%). The male:female ratio was 1.4:1. Seventy-four percent of all neonates had severe disease, compared to only 8% of all adults. Fatal disease occurred in five infants. The reported incidence of enteroviral disease was 10 or more times greater in infants than it was in school-aged children and nearly 100 times greater than in middle-aged adults.

Jenista et al. (3) prospectively followed 586 infants born in Rochester, New York, during the summer of 1981. Infants had throat and rectal cultures done on day 1 of life and weekly until 28 days. Enteroviruses were not isolated on day 1 of life, nor at any time in the 12 infants who were never discharged from the hospital during the first month. Nonpolio enteroviruses were isolated at least one time from 75 (12.8%) infants. Seventy-nine percent of infants who were culture-positive for enterovirus were asymptomatic. During the neonatal period, 24 of 586 (4%) infants were readmitted to the hospital; 17 of the 24 (71%) were diagnosed with suspected sepsis; 14 of the 17 (82%) had an enterovirus isolated from admission viral cultures. Risk factors for enterovirus infection included lower socioeconomic status and lack of breast-feeding.

Abzug et al. (4) reported on 57 infants less than 2 weeks of age referred for possible enteroviral infections based on a clinical diagnosis during a 2-year period. Physicians in metropolitan Denver were encouraged to refer patients who had illnesses compatible with enterovirus infection. Twenty-nine infants had culture-proven enteroviral infections, 23 had illnesses compatible with enteroviral infection, and five had definitively established alternative diagnoses: herpes simplex virus infection (one), bacterial infections (two), and metabolic disorders (two). Of the 29 neonates with proven enteroviral infection, 93% were term and 52% were female. In other reported series, there is usually a male predominance. Exposure to ill contacts with symptoms of viral illness 1 week prior to one week after deliver was frequent—mothers (65%), one sibling (58%), a second sibling (21%), fathers (14%), and other visitors (17%). Onset of symptoms was reported at a mean age of 6.6 days. Neonatal symptoms and signs included fever, irritability, anorexia, lethargy, hypoperfusion, rash, jaundice, and respiratory abnormalities. Laboratory abnormalities included CSF pleocytosis (53%), infiltrate on chest x-ray (38%), transaminase elevation (21%), and thrombocytopenia (14%). Five of the 29 infants had severe disseminated disease (pneumonitis, hepatitis, thrombocytopenia, bleeding, and meningitis) requiring lengthy hospitalizations. No patient died, although two had residual hepatic dysfunction. Severe disease was more likely if symptoms were noted at an early age or maternal symptoms were present at delivery. Absence of fever, tachypnea, lethargy, abdominal distention, hepatomegaly, and positive serum viral cultures were all associated with severe illness.

PATHOGENESIS

Maternal viremia during enteroviral infections occurs commonly. There have been several reported cases of early transplacental infection, but there is no "congenital enterovirus syndrome." The majority of neonatal infections occur late in pregnancy, near the time of delivery, as a result of hematogenous dissemination from the infected placenta or ingestion or aspiration of contaminated maternal vaginal or fecal material at the time of delivery. After local infection of the pharynx, lower alimentary tract, or lungs, the infection progresses to the regional lymph nodes. Several days later a minor viremia occurs, resulting in dissemination of virus to susceptible organ systems: brain, heart, spleen, pancreas, adrenals. Three to 7 days after infection, symptomatic disease is manifest. The primary immune mechanism for recovery is the development of neutralizing serotype-specific antibody. After recovery, neonates may shed enterovirus in the stool for many weeks. Based on murine models and the age distribution of severe disease, it is hypothesized that enteroviral disease is more severe in neonatal mice and human neonates than in older children and adults. The possible mechanisms for the increased susceptibility include a deficiency in neonates to produce interferon, increased concentration of adrenocortical hormones, increased receptor sites for enteroviruses present in neonatal cells, and physiological hypothermia of infancy (5).

DIAGNOSIS

Viruses can be isolated from many sources—throat, nasopharynx, eyes, blood, CSF, feces, urine, and tissue (heart, liver, spleen, pancreas, adrenals). Since many neonates are asymptomatically infected, stool is generally not an ideal source for culture to establish the etiology of symptomatic disease. The most common sites for culture are blood, CSF, and throat.

Initially, nonpolio enteroviruses were isolated in suckling mice. Today, this method is only used in reference laboratories. Tissue culture is currently the diagnostic method of choice. Most virology laboratories use primary monkey kidney (PMK) cells and human diploid fibroblasts (e.g., WI-38). These may be supplemented with rhabdomyosarcoma (RD) cells and Buffalo green monkey (BGM) cells. Unfortunately, the yield of positive cultures in presumptive enteroviral neonatal infections is usually about 50% in excellent virology laboratories. Reasons for failure to isolate virus include obtaining cultures late in disease when CNS and blood cultures have become negative, as demonstrated in studies performing serial cultures, and that inoculated cell lines may not support replication of the particular enterovirus serotype (particularly Coxsackie A). Recently, polymerase chain reaction (PCR) assays have been developed that are more sensitive and rapid than conventional tissue culture.

THERAPY

General Management of Enteroviral Infections

Therapy for systemic enteroviral infections is primarily supportive. The use of steroids in treating myocarditis remains controversial. No antiviral chemotherapeutic agents have reached clinical trials. Most compounds that inhibit enterovirus in tissue culture are too toxic for clinical evaluation.

During an enterovirus outbreak in Massachusetts in the summer of 1979 (6), seven of 194 pregnant women at term (3.6%) had echovirus 11. All of the mothers and infants had detectable neutralizing antibodies to echovirus 11. Four of the seven infants were shedding virus from the respiratory or gastrointestinal tract by 3 days of age. None of these four infants developed any symptoms of enterovirus disease. High serum-neutralizing antibody levels prevent invasive disease but do not necessarily prevent gastrointestinal or respiratory mucosal infection.

Prophylactic Immunotherapy

The use of intramuscularly administered immune serum globulin (ISG) has been advocated for prevention of nosocomial epidemics in neonatal nurseries. The success of such an approach has had mixed results. In a newborn special care unit, Nagington (7) found in the analysis of a small number of cases that none of the mothers whose infants had symptoms and positive cultures had detectable antibodies in prenatal serum, and that of those with asymptomatic babies and positive cultures, two of three had neutralizing antibodies. The same authors, compiling the results of the preceding outbreak and several other outbreaks (8), found negative antibody titers in seven of eight symptomatically infected infants and elevated titers in three of three asymptomatically infected infants. With this information in mind, convalescent antiecho 11 serum specimens (neutralizing titer 1:640), which had been stored at –20°C, were given in two 1-ml injections to a total of three neonates exposed to known echovirus 11. No symptomatic infections were noted in the recipients, and only one asymptomatic infection was noted.

Nagington has also reported the use of normal immunoglobulin (9) in the interruption of another echovirus 11 outbreak. The globulin was known to have neutralizing titer of 1:80. After administration of 250 mg intramuscularly to all infants exposed to a known case of echovirus 11, there were no further cases with positive cultures until after the cessation of the gammaglobulin regimen, whereupon another case occurred, followed by several others. The number of new cases decreased significantly in the weeks after the resumption of gammaglobulin, and eventually no new cases occurred for several weeks until the end of the enterovirus season.

Kinney et al. (10) reported an outbreak of nosocomial echo 11 infection in a Canadian neonatal nursery during the summer of 1983. In an attempt to control the outbreak, ISG was administered. Four infants who received ISG developed echovirus 11 disease. She concluded that ISG administration did not appear to be beneficial. Two possible explanations for the failure of ISG prophylaxis are that it was administered to infants who had already been infected or that the amount of neutralizing antibody present in the ISG was too low to be effective.

Immunotherapy for Chronic Enteroviral Meningitis

Additional evidence for the beneficial effect of serum-neutralizing antibody against enteroviral illness was presented by Mease (11) in the case of a man with X-linked agammaglobulinemia and chronic echo 11 meningitis and myositis. Following one course of intravenous globulin (titer 1:32), he showed clinical improvement, as well as elimination of the echovirus from his CSF. After a repeated course of IV globulin, a muscle biopsy was also culture-negative for virus. Another agammaglobulinemic patient with chronic encephalitis was reported by Weiner (12) in whom the CSF was continually positive for virus in spite of treatment with commercial low-titered gamma globulin. When immune plasma with high antiecho 5 activity was given, virus was eliminated from the blood and CSF.

In Vitro Activity of Immunoglobulin Against Enteroviruses

Dagan et al. (13) have shown that each of several commercially available gammaglobulin preparations which were tested had neutralizing antibodies against a variety of enteroviruses (Coxsackie A9, B1-5; echo 3, 5, 6, 9, 13). The serotypes tested accounted for 60% of the nonpolio enteroviruses reported to the CDC, as published in 1982 (14).

Keyserling et al. (15) evaluated three commercial intravenous immune globulin (IVIG) preparations: Gammagard (ion-exchange adsorption), Gamimune (reduced and alkylated), and Sandoglobulin (acid, pepsin treated) for neutralizing activity against 13 common enteroviral serotypes. IVIG preparations can differ in IgG subclass distribution and biological activity, which might influence the neutralizing potency against enteroviruses. Random lots were obtained from the hospital pharmacy and reconstituted according to the manufacturer's instructions immediately prior to testing. All three IVIG products had neutralizing activity for all viruses tested (Table 1). Titers ranged from 8 (echo 4) to 496 (CB2). Gammagard had slightly higher titers than the other two preparations.

Case Reports of IVIG Therapy

Based on the evidence that commercial lots of IVIG preparations have high neutralizing antibody titers against common enteroviral serotypes circulating in the community, these products have been considered as therapy for severe neonatal enteroviral disease. The use of IVIG in a severely ill neonate with echo 5 was reported by Black et al. at Kaiser Hospital in Oakland, California (16). During 4 days of therapy there was im-

Table 1 Neutralizing Antibody Against Common Enterovirus Serotypes

Virus type	Gammagard	Gamimune	Sandoglobulin
Coxsackie A9	32	16	16
Coxsackie A16	2048	1024	1024
Coxsackie B1	512	256	256
Coxsackie B2	4096	2048	1024
Coxsackie B3	512	256	256
Coxsackie B4	2048	1024	1024
Coxsackie B5	512	256	256
Echo 4	16	8	8
Echo 6	512	256	256
Echo 9	1024	512	512
Echo 11	1024	256	128
Echo 11'	512	64	64
Echo 30	256	128	128

provement in platelet count, liver function, and oxygen requirement. Both liver function and platelet count deteriorated after therapy was discontinued. Improvement occurred again when therapy was resumed, and the child survived without apparent sequelae following a 10-day course.

Johnston et al. (17) reported a disseminated echo 11 infection in a term infant who became ill at day 3 of life. She had pneumonia, hepatitis, meningitis, and disseminated intravascular coagulation. On day 7 of life, a single 1 g/kg dose of IVIG was infused over 3 h. The patient began to improve 2–3 days after the IVIG and was discharged at day 16 of life. The IVIG preparation had a 1:40 titer of antibody against echovirus 11. Six days after the IVIG infusion, the infant's antibody titer was 1:160. It is not known whether the patient's recovery was due to the IVIG infusion or the endogenous production of neutralizing antibody.

Wong et al. (18) reported on a Coxsackie B1 infection in a male term infant who developed symptoms on day 2 of life. He had hepatitis, disseminated intravascular coagulation, pulmonary hemorrhage, pneumonia, myocarditis, and meningitis. On day 5 of life, he received 1 g/kg of IVIG. During the next 4 days, he had progressive liver failure and cardiac failure. He died on day 10, of massive pulmonary hemorrhage.

Valduss et al. (19) reported on a set of twin girls with Coxsackie B1 infection. Both infants became ill on day 3 of life with meningitis and disseminated intravascular coagulation. On day 8 of life, viral cultures were positive for a presumptive enterovirus. Both infants received multiple doses of IVIG at 500 mg/kg/day. Both infants survived and were discharged at day 25 of life.

Prospective IVIG Trial

Abzug et al. (20) conducted a prospective randomized study in 20 neonates < 14 days of age with clinical presentations presumed to be due to enterovirus infection. Enrollment criteria included age ≤ 2 weeks and one of more of the following preliminary diagnoses: meningitis (CSF WBC count $> 50/mm^3$), hepatitis (alanine aminotransferase level > 100 IU/L), myocarditis (abnormal echocardiogram or electrocardiogram), clinical sepsis without evident bacterial focus, or a medical history and findings on physical examination suggestive of enterovirus infection (such as fever, family history consistent with enterovirus infection, viral exanthem). Sixteen infants had positive cultures for an enterovirus (nine in IVIG group, seven in control group). Four had negative cultures (one in IVIG group, three in control group). The treatment group received 750 mg/kg of Gammagard immune globulin intravenous. Two different lots of IVIG were used. Placebo therapy was not administered to the control group. Therapy was administered on admission to the hospital prior to tissue culture confirmation of enteroviral disease. Viral cultures of throat, stool, CSF , serum, and urine were obtained prior to enrollment. Serial cultures of serum and urine were obtained daily for 5 days. Patients were examined daily to monitor the resolution of symptoms.

Enterovirus serotypes isolated included echovirus 6 (IVIG, none; control, two), echovirus 9 (IVIG, one; control, one), echovirus 11 (IVIG, three; control, none), Coxsackie virus B2 (IVIG, one; control, 1), and Coxsackie virus B4 (IVIG, three; control, two). One isolate in the IVIG group was nontypeable; one isolate in the control group was not available for typing or neutralization assays. Eleven of 15 neonates had no measurable neutralizing antibody (< 1:20) against their respective serotype. Sequential cultures demonstrated that eight (50%) of 16 had viremia and seven (44%) of 16 had viruria at some point during the study period. Viremia occurred in five (71%) of seven patients with echovirus infection, compared to only one (14%) of seven patients with Coxsackie B virus infection. All 14 patients who had follow-up serum available 1 or 4 months after enrollment seroconverted or had a ≥2 to fourfold rise in neutralizing antibody to their respective isolates.

Neutralizing titers of the two lots of immune globulin were tested against each patient isolate. Both lots had reciprocal geometric mean titers to all isolates of 439. Neutralizing titers between the two lots were within 1 dilution of each other. Five of the nine patients who were in the treatment arm received IVIG with a titer of ≥1:800 to their isolates. Neutralizing antibody against 14 of 15 isolates was present in the IVIG with a range of 1:100 to 1:3200. No significant differences in positive serum or urine cultures were noted in comparing the IVIG and control groups. If patients were stratified into those who received IVIG containing a titer of ≥1:800, three (60%) of five had positive cultures at study entry and negative cultures on all subsequent days. Six (54%) of 11 patients had positive cultures at enrollment in the control group or who received IVIG with a titer < 1:800. Eight (73%) of 11 had positive cultures after the day of enrollment (Table 2). No significant differences were noted between the IVIG and control groups with respect to days of fever (mean 3.1 vs. mean 4.3), days of symptomatic disease (mean 5.2 vs. mean 4.8), hospital days (mean 10.8 vs. mean 5.6), and residual problems at discharge (22% vs. 14%). IVIG infusions were generally well tolerated. All infants who received IVIG developed endogenous antibody to their isolates as demonstrated in convalescent sera.

This study, limited by small sample size, showed that cessation of viremia and viruria was associated with administration of IVIG containing relatively high neutralizing titers.

CONCLUSIONS

IVIG therapy for enteroviral infections remains controversial. One issue is selecting appropriate patients and initiating therapy early in the course of disease progression,

Table 2 Daily Viral Cultures (serum or urine)

	No. days after entry in study				
	0	1	2	3	4-7
IVIG, neutralization titer ≥1:800	+	−	−	ND	ND
	+	−	−	−	−
	+	−	−	−	ND
	−	−	−	ND	−
	−	−	−	−	ND
IVIG, neutralization titer <1:800	+	+	−	−	−
	+	−	+	−	−
	−	+	−	−	−
	+	+	−	−	ND
No IVIG	+	+	−	−	−
	−	−	+	ND	−
	−	−	−	+	+
	+	+	−	−	−
	+	−	−	ND	−
	−	−	−	ND	−
	−	−	−	−	−

Key: + = virus isolated in tissue culture; − = no virus isolated; ND = culture not done.

prior to serious organ system involvement. Severe illness is associated with maternal disease and early age of presentation. Term infants who manifest symptoms after 2 weeks of age generally have mild disease with no neurological or cardiac sequelae. Neonatal enteroviral infections cannot be differentiated from herpes simplex infections or disseminated bacterial or fungal infections. There is currently no methodology to make a rapid diagnosis. The potential exists to develop PCR techniques that could achieve a rapid diagnosis with the possibility of identifying the particular serotype. Empiric therapy with IVIG may not provide sufficient neutralizing activity for uncommon types or new epidemic strains not previously encountered by the community. Public health surveillance to identify the serotypes circulating early in the enteroviral season would provide data for the selection of prescreened IVIG lots with high neutralizing activity directed against community types or the 5–10 most commonly encountered serotypes.

Future studies with IVIG will require multicenter collaborative trials to enroll sufficient subjects to demonstrate a clinical benefit of therapy. The studies should have sufficient power to evaluate both virological and clinical endpoints. Higher or repeated doses versus a single infusion may provide a better outcome. Until additional information is generated from appropriate prospective randomized trials, routine use of IVIG remains unproven. Therapy should be considered in severely ill neonates with onset of disease in the first few days of life.

REFERENCES

1. Lake AM, Lauer BA, Clark JC, Wesenberg RL, McIntosh K. Enterovirus infections in neonates. J Pediatr 1976; 89:787–791.

2. Morens DM. Enteroviral disease in early infancy. J Pediatr 1978; 92:374–377.

3. Jenista JA, Powell KR, Menegus MA. Epidemiology of neonatal enterovirus infection. J Pediatr 1984; 104:685–690.

4. Abzug MJ, Levin MJ, Rotbart HA. Profile of enterovirus disease in the first two weeks of life. Pediatr Infect Dis J 1993; 12:820–824.

5. Cherry JD. Enteroviruses. In: Remington JS, Klein JO, eds. Infectious Diseases of the Fetus and Newborn. 4th ed. Philadelphia: W. B. Saunders, 1995:405–446.

6. Modlin JF, Polk BF, Horton P, Etkind P, Crane E, Spiliotes A. Perinatal echovirus infection: risk of transmission during a community outbreak. N Engl J Med 1981; 305:368–371.

7. Nagington J, Wreghitt TG, Gandy G, Roberton NRC, Berry PJ. Fatal echovirus 11 infections in outbreak in special-care baby unit. Lancet 1978; ii:725–728.

8. Nagington J. Echovirus 11 infection and prophylactic antiserum. Lancet 1982; i:446.

9. Nagington J, Walker J, Gandy G, Gray JJ. Use of normal immunoglobulin in an echovirus 11 outbreak in a special-care baby unit. Lancet 1983; ii:443–446.

10. Kinney JS, McCray E, Kaplan JE, et al. Risk factors associated with echovirus 11' infection in a hospital nursery. Pediatr Infect Dis 1986; 5:192–197.

11. Mease PJ, Ochs HD, Wedgwood RJ. Successful treatment of echovirus meningoencephalitis and myositis-fasciitis with intravenous immune globulin therapy in a patient with X-linked agammaglobulinemia. N Engl J Med 1981; 304:1278–1281.

12. Weiner LS, Howell JT, Langford MP, Stanton GJ, Baron S, Goldblum RM. Effect of specific antibodies on chronic echovirus type 5 encephalitis in a patients with hypogammaglobulinemia. J Infect Dis 1979; 140:858–863.

13. Dagan R, Prather SL, Powell KR, Menegus MA. Neutralizing antibodies to non-polio enteroviruses in human immune serum globulin. Pediatr Infect Dis 1983; 2:454–456.

14. Moore M. Enteroviral disease in the United States, 1970–1979. J Infect Dis 1982; 146:103–108.

15. Keyserling HL, Torfason EG. Comparison of intravenous gamma globulin preparations in neutralization assays against enteroviruses. In: Program and Abstracts of the 26th Interscience Conference on Antimicrobial Agents and Chemotherapy, New Orleans, LA. Washington, D.C.: American Society for Microbiology, 1986:156. Abstract 328.

16. Black S. Treatment of overwhelming neonatal echo 5 virus infection with intravenous gamma globulin. In: Program and Abstracts of the 23rd Interscience Conference on Antimicrobial Agents and Chemotherapy, Las Vegas, NV. Washington, D.C.: American Society for Microbiology, 1983:140. Abstract 314.

17. Johnston JM, Overall JC Jr. Intravenous immunoglobulin in disseminated neonatal echovirus 11 infection. Pediatr Infect Dis J 1989; 8:254–256.

18. Wong SN, Tam AYC, Ng THK, Ng WF, Tong CY, Tang TS. Fatal Coxsackie B1 virus infection in neonates. Pediatr Infect Dis J 1989; 8:638–641.

19. Valduss D, Murray DL, Karna P, Lapour K, Dyke J. Use of intravenous immunoglobulin in twin neonates with disseminated Coxsackie B1 infection. Clin Pediatr 1993; 32:561–563.

20. Abzug MJ, Keyserling HL, Lee ML, Levin MJ, Rotbart HA. Neonates enterovirus infection: virology, serology, and effects of intravenous immune globulin. Clin Infect Dis 1995; 20:1201–1206.

20

Treatment of Chronic Fatigue Syndrome

Andrew R. Lloyd and Denis Wakefield
Prince Henry Hospital, Sydney, Australia

INTRODUCTION

Chronic fatigue syndrome (CFS) is characterized by unexplained persistent or relapsing fatigue and constitutional symptoms including myalgia and arthralgia, sore throat, headache, and tender glands (1). In addition, unrefreshing sleep and neurocognitive difficulties such as short-term memory impairment and concentration loss are typical (1). The syndrome predominantly affects young adults often following a documented, or an apparent, infective illness (2). Estimates of prevalence in primary care range from 5.9 to 37/100,000 (2,3).

ETIOLOGY

The recent development and refinement of diagnostic criteria for CFS (1,4–6) has been the result of concerted efforts by several research teams to delineate a unique patient group who are likely to share a common underlying pathophysiology. Despite these efforts the etiology of the disorder remains unclear, with immunological (7), virological (8–10), neuroendocrine (11), and psychological (12) hypotheses all under evaluation. Recent evidence from our research suggests that the label of CFS continues to describe a heterogeneous patient group with the primary confounding diagnoses being depression, anxiety, and somatization disorder (13,14). Nevertheless, the major case series (15,16) continue to document significant numbers of patients in whom careful assessment excludes these psychiatric diagnoses (as well as alternative medical conditions), thus supporting the notion of a unique fatigue syndrome of unknown basis.

The rationale for treatment of patients with CFS with intravenous immunoglobulin (IVIG) is based first upon the link with infectious diseases as precipitants for the syndrome, and second upon evidence for disordered cell-mediated immunity in patients with CFS. The data on which these associations have been made are reviewed briefly below.

Infection and CFS

The most obvious link between infection and the onset of CFS comes from the anecdotal histories patients give. These recollections typically describe a "flulike" illness demarcating the patient's prior good health from the subsequent chronic fatigue state. Unfortunately, these associations are frequently retrospective attributions with uncertain validity, as the expected incidence of upper respiratory tract infections in the general population is approximately four annually (17), making chance associations likely. The patient groups reported are also confounded by the selection bias of referral to specialty clinics *because* of the history of an infective illness (17). Recent data from prospective cohort studies confirm both the arguments for—and against—the association between infections and CFS (18–20). In the study reported by Wessely et al. (18), minor infective illnesses such as upper respiratory tract infections were not associated with the advent of chronic fatigue states. Conversely, White et al. (19,20) demonstrated that approximately 10% of individuals followed from serologically documented infection with Epstein-Barr virus (EBV), but not nonspecific upper respiratory tract infections, developed CFS. In approximately half of these CFS cases, neither premorbid nor intercurrent psychiatric morbidity was evident, thus firmly endorsing the notion of a discrete postinfective fatigue syndrome. As yet, studies examining pathophysiological hypothesis in these well-defined cases have not been undertaken.

Evidence has also been sought for direct involvement of recognized, or novel, infectious agents in the pathogenesis of CFS. Prominent amongst the list of agents studied are EBV (21–23), human herpes virus 6 (HHV-6) (24,25), enteroviruses (26,27), a human T lymphotropic (HTLV)-II-like retrovirus (28–30), and spumaviruses (31,32). Overall, no consistent evidence exists for aberrant infection with the more ubiquitous viruses (EBV or enteroviruses), and several studies have refuted early suggestions of retroviral infection (including spumaviruses). Patients with CFS appear to have a substantially higher prevalence of reactivation of HHV-6 infection than do healthy control subjects (24,25). However, as the seroprevalence of HHV-6 in adult populations is almost universal, the significance of this finding to the pathogenesis of CFS is unclear.

Immune Function in Patients with CFS

Studies of cellular immunity in patients with CFS have evaluated the hypothesis that CFS may result from a disordered cell-mediated immune response to viral antigens, with chronic and excessive cytokine production directly mediating fatigue and other symptoms (33). In brief, these studies have demonstrated a significant impairment of in vitro responsiveness of peripheral blood lymphocytes to mitogens such as phytohemagglutinin (16,21,34,35), and reduced natural killer cell cytotoxicity in patients with CFS (34–36), in comparison to healthy control subjects. Increased expression of activation markers on a subset of CD8 T lymphocytes has also been demonstrated (35,37). In addition, altered immune function in vivo evidenced by reduced or absent delayed type hypersensitivity (DTH) skin responses in patients with CFS has been reported (2,16,33). Studies seeking to identify increased blood levels of cytokines in patients with CFS have been predominantly negative (38–40). Serum levels of immunoglobulins in patients with CFS are typically normal, although minor reductions in levels of immunoglobulin G subclasses have been reported (41).

In summary, reasonable evidence has been collected for disturbances in cellular immunity in patients with CFS, not seen in matched patients with depression or healthy control subjects. The magnitude of the alterations in immunity are minor, however, and are not associated with clinically significant consequences such as infection or malignancy. It remains unclear whether these changes are causal in CFS or related to an undefined underlying disease process or other cofactor (7).

TREATMENT WITH INTRAVENOUS IMMUNOGLOBULINS

Despite the considerable limitations of case definitions for CFS and the uncertain pathophysiological basis for the disorder, two published (42,43) controlled trials have evaluated the potential benefit of IVIG therapy for patients with CFS. Two subsequent controlled trials are now awaiting publication (44,45). The proposed justification for these therapeutic trials includes the hypothesis of persistence of viral antigen as a critical defect, and hence provision of neutralizing antibodies in the regimen (43). Alternatively, the pathogenesis of CFS has been proposed to be one of the disordered immunoregulation; hence immunoglobulin therapy was proposed to offer potential benefit by analogy with its use in autoimmune disorders (42,43). Undoubtedly, the trials have also been compassionate efforts to establish useful treatment for a condition without definitive therapeutic options (46).

After anecdotal reports of symptomatic benefit from IVIG in a small number of patients suffering CFS following EBV infection, and a limited trial of intramuscular immunoglobulin (47), our research group conducted an uncontrolled pilot study (48). Twenty-nine patients (66%) were treated with three infusions of IVIG at monthly intervals with a dose of 2 g IgG/kg. Nineteen of these patients (66%) reported symptomatic improvement which appeared to accumulate with consecutive treatments. Accordingly, a controlled trial was undertaken (42).

Independent of this work in Australia, Peterson et al. (43), from Minneapolis, were also conducting a controlled trial of IVIG therapy for patients with CFS. The two studies were ultimately published together and reached opposite conclusions—a beneficial effect in the Australian study, and no benefit beyond placebo in the American trial. The key features of these two studies are summarized in Table 1.

Given the divergent results of these two studies it is appropriate to consider why their conclusions may have differed. First, the dosage and formulation of the immunoglobulin preparations varied. The Australian study chose a continuous infusion regimen at high dose (2 g/kg) of a local preparation based upon the formulation of

Table 1 Published Controlled Trials of IVIG Therapy for Patients With CFS

Study	Sample size	Dosage (IgG)	No. of treatments	Outcome measured at	Outcome measures
Lloyd et al. (42)	49	2 g/kg monthly	3	3 months after 3rd dose	Physician and psychiatrist assessments
Petersen et al. (43)	28	1 g/kg monthly	6	Time of 6th dose	Self-report questionnaires

Gamimune N (Cutter Laboratories, Berkeley, CA), whereas the American group used 1 g/kg of Gammagard (Baxter Healthcare Corp., Glendale, CA). Second, the number of infusions was greater in the American study although the outcome assessment was conducted at the time of the final infusion, without a treatment-free follow-up period, as was chosen for the Australian trial. Finally, the outcome measures were necessarily subjective in both studies with standardized self-report questionnaires used in both, although the Australian study relied predominantly on a masked evaluation of clinical and functional status by a physician and psychiatrist before and after treatment. Of the differences in trial design, the explanation for the discrepant results would seem most likely to lie in the immunoglobulin dosage; although if the postulated mechanism is provision of neutralizing antibodies, this dosage difference is unlikely to be significant. Another likely confounding issue is the nature of the cases themselves, as recent data suggest that the label of CFS describes a heterogeneous patient group, within which subgroups with quite divergent disease processes (e.g., immunological versus somatization disorders) may exist (13,14).

Some of the shared features of the two studies also deserve comment. The patient groups in both studies had a substantial prevalence of immunological disturbances, including immunoglobulin G subclass deficiency (notably IgG_1 and IgG_3 subclasses) as well as T-cell lymphopenia, and in the Australian study, cutaneous anergy was common. Patients in both series had significant functional impairment as a result of their illness. Interestingly, the incidence of adverse effects from the immunoglobulin infusions was significantly greater than that seen in other patient groups receiving identical immunoglobulin regimens. Patients in both studies described an apparent exacerbation of CFS symptoms including headache, fatigue, and myalgia, following each infusion and lasting 1-4 days.

The issue of dosage has been further evaluated by our group in a more recent blinded and controlled trial in which patients were randomly allocated to one of four treatment arms to receive three infusions at monthly intervals of either 2 g/kg, 1 g/kg, 0.5 g/kg, or placebo (1% albumin in 10% maltose solution). Patients were then followed for a further 3 months without additional therapy. Outcome was assessed using standardized self-report measures and investigator-rated assessments of functional capacity on the Karnofsky Performance Scale. The analysis of data from this trial suggests that no significant dose-response relationship exists between IVIG and symptomatic improvement in patients with CFS. It should be noted that in these Australian trials, patients who experienced substantial symptomatic improvement following IVIG have found the symptoms typically recrudesce over 3-6 months after treatment, with "responders" recording benefit again when retreated (42).

The final controlled trial of immunoglobulin therapy for patients with CFS was also conducted in Australia by a pediatric research group (45). This double-blind trial included 70 children aged 12-18 years with CFS diagnosed after the careful exclusion of alternative medical and psychiatric conditions. The mean duration of symptoms prior to therapy was approximately 18 months. The children were randomized to receive placebo or intravenous immunoglobulin infusions in a dosage of 1 g/kg monthly for 3 consecutive months. A significantly better outcome was documented following the immunoglobulin infusions, measured in terms of physical symptom scores, as well as participation in school and social activities. The apparently unique profile of adverse effects previously reported in adult patients with CFS was observed in this study also, with a clear trend of decreasing severity with repeated infusions.

CONCLUSION

Conflicting data exist in relation to the suggestion that IVIG is an active treatment modality for patients with CFS, although these data are inadequate to recommend its routine usage. The benefit observed is typically short-lived and is apparently restricted to an as yet undefined subgroup. No data are available to suggest a possible mechanism for this benefit, including whether specific antibodies directed against the putative viral triggers are a critical component of the immunoglobulin preparation. Given that repeated doses of at least 1 g/kg appear to be required for any benefit to be recorded and that the profile of adverse effects in patients with CFS is substantial, the financial and human cost associated with immunoglobulin therapy currently outweighs the more limited potential for symptomatic relief. Studies directed at elucidating the mechanisms underlying the apparent therapeutic benefit in carefully selected patients with CFS followed from defined infections (e.g., with EBV) with "antigen-specific" immunoglobulin formulations are justified.

REFERENCES

1. Fukuda K, Straus SE, Hickie I, Sharpe MC, Dobbins JG, Komaroff A. The chronic fatigue syndrome: a comprehensive approach to its definition and study. International Chronic Fatigue Syndrome Study Group. Ann Intern Med 1994; 121:953–959.
2. Lloyd A, Hickie I, Boughton CR, Spencer O, Wakefield D. The prevalence of chronic fatigue syndrome in an Australian population. Med J Aust 1990; 153:522–528.
3. Gunn WJ, Connell DB, Randall B. Epidemiology of chronic fatigue syndrome: the Centers for Disease Control Study. Ciba Found Symp 1993; 173:83–93.
4. Lloyd A, Wakefield D, Dwyer J, Boughton C. What is myalgic encephalomyelitis? Lancet 1988; 1:1286–1287.
5. Holmes GP, Kaplan JE, Gantz N, et al. Chronic fatigue syndrome: a working case definition. Ann Intern Med 1988; 108:387–389.
6. Sharpe MC, Archard LC, Banatvala JE, et al. A report—chronic fatigue syndrome: guidelines for research. J R Soc Med 1991; 84:118–121.
7. Lloyd AR, Wakefield D, Hickie I. Immunity and the pathophysiology of chronic fatigue syndrome. Ciba Found Symp 1993; 173:176–192.
8. Straus SE. Studies of herpesvirus infection in chronic fatigue syndrome. Ciba Found Symp 1993; 173:132–145.
9. Behan PO, Behan WMH, Gow JW, Cavanagh H, Gillespie S. Enteroviruses and postviral fatigue syndrome. Ciba Found Symp 1993; 173:146–159.
10. Folkes T, Heneine W, Khan A, Chapman L, Schonberger L. Investigation of retroviral involvement in chronic fatigue syndrome. Ciba Found Symp 1993; 173:160–175.
11. Demitrack MA, Dale JK, Straus SE, et al. Evidence for impaired activation of the hypothalamic-pituitary-adrenal axis in patients with chronic fatigue syndrome. J Clin Endocrinol Metab 1991; 73:1224–1234.
12. Wessely S. the neuropsychiatry of chronic fatigue syndrome. Ciba Found Symp 1993; 173:212–237.
13. Hickie I, Lloyd A, Hadzi-Pavlovic D, Parker G, Bird K, Wakefield D. Can the chronic fatigue syndrome be defined by distinct clinical features? Psychol Med. In press.
14. Wilson A, Hadzi-Pavlovic D, Lloyd A, et al. What is chronic fatigue syndrome: Heterogeneity within an international multicentre study.
15. Manu P, Lane TJ, Matthews DA. Chronic fatigue and chronic fatigue syndrome: clinical epidemiology and aetiological classification. Ciba Found Symp 1993; 173:23–42.

16. Lloyd AR, Wakefield D, Dwyer J Boughton C. Immunological abnormalities in the chronic fatigue syndrome. Med J Aust 1989; 151:122–124.

17. Hotopf MH, Wessely S. Viruses, neurosis and fatigue. J Psychosom Res 1994; 38:499–514.

18. Wessely S, Chalder T, Hirsch S, Pawlikowska T, Wallace P, Wright DJM. Postinfectious fatigue: prospective cohort study in primary care. Lancet 1995; 345:1333–1338.

19. White PD, Thomas JM, Amess J, Grover SA, Kangro HO, Clare AW. The existence of a fatigue syndrome after glandular fever. Psychol Med 1995. In press.

20. White PD, Grover SA, Kangro HO, Thomas JM, Amess J, Clare AW. The validity and reliability of the fatigue syndrome which follows glandular fever. Psychol Med 1995. In press.

21. Strauss SE, Tosato G, Armstrong G, et al. Persisting illness and fatigue in adults with evidence of Epstein-Barr virus infection. Ann Intern Med 1985; 102:7–16.

22. Jones JF, Ray CG, Minich LL, Hicks MJ, Kibler R, Lucas DO. Evidence for active Epstein-Barr virus infection in patients with persistent, unexplained illnesses: elevated anti-early antigen antibodies. Ann Intern Med 1985; 102:1–7.

23. Tobi M, Morag A, Ravid Z, et al. Prolonged atypical illness associated with serological evidence of persistent Epstein-Barr virus infection. Lancet 1982; 1:61–64.

24. Josephs SF, Henry B, Balanchandran N, et al. HHV-6 reactivation in chronic fatigue syndrome. Lancet 1991; 337:1346–1347.

25. Buchwald D, Cheney PR, Peterson DL, et al. A chronic illnes characterized by fatigue, neurologic, and immunologic disorders, and active human herpesvirus type 6 infection. Ann Intern Med 1992; 116:103–113.

26. Yousef GE, Bell EJ, Mann GF, et al. Chronic enterovirus infection in patients with postviral fatigue syndrome. Lancet 1988; 1:146–150.

27. Gow JW, Behan WM, Clements GB, Woodall C, Riding M, Behan PO. Enteroviral RNA sequences detected by polymerase chain reaction in muscle of patients with postviral fatigue syndrome. Br Med J 1991; 302:692–696.

28. Defreitas E, Hilliard B, Cheney PR, et al. Retroviral sequences related to human T-lymphotropic virus type II in patients with chronic fatigue immune dysfunction syndrome. Proc Natl Acad Sci USA 1991; 88:2922–2926.

29. Khan AS, Heneine WM, Chapman LE, et al. Assessment of a retrovirus sequence and other possible risk factors for the chronic fatigue syndrome in adults. Ann Intern Med 1993; 118:241–245.

30. Gow JW, Simpson K, Schliephake A, et al. Search for a retrovirus in the chronic fatigue syndrome. J Clin Pathol 1992; 45:1058–1061.

31. Heneine W, Woods TC, Sinha SD, et al. Lack of evidence for infection with known human and animal retroviruses in patients with chronic fatigue syndrome. Clin Infect Dis 1994; 18(suppl 1):S121–S125.

32. Flugel RM, Mahnke C, Geiger A, Komaroff AL. Absence of antibody to human spumaretrovirus in patients with chronic fatigue syndrome. Clin Infect Dis 1992; 14:623–624.

33. Wakefield D, Lloyd AR. The pathophysiology of myalgic encephalomyelitis. Lancet 1987; 2:918–919.

34. Lloyd A, Hickie I, Hickie C, Wakefield D. Cell-mediated immunity in patients with chronic fatigue syndrome, healthy control subjects and patients with major depression. Clin Exp Immunol 1992; 87:76–79.

35. Landay AL, Jessop C, Lennette ET, Levy JA. Chronic fatigue syndrome: clinical condition associated with immune activation. Lancet 1991; 338:707–712.

36. Klimas NG, Salvato FR, Morgan R, Fletcher MA. Immunologic abnormalities in chronic fatigue syndrome. J Clin Microbiol 1990; 28:1403–1410.

37. Barker E, Fujimura SF, Fadem MB, Landay AL, Levy JA. Immunologic abnormalities associated with chronic fatigue. Clin Infect Dis 1994; 18(suppl 1):S16–S20.

38. Straus SE, Dale JK, Peter JB, Dinarello CA. Circulating lymphokine levels in the chronic fatigue syndrome. J Infect Dis 1989; 160:1085–1086.

39. Chao CC, Janoff EN, Hu SX, et al. Altered cytokine release in peripheral blood mononuclear cell cultures in patients with chronic fatigue syndrome. Cytokine 1991; 3:292–298.

40. Lloyd A, Hickie I, Brockman A, Dwyer J, Wakefield D. Cytokine levels in serum and cerebrospinal fluid in patients with chronic fatigue synrome and control subjects. J Infect Dis 1991; 164:1203–1204.

41. Wakefield D, Lloyd A, Brockman A. Immunoglobulin subclass abnormalities in patients with chronic fatigue syndrome. Pediatr Infect Dis J 1990; 9(suppl 1):S50–S53.

42. Lloyd A, Hickie I, Wakefield D, Boughton C, Dwyer J. A double-blind, placebo-controlled trial of intravenous immunoglobulin therapy in patients with the chronic fatigue syndrome. Am J Med 1990; 89:561–568.

43. Peterson PK, Shepard J, Macres M, et al. A controlled trial of intravenous immunoglobulin G in chronic fatigue syndrome. Am J Med 1990; 89:554–560.

44. Straus SE. Intravenous immunoglobulin treatment for the chronic fatigue syndrome. Am J Med 1990; 89:551–552.

45. Dubois RE. Gammaglobulin therapy for chronic mononucleosis syndrome. AIDS Res 1986; 2(suppl 1):S191–S195.

46. Lloyd A, Wakefield D, Boughton C, Dwyer J. Beneficial effect of high dose intravenous gammaglobulin in the treatment of post-infection fatigue syndrome. Aust NZ J Med 1988; 18(suppl):453. Abstract.

47. Rowe KS. Chronic fatigue syndrome—double blind trial assessing the efficacy of intravenous gammaglobulin in the management of the condition. J Paediatr Child Health 1994; 30:14.

21

Intravenous Gammaglobulin Therapy for Autoimmune Thrombocytopenic Purpura, Neutropenia, and Hemolytic Anemia

James B. Bussel

The New York Hospital–Cornell Medical Center, New York, New York

INTRODUCTION

In 1981 Paul Imbach et al. (1) first reported on the ability of intravenous immunoglobulin (IVIG) treatment to dramatically increase the platelet count of patients with immune thrombocytopenia. In that year in their initial article and one other (2), these investigators also reported that (1) IVIG was ineffective in aplastic thrombocytopenia; and (2) in one patient, IVIG was ineffective if digested (by pepsin) so that few IgG monomers remained, but the same patient then responded to infusion of a different preparation of IVIG containing "intact" IgG.

These salient observations led to a wide variety of clinical studies of the treatment with IVIG of patients with immune thrombocytopenic purpura (ITP). In turn, the surprising efficacy of IVIG in ITP led to its use in a number of other autoimmune and immunologically mediated diseases.

IVIG is now relatively well understood and well defined in the treatment of ITP (better than the use of prednisone) and other immune cytopenias. However, additional focused studies need to be performed not only to refine clinical indications, but also to relate the use of IVIG directly to the specific pathophysiology of ITP.

This review will emphasize the chronology of development of the use of IVIG in the autoimmune cytopenias and the "knowns" versus the "unknowns." It will also focus on dose considerations as well as careful separation of different outcome assessments in measuring efficacy. References and reviews will be cited for those wishing to pursue individual topics in greater detail.

CLINICAL REVIEW: ITP

Imbach et al. used 400 mg/kg/day of IVIG for five consecutive days in children with acute and chronic ITP (1). Patients typically had pretreatment platelet counts <30,000/

μl whereas peak platelet counts were increased to well over 100,000/μl in 12 of 13 cases. Children with acute and chronic disease responded comparably. No curative effect was discernible in children with chronic disease, but this was not systematically pursued at that time. In several patients, the platelet count was maintained at a level of > 100,000/ μl, but this also did not result in a "cure." Later in 1981, Schmidt (3) reported successful treatment using the same dose of IVIG in four adults with acute and chronic ITP. Subsequent studies generally centered on patient subgroups.

Children with Acute ITP

Initial treatment with children with acute ITP used the dosage of 400 mg/kg/day for 5 days. In 1985 Imbach reported the results of a multicenter randomized trial comparing initial IVIG (400 mg/kg × 5 days) with initial prednisone (2 mg/kg × 3 weeks) in more than 100 patients (4). The platelet increase was more rapid in the IVIG arm, and more patients achieved remission sooner in that arm. However, no curative effects could be ascribed to IVIG: the number of patients with persistent ITP 6 months from diagnosis was approximately the same in each arm. This was not truly a negative result in that a minimum of 300 children would have had to have been entered in each arm in order to be able to demonstrate a 50% reduction of the 10–20% incidence of chronic disease expected in ITP of childhood.

Beginning in 1983 our center used a dose of 1 g/kg/day for 1–3 days depending on response in children at presentation of their ITP. This study, published in 1985 (5), demonstrated that most children with acute ITP would only require a single dose of 1 g/kg IVIG to achieve a substantial platelet increase whether or not they had previously received steroids. This study first raised the issues of dose delivery at a higher dose per day and in a lower total dose. This finding was later confirmed by Blanchette et al. in 1993 (6).

Paul Imbach subsequently reanalyzed the 1985 trial and suggested that two-thirds of the responders to IVIG at the dose for 400 ml/kg for 5 days required only 400 mg/kg for 2 days. This was based on their platelet counts having increased to over 30,000/μl by the morning of their third treatment and their never requiring further treatment.

Blanchette and the Canadian Pediatric ITP group recently completed two randomized trials addressing these issues. The first compared IVIG, prednisone, and no treatment (6). In discussing this, it is important to emphasize that Imbach's controlled trial in Switzerland, Austria, and Germany of IVIG compared to prednisone without a no-treatment control group was a follow-up to a posthumously published trial by Sartorius et al. (7), which demonstrated that on prednisone the platelet count increased more rapidly than it increased without treatment. At least six other trials have demonstrated similar findings: prednisone results in a faster platelet increase than no treatment in children with acute ITP at diagnosis (references listed and reviewed in Ref. 5). Therefore, the Swiss investigators did not feel it was appropriate to include a no-treatment arm.

Blanchette's study demonstrated that the IVIG and prednisone therapies increased the platelets more rapidly than no treatment (6). However, the difference between the IVIG and prednisone arms was not as great as in the Imbach study (4), possibly because the arms were smaller in size or more likely because the prednisone dose was greater: 4 mg/kg/day, instead of 2 mg/kg/day in the Imbach study.

Subsequently, the 1994 controlled trial by the same group (8) addressed additional questions: What was the relative effect of IV anti-D, and what was the advantage of higher-dose compared to lower-dose IVIG (there were two IVIG arms comparing 2 days of 1 g/kg vs. a single day of 0.8 g/kg). Again, these patients were all children with acute ITP at diagnosis. There were 34–39 patients per arm. The IVIG and the prednisone arms increased the platelet count significantly, but marginally faster than the anti-D arm. The higher-dose IVIG arm did not increase the platelet count significantly faster than the lower-dose IVIG arm, as had been suggested in our initial study (5) and in an unpublished study by Fischer.

Only one study systematically addressed the treatment of children with acute ITP, but *not* at diagnosis. In these 21 patients, results appeared to be dramatic, with over half of the patients never requiring any additional treatment after the initial 2 g/kg IVIG (9).

In summary, therefore, for children with acute ITP at least 80% will respond to 0.8–1.0 g/kg/day IVIG administered over 1–2 days. In this case the target of response is a platelet count greater than 20,000–50,000/µl as soon as possible. Additional patients, not responsive to the lower-dose (initial) regimens, may respond to continued, higher total doses of IVIG up to a total of 3 g/kg (5), but this has not been prospectively validated. Specifically, no study has selected nonresponders after a single dose and compared further treatment with no further treatment. Nonetheless, with or without additional doses, the overall response rate is at least 80–90% based on the platelet count to determine response. The exact number of responses will vary somewhat depending on the level of platelet count required and the day on which the platelet count is required to be at that level.

Children with Chronic ITP

Early studies of children with chronic ITP suggested that IVIG was equally effective in acutely increasing the platelet count in these patients, as in the children with acute ITP. In several sites totaling >10 patients, the IVIG effect was equally present in children who had undergone but failed splenectomy. However, IVIG was not obviously curative, and the platelet increases seen were typically transient. Nonetheless, anecdotally there were patients in whom, after a single infusion or more commonly a series of infusions, the platelet count remained substantially elevated if not normal as compared to baseline (10). However, this type of response could not be distinguished from the natural tendency of children with chronic ITP to spontaneously improve.

Two single-arm studies totaling more than 50 patients have been completed in children with chronic ITP to investigate whether or not repeated infusion of IVIG might in fact be beneficial and have lasting effects (9,10). One of the pilot studies at our center in the United States enrolled 29 patients who already had chronic ITP. Twenty-five patients initially responded to IVIG and were able to continue on maintenance. Approximately two-thirds of these patients were able, with repeated infusions of IVIG for up to 2 years, to permanently avoid splenectomy. Medical decision analysis, using a then appropriate cost of $37/g IVIG, suggested that "saving a life" from overwhelming postsplenectomy sepsis by repeated infusion of IVIG for up to 2 years would cost approximately $500,000 per life saved. Since IVIG costs less in smaller patients, it was considered the treatment of choice in preference to splenectomy in children <6 years of age. At current (lower) costs of IVIG in the U.S., IVIG would be the treatment of choice in children with chronic ITP up to 10 years of age (10).

Similar results were published at approximately the same time from Switzerland (9A). This study found that approximately 50% of patients with chronic ITP, treated as needed with IVIG for up to 2 years from initiation of IVIG, would ultimately be able to avoid splenectomy.

Neither of these studies had other than historical controls for reference. There was no specific control group because the great majority of these patients would "normally" have undergone splenectomy rather than persist with the toxicity of prolonged corticosteroid therapy. Therefore, notwithstanding the similarity of the results of the two studies and notwithstanding the apparent difference of these results from what would have been expected according to the natural history, these were not controlled trials and do not prove, although they suggest, that there is a curative effect of repeated infusions of IVIG. A similar-size pilot study from Canada reported similar results with IV anti-D (11). A current multicenter study of IVIG and other therapies may address these issues more definitively.

In summary, IV infusions of gammaglobulin can reliably increase the platelet count dramatically in the great majority of children with chronic ITP. Two studies have raised the possibility of a curative effect, but there has been no clear-cut documentation of any such effect by a controlled trial.

Adults with Acute ITP

Initial treatment of adults with acute disease was first reported by Schmidt et al. describing two patients in 1981 (3) and then amplified by Newland et al. in 1983 as a much larger series (12). Platelet responses were similar to those of children when using similar doses of IVIG, but the peak platelet counts were not quite as great as in children nor was the percentage of responders as great. These studies were summarized in 1988 (13).

Newland reported the successful use of 0.4 g/kg/day for 3 days in adults with acute disease. This was the initial primary dose modification that was attempted in any of the ITP treatment series of adults. Studies that were only recently published also demonstrated that lower total doses of IVIG than 2 g/kg might suffice to produce substantial platelet increases in adults as well as children (14).

Only one study, by Bierling's group (15), directly addressed the possibility of cure in adults with acute ITP. Adults received an initial dose of 2 g/kg followed by infusions of 1 g/kg/dose administered monthly as long as the platelet count was <50,000/µl for a total of 6 months. A surprisingly high percentage, approximately one-third, of the enrolled patients were cured and required no further therapy. Specifically, these patients, six of 18, did not require splenectomy. This would be a far higher number than we would expect from the natural history of "acute ITP" in adults, but the overall numbers were small. No other studies have followed up this salient finding.

In summary, adults with acute ITP also responded well acutely to IVIG. Whether or not the responses, both in percentage of responders and in the mean platelet increase, are as high as those seen in children remains open to debate. Note that children with acute ITP at diagnosis may be entering remission in any event, so that part of their platelet increase may not be treatment-related, which complicates interpretation.

Adults with Chronic ITP

There has only been one extensive study of IVIG treatment in adults with chronic ITP (16). This study included mainly chronic refractory splenectomized patients, representing 30 of the 40 patients in the study. The findings of this study were:

1. 39 of 40 patients responded acutely to the infusion of 2 g/kg of IVIG with a mean platelet increase well over 100,000/μl.
2. Approximately two-thirds of the 30 splenectomized patients had their platelet counts maintained by repeated infusions of 1 g/kg administered as needed, seemingly indefinitely.
3. Approximately one-third of the patients eventually became refractory to IVIG in that they no longer had a platelet increase following infusion. In 10 of these 11 cases, this was after response to the initial infusion, occurring within 2 weeks to 3 months of starting treatment. In fact, the mean initial platelet increase of the 10 patients who initially responded and eventually became refractory was greater than 100,000/μl. Even in retrospect, there was no clear explanation for the sudden onset of refractoriness. Several of these patients were entered in a trial of combined plasmapheresis and IVIG with good but transient responses, suggesting that increased antiplatelet antibody levels were being lessened by the pheresis, allowing the IVIG to regain its effectiveness (17).
4. Approximately one-third of the patients improved enough after an average of 10 infusions of 60 g/infusion to no longer require any therapy by maintaining a platelet count greater than 20,000–30,000/μl without significant hemorrhage. In view of the presumed lack of expected improvement in this group of patients already refractory to splenectomy, this appeared to be a very significant improvement, again implying a curative effect. However, confirmation has not been obtained from either another single arm trial or from a controlled trial.

An additional study explored the dose in maintenance treatment. The above study had utilized essentially 1 g/kg/infusion. Comparing 1 g/kg in maintenance with 0.5 g/kg as single infusions demonstrated that while the higher dose resulted in a higher peak platelet count, the interval between infusions was not different (17).

In summary, chronic refractory patients will usually respond to IVIG with an acute platelet increase. Our anecdotal experience suggests that the addition of high-dose IV steroids with IVIG may be useful. A number of these patients may respond initially to IVIG and then cease responding to subsequent infusions. The amount of IVIG needed to have any curative effect, if any such effect exists, is very large (? 600 g), making this not a practicable approach to patient treatment if viable alternatives exist. At present, no clearly proven "curative" alternatives exist despite small pilot studies that have had encouraging results.

Special Patient Groups

HIV-Related Thrombocytopenia

Another group receiving treatment to increase the platelets with IVIG is patients with HIV-related thrombocytopenia. The exact pathophysiology of their disease is incompletely understood. It appears that there is a component of decreased platelet production (18); however, some of their disease resembles classic ITP in being autoimmune in nature. It is generally believed that the earlier the stage of the patient—i.e., asymptomatic with only isolated thrombocytopenia—the greater the chance that the autoimmune component will dominate. In these patients, the response to IVIG is like that seen in a patient with classic ITP. In contrast, a patient with pancytopenia, opportunistic infections, systemic symptoms, hepatosplenomegaly, and/or lymphadenopathy will respond substantially less well to IVIG, or any treatment of ITP, since their more endstage disease typically involves marrow platelet production failure.

These concepts remain to be prospectively validated by specific data designed to address these points. For example, it may be that a specific variable such as pancytopenia is the most important finding and that the other listed clinical variables add little to the determination of IVIG response. Certain opportunistic infections may matter more than others in this regard, especially if steroids were used as the initial treatment of the HIV-ITP and resulted in an opportunistic infection (e.g., esophageal candidiasis) not reflective of the true state of the HIV.

Depending on the series and the patient population, a higher or lower number of patients will respond to IVIG (19,20). Overall, it is our impression that a higher percentage of patients with HIV-related thrombocytopenia are refractory to IVIG treatment than are patients with classical ITP. Also, it is likely that a higher percentage of treated HIV-ITP patients will develop tachyphylaxis after initial response to IVIG treatment.

A special issue within this patient group involves the hemophiliac patients with HIV-ITP. At least one article has documented a substantially higher incidence of intracranial hemorrhage in these patients (21). We have seen two intracranial hemorrhages (ICH) in nonhemophiliac, HIV-ITP patients both of whom had very low platelet counts at the time; one walked accidentally into a door and hit it with his forehead. Nonetheless, the hemophiliacs are at a higher risk for ICH because of their dual bleeding disorders. Furthermore, there may be an additional effect of chronic infection with hepatitis C. In our pilot series, the hemophiliac patients responded particularly well to IVIG (19). If there is a delay in providing treatment with IVIG, these patients can receive prophylactic infusions with clotting factor concentrate (VIII or IX) to diminish the risk of acute hemorrhage until the platelet count increases.

In summary, patients with HIV-ITP also are responsive to IVIG treatment for acute platelet increases. However, the further advanced the HIV disease, the less well the patients will do and the more likely they will be to stop responding to treatment if they responded previously. We believe that IV anti-D is probably more effective in increasing and maintaining the platelet count, for unclear reasons, in this patient group (21A).

Immune Thrombocytopenia in Pregnancy

IVIG is useful in the treatment of immune thrombocytopenia in pregnancy. There are two types of problems with totally different patterns of usage of IVIG: autoimmune (ITP), and alloimmune (AIT). *In ITP, the primary treatment issue is the mother herself. In AIT, the primary issue is treatment of the mother for the sake of the fetus.*

For women with ITP who are pregnant (autoimmune disease), IVIG, whether or not combined in some fashion with steroids, is usually sufficient, with repeated infusions as needed, to maintain a platelet count greater than 30,000/μl. This allows the avoidance of any significant bleeding including miscarriage. Management should allow the use, in at least 99% of cases, of only IVIG and prednisone during the pregnancy.

Several features are unique to ITP in pregnancy. First, the ITP may fluctuate in severity during the pregnancy. It will not automatically get worse and may in fact improve. It may worsen and then ameliorate. It may be stable throughout the great majority of the pregnancy and then acutely worsen late in the third trimester. Second, delivery is often like "splenectomy" in producing the former condition of the ITP. If the ITP was difficult to treat during the pregnancy, treatment is typically required for only a finite period of time. Finally, splenectomy is to be considered as the treatment of absolutely last resort. Even during the optimal time period for the operation, the second trimester, the risks to the fetus and to the pregnancy are relatively high. We have not performed one at our institution for more than 10 years and would do anything possible, including weekly IVIG, to avoid it while the patient is pregnant.

A number of case reports on the treatment of ITP in pregnancy exist. IVIG has been shown to be as effective in ITP in pregnancy in acutely increasing the platelet count (22), as it is in nonpregnant patients. However, there are some women whose ITP becomes progressively more refractory to treatment during pregnancy, and they then require very frequent treatment. Steroids are the other primary adjunct, but long-term administration of high doses is fraught with complications: renal stones, diabetes, hypertension, etc. First-trimester use may be teratogenic for cleft lip/palate, although this remains uncertain.

Combinations of IVIG at 1 g/kg/infusion with either high-dose alternate-day prednisone or with 20 mg or less daily will be effective in the majority of patients (23). The platelet count usually has to be maintained only at a level $\geq 30,000/\mu l$. There is no increased fetal loss rate from the ITP per se if these counts are maintained.

IVIG is also very useful in pregnant women to acutely increase the platelet count if required for procedures. If such a procedure was an amniocentesis, this does not have a high risk of bleeding, and the timing of it can be scheduled. However, a patient may be planning a vaginal delivery whenever labor begins; then a persistently higher platelet count is desired. This can make treatment with IVIG difficult if a count $> 100,000/\mu l$ is required in order to allow for epidural anesthesia. In this setting, it may be easier to treat with steroids and rapidly taper to 20 mg prednisone per day in order to continuously maintain the platelet count at the desired level—i.e., $> 100,000/\mu l$.

There is only one study that even anecdotally addresses the potential effects of IVIG administered to the mother on the fetal platelet count. In this study, there was no apparent effect in a very small number of patients who underwent fetal blood sampling to determine the fetal platelet count and then had a repeat count, usually after birth, to assess the efficacy of the IVIG (24). Other studies have reported the neonatal platelet count after maternal treatment with the expectation of neonatal thrombocytopenia. More recent demonstration of the relatively low rate of severe neonatal thrombocytopenia in infants of mothers with ITP has emphasized the need for documentation of fetal thrombocytopenia prior to treatment (24–28). Moreover, recent studies have suggested that the risk of fetal blood sampling is not warranted in ITP because of the absence of proven antenatal ICH and the generally low overall risk of ICH (approximately 1%) (22,24–28).

In contrast to ITP in pregnancy, alloimmune thrombocytopenia is a more severe disease, as reflected in the important risk of antenatal fetal intracranial hemorrhage

(29,30). Alloimmune thrombocytopenia is a result of parental platelet antigen incompatibility, most commonly PlA1. As a result of the maternal immune response, fetal thrombocytopenia occurs which is typically severe: *in nearly 50% of our more than 100 cases, the fetal platelet count was < 20,000/μl* (31).

In view of the substantial risk of antenatal hemorrhage, we initiated studies more than 10 years ago in which we infused IVIG weekly to the mother starting as early as 20 weeks of gestation after a fetal blood sampling documented fetal thrombocytopenia in order to increase the fetal platelet count and thereby prevent antenatal intracranial hemorrhage (32). This treatment program appears to be quite effective; a detailed description and discussion of it is beyond the scope of this review, but is discussed elsewhere (31–35). Our most recent study, with 55 patients, brought to a total of 73 patients the number we have enrolled in completed studies. We have enrolled more than 25 additional patients in our newest study, as of 3/1/96. A discussion of the most controversial issues affecting diagnosis and management of alloimmune thrombocytopenia is in a review article in *Maternal Fetal Medicine* (35). The highlights are:

1. IVIG alone in a dose of 1 g/kg/week increases the fetal platelet substantially in the majority of patients.
2. Depending on the definition of a response, the response rate was 59–85% in these studies comprising 73 patients.
3. Two cases of fetal ICH while on IVIG treatment have occurred (36). One was ours and was the only one in more than 100 total cases.
4. There is an increased rate of fetal hemorrhage at the time of fetal blood sampling if the fetal platelet count is < 30,000/μl (37). Therefore, we currently recommend giving maternal platelet concentrates at the time of sampling to thrombocytopenic fetuses. In practice, this may mean giving 2–3 ml platelet concentrate while awaiting the result of the fetal platelet count.
5. The serological diagnosis of AIT is not always straightforward, but DNA-based technology is now available on a routine basis from, for example, the platelet antibody laboratory of the Blood Center of Southeastern Wisconsin.
6. In patients unresponsive to IVIG, low-dose steroids (i.e., 1.5 mg dexamethasone per day) add no additional benefit, but high-dose steroids (i.e., 60 mg prednisone per day or 1 mg/kg/day) in combination with continued IVIG are effective in substantially increasing the fetal platelet count in > 50% of IVIG nonresponders.

Our conclusions based on the above information are that IVIG is effective in increasing the fetal platelet count and should therefore be the first line of treatment prior to weekly fetal platelet transfusion, which should be reserved for truly refractory cases. We believe that fetal blood sampling needs to be utilized to monitor cases because of the incomplete response rates, the possibility of antenatal ICH, and the ability to intensify therapy in nonresponders with the addition of high-dose prednisone and even weekly platelet transfusions until elective early delivery is possible.

In contrast to considerations of the morbidity and mortality of fetal thrombocytopenia, which apply primarily to alloimmune cases, treatment of neonatal thrombocytopenia secondary to either alloimmune or autoimmune disease is relatively straightforward. Studies by Mueller-Eckhardt et al. (38) and Ballin et al. (39), among others, suggest that IVIG is the mainstay of therapy for an affected newborn. Platelet transfusions can be given, especially in alloimmune thrombocytopenia, in which concentrated maternal platelets tend to be an extremely effective form of therapy. In addition, the importance of a cranial ultrasound examination or other radiological testing to demonstrate or exclude intracranial hemorrhage cannot be neglected and is absolutely crucial to appropriate care. The results of the cranial ultrasound will determine the intensity of therapy since *babies can have silent—i.e., clinically totally asymptomatic—intracranial hemorrhage* with, especially, alloimmune thrombocytopenias (40). This includes babies who feed well and whose anterior fontanelle is both soft and flat.

Typically, treatment of the thrombocytopenic neonate would be given only until the platelet count is greater than 20,000–50,000/μl, and then the platelet count would be monitored until it became normal (41). Because steroids have never been clearly validated as an effective treatment in this situation and because of the greater risk of sepsis in the neonate on high-dose steroids, the treatment of choice is IVIG usually in doses of 1 g/kg/day. If ICH is documented, however, platelet transfusions, usually initially random, would be used and IVIG infusions and steroids would aim to maintain a platelet count > 100,000/μl for at least 2 weeks.

Alloimmune Thrombocytopenia Secondary to Platelet Transfusions

Another area of usage of intravenous gammaglobulin is in the *allosensitized* patient who has become refractory to platelet transfusions. The use of IVIG occurs in the setting of a patient with a malignancy who has received and continues to require platelet transfusions. It appears that the administration of sufficiently large amounts of IVIG may have a minor beneficial effect in certain cases (42). IVIG is clearly not a front-line therapy in these patients. Therapeutic efforts have appropriately been focused primarily toward decreasing the incidence of sensitization, especially by leukodepletion via filtration, and also by the use of autologous frozen platelets.

Additional Comments

The adjunctive effects of corticosteroids, administered with IV gammaglobulin, have never been prospectively validated in patients with ITP (43). Specifically, the additional efficacy of high-dose IV steroids on the platelet response to IVIG remains unproven. Anecdotally, the fact that certain patients respond substantially better to corticosteroids than to IVIG also suggests that combined therapy should be better than IVIG alone. Moreover, the effect of IV or high-dose oral steroids on minimizing postgammaglobulin headaches, while also unproven, appears very likely. This is important in a situation in which the sudden onset of a substantial headache in a severely thrombocytopenic patient is a medical emergency and ICH must be excluded immediately.

The recent outbreaks of hepatitis C transmitted by IVIG in the United States and Europe (44) has resulted in establishing that IVIG must undergo a viral inactivation step. Currently, the principal method of viral inactivation, as with factor VIII concentrates, is solvent-detergent treatment. Considerable information exists as to the safety and efficacy of this treatment. Solvent-detergent treatment was developed for factor VIII concentrates and used initially in 1987. The results have been dramatic: no hemophiliac treated with a solvent-detergent concentrate has ever developed hepatitis B, C, HTLV1, or especially HIV. The more limited data available for IVIG treatment are equally unanimous (45). In addition, the two viruses that almost certainly have been transmitted in solvent-detergent-treated factor VIII concentrates, hepatitis A and parvovirus B19, have never been transmitted by IVIG because the antibody titers against these viruses in IVIG are more than sufficient to neutralize them. The record of safety with solvent-detergent-treated IVIG is therefore quite impressive: no failures have ever been documented.

Our data, published in 1995 in Postgraduate Medicine (45) and in Immunologic Investigations (14), demonstrate that solvent-detergent treatment of IVIG does not impair the efficacy of IVIG. Efficacy has not been as well studied as safety, but there are data available derived from essentially three sources. When solvent-detergent-treated IVIGs (Venoglobulin S and Melgam) were used to treat patients with ITP, the results were indistinguishable from that seen with other IVIGs. When the same product was compared with solvent-detergent-treated and nontreated preparations (Venoglobulin S and Venoglobulin I), the mean platelet increases in sequential studies showed that the solvent-detergent product was at least as good as its nontreated counterpart. This comparison included controlling for chronic patients and for adults versus children.

Finally, data were compared in two ways with the WinRho preparation of IV Anti-D (see below) in its solvent-detergent-treated and non-solvent-detergent-treated forms. IV Winrho is used for the treatment of ITP, and opsonizing red cells is crucial; therefore, the Fab portion of the IgG molecule is particularly important. Large numbers of initial infusions were compared (approximately 160 patients vs. approximately 90 patients) and also 10 patients had specifically randomized pairs of infusions using solvent-detergent-treated and non-solvent-detergent-treated preparations. In both comparisons, the Winrho and the WinrhoSD were very similar in their platelet and hemoglobin effects, indicating that the solvent-detergent process had no adverse effect on efficacy (46). This is of particular interest in view of previous accumulated data showing that so-called modified IVIGs are clearly less effective than so-called unmodified IVIGs in the treatment of ITP (13).

A number of hyperimmune IVIGs exist, including anti-VZ, anti-*Pseudomonas*, and anti-HIV; there are others under development, but the only one relevant at the present time to the treatment of ITP is anti-D (46). This usage has been covered elsewhere in greater detail, but a summary includes the following:

1. It is only effective in Rh+ patients who have not been splenectomized.
2. Platelet counts do not increase as fast as they do following IVIG, nor do they increase to as high a level.
3. HIV patients respond well (46,47). Occasionally, patients with HIV-related thrombocytopenia will respond to anti-D when they did not respond to IVIG.
4. Hemoglobin level will typically drop up to 1 g/dl. Rarely are the increases more than 2 g/dl. In either case the decrease is transient and will return to or near baseline within 2–3 weeks.
5. This is a treatment for the typical patient, not for the patient who is refractory to other treatments.
6. IV anti-D is ideal for patients requiring maintenance treatments to keep their counts at a safe level (see sections on IVIG above). This could be appropriate for children or HIV-infected patients.
7. Anti-D can be infused in 2–5 min at much less cost than a comparable treatment of IVIG.

Mechanism of Action of IVIG in ITP

The mechanism of effect on the platelet count in the treatment of ITP with IVIG is quite complex and discussed extensively in another chapter of this volume. Multiple mechanisms of effect are probably operative, and they occur to a different extent in different patients. The only universally agreed-upon, unequivocally documented mechanism of effect of IVIG in ITP is so-called Fc receptor blockade (48,49). In addition to studies with IVIG, the use of a monoclonal anti-FcRIII infusion (50), the efficacy of IV anti-D, and the recent demonstration of efficacy of the Fc piece of IVIG (51) all strongly support the in vivo importance of Fc receptor blockade. This in turn strongly suggests that Fc receptor blockade is an important component of the IVIG effect.

AUTOIMMUNE NEUTROPENIA

Autoimmune neutropenia in children is typically a disease of young infants and children less than 4 years of age (52,53). It is probably by far the commonest cause of an isolated severe neutropenia in infants and toddlers. The differential diagnosis includes Kostman's syndrome, a viral or medication-induced marrow suppression, and cyclic neutropenia. Kostman's syndrome is rare but usually characterized by more severe infectious problems than the other entities. Cyclic neutropenia is confusing because it requires a fixed periodicity and a cycling that is independent of whether a nadir infection occurs. Infectious suppression of the marrow resulting in neutropenia is particularly common in this age group. The normal differential of an infant at 1 year of age has as little as 20–25% neutrophils, and a normal absolute neutrophil count (ANC) may therefore be as low as 1000/µl (20% of a WBC of 5000/µl). ANCs between 500 and 1000/µl should be viewed suspiciously, but testing needs to be repeated prior to making an assumption of disease. Almost all infants with autoimmune neutropenia will usually have ANCs <500/µl.

Choosing whom to treat involves making the diagnosis, since neutrophil antibodies are not widely available, not very specific (52), and probably not necessary in the majority of cases. A patient should be thought of as likely to have autoimmune neutropenia if he or she:

1. Is between 6 and 18 to 24 months of age
2. Has a normal white count
3. Has a percent of neutrophils less than 5%
4. Has no abnormalities of the CBC other than coincident ones—i.e., thalassemia trait
5. Has no hepatosplenomegaly or noninfectious adenopathy to a degree that is abnormal for age
6. Has a history of being basically well and growing normally, whether or not intermittent minor infections have occurred.

This last criterion is intended to exclude sicker patients with serious infections who will be found to have Kostman's syndrome. As with ITP, a bone marrow examination is not required in the great majority of patients. If performed, the marrow in autoimmune neutropenia should reveal a myeloid hyperplasia. Occasionally there are arrests at the myelocyte or even promyelocyte stage of the marrow. Similarly, the marrow in

Kostman's syndrome may not reveal the absence or hypoplasia of myeloid precursors, but may indicate an arrest at the myelocyte or promyelocyte stage.

There are at least three series, each of which has reported more than 50 children with autoimmune neutropenia, emphasizing how common it is (52–54). These series have all documented the lack of life-threatening infections, which is helpful in considering the diagnosis but confusing in regard to deciding when to treat. Sepsis in these patients is virtually unheard of despite neutrophil counts that are frequently less than 200/μl. Meningitis may never have been reported in these patients. The series by Bux and Mueller-Eckhardt (53) focused on the incidence of proven pneumonia, but even this is distinctly uncommon, occurring in 10% or less of all infants. On the other hand, perirectal and other superficial, i.e., breast, abscesses in young girls are not rare, and chronic recurrent otitis media is also frequent (55). The latter may result in hearing loss and speech delay. Long-term studies have not been conducted to define the true incidence of this complication. Similarly, there are no reports of chronic gingivitis and the loss of teeth, but this may also be underreported with lack of follow-up; it is an important problem in Kostman patients.

In autoimmune neutropenia, typically there is spontaneous resolution of the neutropenia in approximately 90% of children by the age of 4. This is similar to the high incidence of spontaneous improvement of children with ITP, although autoimmune neutropenia is rare after the age of 2 years, whereas ITP is seen in children of all ages. In turn, this has implications for long-term toxicity; for example, gingivitis, if it occurs, will probably heal. Therefore, our current indications for treatment of such infants are:

1. A chronic or recurring infection in a specific area
2. An abscess
3. Prophylaxis for surgery
4. Protection of hardware, e.g., fever occurring in a child with autoimmune neutropenia who has a VP shunt or a central catheter

Speech delay or hearing loss would fall under (1), in which there would certainly be a chronic or persistent otitis media.

In 17 of our 20 treated cases, infusions of two doses of 1 g/kg IVIG resulted in an extremely rapid and dramatic increase in the ANC of > 1000/μl within 24–48 h. In certain cases, abscesses or lymphadenitis improved dramatically overnight without significant change in the neutrophil count, implying that the neutrophils had increased and were attacking the abscess. In certain chronic-recurrent infections, e.g., otitis media, prophylactic antibiotics may be warranted. The usual cost discrepancy between standard supportive therapy and therapy with IVIG is greatly diminished but not eliminated in autoimmune neutropenia because of the small size of these infants. For example, if the typical size of a patient is 10 kg, infusion with two doses of 1 g/kg only involves 20 g, which may cost only $500–1000. If this shortens a hospitalization by 1 day, there is a trade-off in terms of cost, and the patient may achieve a clear medical benefit in addition (55).

There are insufficient data as of yet to predict which infants will and which will not respond to therapy. In our experience, one of our three nonresponders had a predominantly IgM-mediated autoimmune neutropenia.

An infrequent issue is the need for maintenance treatment. Most patients requiring treatment can receive it as a single course. This will almost always suffice to clear up the specific infection so that even if the ANC becomes low again, there will not be a clear indication for repeated treatment. Furthermore, we have seen a high incidence of IgG_2 deficiency in these patients, and infusion of IVIG may therefore help with more than one immunodeficiency. The ANC typically will not remain increased for long following treatment: usually it is again $< 500–1000/\mu l$ by 7–14 days. If repeated treatment is required, however, tachyphylaxis seems common in our limited experience. In the two situations in which repeated infusions were administered, we gave 1.5 g/kg infusion of IVIG combined with IV solumedrol 30 mg/kg as a single, same-day infusion to ensure continued effect.

There are older patients with autoimmune neutropenia who are likely to be adolescents with hepatosplenomegaly and a neutropenia that may resemble Felty syndrome: neutropenia, rheumatoid arthritis, and splenomegaly. These patients respond well in the short term to steroid treatment, do not generally respond well to splenectomy (although this is a possible treatment), and generally do not respond at all to IV gammaglobulin. These patients are most readily distinguished from infant autoimmune neutropenia by age, leukopenia rather than isolated neutropenia, splenomegaly, and possibly other systemic signs and symptoms. Treatment is either to leave them alone, put them on minimal daily or alternate steroids, or use G- or GM-CSF. Use of the latter (growth factors) may exacerbate the splenomegaly; this requires careful monitoring. IVIG can be tried, but is almost uniformly unsuccessful.

Scattered cases exist of adults with pure autoimmune neutropenia. The small number reported to respond to IV gammaglobulin resemble infants with autoimmune neutropenia in certain features: neutropenia rather than leukopenia, otherwise normal CBC, and no significant adenopathy or hepatosplenomegaly. However, unlike the idiopathic transient cases in the infants, the reported adults tend to have clinically evident predispositions: hypogammaglobulinemia or systemic lupus erythematosus. However, these cases are rare compared to the overall number of adults with neutropenia (references reviewed in Ref. 55).

In summary, autoimmune neutropenia responsive to IV gammaglobulin is common only in small infants and children less than 0.5–4 years of age. Many of these patients do not require any treatment in view of their relatively benign natural history. Approximately one-fourth to one-half of these children may be treated for one of the four indications listed above or other individual problems of similar types. If treatment is required, one to three infusions of IVIG will usually dramatically increase the neutrophil count and help to clear up any infection. Maintenance treatment may be difficult if required, because of the development of tachyphylaxis.

AUTOIMMUNE HEMOLYTIC ANEMIA

Treatment with IVIG of patients with autoimmune hemolytic anemia (AIHA) has met with considerably less success than has the use of IVIG in the immune cytopenias described above. Recently we incorporated a series of our own patients comprising more than 30 individuals and pooled data from the literature from published series of more than 30 patients. This meta-analysis summarized results of treatment in over 70 patients and included many of the treatment references (56). Several items of interest emerged:

1. If a response was defined as an increase in hemoglobin of > 2 g/dl within 10 days of initiation of treatment, only 39% of the patients responded to treat-

ment with IVIG. This is particularly striking since most of the patients received concomitant steroid therapy.

2. Six of the 11 children responded. While this is not statistically different from the response rate seen in adults, it suggests, as with ITP and autoimmune neutropenia, that children may be more responsive than adults to IVIG treatment of AIHA.

3. The presence of hepatomegaly or of splenomegaly had a surprising, prominent effect on IVIG response. The presence of hepatomegaly was the strongest *positive* predictive factor of response to IVIG. Conversely, patients who had splenomegaly responded very poorly to IVIG. Those with hepatosplenomegaly acted like those with hepatomegaly. The pathopysiological reason(s) for this striking dichotomy remain to be clarified.

4. Higher-dose IVIG (1 g/kg/day $\times$ 5 days) could not be demonstrated to have a beneficial effect.

In general, it seems that the use of IVIG should be restricted to certain situations for patients with AIHA:

1. Children
2. Presence of hepatomegaly
3. (?) difficulty maintaining intravascular volume (the IVIG seems to stabilize the patient when the hemoglobin is very low)
4. (?) To protect red cells that are going to be transfused (57)

HEMOLYTIC DISEASE OF THE FETUS AND NEWBORN

Rh disease (hemolytic disease of the fetus and newborn; i.e., erythroblastosis fetalis) has also been the subject of treatment with IVIG. There is a controversy regarding administration of weekly IVIG to the pregnant woman with anti-D. The background for this controversy is described at least in part in the section on treatment of the fetus with alloimmune thrombocytopenia. One school of thought, voiced by Rewald and Suringar, is that IVIG is beneficial *provided* fetal blood sampling is not attempted. Sampling is likely to cause transplacental hemorrhage, and Rewald and Suringar feel that this may offset the IVIG effect (58). Our study of weekly maternal infusion of IVIG, which included fetal blood sampling, saw no benefit of IVIG treatment, unlike what we have reported in the parallel platelet disease, alloimmune thrombocytopenia (59). Unfortunately, without fetal blood sampling, it is extremely difficult to document an IVIG effect since the degree of fetal anemia is unknown and can only be the subject of speculation based on the previous sibling(s).

One controlled trial exists on the effect of IVIG on the newborn with Rh disease (60). The most prominent effect in this placebo-controlled trial was to slightly but significantly decrease the peak bilirubin. This allowed for significantly less exchange transfusions. It would seem that administering IVIG to anyone with present or anticipated jaundice secondary to an immune hemolytic anemia might be useful in this setting. However, it has not yet become common practice.

CONCLUSIONS

In summary, IVIG is a useful treatment in a number of types of immune cytopenias. There are a number of reasons that there is not more widespread usage of IVIG. The most obvious is the cost. Another is the usually temporary effect. Also, the amount of time required for each infusion, the possible requirement for more than one infusion, and the propensity for postinfusion headaches all also contribute as disincentives to treatment—the last especially from the patient's viewpoint. The reasons to use IVIG are relatively obvious: rapid, often dramatic response; lack of long-term side effects (with viral inactivation of the IVIG); lack of any very serious acute side effects; and multiple potential types of beneficial effect.

More double-blind, placebo-controlled trials are required to better define the advantages and disadvantages of IVIG in specific patient populations so that clinicians can make more informed decisions. Many of these areas involve disease states not covered in this review but discussed in other chapters in this volume. However, hematological areas requiring better study abound. Examples include, but are not limited to, trials to:

1. Determine whether or not there is a curative effect of IVIG in the treatment of ITP
2. Confirm the findings in autoimmune hemolytic anemia, especially regarding the predictive effects of hepatosplenomegaly
3. Examine the additive role, if any, of steroids with IVIG in increasing the platelet count in ITP
4. Integrate the use of IVIG, steroids, and fetal sampling into the optimal management of fetal alloimmune thrombocytopenia

REFERENCES

1. Imbach, P, Wagner HP, Berchtold W, et al. Intravenous immunoglobulin versus oral corticosteroids in acute immune thrombocytopenic purpura in childhood. Lancet 1985; ii:495–498.
2. Imbach P, Barandun S, Baumgartner C, Hirt A, Hofer F, Wagner HP. High-dose intravenous gammaglobulin therapy of refractory, in particular idiopathic thrombocytopenia in childhood. Helvetica Pediatr Acta 1981; 36(1):81–86.
3. Schmidt RE, Budde U, Schafer G, et al. High-dose intravenous gammaglobulin for idiopathic thrombocytopenic purpura. Lancet 1981; 2:475. Letter.
4. Imbach P, Wagner HHP, Berchtold W, et al. Intravenous immunglublin versus oral corticosteroids in acute immune thrombocytopenic purpura in childhood. Lancet 1985; ii:1:464–468.
5. Bussel JB, Goldman A, Imbach P, Schulman I, Hilgartner MW. Treatment of acute ITP of childhood with intravenous infusions of gammaglobulin. J Pediatr 1985; 106(6):886–890.
6. Blanchette VS, Luke B, Andrew M, et al. A prospective, randomized trial of high-dose intravenous immune globulin G therapy, oral prednisone therapy, and no therapy in childhood acute immune thrombocytopenic purpura. Pediatric pharmacology and therapeutics. J Pediatr 1993; 123:989–995.
7. Sartorius JA. Steroid treatment of idiopathic thrombocytopenia in children: preliminary results of a randomized cooperative study. Am J Pediatr Hematol Oncol 1984; 6:165.
8. Blanchette V, Imbach P, Andrew M, et al. Randomized trial of intravenous immunoglobulin G: intravenous anti-D and oral prednisone in childhood acute immune thrombocytopenic purpura. Lancet 1994; i:703–706.
9. Bussel J. Management of infants of mothers with immune thrombocytopenic purpura. J Pediatr 1988; 113(3):497–499.
9a. Imholz B, Imbach P, Baumgartner C, et al. Intravenous immunoglobulin (i.v. IgG) for previously treated acute or for chronic idiopathic thrombocytopenic purpura (ITP) in childhood: a prospective multicenter study. Blut 1988; 56:63–68.

10. Hollenberg, PJ, Subak LL, Ferry JJ, Bussel JB. Cost-effectiveness of splenectomy versus intravenous gammaglobulin in treatment of chronic immune thrombocytopenia purpura in children. J Pediatr 1988; 112:530–539.

11. Andrew M, Blanchette VS, Adams M, et al. A multicenter study of the treatment of childhood chronic idiopathic thrombocytopenic purpura with anti-D. J Pediatr 1991; 120:522–527.

12. Newland AC, Treleaven JG, Minchinton RM, Water AH. High-dose intravenous IgG in adults with autoimmune thrombocytopenia. Lancet 1993; i:83–87.

13. Bussel JB, Pham LC. Intravenous treatment with gammaglobulin in adults with immune thrombocytopenic purpura: review of the literature. Vox Sang 1987; 52:206–211.

14. Bussel JB, Szatrowski TP. Uses of intravenous gammaglobulin in immune hematologic. Immunol Invest 1995; 24:451–456.

15. Godeau BS, Lesage M, Divine V, et al. Treatment of adult chronic autoimmune thrombocytopenic purpura with repeated high-dose intravenous immunoglobulin. Blood 1993; 82(5):1415–1421.

16. Bussel J, Pham LC, Aledort L, Nachman R. Maintenance treatment of adults with chronic refractory immune thrombocytopenic purpura using repeated intravenous infusions of gammaglobulin. Blood 1988; 72(1):121–127.

17. Bussel JB, Fitzgerald-Pedersen J, Feldman C. Alternation of two doses of intravenous gammaglobulin in the maintenance treatment of patients with immune thrombocytopenic purpura. Am J Hematol 1990; 33:184–188.

18. Ballem P, Belzerg A, Devine D, et al. Kinetics studies of the mechanism of thrombocytopenia in patients with human immunodeficiency virus infection. N Engl J Med 1991; 327–1779–1784.

19. Bussel J, Haimi JS. Isolated thrombocytopenia in patients infected with HIV: treatment with intravenous gammaglobulin. Am J Hematol 1988; 28:79–84.

20. Laurian Y, Le Bras P, Ellrodt A, Alvin P. Immune thrombocytopenia gammaglobulin and seropositivity to the human T-lymphotropic virus type III. Ann Intern Med 1996; 105(1):145–146.

21. Ragni M, Bontempo FA, Myers DJ, Kiss JE, Oral A. Hemorrhagic sequelae of immune thrombocytopenic purpura in human immunodeficiency virus-infected hemophiliacs. Blood 1990; 75(6):1267–1272.

21a. Scaradavou A, Woo B, Woloski BMR, et al. Intravenous anti-D treatment of immune thrombocytopenia purpura: Experience in 272 patients. Blood 1997; 89(8):2689–2700.

22. Wenske C, Gaedicke G, Kuenzlen E, et al. Treatment of idiopathic thrombocytic purpura in pregnancy by high-dose intravenous immunoglobulin. Blut 1983; 46(6):347–353.

23. Bussel JB, Berkowitz RL, Lynch L, et al. Antenatal management of alloimmune thrombocytopenia with intravenous immunoglobulins: A randomized trial of the addition of low-dose steroid to intravenous gammaglobulin. Am J Obstetr Gynecol 1996; 174:1414–1423.

24. Kaplan C, Daffos F, Forestier F, et al. Fetal platelet counts in thrombocytopenic pregnancy. Lancet 1990; 336:979–982.

25. Burrows RF, Kelton JG. Pregnancy in patients with idiopathic thrombocytopenic purpura: assessing the risks for the infant at delivery. Obstet Gynecol Survey 1993; 48(12):781–788.

26. Burrows RF, Kelton J. Fetal thrombocytopenia and its relation to maternal thrombocytopenia. N Engl J Med 1993; 329(20):1463–1466.

27. Bussel JB, Druzin ML, Cines DB, Samuels P. Thrombocytopenia in pregnancy. Lancet 1991; 337:251.

28. Samuels P, Bussel JB, Braitman L, et al. Estimation of the risk of thrombocytopenia in the offspring of pregnant women with presumed immune thrombocytopenic purpura. N Engl J Med 1990; 323:229–235.

29. Herman JH, Jumbelic MI, Ancona RJ, Kickler TS. In utero cerebral hemorrhage in alloimmune thrombocytopenia. Am J Pediatr Hematol Oncol 1986; 8:312–317.

30. Kramer K, McFarland J, Kaplan C, Alvarez O, Bussel J. Bedside clinical diagnosis of alloimmune thrombocytopenia. Submitted.

31. Bussel J, Zabusky M, Berkowitz R, Lynch L, McFarland J. New insights into the natural history of alloimmune thrombocytopenia. N Engl J Med, in press.

32. Bussel JB, Berkowitz RL, McFarland JG, Lynch L, Chitkara U. Antenatal treatment of neonatal alloimmune thrombocytopenia. N Engl J Med 1988; 319:1374–1378.

33. Lynch L, Bussel JB, McFarland JG, Chitkara U, Berkowitz RL. Antenatal treatment of alloimmune thrombocytopenia. Obstet Gynecol 1992; 80:67–71.

34. Lescale KB, Eddleman KA, Cines B, et al. Antiplatelet antibody testing in the thrombocytopenic pregnant women. Am J Obstet Gynecol, 1996. In press.

35. Bussel JB, Skupski D. Fetal alloimmune thrombocytopenia: controversies in laboratory diagnosis and clinical management. Maternal Fetal Med 1996; 5:281–292.

36. Kroll H, Kiefel V, Giers G, et al. Maternal intravenous immunoglobulin treatment does not prevent intracranial hemorrhage in fetal alloimmune thrombocytopenia. Transfus Med 1994; 4:293–296.

37. Paidas MJ, Berkowitz RL, Lynch L, et al. Alloimmune thrombocytopenia: fetal and neonatal losses related to cordocentesis. Am J Obstet Gynecol 1995; 172:475–479.

38. Mueller-Eckhardt C, Keifel V, Grubert A, et al. 348 Cases of suspected neonatal alloimmune thrombocytopenia. Lancet 1989; 1:363–365.

39. Ballin A, Andrew M, Ling E, Perlman M, Blanchette V. High-dose intravenous gammaglobulin therapy for neonatal autoimmune thrombocytopenia. J Peds 1988; 112(6):789–792.

40. Bussel JB, Tanli S, Peterson HC. Favorable neurological outcome in 7 cases of perinatal intracranial hemorrhage due to immune thrombocytopenia. Am J Pediatr 1991; 13(2):156–159.

41. Bussel JB, Kaplan C, McFarland JG, Working Party on Neonatal Immune Thrombocytopenia of the Neonatal Hemostasis Subcommittee of the Scientific and Standardization Committee of the ISTH. Recommendations for the evaluation and treatment of neonatal autoimmune and alloimmune thrombocytopenia. Thrombos Hemostas 1991; 65(5):631–634.

42. Kickler T, Braine HG, Piantoadosi S, Ness PM, Herman JH, Rothko K. A randomized, placebo-controlled trial of intravenous gammaglobulin in alloimmunized thrombocytopenic patients. Blood 1990; 75(1):313–316.

43. Hara T, Miyazaki S, Yoshida N, et al. High doses of gammaglobulin and methylprednisolone therapy for idiopathic thrombocytopenic purpura in children. Eur J Pediatr 1985; 144:240.

44. Bjoro K, Stig F, Zhibing Y et al. Hepatitis C infection with patients with primary hypogammaglobulinemia after treatment with contaminated immune globulin. N Engl J Med 1994; 331:1607–1611.

45. Bussel JB, Horowitz B, James W. Solvent/detergent treatment of intravenous gammaglobulin: rhyme and reason. Immunoglobulin therapy. Viral Transmission Safeguards. Postgrad Med 1995; Winter.

46. Bussel JB, Graziano JN, Kimberly RP, Pahwa S, Aledort L. IV anti-D treatment of immune thrombocytopenic purpura: analysis of efficacy, toxicity, and mechanism of effect. Blood 1991; 77:1884–1893.

47. Oksenhendler E, Bierling P, Brossard Y, et al. Anti-Rh immunoglobulin therapy for human immunodeficiency virus-related immune thrombocytopenic purpura. Blood 1988; 71(5):1499–1502.

48. Bussel J, Kimberly R, Inman R, et al. Intravenous gammaglobulin treatment of chronic idiopathic thrombocytopenic purpura. Blood 1983; 62:480.

49. Fehr J, Hoffman V, Kappeler U. Transient reversal of thrombocytopenia in idiopathic thrombocytopenia purpura by high-dose intravenous immunoglobin. N Engl J Med 1982; 306:1254–1258.

50. Clarkson SB, Bussel JB, Kimberly RP, Valinsky J, Nachman RL, Unkeless JC. Treatment

of refractory immune thrombocytopenia purpura with an anti-Fc receptor antibody. N Engl J Med 1986; 314(19):1236–1239.

51. Debre M, Bonnet MC, Fridman WH, et al. Infusion of Fcγ fragments for treatment of children with acute immune thrombocytopenic purpura. Lancet 1993; 342:945–949.

52. Lalezari P, Khorshidi M, Petrosova M. Autoimmune neutropenia of infancy. J Pediatr 1986; 109:764–769.

53. Bux J, Mueller-Eckhardt C. Autoimmune neutropenia. Semin Hematol 1992; 79:728–733.

54. Conway LT, Clay ME, Kline WE, Ramsay NKC, Krivit W, McCullough J. Natural history of primary autoimmune neutropenia in infancy. Pediatrics 1987; 79:728–733.

55. Dunkel I, Bussel JB. New developments in the treatment of neutropenia. Am J Dis Child 1993; 147:994–1000.

56. Flores G, Cunningham-Rundles C, Newland A, Bussel JB. Treatment of autoimmune hemolytic anemia with intravenous gammaglobulin. Am J Hematol 1994; 44:237–242.

57. Baumann MA, Menitove JE, Aster RH, et al. Mechanism of thrombocytopenia purpura with single-dose gammaglobulin infusion followed by platelet transfusion. Ann Intern Med 1984; 104:808.

58. Rewald E, Suringar F. Substitutive-inhibitory gamma globulin therapy as prevention of stillbirth in Rh incompatibility. Acta Haematol 1965; 34:208–214.

59. Chitkara U, Bussel J, Alvarez M, Lynch L, Meisel RL, Berkowitz RL. High-dose intravenous gamma globulin: does it have a role in the treatment of severe erythroblastosis fetalis? Obstet Gynecol 1990; 76:703–708.

60. Rubo J, Albrecht K, Lasch P, et al. High-dose intravenous immune globulin therapy for hyperbilirubinemia caused by Rh hemolytic disease. J Pediatr 1992; 1(21):93–97.

22

Use of IVIG in Kawasaki Syndrome

Marian E. Melish

University of Hawaii and Kapiolani Medical Center for Women and Children, Honolulu, Hawaii

INTRODUCTION

Kawasaki syndrome (KS) is an acute, febrile, generally self-limited, multisystem vasculitis of unknown etiology primarily affecting young children. Since its first description in 1967 by Dr. Tomisaku Kawasaki of Tokyo, it has been recognized in children of all racial groups on all continents (1,2). Originally described as "benign mucocutaneous lymph node syndrome," it was quickly recognized that serious and even fatal involvement of the coronary arteries was a common feature (3). In the quarter century since its first description, much has been learned about the clinical features, natural history, pathology, and the epidemiology of the disease, although the etiology of the disease has remained undiscovered despite extensive search. Despite our ignorance of the etiology, IVIG has proven to be a remarkably effective therapy, resulting in rapid clinical improvement and a marked reduction in the incidence of coronary artery abnormalities.

CLINICAL FEATURES

Acute Illness

The onset is typically abrupt with the sudden occurrence of high fever which is followed in 1-3 days by the appearance of the diagnostic clinical features described by Dr. Kawasaki (Table 1). By day 5 of illness, the feverish child with the typical course presents a striking picture: the conjunctivae show discrete vascular injection; the lips are reddened, cracked, and often scabbed or bleeding; there is a dramatic bright red rash which may take multiple forms; and the hands and feet are swollen and tender with a diffuse red to purple discoloration of the palms and soles. Approximately 50% of the patients have marked enlargement of cervical lymph nodes which are often tender and erythematous but which do not suppurate. The associated features of the illness attest to the multisystem involvement (Table 2). Despite the involvement of mucous membranes, joints, liver, and the gastrointestinal system, the only severe or permanent damage occurs in the cardiovascular system. Kawasaki syndrome is basically self-limited

Table 1 Principal Diagnostic Criteria for Kawasaki Syndrome

Five of the six criteria are required to make a secure diagnosis:
Fever
Conjunctival injection
Changes in the mouth
    erythema, fissuring and crusting of lips
    diffuse oropharyngeal erythema
    strawberry tongue
Changes in the peripheral extremities
    Induration of the hands and feet
    Erythema of the palms and soles
    Desquamation of the finger and toe tips 2 weeks after onset
Erythematous rash
Enlarged cervical lymph node mass (>1.5 cm diameter)

with the resolution of the acute inflammatory symptoms and laboratory abnormalities within a 3-month period. Damage sustained by the cardiovascular system during the acute phase may be persistent and able to cause problems in later life.

Cardiovascular Involvement

The spectrum of cardiovascular involvement includes inflammatory pancarditis, coronary artery inflammation with coronary artery aneurysms, and systemic artery abnormalities.

Inflammatory Pancarditis

This may be manifest as pericardial effusion, congestive heart failure, and valvular insufficiency in the acute phase. Some degree of myocardial dysfunction has been documented in all cases by special echocardiographic studies (4) and some degree of inflammation in all cases by routine myocardial biopsy (5).

Table 2 Associated Clinical
Features of Kawasaki Syndrome
(in order of frequency)

Pyuria and urethritis
Arthritis and arthralgia
Myocardopathy
Pericardial effusion
Aseptic meningitis
Diarrhea
Abdominal pain
Coronary artery abnormalities
Obstructive jaundice
Hydrops of the gallbladder
Myocardial infarction

Coronary Artery Inflammation

Coronary artery abnormalities documented by echocardiography or angiography at approximately 1 month after onset are seen in 20–40% of unselected cases in multiple series. In children who develop coronary artery abnormalities, the first sign of coronary dilation appears on day 10 (mean) but may be apparent as early as illness day 7. Approximately 5–10% of patients with abnormalities at 1 month have mild changes which appear to resolve by 2 months after onset (transient dilation). This leaves approximately 15–20% of patients with significant abnormalities which persist at or beyond 2 months. These coronary abnormalities can be subdivided by size as small (3–4 mm), moderate (5–7 mm), or giant (>8 mm). Small and some moderate aneurysms may undergo regression over the next few years with restoration of a normal lumen size as demonstrated by repeat echocardiography or angiography. Dynamic studies, however, show that the areas of former aneurysm do not dilate normally in response to exercise or drugs. Thus, the normally elastic artery segment has been transformed into a rigid pipe (6). Patients whose aneurysms persist beyond 2 years are at risk for stenosis which generally develops at the inlet or outlet of the aneurysm. The giant aneurysm is the most serious coronary complication. Turbulent flow within the large saccular or fusiform structure results in ideal conditions for thrombosis and resultant myocardial infarction or sudden death in the first few months after onset (7). Coronary artery stenosis is a frequent result over the subsequent 10–15 years (8). Chronic myocardial ischemia may occur in the long term.

Systemic Artery Inflammation

This may result in the development of aneurysms and stenosis in multiple sites. Peripheral artery aneurysms are nearly always associated with large aneurysms of the coronary system. They are most often asymptomatic and remain undiscovered or present as painless pulsatile masses in the axilla or groin. Complications of peripheral ischemia or gangrene affecting the digits or the limbs are encountered very rarely in the acute phase (9). Involvement of the renal artery is almost always asymptomatic in the acute phase but may result in renovascular hypertension in later life.

PATHOLOGY OF KAWASAKI SYNDROME

The pathological features of Kawasaki syndrome vary depending on the duration of illness (10).

Early Deaths Acute Phase (First 10 Days of Illness)

Death during the first 10 days of illness has been rare and appears to be most often the result of arrhythmias. The small number of patients who have had postmortem examinations at this early stage have an intense acute inflammatory infiltrate with a polymorphonuclear cell predominance throughout the heart. The pericardium, endocardium, and valve leaflets are densely infiltrated. The myocardial fibers are intact but separated by inflammatory cells. Vessels within the myocardium are surrounded by edema and inflammatory infiltrate. There is enhanced inflammation in the sinus node, the A-V node, and the conduction system. The adventitia and vasa vasorum of the coronary arteries and the aorta are intensely inflamed. The intima shows patchy areas of proliferation with edema and inflammatory cells. The media is generally intact with little or no infiltration, although some attenuation of elastic fibers may be seen. The coronary arteries have generally been of normal caliber and free of thrombosis in cases dying at this stage.

Death During the Subacute Phase (Days 11–60)

During this period there is a steady decrease in the intensity of the pancarditis and vascular inflammatory infiltrate in the arteries. The predominance of polymorphonuclear cells in the infiltrate diminishes and mononuclear cells become dominant, followed by resolution of the infiltrate. Extensive damage to the internal elastic lamina and degeneration of the medial layer of the involved arteries is associated with the development of saccular, fusiform, or diffusely dilated aneurysms. The proximal portions of the left and right main coronary arteries and the left anterior descending and the left circumflex coronary arteries near their bifurcation are most often and most seriously involved. The cause of death is usually acute thrombosis within the most involved artery segments. Rupture of aneurysm is extremely rare. There is similar but usually less intense and less extensive involvement of medium-size muscular arteries elsewhere in the body.

Late Death (Months to Years After Onset)

Death during this phase may be due to acute myocardial infarction secondary to thrombosis or may be due to chronic myocardial ischemia. Children with prior myocardial infarction are at greatest risk for a fatal outcome with subsequent cardiac events. There is little inflammation in the heart or the coronaries associated with late death. There are chronic damage to the arteries with patchy remodeling of the vessels, intimal hypertrophy, roughened intimal surface, evidence of prior thrombosis and recanalization, and the development of stenosis. The vessel walls show evidence of calcification ranging in severity from small deposits to extensive circumferential infiltration. There is evidence of extensive disruption in the elastic lamina. Bizarre remodeling of the vessel with the development of multiple lumens in areas of prior giant aneurysms has been encountered. The myocardium may show evidence of both recent and old infarction with subsequent fibrosis.

EPIDEMIOLOGY

Kawasaki syndrome is overwhelmingly a disease of young children. The peak age affected is between ages 1 and 2 years. Fifty percent of cases are less than 2 years; 80% are less than 5 years. Cases are rarely encountered less than 3 months or over 12 years. Males outnumber females by a ratio of 1.5:1.

The disease is most common in Japan and Hawaii, where the annual incidence is of 50-90 cases/100,000 children <5 years. Active surveillance among children's hospitals in the United States has suggested that the minimum U.S. incidence is 10/100,000 children <5 (11), although passive surveillance indicates a rate of only 1.4/100,000 children <5 (12). The incidence rates show marked variation by ancestry even among children residing in the same community. In Hawaii the annual incidence per 100,000 children <5 is 145 for children of unmixed Japanese and Korean ancestry, 80 for Chinese, 25 for Philippino and part Polynesian, 20 for African-American, and nine for children of unmixed European ancestry. These rates are similar to those recorded among other areas with active surveillance: for children of Japanese ancestry living in Japan (13), Chicago (14), and Washington state (15), and for children of European ancestry living in Chicago, Los Angeles (16), Ontario, Quebec (17), Finland (18), Sweden (19), and southwestern Germany.

Communitywide outbreaks during which the annualized incidence is markedly elevated over a period of several months have been recorded in Japan (20), Korea (21), and North America (22). In Japan, at least one national pandemic has occurred, but in North America there has been little evidence of spread from one geographic area to another. Outbreaks tend to be communitywide with no evidence of point source exposure or association with any particular group, school, or event. Epidemics have tended to occur in the winter and spring months, although there is no strong seasonal distribution of endemic cases in either temperate or subtropical zones.

There is no strong urban-rural differential and no evidence for an animal or insect vector. Several case control investigations in the U.S. have shown an association of cases with exposure to a small area of freshly shampooed carpets or to a body of water in the neighborhood of the home (23). Other studies have shown no such association. Recall bias may explain the apparent associations of cases with these relatively frequent, generally unremarkable exposures. In any case, the biological significance of any such association remains obscure. Initially a house dust mite association was proposed to explain a connection with carpet shampooing. However, exposure to mites and possession of antimite antibodies has been found to vary with climate and geographic area, but not between cases and controls within the same community.

ETIOLOGY

The etiology of Kawasaki remains unknown despite extensive search. The clinical features of the disease, its acute self-limited nature, its virtual restriction to young children, the regular occurrence of communitywide epidemics, and the lack of important epidemiological associations with foods, animals, insects, chemicals, vaccines, or drugs suggest that the disease is caused by a human-associated microbial agent which spreads widely among children resulting in widespread immunity early in life in most who encounter it and expressed disease in only a few. Examples of etiological agents that fit this epidemiological pattern are provided by *H. influenzae* type b among bacteria and by human herpesvirus 6 among viruses. Among the agents that have been proposed but ultimately disproved as the elusive etiological agent are a novel retrovirus (25), proprionbacterium acnes possessing a mutant toxin (26), the staphylococcal superantigen toxic shock syndrome toxin-1 (27), Epstein-Barr virus (28), various streptococci, and parvovirus B19.

IMMUNOLOGICAL FEATURES AND PATHOGENESIS

There is considerable evidence for generalized activation of the immune system in Kawasaki syndrome. Patients with the disease generally have a normal infection history with no suggestion of past or recent depressed immune responses or prodromal illness. During the various phases of illness there are characteristic changes in T cells, B cells, immunoglobulins, monocytes, macrophages, and cytokines.

T cells show characteristic changes in their subpopulation distribution in the circulation during the course of illness. During the acute early phase there is a substantial decrease in the number and percentage of CD8+ (T8) cells with a normal or only slightly shifted amount of CD4+ (T4) cells, usually resulting in a slight decrease in total T cells (29,30). T cells from patients with acute Kawasaki syndrome stimulate normal donor b cells to produce immunoglobulins, indicating that the populations shifts in T cells have a functional component. Over the course of 2–3 months, the T8 cells increase gradually to the normal absolute number and percentage of T cells (31). Some studies have shown activation markers on the T-cell surface including increased HLA-DR and sIL-2R expression in the acute stage (32). There are conflicting reports about the expression of V-beta families on the T-cell receptor. A report demonstrating a very modest expansion of the V-beta 2 and V-beta 8 families has not been confirmed by several other groups using newer and more quantitative assays (33,34). There is an increase in circulating B cells spontaneously secreting immunoglobulins late in the first week and continuing during the first month of illness. Although total IgG levels are initially low for age, by day 7 of illness they have reached normal levels. A rise in all immunoglobulin classes is seen from weeks 1 to 3 of illness followed by a convalescent fall. A variety of autoantibodies have been described during the course of the disease, most notably antibodies to native vascular endothelium and to endothelium, expressing novel antigens after being exposed to the cytokines TNF and IL-1 (35). Modest quantities of circulating immune complexes peaking in weeks 2 and 3 of illness are characteristically found without evidence of significant complement depletion (36).

A marked increase of cytokines including TNF, IL-1, IL-6, and IFN-γ is found in the circulation during the acute phase of the illness (32).

TREATMENT WITH IVIG

Studies Comparing IVIG and ASA with ASA Alone

IVIG was first employed in the treatment of Kawasaki syndrome by Furusho et al., who applied the regimen used in the treatment of idiopathic thrombocytopenia purpura to a group of patients with KS (37). The rationale for this attempt was that immunological mechanisms are known to play a part in both diseases. In the first clinical trial of the effect of IVIG, 45 patients were randomized to treatment with aspirin (ASA) alone at a dose of 30–50 mg/kg in three divided doses. The comparison group was randomized to receive IVIG 400 mg/kg/day for 5 days (total dose 2 g/kg) in addition to ASA as above. The IVIG preparation used in this study was a sulfonated intact gammaglobulin, "Venilon" (Teijin Ltd., Japan), which was prepared from plasma collected in North America (majority source) and Japan. The mean ages of the patients, the sex distribution, and the initial laboratory studies were similar in the two groups. The mean duration of symptoms before treatment was similar at 5.2 days. The primary outcome criterion was the cumulative incidence of coronary artery abnormalities (CAA) in the two groups. Echocardiograms were performed three times a week for 60 days after the onset of disease. Any abnormality, even a transient dilation, was diagnosed as a CAA using the criterion that coronaries with a diameter of >3 mm or more than 1.5 times the adjacent vessel diameter were abnormal. The resulting cumulative incidence of abnormalities by 30 days was 19/45 (42%) in the ASA group and 6/40 (15%) in the IVIG and ASA group ($p = <.01$). No new lesions were encountered between 30 and 60 days in either group, but regression of abnormalities was noted among those with previous CAA. The point prevalence of CAA at 60 days was 14/45 (31%) in the ASA group and 3/40 (8%) in the IVIG and ASA groups.

The U.S. Multicenter Kawasaki Syndrome Study Group has conducted two multicenter randomized controlled trials of IVIG treatment for KS (38). The first trial compared patients given ASA alone at an anti-inflammatory dose of 100 mg/kg until day 14 of illness, with patients given the same dose of ASA and IVIG 400 mg/kg/day for four consecutive days (1.6 g total dose). Echocardiograms were performed and interpreted according to a uniform predetermined protocol. Each patient had echocardiograms at enrollment, 2 weeks and 7 weeks after study entry. The primary outcome criterion in this study was the presence of CAA on echocardiograms at 2 weeks and 7 weeks. Because echocardiogram interpretation has subjective aspects, all echocardiograms were read by two echocardiographers from centers other than the one where the patient was hospitalized. These echocardiographers performed "blinded readings" without knowledge of the treatment assignment or of the clinical course of the subject patient. In case of disagreement, a third echocardiographer (tie breaker) was asked to resolve the matter. The patients were well matched in this study according to age, sex, ethnic origin, presence of fever at enrollment, white blood cell count, platelet count, acute phase reactants, and initial echocardiogram. The coronary artery outcome was determined at 2 weeks and 7 weeks after treatment. At 2 weeks, 23% of children in the ASA-alone group had CAA compared with 8% in the ASA plus IVIG group. This is an adjusted relative prevalence of .33 for IVIG. At 7 weeks 17% of the ASA alone group had CAA compared with 4% for IVIG plus ASA. This is an adjusted relative prevalence of .55 for IVIG. These differences were statistically significant by Fisher Exact and by Mantel-Haenzel statistics. IVIG was found to have a statistically significant effect on the degree and duration of fever as well as on laboratory measures of inflammation (white blood cell count, granulocyte count, and alpha-1 antitrypsin).

Furusho *et al.* carried out another controlled trial comparing ASA 30–50 mg/kg/day with the same ASA dose and IVIG 200 mg/kg × 5 days (total dose 1 g/kg), with a third group receiving 200 mg/kg/day × 5 days without ASA. The rates for CAA for both IVIG groups were similar, and both were statistically significantly lower than for ASA alone at all stages in the follow-up period: <30 days, 30 days, 2 months, 6 months, and 1 year (39).

Ogino *et al.* reported a statistical reduction in CAA at 30 days in a cohort of patients treated with 400 mg/kg IVIG (total dose 1.2 g/kg) and ASA compared with a group treated with ASA alone (40).

Thus, all studies utilizing direct comparison of sufficient numbers of patients treated with ASA alone with patients treated with IVIG at a total dose of at least 1 g/kg have demonstrated a reduction in the proportion of IVIG-treated patients with CAA. Some studies have also noted an effect of IVIG on the height and duration of fever and on laboratory measures of inflammation.

Dose Comparison Studies

A dose of 100 mg/kg of IVIG given once has been found to be ineffective in reducing the rate of CAA development compared to ASA alone (41). A dose of 100 mg/kg/day for 5 days (total dose 500 mg/kg) has been used in two studies. As compared with ASA-treated patients studied with the same protocol for evaluating and measuring CAA, one study showed no efficacy for IVIG at this dose (39), while the other showed a modest decrease in CAA which was inferior to that of patients treated with 400 mg/kg/day for 5 days (total dose 2 g/kg) by direct comparison (41). With the clinical trial evidence available to date, total doses of <1 g/kg IVIG have been proven to be either ineffectual or inferior to higher doses.

A large prospective trial multicenter trial involving 549 KS patients compared 400 mg/kg/day IVIG in four daily doses (total dose 1.6 g/kg) to a single dose of 2 g/kg. The single large dose was demonstrated to be superior to the 4-day dose regimen in frequency and severity of CAA, duration of fever, and laboratory indices of acute inflammation. The serum IgG profile of patients treated with either dose was similar when measured at 4 days, 2 weeks, and 7 weeks after the start of treatment. The large single dose of IVIG given over 10 h was equally safe as the 4-day regimen including the frequency of new or worsening heart failure. All adverse effects were transient, and none required discontinuation of IVIG therapy (42).

Another study involving 108 KS patients selected for severity by means of a clinical scoring system compared a regimen of 400 mg/kg/day for 5 days (total dose 2 g/kg) with a single dose of 2 g/kg. As in the large U.S. multicenter trial, the frequency of CAA and the duration of fever were lower in the single infusion group. The single infusion therapy was equally safe (43).

The experience with a single large 2 g/kg dose of IVIG represents the optimal results obtained to date among the clinical trials of IVIG therapy for KS. Unpublished results from the U.S. Multicenter trial and from a trial comparing high- and low-dose ASA therapy as an adjunct to 2 g/kg single infusion therapy, indicate that approximately two-thirds of patients will be afebrile within 24 h and that 90% will be afebrile by 48 h after completing IVIG infusion. The patients who develop CAA despite IVIG are found overwhelmingly among those with persistent or recrudescent fever. Therefore, further therapy for this group of clinical failures is needed.

A meta-analysis has reviewed multiple reports of the outcome of patients treated with ASA or IVIG or both. The authors concluded that IVIG in total doses of at least 1 g/kg administered with some dose of ASA is superior to therapy with IVIG at total doses of <1 g/kg or ASA alone in reducing the frequency of CAA. The study also suggested that single, high-dose IVIG was superior to multiple-dose IVIG. The usual problems with meta-analysis are here compounded, as the technique, timing, and interpretation of echocardiograms were not uniform in the various studies. Nevertheless, the conclusions of the meta-analysis can be amply supported by a literature review without the statistical techniques of meta-analysis (44).

Product Comparisons

There is only one study comparing a pepsin-treated IVIG product with intact IVIG. The doses used in these comparison trials were either subeffective (100 mg/kg × 1) or marginally effective (100 mg/kg × 5), so it is difficult to draw any firm conclusions. In the trial at the 100 mg/kg × 5 dose level, there were fewer definite aneurysms in the patients treated with intact IVIG than with either ASA alone or pepsin-treated IVIG, although the frequency of total CAA was not significantly reduced compared with pepsin-treated IVIG (41).

There are significant-differences in purification and preparation procedures among different products of intact IVIG. To date no direct comparison trials have been carried out. A retrospective multicenter product comparison involving nine North American centers using multiple brands of IVIG commercially available in the United States failed to show any differences in frequency of CAA or persistence of fever among patients treated by medical centers experienced in the care of children with KS. This study had significant limitations, as it was retrospective; it had limited power to discriminate among brands due to small numbers studied, and there was an overall low frequency of adverse outcomes of CAA and persistent fever. Therefore, very large numbers of patients would be required to show a small difference in efficacy between brands. The Immuno brand was the preparation used most often in these centers. By combining all other brands and comparing the outcome across centers with that of the Immuno brand, there was no significant difference in clinical outcome or CAA. Although there was no difference in efficacy demonstrated in this survey, there were clear differences in the frequency of minor and moderate adverse reactions during IVIG infusions. These adverse reactions included chills, hyperpyrexia, hypotension and hypertension, and dysphoric reactions (45). The efficacy and safety experience with the Immuno brand in this retrospective study did not differ from the earlier experience with the same brand in the Phase II U.S. Multicenter Trial (42).

A smaller, two-center prospective study designed to search for adverse effects compared the Immuno product, Iveegam, with the Alpha Therapeutics Product, Venoglobin I. This study, with a sample size of 45 per group, found no differences in efficacy in regard to fever and CAA but found that the Venoglobin I had a significantly higher frequency of minor, infusion-related adverse effects, principally chills (46).

By contrast, a prospective study at a single center showed a significant difference in the rate of CAA comparing patients treated with the Immuno brand (7.4% CAA at 42–49 days) with the Canadian Red Cross preparation (20.3% CAA to 42–49 days) (47). This latter product is produced by Cutter laboratories from plasma supplied by the Canadian Red Cross blood bank and is not commercially available, but is intended to be used across Canada for patients covered by the Canadian provincial health insurance schemes. This lack of efficacy associated with the Canadian product may be reflected in another study of the epidemiology of KS in Ontario and Quebec, which found no decrease in the frequency of CAA in patients treated with IVIG and found similar rates of CAA in 1990–1994, as had been recorded in the period before IVIG became available (17). This disappointing efficacy in a population-based study differs from the US experience whether recorded by the passive surveillance maintained by the U.S. Centers for Disease Control (12) or recorded by active surveillance in the centers of the U.S. Kawasaki syndrome study group (45).

ASA as Adjunctive Therapy to IVIG for KS

Early awareness of the inflammatory and rheumatic aspects of KS as well as the universal occurrence of thrombocytosis prompted the use of ASA on an empirical basis. Various doses of ASA have been used: (1) low "antiplatelet"—3–10 mg/kg/day; (2) medium "antipyretic"—30 mg/kg/day in 3–4 divided doses; and (3) high "anti-inflammatory"—100 mg/kg/day or more. While there have been no clinical trials comparing the use of ASA at any dose with a placebo, many clinicians felt that the early administration of ASA improved the resolution of fever and possibly of arthritis. Thus, in the era prior to the studies demonstrating efficacy of IVIG, ASA therapy had become standard therapy for KS. For this reason all but one trial of IVIG to date have also provided ASA at some dose either alone or as an adjunct to IVIG. We have recently concluded a multicenter trial in which all patients received 2 g/kg of IVIG. Patients were randomized into two groups: (1) to receive either ASA at an antiplatelet dose of 3–8 mg/kg/day in a single dose, or (2) to receive ASA at an anti-inflammatory dose of 100 mg/kg/day in four divided doses. We found no difference in efficacy for CAA between the two groups. Fever resolution was significantly faster and more complete with in the high-dose ASA group. There were fewer episodes of recrudescence of disease in the high-dose ASA group. There was no evidence of increased adverse reactions of any type in the high-dose ASA group. There was no clinical evidence of salicylate toxicity or bleeding episodes, and the resolution of initial liver enzyme elevations was equal in the two groups. We have therefore concluded that IVIG therapy should be accompanied by ASA 100 mg/kg/day through day 14 of illness in order to reduce duration of fever and shorten hospitalization (48).

THERAPEUTIC RECOMMENDATIONS

As soon as KS can be diagnosed (preferably in the first 7 days after onset), the patient should be given IVIG 2 g/kg and be started on ASA 100 mg/kg/day in four divided doses every 6 h. Baseline EKG and echocardiogram should be performed. It is critically important that the echocardiogram be performed at a center that has experience in imaging the coronary arteries in children. Echocardiographers inexperienced in the evaluation of children with KS may overlook CAA or fail to visualize the coronary artery system in an optimal manner. Patients who have persistent or recurrent fever 48 h or more after completing their IVIG infusion may receive another 2 g/kg infusion. These patients may also benefit from having their ASA dose increased to achieve a serum salicylate level of 18–30 mg/dl until fever is controlled. Considerable effort should be expended in controlling the fever, as CAAs are more likely in those with persistent or recurrent fever. Patients should be hospitalized until fever has been absent for 24 h and then discharged with careful follow-up care to detect recurrent fever and/or rash. Recurrent illness is unlikely to occur beyond 21 days from onset of fever. High-dose ASA should be continued through 14 days from onset, after which it can be reduced to 3–8 mg/kg/day if fever has been controlled. Echocardiograms should be repeated approximately 1 week and 3–4 weeks after treatment is started. If an echocardiogram of good quality is normal at 3–4 weeks after therapy, CAA will not develop later. An antiplatelet dose of ASA may be discontinued 2–3 months from onset in those without CAA.

Patients with CAA at 3–4 weeks should continue low-dose ASA indefinitely. These patients will require follow-up echocardiograms at 2 months after therapy and will need to be followed by a pediatric cardiologist who is experienced in the care of KS. Patients with giant coronary aneurysms will require consideration of more potent anticoagulant therapy and will require coronary angiography at some time in the future. Exercise thallium scintigraphy is the most sensitive measure other than angiography for discovering stenotic lesions, and can be used in the care of all children with CAA due to KS when they are old enough to cooperate. Occasional patients with severe CAA and stenosis or ischemia may benefit from coronary angioplasty or coronary artery bypass grafting.

THERAPEUTIC PROBLEMS

Therapy for Patients Encountered Late in the Illness

There are no clinical studies to provide guidance for the care of patients encountered late in the illness. Coronary artery abnormalities may be well established by day 10 of illness, so every effort should be directed toward early diagnosis and early referral for IVIG therapy. In most areas where there is active clinical research in KS, there are too few patients who are encountered late to allow the initiation of a controlled trial. Lacking guidance from a clinical trial the following considerations seem reasonable. If patients encountered late (day 10) are still febrile, IVIG therapy may be indicated to hasten resolution of inflammation and to prevent or minimize further vascular damage. If coronary abnormalities are present when the patient is diagnosed between days 10 and 30 of illness, whether or not the patient is still febrile, IVIG therapy may attenuate the vasculitic process and minimize further artery damage. If, however, the patient is afebrile and the echocardiogram is normal, there may be no clinical advantage to starting IVIG therapy for the "missed diagnosis" patient encountered between days 10 and 30 of illness. It is unlikely that any IVIG therapy will benefit the afebrile patient encountered after day 30 of illness.

Therapy for the Patient with Incomplete or Atypical Manifestations

In the absence of any pathognomonic diagnostic test for KS, the diagnosis must be made by adherence to clinical criteria, exclusion of other possible diagnoses, and the presence of some nonspecific but compatible clinical laboratory features. When the elusive etiological agent is finally discovered, it is almost certain that patients will be found who are infected with the same agent and who are at risk for CAA and who will benefit from IVIG therapy. At present we know that there are some children who have mild or incomplete clinical manifestations who nevertheless develop CAA typical of KS. There are also patients who manifest all of the diagnostic criteria, but who may have atypical features which suggest alternate diagnoses. For example, children who present with very severe lymphadenitis may be treated intensively with antibiotics; after rash develops, antibiotics are changed, a diagnosis of drug hypersensitivity is made, but the true diagnosis of KS is not considered for many days despite typical manifestations. This pattern of failure to consider KS despite compatible clinical features is also a problem for children presenting with severe polyarticular arthritis, for those presenting with aseptic meningitis, and for some children whose age is less typical (over 6 years or under 3 months). In order to prevent CAA, clinicians must be prepared to consider the possibility of KS in any febrile child whose illness is unexplained to an administer IVIG to certain patients who have fever, incomplete clinical features of KS, and compatible laboratory manifestations including elevated white blood cell count, elevated absolute granulocyte count, elevated acute phase reactants, progressive thrombocytosis, and, in some cases, abnormal liver function tests and sterile pyuria.

MECHANISM OF ACTION OF IVIG

As with so many other aspects of this fascinating disease, the mechanism of action of IVIG remains undiscovered. The resolution of fever, rash, conjunctival injection, and adenopathy is so extraordinarily rapid that over half of cases become afebrile and appear nearly normal by the end of the 10-h infusion. Many clinicians have noted that this resolution is more rapid than the clinical improvement that occurs when treating pneumococcal pneumonia with penicillin, a disease known to respond unusually rapidly to therapy. IVIG therapy is temporally associated with rapid improvement in left ventricular contractility and function in all treated patients (49). IVIG therapy is also known to result in reduction in B-cell activation, more rapid return of T suppressor cells to normal, and rapid reduction in cytokine secretion (50). Skin biopsy studies before and after IVIG show disappearance of endothelial cell activation antigens in vessels after therapy (51). Prompt reversal of cytokine elaboration and other aspects or immune activation impacting endothelial cell function and antigen expression provide an attractive explanation for the as yet unknown mechanism of action of IVIG. Other theories include nonspecific downregulation of immunoglobulin production by a negative feedback mechanism, specific immunoglobulin neutralization of the unknown etiological agent or toxin, Fc receptor blockade, and nonspecific blockade of an attachment site on the vascular endothelium for immune complexes or harmful autoantibodies.

REMAINING PROBLEMS

The cause of KS remains unknown; therefore, secure diagnostic tests are still unavailable. Once the etiological agent is discovered, it may be possible to design some means of prophylaxis and more rational therapy. Until that time, however, IVIG has proven to be a most effective means of therapy. Applied optimally in a single high dose of 2 g/kg to all children with a compatible clinical picture, IVIG can prevent most severe cardiac morbidity. In Japan, where a suboptimal therapeutic dose (200 mg/kg/day × 5 days) has been deemed the official standard of care, there has been no decline in the rate of CAA reported to nationwide surveys. Although several brands of intact IVIG available in the United States and Japan appear to be effective in preventing CAA, very few product comparison data are available. The sobering experience in Ontario and Quebec, which has demonstrated that the officially sanctioned Canadian product may have limited efficacy, indicates the urgency of the need to compare products in well-designed clinical trials and to understand the mechanism of action of IVIG.

REFERENCES

1. Kawasaki T. Acute febrile mucocutaneous lymph node syndrome. Jpn J Allergy 1967; 16:178–222.
2. Yanagawa H. Comments on global epidemiology of Kawasaki disease. In: Kato H, ed. awasaki Disease. 1995. New York: Elsevier Science,
3. Kawasaki T, Kosaki F, Okawa S, et al. A new infantile febrile mucocutaneous lymph node syndrome (MLNS) prevailing in Japan. Pediatrics 1974; 54:271–276.
4. Newberger JW, Sanders SP, Burns JC, et al. Left ventricular contractility and function in Kawasaki syndrome: effect of intravenous gamma globulin. Circulation 79 1989; 79:1237–1746.
5. Yutani C, Go S, Kamiya F, et al. Cardiac biopsy of Kawasaki disease. Arch Path Lab Med 1981; 105:470–473.

6. Sugimura T, Kato H, Inoue O. Vasodilatory response of the coronary arteries after Kawasaki disease: evaluation by intracoronary injection of isosorbide dinitrate. J Pediatr 1992; 121:684–688.

7. Kato H, Ichinose E, Kawasaki T. Myocardial Infarction in Kawasaki disease: clinical analyses in 195 cases. J Pediatr 1986; 108:923–927.

8. Kamiya T, Suzuko A, Ono Y, et al. Angiographic follow-up study of coronary artery lesion in the cases with a history of Kawasaki disease—with a focus on the follow-up more than 10 years after the onset of the disease. In Kato H, ed. Kawasaki Disease. New York: Elsevier Science, 1995:569–573.

9. Kato H, Inoue O, Akagi T. Kawasaki disease: cardiac problems and management. Pediatr Rev 1988; 9:209–217.

10. Fujiwara H, Hamashima Y. Pathology of the heart in Kawasaki disease. Pediatrics 1978; 61:100–107.

11. Taubert KA, Rowley AH, Shulman ST. A 10 year (1984–1993) United States hospital survey of Kawasaki disease. In: Kato H, ed. Kawasaki Disease. New York: Elsevier Science, 1995:34–38.

12. Khan AS, Holman RC, Clarke MJ, et al. Kawasaki Surveillance United States 1991–1993. In: Kato H, ed. Kawasaki Disease. New York: Elsevier Science, 1995:80–84.

13. Yashiro M, Nakamura Y, Hirose K, Yanagawa H. Surveillance of Kawasaki disease in Japan, 1984–1994. In: Kato H, ed. Kawasaki Disease. New York: Elsevier Science, 1995.

14. Shulman ST, McAuley JB, Pachman LM, et al. Risk of coronary abnormalities due to Kawasaki disease in an urban area with small Asian populations. Am J Dis Child 1987; 141:421–425.

15. Dykewicz CA, Davis RL, Khan AS, et al. Kawasaki syndrome in Washington state, 1985–1989. In: Takahashi M, Taubert K, eds. Proceedings of the Fourth International Symposium on Kawasaki Disease. New York: American Heart Association, 1993:10–15.

16. Mason WH, Schneider T, Takahashi M. The epidemiology and etiology of Kawasaki disease. Cardiol Young 1991; 1:196–205.

17. McCrindle BW, Newman A, Rose V, et al. Kawasaki disease in Ontario and Quebec, Canada, 1990–1994. In: Kato H, ed. Kawasaki Disease. New York: Elsevier Science, 1995:62–68.

18. Salo E. Epidemiology of Kawasaki disease in Finland. In: Kato H, ed. Kawasaki Disease. New York: Elsevier Science, 1995:48–52.

19. Schiller B, Elinder G, Fasth A, Bjorkhem G. Kawasaki disease in Sweden—incidence and clinical features. In: Kato H, ed. Kawasaki Disease. New York: Elsevier Science, 1995:39–47.

20. Yanagawa H, Nakamura Y, Kawasaki T, et al. Nationwide epidemic of Kawasaki disease in Japan during winter of 1985–86. Lancet 1986; 2:1138–1139.

21. Lee DB. Epidemiologic survey of Kawasaki syndrome in Korea (1976–1984). J Cath Med Coll 1985; 38:13–19.

22. Dean AG, Melish ME, Hicks RV, et al. An epidemic of Kawasaki syndrome in Hawaii. J Pediatr 1982; 100:552–557.

23. Rauch AM. Kawasaki syndrome: clinical review of US epidemiology. In: Shulman S, ed. Kawasaki Disease. New York: Alan R. Liss, 1987:33–44.

24. Glode MP, Brogden R, Joffe LS, et al. Kawasaki syndrome and house dust mite exposure. Pediatr Infect Dis J 1986; 5:644–648.

25. Burns JC, Geha RS, Schneeberger EE, et al. Polymerase activity in lymphocyte culture supernatants from patients with Kawasaki disease. Nature 1987; 323:814–816.

26. Kato H, Inoue O, Koga Y, et al. Variant strain of *Propionibacterium* acnes: a clue to the etiology of Kawasaki disease. Lancet 1983; 2:1383–1387.

27. Marchette NJ, Cao XX, Kihara S, Melish ME. Staphylococcal toxic shock syndrome toxin-1, one possible cause of Kawasaki syndrome? In: Kato H, ed. Kawasaki Disease. New York: Elsevier Science, 1995:149–155.

28. Marchette NJ, Melish ME, Hicks RV, et al. Epstein-Barr virus and other herpesvirus infections in Kawasaki syndrome. J Infect Dis 1990; 161:680–684.

29. Leung DYM, Collins T, LaPierre KA, et al. Immunoregulatory T cell abnormalities in mucocutaneous lymph node syndrome. J Immunol 1983; 130:2002–2004.

30. Laxer RL, Schaffer FM, Myones BL, et al. Lymphocyte abnormalities and complement activation in Kawasaki disease. Prog Clin Biol Res 1987; 250:175–180.

31. Barron K, DeCunto C, Montalvo J, et al. Abnormalities of immunoregulation in Kawasaki syndrome. J Rheumatol 1988; 15:12–43.

32. Matsubara T, Furukawa S, Yabuta K. Serum levels of tumor necrosis factor, interleukin 2 receptor and interferon-gamma in Kawasaki disease involved coronary-artery lesions. Clin Immunol Immunopathol 1990; 56:29–35.

33. Abe J, Kotzin BL, Meissner C, et al. Characterization of T cell repertoire changes in Kawasaki disease. J Exp Med 1993; 177:791–799.

34. Pietra BA, De Inocencio J, Giannini EH, et al. T cell receptor Vbeta family repertoire and T cell activation markers in Kawasaki disease. J Immunol 1994; 153:1881–1888.

35. Leung DYM, Geha RS, Newburger JW, et al. Two monokines, interleukin-1 and tumor necrosis factor, render cultured vascular endothelial cells susceptible to lysis by antibodies circulating during Kawasaki syndrome. 1995; 164:1048–1065.

36. Mason WH, Jordan SC, Sakai R et al. Circulating immune complexes in Kawasaki syndrome. Pediatr Infect Dis 1985; 4:48.

37. Furusho K, Nakano H, Shinomiya K, et al. High-dose intravenous gammaglobulin for Kawasaki disease. Lancet 1984; 2:1055–1057.

38. Newburger JW, Takahasi M, Burns JC, et al. The treatment of Kawasaki syndrome with intravenous gamma globulin. N Engl J Med 1986; 315:341–347.

39. FuroshoK, Kamiya T, Nakano H, et al. Intravenous gamma globulin for Kawasaki disease. Acta Paediatr Jpn 1991; 33:799–804.

40. Ogino H, Ogawa M. Harima Y, et al. Clinical evaluation of gamma-globulin preparations for the treatment of Kawasaki disease. Prog Clin Biol Res 1987; 260:555–556.

41. Harada K. Intravenous gamma globulin in Kawasaki disease. Acta Paediatr Jpn 1991; 33:805–810.

42. Newburger JW, Takahashi M, Beiser AS, et al. A single intravenous infusion of gamma globulin therapy as compared with four infusions in the treatment of acute Kawasaki syndrome. N Engl J Med 1991; 324:1633–1639.

43. Sato N, Sugimura T, Ahagi T, et al. Selective gammaglobulin treatment in Kawasaki disease: Single 2 g/kg or 400 mg/kg/day for 5 days? In: Kato H, ed. Kawasaki Disease. New York: Elsevier Science, 1995:332–338.

44. Durongpisitkul K, Gururaj VJ, Park JM, Martin CF. The prevention of coronary artery aneurysms in Kawasaki disease: a meta-analysis on the efficacy of aspirin and immunoglobulin treatment. Pediatrics 1995; 96:1057–1061.

45. Burns JC, Glode MP, Capparelli E, Brown JA, Newberger JA. Intravenous gammaglobulin treatment in Kawasaki syndrome: are all brands equal? In: Kato H, ed. Kawasaki Disease. New York: Elsevier Science, 1995:296–300.

46. Rosenfeld EA, Shulman ST, Carydon KE, et al. Comparative safety and efficacy of two immune globulin products in Kawasaki disease. In: Kato H, ed. Kawasaki Disease. New York: Elsevier Science, 1995:291–295.

47. SilvermanED, Huang C, Rose V, et al. IVGG treatment of Kawasaki disease: are all brands equal? In: Kato H, ed. Kawasaki Disease. New York: Elsevier Science, 1995:301–304.

48. Melish ME, Takahashi M, Shulman S. ASA as an adjunct to IVIG in the treatment of Kawasaki syndrome. 1996. In preparation.

49. Newberger JW. Myocardial function in Kawasaki disease. Circulation.

50. Leung DY, Burns JC, Newburger JW, Geha RS. Reversal of lymphocyte activation in vivo in the Kawasaki syndrome by intravenous gammaglobulin. J Clin Invest 1987; 79:468–472.
51. Leung DYM. Immunomodulation by intravenous immune globulin in Kawasaki disease. J Allergy Clin Immunol 1989; 84:588–594.

23

Juvenile Rheumatoid Arthritis

Thomas A. Griffin and Edward H. Giannini
Children's Hospital Medical Center, University of Cincinnati College of Medicine, Cincinnati, Ohio

OVERVIEW

Juvenile rheumatoid arthritis (JRA) is defined as persistent arthritis of at least 6 weeks' duration in one or more joints with all other causes excluded and with onset before the 16th birthday (1). JRA can be classified into three subtypes: systemic, polyarticular, and pauciarticular. Systemic JRA is characterized by persistent intermittent fevers with or without rheumatoid rash or extra-articular involvement. Patients without systemic features are classified as polyarticular or pauciarticular based on the number of joints involved over the course of the disease, with polyarticular JRA involving five or more joints.

JRA is associated with abnormalities of the immune system, including alterations of immunoglobulin and cytokine levels and both B lymphocyte and T lymphocyte numbers and functions (2). The involvement of the immune system in the pathogenesis of JRA appears to be multifactorial and heterogeneous. Therefore, efficacy of immunomodulatory treatment of JRA may vary depending on the subtype and the individual. Medications that have been used include nonsteroidal anti-inflammatory drugs, slow-acting antirheumatic drugs, cytotoxic drugs, methotrexate, and corticosteroids. Methotrexate is currently the most efficacious agent for suppressing articular disease without significant risk (3). Corticosteroids are often required to control severe systemic manifestations of systemic JRA. Unfortunately, long-term use of corticosteroids can produce severe side effects. None of these medications are curative, and their beneficial impact on long-term outcome is uncertain. This has prompted the search for more efficacious and less toxic immunomodulatory agents to use in the treatment of JRA.

OPEN TRIALS OF IVIG IN JRA

Intravenous immunoglobulin (IVIG) was considered a potential therapy for JRA based upon several observations. First, arthritis associated with certain hypogammaglobulinemias may be responsive to immunoglobulin replacement (4). Second, IVIG is effective in treating other autoimmune diseases of childhood, such as Kawasaki's disease (5) and idiopathic thrombocytopenic purpura (6). Third, a severely affected patient with JRA appeared to improve after receiving gammaglobulin for varicella prophylaxis (7).

The first published report of the use of IVIG in the treatment of JRA was by Groothoff and Van Leeuwen in 1988 (8). They described a patient with systemic JRA who for 3 years had responded only to corticosteroids. Many standard therapies, including cytotoxic drugs, were of no benefit. Unfortunately, corticosteroids caused severe osteoporosis with vertebral fractures and had to be withdrawn. IVIG in high doses was tried as an alternative, and this produced dramatic results (Fig. 1). Fever, rash, and arthritis responded rapidly. Unfortunately, control of disease required repeated infusions, and long-term remission without IVIG was not achieved.

The results of two open trials using IVIG in the treatment of JRA were subsequently published (9,10). Silverman et al., in 1990, described the response of eight patients with systemic JRA to monthly infusions of IVIG at 1 g/kg/day for 2 consecutive days. One patient was treated for 13 months, another 10 months, and the rest 6 months. Their response at completion of IVIG therapy is summarized in Table 1. Seven patients were felt to be "responders" by having significant improvement in at least one outcome measure. Interestingly, serum IgG levels decreased in the responders but not in the single "nonresponder." Peripheral blood mononuclear cells obtained from responders within 24 h of an IVIG infusion had decreased in vitro IgG production (mean decrease 53%) and had normalization of immunoglobulin production in response to interleukin-2 (IL-2) (11). This suggested that regulation of immunoglobulin production may partially account for the action of IVIG in these patients. The overall results of this trial suggest that IVIG may improve both articular and systemic features of systemic JRA in the short term. No side effects were reported in this trial.

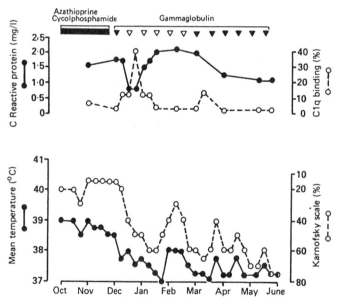

Figure 1 Clinical course of disease as indicated by C-reactive protein and C1q binding concentrations, mean body temperature, and quality of life according to Karnofsky scale (10% = very ill and wholly dependent on outside help; 80% = only few interferences with activities of daily living) during treatment with gamma globulin from October 1986 to June 1987. ▼ = 60 g in 5 days; ▽ = 24 g in 1 day.

Table 1 Responders to Open Trials of IVIG in Systemic JRA

Outcome measure	Silverman (9)	Prieur (10)
Improved physician global assessment	6/7 (86%)	ND[a]
Decreased number of days with fever	6/7 (86%)	6/10 (60%)
Disappearance of rash	3/6 (50%)	1/7 (14%)
Resolution of organomegaly	4/4 (100%)	1/5 (20%)
≥30% decreased active joint count	4/8 (50%)	5/9 (56%)
≥25% improved or normalized lab values	23/31 (74%)	20/25 (80%)
≥50% reduced or discontinued steroids	7/7 (100%)	1/10 (10%)

[a]ND, not determined.

Prieur et al., in 1990, described the response of 16 patients with JRA (13 systemic; three polyarticular) to treatment with high-dose IVIG for up to 4 years. IVIG was discontinued within 1 year in six patients because of possible side effects or lack of efficacy. Putative side effects of IVIG included vasculitic rash, urticaria, and proteinuria/hematuria. IVIG was totally ineffective in three systemic JRA patients. The response of the systemic JRA patients at completion of IVIG therapy is summarized in Table 1. Only one patient had complete resolution of systemic features and did not require the addition of other medications, particularly corticosteroids. Unfortunately, that patient had onset of arthritis while on IVIG. Both of the patients with polyarticular JRA who were treated long term had complete resolution of their arthritis by the end of the trial. Long-term follow-up after IVIG (3.25–7.25 years) was reported in 14 patients (eight treated >1 year). There was no difference in the functional status of those treated more or less than 1 year, and most still had progressive polyarthritis requiring anti-inflammatory therapy. The overall results of this trial suggest that, although IVIG may provide some short-term benefit, it does not appear to significantly alter the long-term outcome of JRA.

Recently, long-term follow-up of 27 patients with systemic JRA treated with high-dose IVIG for 2–54 months was reported by Uziel et al. (12). Six months after starting IVIG, 20 patients had either at least a 50% reduction in number of days with fever and/or prednisone dose (19 patients) and/or at least a 50% reduction in the number of active joints (nine patients). At last follow-up (7–75 months), 11 of the 20 responders were in remission, though four were still on IVIG. Of concern was the fact that three of the patients treated with IVIG developed another autoimmune disease (systemic lupus erythematosus, membranous nephropathy, or vasculitis).

Several other small trials and case reports regarding the use of IVIG in JRA have been published. Weekly low-dose IVIG (40–50 mg/kg) was beneficial in treating articular flares in three patients with longstanding JRA (13). High-dose IVIG (2 g/kg) every 3 weeks was not efficacious in five patients with systemic JRA (14). IVIG was beneficial in sparing corticosteroids in three patients with systemic JRA (15). Finally, IVIG suppressed both systemic and articular features of systemic JRA in two patients (16).

The open trial experience with IVIG in JRA suggests that it may be beneficial in some patients, particularly in controlling severe systemic features and sparing corticosteroids. Unfortunately, JRA has a variable clinical course with spontaneous remission occurring in a significant proportion of patients. Therefore, no definitive conclusions can be made from the open trial experience.

RANDOMIZED PLACEBO-CONTROLLED TRIALS

Because of uncertain benefit and significant expense, randomized multicenter double-blinded placebo-controlled trials of IVIG in both systemic and polyarticular JRA were undertaken to determine efficacy and safety.

In 1994, Silverman et al. published the results of a randomized placebo-controlled trial of IVIG in systemic JRA (17). Thirty-one patients with severe, refractory disease were enrolled. Patients received infusions of 1.5 g/kg of either IVIG or placebo (0.1% albumin) every 2 weeks for 2 months and then monthly for 4 months. Fourteen patients discontinued prematurely from the study—seven from each treatment group. Twelve of these discontinued due to insufficient therapeutic effect. IVIG appeared to have relatively good short-term safety in systemic JRA. Adverse effects experienced in this study included brief episodes of chills, fever, emesis, and headaches in three patients, and severe nonviral hepatitis in one patient, which resolved without complication after discontinuing IVIG.

Twenty-nine patients were included in the intent-to-treat efficacy subset. Their response at completion of the study is summarized in Table 2. The number of patients was inadequate for sufficient statistical power to detect significant differences between the two groups with regard to any of the outcome measures, including the modest difference in the physician global assessment. Of particular interest was the inability of IVIG to spare corticosteroids. Several patients in each group had impressive improvements in systemic features, perhaps reflecting the natural history of systemic JRA rather than effective treatment. Articular involvement showed little change in both groups. In view of the small sample size and lack of dramatic differences between the two groups, the study was considered nondefinitive.

Recently, an open trial followed by a randomized, blinded-withdrawal, placebo-controlled trial of IVIG in polyarticular JRA was completed (18). Twenty-five patients who were candidates for second-line therapy or who had inadequate disease control with second-line therapy were enrolled in the open, noncontrolled phase. Patients received 1.5-2.0 g/kg of IVIG (100 g max) every 2 weeks for 2 months and then monthly for up to 4 more months. Beginning at month 3, those who met criteria for "clinically important improvement" were randomized to receive four monthly infusions of either IVIG or placebo in the double-blind phase. Only mild, transient adverse effects occurred (headache, dizziness, nausea and vomiting, diarrhea, tachycardia, fatigue, and chills), again suggesting that the short-term safety of IVIG in JRA is excellent.

Nineteen of the 25 patients achieved "clinically important improvement" during the open phase, defined as at least a 25% improvement in at least two of three primary

Table 2 Responders to Placebo-Controlled Trial of IVIG in Systemic JRA

Outcome measure	IVIG	Placebo
Improved physician global assessment	7/14 (50%)	4/15 (27%)
Decreased number of days with fever	11/12 (92%)	10/14 (71%)
Disappearance of rash	4/7 (57%)	4/10 (40%)
Resolution of organomegaly	3/3 (100%)	6/7 (86%)
≥30% decreased active joint count	7/14 (50%)	7/15 (47%)
≥25% improved or normalized lab values	14/47 (30%)	22/48 (46%)
≥50% reduced or discontinued steroids	0/3 (0%)	1/5 (20%)

outcome measures (number of active joints, overall severity score, physician global assessment). Ten were randomized to continue with IVIG, and nine were discontinued from IVIG and given placebo. Within 3 months, two of the IVIG treated patients and five of the placebo-treated patients had "clinically important worsening," defined as at least a 25% worsening in at least two of three outcome measures. These results, in which placebo-treated patients had rapid loss of efficacy, suggest that the duration of effect in polyarticular JRA is limited. Important observations made during the open phase were that response to IVIG was unlikely if it did not occur within 4 months (17 patients responded within 4 months), and patients with disease duration less than 3 years were more responsive than those with disease duration >5 years (13/15 vs. 6/10). This study did not address issues of long-term safety or efficacy.

CURRENT RECOMMENDATIONS

There are no definitive recommendations regarding the use of IVIG in JRA. In the treatment of systemic JRA, efficacy of high-dose IVIG has been difficult to demonstrate, though it may have suppressed severe systemic features and spared corticosteroids in individual patients. Predictors of response have yet to be identified. Therefore, a trial of IVIG may be warranted in a patient with unremitting or steroid-dependent systemic JRA, but the likelihood of response is unpredictable.

Two other factors involved in the decision to use IVIG are safety and cost. IVIG appears to be relatively safe compared to alternatives such as corticosteroids and cytotoxic drugs. Long-term safety of IVIG is less certain, as several patients treated with IVIG developed other autoimmune diseases, which may be associated with immune complex formation and may have been triggered by IVIG treatment. Cost can also be a significant limiting factor. At our institution the cost of 50 g IVIG is $3100. Therefore, IVIG should be reserved for patients with severe systemic JRA in whom standard treatments are ineffective and/or disease suppression is corticosteroid-dependent, and for whom IVIG is economically feasible. IVIG should be continued on a long-term basis only in patients with significant response within 4–6 months and should be given only as frequently as needed for disease control. Patients should be closely monitored for the appearance of other autoimmune diseases, particularly vasculitis and nephropathy, and IVIG should be discontinued if such develops.

Recommendations regarding the use of IVIG in polyarticular JRA are even less definitive. The short-term efficacy of IVIG in polyarticular JRA appears to be of limited duration, and patients with longstanding disease are less responsive than those with short disease duration. Unlike severe systemic JRA, disease activity of polyarticular JRA can often be suppressed with relatively safe medications, such as methotrexate. Therefore, the rationale for using IVIG as an alternative treatment for polyarticular JRA is less compelling. Nevertheless, there are individuals with unremitting disease that cannot be controlled by standard treatments who may benefit from IVIG therapy.

THE FUTURE

The role of IVIG in the treatment of JRA is evolving. Studies to date do not support the use of IVIG in all patients with severe systemic or polyarticular JRA. Further studies are needed to support its use in selected individuals. Protocols for high-dose IVIG administration in JRA were derived from those used in other autoimmune diseases. The efficacy of IVIG in JRA may be increased by protocol alterations such as higher dosing, shorter dosing intervals, or adjustment of the protocol relative to the patient's response. Likewise, efficacy may be increased by identifying predictors of positive response. Candidate predictors include disease duration, serum IgG level, and the presence of an underlying immunodeficiency. We recently observed a dramatic response to IVIG in a patient with systemic JRA and IgG subclass 1 deficiency. IVIG may also have a role in the treatment of acute JRA crises such as pneumonitis (19), pericarditis, and coagulopathy/encephalopathy. Studies to investigate these possibilities should include pharmacoeconomic analyses and surveillance for both short-term and long-term safety.

ACKNOWLEDGMENTS

This work was supported in part by the Children's Hospital Research Foundation and the Schmidlapp Foundation.

REFERENCES

1. Brewer EJ, Bass J, Baum J, et al. Current proposed revision of JRA criteria. Arthritis Rheum 1977; 22(suppl):195–202.
2. Lang BA, Shore A. A review of the current concepts on the pathogenesis of juvenile rheumatoid arthritis. J Rheumatol 1990; 17(suppl 21):1–15.
3. Giannini EH, Brewer EJ, Kuzmina N, et al. Methotrexae in resistant juvenile rheumatoid arthritis. Results of the U.S.A.-U.S.S.R. double-blind, placebo-controlled trial. N Engl J Med 1992; 326:1043–1049.
4. Webster ADB, Loewi G, Dourmashkin RD, Golding DN, Ward DJ, Asherson GL. Polyarthritis in adults with hypogammaglobulinemia and its rapid response to immunoglobulin treatment. BMJ 1976; 1:1314–1316.
5. Newburger JW, Takahashi M, Baiser AS, et al. A single intravenous infusion of gamma globulin as compared with four infusions in the treatment of acute Kawasaki syndrome. N Engl J Med 1991; 324:1633–1639.
6. Blanchette VS, Luke B, Andrew M, et al. A prospective, randomized trial of high-dose intravenous immune globulin G therapy, oral prednisone therapy, and no therapy in childhood acute immune thrombocytopenic purpura. J Pediatr 1993; 123:989–995.
7. Gelfand EW. The use of intravenous immune globulin in collagen vascular disorders: a potentially new modality of therapy. J Allergy Clin Immunol 1989; 84:613–616.
8. Groothoff JW, Van Leeuwen EF. High dose intravenous gammaglobulin in chronic systemic juvenile arthritis. BMJ 1988; 296:1362–1363.
9. Silverman ED, Laxer RM, Greenwald M, et al. Intravenous gamma globulin therapy in systemic juvenile rheumatoid arthritis. Arthritis Rheum 1990; 33:1015–1022.
10. Prieur AM, Adleff A, Debre M, Boulate P, Griscelli C. High dose immunoglobulin therapy in severe juvenile chronic arthritis: long-term follow-up in 16 patients. Clin Exp Rheum 1990; 8:603–609.
11. Silverman E, Isacovics B, Schneider R, Dosch HM, Laxer R. Effect of intravenous gamma globulin on immunoglobulin production in systemic onset juvenile arthritis. Arthritis Rheum 1988; 31(suppl):S27. Abstract.
12. Uziel Y, Laxer R, Schneider R, Silverman ED. Intravenous immunoglobulin therapy in systemic juvenile arthritis: A follow up study. J Rheumatol 1996; 23:910–918.

13. Savery F. Intravenous immunoglobulin treatment of rheumatoid arthritis-associated immunodeficiency. Clin Ther 1988; 10:527–529.
14. Hiemstra I, de Graeff-Meeder ER, Zegers BJM, Kuis W. Efficacy of intravenous immunoglobulin in systemic juvenile chronic arthritis. Clin Exp Rheum 1989; 7:457. Abstract.
15. Falcini F, Taccetti G, Trapani S, Tafi L, Volpi M. Growth retardation in juvenile chronic arthritis patients treated with steroids. Clin Exp Rheum 1991; 9(suppl 6):37–40.
16. Horneff G, Wahn V. Immunomodulating therapy of systemic juvenile rheumatoid arthritis: administration of high-dose intravenous gamma globulin. Infusionsther Transfusionsmed 1993; 20(suppl 1):121–126.
17. Silverman ED, Cawkwell GD, Lovell DJ, et al. Intravenous immunoglobulin in the treatment of systemic juvenile rheumatoid arthritis: a randomized placebo controlled trial. J Rheumatol 1994; 21:2353–2358.
18. Giannini EH, Silverman ED, Lovell DJ, et al. Intravenous immunoglobulin in the treatment of polyarticular juvenile rheumatoid arthritis. A phase I/II study. J Rheumatol 1996; 23:910–918.
19. Yoshinaga H, Koike R, Maruyama T. Still's disease relapse with severe pneumonitis after prolonged remission. Intern Med 1993; 32:902–905.

24

Intravenously Administered Gammaglobulin for the Prevention or Modulation of Insulin-Dependent Diabetes Mellitus

John M Dwyer and Stephen Colagiuri
The University of New South Wales, Sydney, Australia

INTRODUCTION

Insulin-dependent diabetes (IDDM), sometimes referred to as type 1, or juvenile-onset diabetes, is an autoimmune disease (1). It frequently occurs in individuals or families where diabetes and other autoimmune endocrinopathies are common. Associated autoimmune diseases include pernicious anemia, myasthenia gravis, and juvenile rheumatoid arthritis (2). Paraphenomena such a vitiligo and premature graying of the hair are well-recognized associates.

IDDM can occur at any age and despite meticulous management 7% of those affected will die within the first decade of the diagnosis being confirmed (3). After 15 years many patients with this form of diabetes have developed severe complications such as blindness, renal failure, cardiovascular disease, and peripheral and autonomic neuropathies. Limb amputations are frequently required. Fifty percent die within 30–40 years of the clinical onset of their diabetes. It is clear that better management strategies are needed (4).

GENETICS OF IDDM

The finding of islet cell antibodies (ICA) in the serum of 70–90% of patients with recently diagnosed IDDM provides evidence of an ongoing autoimmune process. First-degree relatives of IDDM patients have an increased incidence of islet cell antibodies, and the presence of these molecules may help predict future or subclinical beta cell dysfunction and therefore impending IDDM (5). Those patients with the highest titers of islet cell antibodies are most likely to develop IDDM. Insulin autoantibodies among unaffected relatives of a patient with IDDM are frequently associated with the presence of islet cell antibodies. Relatives with both islet cell and insulin autoantibodies frequently have impaired insulin responses and are more likely to progress to IDDM than are those with only one type of autoantibody (6).

A genetic basis for IDDM has been established in humans with a demonstration that 95% of patients (compared to 45% of the normal Caucasian population) express on antigen-presenting cells the class II MHC gene products DR3 and/or DR4. The expression of DR2 is decreased on the cells of patients with IDDM, and it is more likely that monozygotic twins who express DR3 and DR4 will both develop diabetes if one does (7). It now appears that two genes are involved in the development of IDDM— one linked to the DR3, and one to the DR4 alleles. In individuals developing IDDM who are both DR3- and DR4-positive, C-peptide levels fall more rapidly, and there is an accelerated destruction of beta cells in the pancreas (8).

The destruction of beta cells by autoimmune mechanisms may occur very rapidly; infants can present with clinical diabetes. On the other hand, it is not uncommon for the destruction of sufficient beta cell mass to produce clinical diabetes to take 10 years or more (9).

ENVIRONMENTAL FACTORS AND IDDM

It is likely that environmental factors trigger the accelerated phase of beta cell destruction by immunological processes that lead to clinically overt diabetes. Viral infections are suspected to be but are not clearly established as major triggering factors. Coxsackie virus type B4, for example, can be diabetogenic, and it is of interest that 20% of patients with congenital rubella develop IDDM (10).

IMMUNOPATHOGENESIS OF IDDM

Anti-islet cell antibody secretion proceeds the development of clinical disease. However, the pathology features a strong infiltration of mononuclear cells into the beta cell area of the pancreas, with the majority of the infiltrating cells being activated (DR+) T cells (11). Studies in animal models of diabetes (see below) indicate that it is not possible to transfer diabetes with islet cell or insulin antibodies but that it is possible to transfer the disease with T cells from an IDDM animal. It thus seems highly likely that cell-mediated rather than humoral immune mechanisms are responsible for the destruction of the beta cells that results in IDDM (12).

Induction of the expression of major histocompatibility (MHC) gene products required for immune activation on the surface of islet cells is a prominent early feature of the pathological process involving the beta cell in IDDM. In vitro observations would suggest that increased activity of both alpha and gamma interferon in the islets of the pancreas may be responsible for the upregulating of these molecules, which increases the likelihood of beta cells becoming targets for an immunological response (13). Other cytokines such as interleukin-1 (IL-1) and tumor necrosis factor (TNF) are also implicated in the pathophysiology of IDDM (14). Indeed IL-1 was the first cytokine reported to impair islet cell function, though the IL-1 effect is mediated without altering the expression of MHC molecules on the surface of the islet cells. TNF and interferon gamma, when combined, have been shown in vitro to have a similar effect on islet cell function and integrity while either agent alone upregulates expression of class I MHC molecules; in combination, they induce the expression of class II MHC products on the surface of islet cells. TNF has been shown to markedly potentiate the cytotoxic effects of IL-1 on beta cells (15).

It does seem plausible that in genetically predisposed individuals an environmental insult such as a viral infection in the area of the islets of Langerhan results in an abnormal and potentially fatal upregulation of the MHC class I and class II molecules required for antigen presentation to inducer and cytotoxic T lymphocytes. Direct cytotoxic effects mediated by CD8-bearing T lymphocytes and indirect toxic effects from numerous cytokines released by macrophages and lymphocytes probably lead to the slow but ultimate destruction of all beta cell function. Antigen presentation to B lymphocytes leads to the production of antibodies that are predictors rather than predators in this scenario.

ANIMAL MODELS FOR IDDM IN HUMANS

The bio-breeding BB/w rat provides an excellent laboratory model for IDDM. These rats become spontaneously diabetic and develop metabolic and immunological defects that are similar to those noted in humans with this disease. Diabetes developing in the BB/w rat was first described in 1977 (16). The diabetic syndrome has been extensively characterized, and 60–80% of the BB/w rats will develop IDDM between 60 and 120 days of life (17).

BB/w rats have mild insulinitis without significant elevations of their circulating blood glucose level before severe destruction of the beta cells of their pancreas leads to clinically obvious diabetes. Male and female rats are affected equally. Inbreeding, now beyond the 17th generation, provides sublines genetically identical in every way except that they do not develop diabetes (18). The development of this latter strain has been important in attempts to understand the immunopathogenesis involved.

In contradistinction to the situation with human diabetes, there does not appear to be a role for environmental factors in the initiation of diabetes in BB/w rats. The abnormalities develop equally well in a germ-free environment. Prior to the development of hyperglycemia and ketoacidosis, the beta cells of the pancreas are infiltrated by T lymphocytes. The severity of the metabolic disorder is directly proportional to the intensity of this lymphocytic attack. While it is unusual to detect any abnormalities in the thymus gland, the T cell areas of the spleen and lymph nodes of the BB/w rat are hypocellular. There is an increased occurrence of B cell lymphomas in these animals.

In a manner analogous to human diabetes, at least two genes are involved in the development of diabetes in the BB/w rat (19). Unlike in human diabetes, this gene is responsible for predisposing animals not only to the development of IDDM but also to a profound T cell lymphopenia. The activity of a second gene linked to the histocompatibility region of the rat is also necessary for the development of diabetes.

PREVENTING DIABETES IN BB/w RATS BY IMMUNOMANIPULATION

The development of IDDM in BB/w rats can be prevented by most immunosuppressive techniques. Thus treatment with cyclosporin A, neonatal thymectomy, nodal irradiation, antilymphocyte serum, and total body irradiation will all prevent IDDM developing in this susceptible animal (20,21).

Of particular relevance has been the demonstration that immunomodulation rather than immunosuppression can affect the natural history of diabetes in the BB/w rat. The diabetic syndrome will develop in normal nondiabetes-prone BB/w rats and nude mice following the transfer of spleen or blood lymphocytes from BB/w rats. Such studies strongly suggest that T cells can initiate an insulinitis without requiring the presence of any abnormal foreign antigenic determinants on the beta cells of the pancreas. In contradistinction, diabetes can be prevented from developing in the BB/w rat by bone marrow transplantation, blood transfusions, and blood or splenic cell transfusion from rats not prone to develop diabetes. The administration of dialyzable leukocyte extracts obtained from BB rats not prone to diabetogenesis can also prevent disease (22). These findings all suggest that stimulation of immunoregulatory T cells in BB/w rats before diabetes becomes clinically obvious can prevent beta cell destruction.

IMMUNOMANIPULATION TO PREVENT IDDM IN HUMANS

At the time of the onset of clinically significant IDDM in humans, approximately 20% of the beta cell mass remains (23). Treatment with insulin is known to suppress for varying periods the continuation of the autoimmune process producing what is known as a "honeymoon effect." During this stage, C-peptide levels increase and insulin requirements decrease. C-peptide is a fraction of one of the insulin chains and provides a valuable method for monitoring beta cell function in humans.

As it seems likely that maneurves that would successfully maintain the integrity of the remaining beta cell mass present when clinically obvious IDDM develops might facilitate the maintenance of glucose homeostasis and minimize the common complications of IDDM, there has been much interest in recent years in preserving these potentially important beta cells. Immunosuppressive techniques including the use of azathioprine and cyclosporin A have been shown to be successful in preserving beta cell function, but only at the expense of the significant side effects associated with immunosuppression (24,25).

Given the evidence that it is possible to prevent beta cell destruction in animal models by immunomanipulative techniques that do not feature immunosuppression, it seems reasonable to attempt to preserve the remaining beta cell mass in humans with recently diagnosed IDDM by immunomanipulative techniques. We have attempted to do this using dialyzable leukocyte extracts (transfer factors) since these low-molecular-weight molecules have been successful in minimizing the onset of diabetes in the BB/w rat model and intravenously administered immunoglobulin G (IVIG). IVIG has successfully suppressed autoimmune aggression in numerous autoimmune diseases, and the mechanisms involved are multifactorial (26). They include the neutralization of autoantibodies by anti-idiotypic antibodies present in pooled preparations of human IVIG, the activation of suppressor T cell mechanisms, and the downregulation of the production of numerous cytokines. All of these mechanisms could be relevant to modulating the autoaggression destroying the beta cells of the pancreas in patients with IDDM.

Table 1 Clinical Details of Subjects Studied

	Placebo	Gammaglobulin	Transfer factor
Number	17[a]	17	18
Gender (F:M)	4:13	10:7	6:12
Age (yr)	17.6 ± 7.1	16.6 ± 7.8	15.4 ± 7.9
Duration diabetes (days)	176 ± 107	155 ± 148	171 ± 196
Body mass index	20.9 ± 5.4	19.9 ± 4.5	19.5 ± 3.3
Insulin dose (U/kg/day)	0.42 ± 0.29	0.40 ± 0.22	0.36 ± 0.18
HbA_{1c} (%)	7.7 ± 1.8	8.1 ± 2.8	7.5 ± 2.1

[a]Numbers refer to mean ± SD.

USE OF IVIG IN CHILDREN AND ADULTS WITH IDDM

There have been a number of reports of the use of IVIG in IDDM involving small numbers of patients with variable results (27,28). We conducted a trial of IVIG therapy in children and adults with IDDM over a period of 2 years utilizing a randomized and controlled protocol which also examined the effect of dialyzable leukocyte extracts on the natural course of IDDM (29) (Tables 1–4).

Patients

A total of 52 patients with IDDM were randomized into three arms of the study. Seventeen patients were treated with IVIG, and another 17 were treated with dialyzable leukocyte extracts (DLE); 18 patients were treated with placebo and served as a control group. All patients were aged between 3 and 30 years at the time of recruitment. Two subgroups of patients were studied. Group 1 involved patients who began treatment within 3 months of diagnosis of their diabetes, while group 2 involved subjects who had clinically overt diabetes for between 3 months and 2 years but were using an insulin dose of ≤0.5 units/kg/day. To be eligible, this group of patients were required to be able to secrete C-peptide in response to glucagon and a meal ≥10th centile of normal controls. The clinical details of the subjects are shown in Table 1. The three groups were similar in age, duration of diabetes, body mass index, daily insulin dose, and initial glycosylated hemoglobin.

Table 2 Insulin Dose and Glycated Hemoglobin During First 12 Months of Study

Months	Insulin dose (U/kg/day)			Glycated hemoglobin (%)		
	Placebo	IVIG[a]	TF[b]	Placebo	IVIG[a]	TF[b]
0	0.42 ± 0.29	0.40 ± 0.22	0.36 ± 0.18	7.7 ± 1.8	8.1 ± 2.8	7.5 ± 2.1
2	0.43 ± 0.23	0.41 ± 0.25	0.40 ± 0.16	7.7 ± 1.3	7.5 ± 2.1	7.1 ± 2.8
6	0.50 ± 0.22	0.48 ± 0.22	0,43 ± 0.24	7.5 ± 1.7	8.1 ± 2.2	8.2 ± 2.7
12	0.60 ± 0.20	0.55 ± 0.22	0.58 ± 0.23	8.7 ± 1.8	8.8 ± 2.3	8.1 ± 2.9

Numbers refer to mean ± SD.
[a]Gammaglobulin therapy group.
[b]Transfer factor therapy group.

Table 3 Fasting and Stimulated C-Peptide Responses During First 12 Months of Study

Months	Fasting C-peptide (pmol/ml)			Stimulated C-peptide (pmol/min/ml)[a]		
	Placebo	IVIG[b]	TF[c]	Placebo	IVIG[b]	TF[c]
0	0.32 ± 0.03	0.22 ± 0.03	0.29 ± 0.03	35.4 ± 7.7	48.7 ± 9.4	39.2 ± 9.2
2	0.24 ± 0.04	0.23 ± 0.03	0.26 ± 0.03	35.7 ± 6.3	31.3 ± 8.3	34.2 ± 8.1
6	0.24 ± 0.04	0.18 ± 0.02	0.23 ± 0.04	21.7 ± 5.5	33.6 ± 11.2	26.0 ± 6.9
12	0.12 ± 0.02	0.14 ± 0.04	0.18 ± 0.04	14.8 ± 3.8	24.8 ± 8.9	24.4 ± 5.7

Numbers refer to mean ± SEM.
[a]Area above baseline following glucagon and meal stimuli.
[b]Gammaglobulin therapy group.
[c]Transfer factor therapy group.

Protocol

Treatment was administered every 2 months for the duration of the study. IVIG was given in a dose of 2 g/kg body weight in divided doses on 2 consecutive days. The IVIG was infused over 6–10 h each day. The other two groups received an intramuscular injection of either saline (control group) or DLE at a dose of 1 IU, which is the amount extracted from 5×10^8 peripheral blood leukocytes. The investigators and patients were blinded to treatment in the two groups receiving the intramuscular injection. No blinded control was used for the IVIG, as this was not considered ethical or practical. Assessments were performed at entry and then at 2, 6, 12, 18, and 24 months. Insulin dose and glycosylated hemoglobin were also recorded.

Clinical Assessment

Complete remissions from diabetes were sought. A complete remission was defined as a situation wherein a patient did not require any insulin or oral hypoglycemic agents

Table 4 Side Effects Associated with Gammaglobulin Therapy

Side effect	Mild	Moderate	Severe	Total
Headache	42	30	6	78
Nausea	25	15	0	40
Lethargy	29	10	0	39
Pyrexia	16	15	0	31
Vomiting	14	10	1	25
Edema	20	0	0	20
Generalized ache	18	0	0	18
Dyspnea	13	0	0	13
Anorexia	5	1	0	6
Rash	2	0	0	2
Periorbital swelling	0	1	0	1

Numbers represent percentages.

and had verified blood glucose readings below 10 mmol/L while consuming a diet appropriate for age.

Beta Cell Function

Beta cell function was assessed by a combined sequential glucagon meal test. After an overnight fast and without insulin administration prior to the test, subjects were given 10 μg/kg glucagon intravenously. The C-peptide response was measured for 120 min, after which a standard meal was administered and the C-peptide response followed for a further 180 min.

Laboratory Analysis

C-peptide was measured by radioimmunoassay with antiserum M1221 (Novo, Bagsvaerd, Denmark). The detection limit of the assay was 0.06 pmol/ml. Glycosylated hemoglobin was measured by HPLC using a standard assay (normal range, 3.9–7.4%).

Results

Only four patients on the IVIG treatment group completed 2 years of the study, compared to eight in the placebo group and 10 in the DLE group. Because of the low continued participation rates, only status for the first 12 months of the study is analyzable.

No patient in the IVIG or control groups experienced a complete remission from diabetes. Two patients in the DLE group were in remission at the time of entry to the study. The remissions did not last for more than 3 months in either of the subjects. There were no differences in diabetes control or insulin dose requirements during the study. Insulin dose increased steadily in all three groups over the first 12 months of the study. Similarly, glycosylated hemoglobin showed a slight increase over the 12-month period in all three groups. Fasting C-peptide decreased significantly over the 12 months, with the decline being similar in the three groups. The stimulated C-peptide response also declined over the study period to a similar extent in all the treatment groups.

Side Effects

Side effects were common in the gammaglobulin-treated group. The most common side effects were headaches 78%, nausea 40%, lethargy 39%, pyrexia 31%, vomiting 25%, and edema 20%. One subject developed severe side effects which required overnight hospitalization. The common occurrence of side effects was one of the major reasons for the declining participation rate over the course of this study in the IVIG-treated group. As is usual with IVIG therapy, some of the side effects were related to the rate of infusion, but there is no doubt that some children had moderately severe side effects for other reasons. There seems to be no way to avoid the emotionally charged atmosphere associated with conducting this type of research when parents and at least some older children are desperately anxious to have the protocol succeed. Understandably, parental tolerance of even mild side effects associated with IVIG is proportional to signs of success with the approach being taken.

DISCUSSION

This study failed to show a clear beneficial effect of IVIG therapy on the natural course of IDDM. IVIG therapy did not result in any clinical remissions. The declines in beta cell function in terms of both fasting and stimulated C-peptide levels were similar in the control and IVIG-treated group.

A limitation to this study was the mixed groups of patients studied, which included both newly diagnosed patients as well as those with established IDDM. Most studies of immunotherapy have shown that a beneficial response is more likely to be observed in patients who commence treatment soon after diagnosis. In our study the beta cell function was significantly greater in newly diagnosed patients, providing a better chance of treatment. However, perhaps due to small numbers, no benefits of IVIG therapy were demonstrable in the subgroup of subjects treated within 3 months of diagnosis.

OTHER STUDIES

There have been relatively few studies of the use of IVIG in IDDM. Treatment protocols and assessments have varied, and some studies have lacked a matched control group and have produced variable results. Preservation of some C-peptide secretion in some IVIG-treated children compared with a group of conventionally treated children was reported in 1986 (27). However, two additional studies failed to show any significant benefits after 12 months in a total of 14 children compared with a matched group that did not receive IVIG treatment (28,30). A transient beneficial effect in eight IDDM subjects recently treated with IVIG compared to the matched untreated group in terms of insulin dose and fasting C-peptide levels was reported, but this effect was lost after 2 years (31).

In summary, these additional studies have failed to show a clinically worthwhile and lasting effect of IVIG in people with established IDDM.

CONCLUSIONS

With currently safe techniques for manipulating autoaggressive immune responses to beta cell determinants, preliminary studies do not support the conduct of a major trial using IVIG in children in whom IDDM has just become clinically apparent. This opinion could change, however, if the antigenic determinants that provide targets for the autoaggression and the cytokines involved could be better identified. The goal of maintaining some beta cell function in newly diagnosed cases of IDDM is an important one.

Perhaps of greater interest is the potential to prevent the onset of serious autoimmune damage to the beta cells of the pancreas with IVIG and other techniques once methods to accurately diagnose the prediabetic state become reliable (32). Certainly in the animal models referred to above, it has been far simpler to manipulate the immune response and call off autoaggression earlier rather than later in the natural history of the immunopathogenesis.

REFERENCES

1. Eisenbarth GS. Type 1 diabetes mellitus. A chronic autoimmune disease. N Engl J Med 1986; 314(21):1360–1368.
2. Rudolf MCJ, Genel M, Tamborlane WV, et al. Juvenile rheumatoid arthritis in children with diabetes mellitus. J Pediatr 1981; 99:519–524.
3. Skyler JS. Immune intervention studies in insulin-dependent diabetes mellitus. Diabetes/Metab Rev 1987; 3(4):1017–1035.
4. Pozzilli P. Immunotherapy in type 1 diabetes. Diab Med 1988; 5(8):734–738.
5. Atkinson MA, Maclaren NK, Riley WJ, et al. Are insulin antibodies markers for insulin dependent diabetes mellitus? Diabetes 1986; 35:894.
6. Riley WJ, Maclaren NK, Spillar RP, et al. The use of islet cell antibodies in identifying 'pre-diabetes.' In: Larkins R et al., eds. Diabetes. Proceedings of 13th International Diabetes Federation, 1988:266.
7. Rossini AA, Mordes JP, Like AA. Immunology of insulin dependent diabetes mellitus. Annu Rev Immunol 1985; 3:289.
8. Srinkant S, Ganda OP, Radizadeh A, et al. First-degree relatives of patients with type 1 diabetes: islet cell antibodies and abnormal insulin secretion. N Engl J Med 1985; 313:461.
9. Gorsuch AN, Spencer KM, Lister J, et al. Evidence for a long pre-diabetic period in type 1 (insulin dependent) diabetes mellitus. Lancet 1981; ii:1363.
10. Foulis AK, Farguharson MA, Meagher A. Immunoreactive alpha-interferon in insulin secreting B cells in type 1 diabetes mellitus. Lancet 1987; ii:1423.
11. Campbell IL, Wong GHW, Schrader JW, et al. Interferon-delta enhances the expression of the major histocompatibility class I antigens on mouse pancreatic beta cells. Diabetes 1985; 34:1205.
12. Campbell IL, Harrison LC. Interaction of cytokines with the pancreatic beta cell. In: Larkings et al., eds. Diabetes. Proceedings of 13th International Diabetes Federation, 1987:101.
13. Harrison LC, Campbell IL, Allison J, et al. MHC molecules and B cell destruction. Diabetes 1989; 38:815.
14. Mandrup-Poulsen T, Bendtzen K, Nerup J, et al. Affinity-purified human interleukin 1 is cytotoxic to isolated islets of Langerhans. Diabetologia 1986; 29:63.
15. Mendrup-Poulsen T, Bendtzen K, Dinarello CA, Nerup J. Human tumour necrosis factor potentiates human interleukin 1 mediated rat pancreated B cell cytotoxity. J Immunol 1987; 139:4077.
16. Nakhooda AF, Like AA, Chappell CI, et al. The spontaneously diabetic Wister rat. Metabolic and morphologic studies. Diabetes 1977; 26(2):100–112.
17. Poussier P, Nakhooda AF, Grose M, et al. Arginine-induced glucagon secretion in the spontaneously diabetic BB Wistar rat. Metab Clin Exp 1983; 32(5):487–491.
18. Poussier P, Nakhooda AF, Sima AA, et al. Passive transfer of insulitis and lymphopenia in the BB rat. Metal Clin Exp 1983; 32(suppl 1):73–79.
19. Colle E, Guttman RD, Seemayer TA, et al. Spontaneous diabetes mellitus syndrome in the rat. IV. Immunogenetic interactions of MHC and non-MHC components of the syndrome. Metab Clin 1983; 32(suppl 1):54–61.
20. Yale JF, Marliss EB. Altered immunity and diabetes in the BB rat. Clin Exp Immunol 1984; 57:1–11.
21. Stiller Cr, Laupacis A, Keown PA, et al. Cyclosporine: action, pharmacokinetics and effect in the BB rat model. Metab Clin Exp 1983; 32(suppl 1):69–72.
22. Dwyer JM, Colagiuri S, Leong G, et al. A controlled trial of dialyzable leukocyte extracts (DLE) in the management of newly diagnosed insulin dependent diabetes mellitus. In: Fujisawa T, Sasakawa S, Iikura Y, Komatsu F and Yamaguchi Y, eds. Recent Advances in Transfer

Factor and Dialyzable Leukocyte Extracts. Proceedings of the 7th International Congress on Transfer Factor, 1991. Maruxen Co. Ltd., Tokyo, Japan.

23. DCCT Research Group. Effects of age, duration and treatment of insulin-dependent diabetes mellitus on residual beta cell function: observations during eligibility testing for the diabetes control and complications trial (DCCT). J Clin Endocrinol Metab 1987; 65:30-36.

24. Harrison LC, Colman PG, Dean B, Baxter R, Martin FIR. Increase in remission rate in newly diagnosed type 1 diabetic subjects treated with azathioprine. Diabetes 1985; 34:1306-1308.

25. Canadian-European Randomised Control Trial Group. Cyclosporin-induced remission of IDDM after early intervention. Diabetes 1988; 37:1574-1581.

26. Dwyer JM. Manipulating the immune system with immune globulin. N Engl J Med 1992; 326(2):107-116.

27. Heinze E, Zuppinger K, Thon A, et al. Gammaglobulin therapy in type 1 diabetes mellitus. In: Laron Z, Karp M, eds. Pediatr Adolesc Endocr Future Trends Juvenile Diabetes. Basel: Karger 1986; 15:362-370.

28. Pocecco M, De Campo C, Cantoni L, et al. Effect of high doses intravenous IgG in newly diagnosed insulin dependent diabetes. Helv Paediatr Acta 1987. 42:289-295.

29. Leong G, Thayer Z, Antony G, et al. High dose intravenous immunoglobulin therapy for insulin-dependent diabetes mellitus. In: Immunotherapy with intravenous immunoglobulins, P Imbach (ed). Proceedings of the Intravenous Immunoglobulin Symposium Interlaken. Harcourt Brace Jovanovich, 1991.

30. Lorini R, Lombardi A, Cortona L, et al. Gammaglobulin therapy in newly diagnosed children with type 1 diabetes mellitus. International Study Group of Diabetes (ISGD) Bulletin 1987; 17:48. Abstract.

31. Galluzo A. The influence of high dose immunoglobulins on newly diagnosed type 1 diabetes patients. International Symposium on Immunoglobulins in Endocrine Autoimmunity, Bingen, Germany, 1995.

32. Vardi P, Dib S, Tuttleman J, et al. Competitive insulin autoantibody assay. Prospective evaluation of subjects at high risk for development of type 1 diabetes mellitus. Diabetes 1987; 36:1286.

25

Advances in the Treatment of Alloimmune-Mediated Platelet Disorders with Intravenous Immunoglobulin

Thomas S. Kickler

Johns Hopkins University School of Medicine, Baltimore, Maryland

INTRODUCTION

Platelet destruction by alloantibodies is an important and frequently encountered clinical problem in both adult and pediatric hematology. Alloantibody formation to platelet antigens leads to three principal conditions of immune-mediated platelet destruction: platelet transfusion refractoriness in platelet transfusion recipients; posttransfusion purpura; and neonatal alloimmune thrombocytopenia (1).

Our understanding of the alloimmune-mediated platelet disorders has undergone rapid changes in the last decade. These advances have had broad implications in our understanding of basic immunohematological mechanisms and in leading to new insights concerning platelet biology. Contributing to these advances has been the immunogenetic, biochemical, and molecular characterization of platelet alloantigens that are carried on functionally important platelet membrane proteins. Besides these advancements, the introduction of intravenous gammaglobulin has led to significant improvement in the management of these conditions (2,3).

The purpose of this review is to discuss the conditions mediated by platelet alloantibodies and to provide a perspective on the use of intravenous immunoglobulin in these different clinical situations. A description of the clinical disorders, pertinent platelet immunology, and therapeutic options will be given. With these considerations in mind, one will discern the potentially important adjunctive role of intravenous immunoglobulin in alloimmune-mediated platelet disorders. Included in this review are only those clinical trials where there is described a study design involving more than 10 patients. No attempt is made to discuss the many case reports supporting the use of high-dose intravenous gammaglobulin in alloimmune-mediated thrombocytopenia.

PLATELET ALLOANTIGEN SYSTEMS

The well-characterized platelet antigens include those shared with other cells and those restricted to platelets (the human platelet antigens or the platelet-specific antigens). The

ABH antigens are found on platelets but appear largely to be passively absorbed from plasma. Antibodies to ABH antigens are not important causes of platelet destruction. The class I HLA-A and HLA-B antigens are found on platelets. Antibodies to these antigens account for the major cause of alloimmune-mediated platelet transfusion refractoriness in thrombocytopenic patients receiving platelet transfusion. Approximately 20% of leukemic patients who receive platelet transfusions during induction chemotherapy become alloimmunized to class I HLA antigens (4,5).

The human platelet antigens or platelet-specific antigens are the principal antigenic determinants causing neonatal alloimmune thrombocytopenia and posttransfusion purpura. Alloimmunization to these antigens occurs in 10% of platelet transfusion recipients. The first recognized and the most important platelet specific antigen system is the PI^A system. Alloimmunization to PI^{A1} accounts for the majority of cases of neonatal alloimmune thrombocytopenia and posttransfusion purpura (6).

PLATELET TRANSFUSION REFRACTORINESS

Alloimmunization to HLA antigens is the principal cause of immune-mediated platelet transfusion refractoriness. Alloimmunization may develop in 25–50% of leukemic patients or patients with solid tumors receiving intensive chemotherapy and multiple transfusions. As many as 80% of patients with aplastic anemia may become alloimmunized. Leukemic patients who are undergoing induction chemotherapy and who become alloimmunized usually do so by the third week of transfusion support.

Specific identification of alloimmunization can be done by measurement of HLA antibodies using lymphocytotoxicity testing. Serial lymphocytotoxic antibody measurements are helpful in the management of alloimmunized patients. Some patients may have decreases or a loss of lymphocytotoxic antibody, either permanently or transiently, and can be successfully transfused with platelet concentrates (4).

Platelet Transfusion Therapy for Alloimmunized Patients

Once it is determined that a patient is alloimmunized, the following guidelines are used in selecting platelets for the alloimmunized patient:

1. If HLA-identical platelets are unavailable, platelets from donors whose HLA types are serologically cross-reactive with the recipient may be substituted.
2. Matching for antigens of the HLA-C locus is not necessary.
3. Mismatching for some HLA-B locus antigens that are weakly expressed on platelets is acceptable for some donor-recipient pairs.
4. If cross-reactive platelets are ineffective for some patients, attention to linked HLA specificities may be important (i.e., BW4/BW6).
5. Although expressed on platelets, ABO matching is less critical than HLA matching.
6. Platelet cross-matching.

Clinically, one can assess the response of a platelet transfusion by measuring the increment in the platelet count over time. The posttransfusion platelet response should be calculated on the basis of the patient's body surface area and corrected for the number of platelets transfused. The corrected platelet count increment is calculated using the following formula:

$$\text{Correct count increment} = \frac{(\text{Pretransfusion count} - \text{Posttransfusion count}) \times \text{body surface area/mm}^2}{\text{Number of platelets} \times 10^{11}}$$

In general, a successful corrected count increment should be greater than 7500 within 1–60 min of a transfusion and greater than 4500 if measured 18–24 h after transfusion. Refractoriness to platelet transfusions may be on either an immune or nonimmune basis. The nonimmune causes of platelet transfusion failures include sepsis, fever, splenomegaly, disseminated intravascular coagulation, graft rejection, and loss of platelet viability during processing and storage of the platelet transfusion.

When compatible platelets are unavailable for the alloimmunized patient, a variety of approaches have been tried. Splenectomy has been tried and found to be ineffective. It should be considered a potentially dangerous undertaking in someone who is alloimmunized. Corticosteroids have no role in preventing alloantibody-mediated platelet destruction. Plasmapheresis requires numerous exchanges of the patient's total blood volume to reduce antibodies so that transfusion outcome is improved. This maneuver should not be considered a simple or completely effective undertaking.

Intravenous Immunoglobulin in Managing Platelet Transfusion Refractoriness

There have been at least four clinical trials evaluating the usefulness of intravenous immunoglobulin (IVIG) in the amelioration of platelet transfusion refractoriness caused by antibodies to class I HLA antigens. The differing results of these studies may relate to clinical condition of the patient, qualitative and quantitative differences in the alloantibodies, and differences in the degree of HLA-matched platelets being transfused, as discussed above. It should also be pointed out that none of the study groups had large numbers of patients and only one was placebo-controlled. These types of studies are difficult to conduct since the patients are frequently quite ill and can be refractory to transfusions on the basis of nonimmune factors. These considerations should be kept in mind when interpreting the results of the following clinical trials and in reconciling the different outcomes reported.

In one of the earliest series reported by Schiffer and co-workers, they studied the administration of immune globulin to 11 alloimmunized leukemic patients under different conditions that included not only intravenous administration but also incubation with the platelets prior to transfusion (7). Either random donor or partially HLA-matched platelet transfusion were administered during or the day after intravenous immunoglobulin infusion. No patient had an improvement in the 1-h posttransfusion platelet count increments. In a subsequent study from this group of investigators, Lee and co-workers studied the use of intravenous immunoglobulin in seven alloimmunized patients, who most likely had antibodies to HLA antigen of apparent public specificity. When HLA-matched platelets were transfused prior to treatment, these patients had excellent transfusion outcomes, showing that the patients were clinically alloimmune-refractory. Following the 5-day administration of IVIG at a dose of 0.4 mg/kg/day, Lee et al. reported that in two of seven patients lymphocytotoxic antibodies decreased. Borderline acceptable platelet increments were seen at 1 h posttransfusion. They took efforts to exclude the possibility of nonimmune-mediated platelet destruction following these test transfusions. The authors of this study did not believe that they were able to conclude that IVIG benefited their patients (8).

Despite the unpromising results of these studies, subsequent studies were able to show in some patients benefit that at least reached statistical significance. In a well-studied group of patients, Ziegler and co-workers presented more positive findings. In 1987 they first presented findings that suggested that high-dose intravenous gammaglobulin improves the response to pheresis platelets (9). A more recent study by this investigator extended Ziegler's earlier findings. In an attempt to improve platelet transfusion responses, IVIG was administered to 19 patients who were refractory to random and best available HLA-matched platelets. A response to intravenous immunoglobulin was defined as two or more successive transfusions of HLA-matched products that provided recoveries greater than 30%. Thirteen of 19 (68%) patients responded to therapy at a median time of 7 days after initiation of intravenous immunoglobulin (range 2–17 days). Baseline platelet-associated IgG levels were elevated in both the responders and the nonresponders. Post-therapy, platelet-associated IgG levels remained unchanged in the nonresponders but were decreased significantly ($P < .05$) in the responders. The latter levels were similar to those measured in a series of 36 transfusion-responsive patients. This decline in platelet-associated immunoglobulin was not explained by differences in lymphocytotoxic antibodies after therapy (10).

Moreover, a high degree of alloimmunization was associated with a poorer response to IVIG. Only two of eight patients with lymphocytotoxic antibody of $>85\%$ were responders. By contrast, improved transfusion outcomes were seen uniformly in patients with lymphocytotoxic antibody levels $\geq 85\%$. Improved recoveries were obtained using compatible but not incompatible platelets. The median increment (% predicted) with compatible platelets before therapy was 6.0%. Post-IgG, median recoveries were 37.0 %, $P < .001$. These findings suggest that the response to intravenous gammaglobulin may depend on the type of HLA antibody present.

Kickler and co-workers performed a randomized, placebo-controlled clinical trial investigating the use of IVIG in alloimmunized thrombocytopenic patients (11). In this trial intravenous immunoglobulin was administered at a dose of 400 mg/kg for 5 days. An incompatible platelet transfusion from the same donor was used before and after the patient received study drug or placebo. Seven patients received IVIG, and five received placebo Although platelet recovery in 1–6 was satisfactory in five patients after IVIG treatment, 24-h survival was not improved in most of these patients. It could not be excluded that this poor 24-h survival was unrelated to nonimmune causes of shortened platelet survival. None of the placebo group achieved satisfactory 1-h platelet corrected count increments. By t-test, the posttreatment mean values 1 h after transfusion were significantly greater than in the control group. Using a regression model to adjust for any distributional assumptions of the study population, the parameter estimate for immunoglobulin treatment was positive. This indicated that intravenous immunoglobulin may improve 1-h platelet recovery. These studies also suggest that the kinetics of platelet survival may be affected by IVIG. It is likely that if additional platelets were administered, severe thrombocytopenia may be corrected in these patients. Furthermore, the authors suggest that this approach may permit the performance of invasive procedures.

In summary, it appears that when pheresis platelets are administered, IVIG can affect the kinetics of platelet survival. Further studies are needed to determine the safety of this approach in larger numbers of patients.

NEONATAL ALLOIMMUNE THROMBOCYTOPENIA

Neonatal alloimmune thrombocytopenia, caused by fetal maternal incompatibility of platelet alloantigens, is a well-recognized cause of neonatal thrombocytopenia. In neonatal alloimmune thrombocytopenia immunization of the mother by human platelet antigens on the fetus's platelets occurs (1,12). The transplacental transfer of antibody leads to thrombocytopenia in the fetus and newborn. The antigen most commonly implicated is PI[A1], with other antigens such as Bak[a] and Br[a] also being frequently implicated.

In a carefully performed Canadian study, Blanchette and co-workers documented eight cases of neonatal alloimmune thrombocytopenia out of 8197 admissions to a single neonatal intensive care unit (13,14). In contrast to Rh hemolytic disease of the newborn, neonatal alloimmune thrombocytopenia may affect firstborn infants. Between 20% and 59% of cases of neonatal alloimmune thrombocytopenia occur in the firstborn. Since a child of a primigravida woman may be affected and prenatal screening for platelet alloantibodies is not routinely done, appropriate prenatal management is often not performed, resulting in serious bleeding complications in approximately 20% of these infants. Central nervous system hemorrhage is a well-recognized complication of neonatal alloimmune thrombocytopenia that may occur in utero, during delivery, or postnatally. Approximately 20% of cases of neonatal alloimmune thrombocytopenia will be complicated by intracranial hemorrhage, with 50% occurring in utero. Intracranial bleeding may occur as early as the first trimester (1,15,16).

Children subsequently born to the same couple with a previously affected child are also likely to be affected, although this generalization depends on the zygosity of the father for the immunizing platelet alloantigen. In these second-born infants, obstetricians are aware of the possibility of thrombocytopenia and can take the preventive measures described below.

Patient Management

Postnatal Platelet Transfusions

Since blood centers do not generally maintain pools of donors typed for platelet-specific antigens, the mother is generally used as the platelet donor. Transfusion of 1 unit of platelets may be sufficient to increase the platelet count above 200,000/µl. Some babies may have shortened survival particularly if bleeding is severe. In these cases daily platelet transfusions may be required. If maternal platelets are used, they should be washed to remove any antibody to the infant's antigens (1,12).

Antenatal Platelet Transfusions

Since intrauterine bleeding may occur, in utero platelet transfusions by percutaneous umbilical sampling have been employed (17). This approach was originally proposed as a method of allowing safe delivery and was used immediately before delivery. More recently investigators have advocated giving weekly platelet transfusions until an early delivery is feasible to prevent possible intrauterine bleeding. Percutaneous umbilical sampling may produce trauma that in a thrombocytopenic fetus is life-threatening. Therefore, there is a great deal of interest in noninvasive methods of managing the thrombocytopenic fetus. At present, steroids and IVIG are the only available forms of therapy that can be given to the mother that avoid any invasive procedures to the fetus.

Postnatal Intravenous Gammaglobulin

In anecdotal reports, intravenous gammaglobulin has been reported useful both antenatally and postnatally in neonatal alloimmune thrombocytopenia. The usual dose of intravenous gammaglobulin is 0.4 g/kg/day for 5 days or 1 g/kg/day for 2 days. A response is usually seen within 48 h with the count rising to above 50,000/μl. Occasionally, subsequent doses of intravenous gammaglobulin are required. It is unclear whether intravenous therapy alone is preferable to simply transfusing maternal platelets. Certainly if maternal platelets are not available, intravenous gammaglobulin should be used. In the more persistent or severe cases of neonatal alloimmune thrombocytopenia, intravenous gammaglobulin may be of benefit in reducing the duration of thrombocytopenia. If platelet transfusions are needed and platelets lacking the offending antigen are not available, intravenous gammaglobulin may prolong the survival of transfused platelets.

Antenatal Intravenous Immunoglobulin

Antenatal IVIG has been given to alloimmunized mothers to protect the fetus from maternal platelet alloantibodies (20,21). Lynch and co-workers have antenatally treated mothers who are immunized to platelet-specific antigens (21). Eighteen women who had previously delivered infants with severe alloimmune thrombocytopenia were treated with weekly infusions of intravenous gammaglobulin from the diagnosis of fetal thrombocytopenia until birth; nine were also treated with corticosteroids. The dose of immune globulin was 1.0 g/kg/week. There were no intracranial hemorrhages in the treated fetuses, compared with 10 cases among the 21 untreated siblings (48%). Only three treated fetuses, compared with 16 of 20 untreated siblings, had platelet counts of less than 30,000/μl, with no bleeding complications. These investigators concluded that treatment of fetuses with alloimmune thrombocytopenia using weekly gammaglobulin effectively improves the fetal platelet count and prevents intracranial hemorrhage. One case report, however, documents that IVIG treatment may not prevent intracranial hemorrhage in fetal alloimmune thrombocytopenia (22).

In a second large study, Murphy and co-workers investigated the use of antenatal immunoglobulin (23). They studied 15 pregnancies of 11 women who had previously affected infants with alloimmune thrombocytopenia due to anti-PI[A1]. The antenatal management included fetal platelet transfusions and maternal steroids and/or high-dose IVIG. In the first pregnancy, intracranial hemorrhage occurred between 32 an 35 weeks' gestation, before any treatment had been given, emphasizing the need for earlier intervention. Five of the 14 subsequent pregnancies in this study were considered to be severely affected (severe hemorrhagic complications in a previous infant and initial fetal platelet count < 20,000/μl in this study); four were managed successfully with weekly fetal platelet transfusions started between 18 and 29 weeks and continued until delivery at 33–35 weeks, and one severely affected case who was referred at 36 weeks was managed successfully with a single platelet transfusion prior to delivery. Five pregnancies were considered to be mildly affected (previous infants were unaffected by severe bleeding and initial fetal platelet count $> 50,000/\mu l$ in this study). The platelet counts were maintained in one case with steroids and in three with immunoglobulin without the need for repeated platelet transfusions, but in the fifth the fetal platelet count fell despite steroids and immunoglobulin and serial platelet transfusions were required. Four pregnancies were unsuccessful: two pregnancies were terminated after severe intracranial hemorrhage occurred at an early stage before fetal blood sampling had been carried out; one fetus died after the mother had a severe fall despite the successful initiation of fetal platelet transfusions; and one died due to a cord hematoma that occurred at the time of the initial fetal blood sampling. The optimal management of neonatal alloimmune thrombocytopenia to reduce the risk of antenatal intracranial hemorrhage remains uncertain. Steroids and immunoglobulin may be effective in some mildly affected cases, but serial fetal platelet transfusions are the preferred therapy for those who are severely affected.

Direct fetal administration has not been extensively evaluated. In two well-studied fetuses, this approach was not successful (24). It is not clear whether the direct administration offers any advantage. It could be argued that if invasive fetal sampling is performed it might be more prudent to proceed with a platelet transfusion prepared from the mother's platelets or another source of compatible platelets. Some fetal-maternal specialists may actually argue that antenatal sampling of thrombocytopenic fetuses should not be done if compatible platelets are not available should acute hemorrhage should occur during the procedure. Furthermore, we do not know the acute or chronic effects of intravenous immunoglobulin to the fetus.

POSTTRANSFUSION PURPURA

The syndrome of posttransfusion purpura was initially described by Shulman and coworkers (1). This disorder was first described in patients who were PI^{A1}-negative although other platelet-specific antigens have since been implicated. Thrombocytopenia occurs after transfusion with PI^{A1}-positive blood in individuals previously sensitized by pregnancy or transfusion. With development of thrombocytopenia, anti-PI^{A1} is found in the patient's blood.

Clinical Features of Posttransfusion Purpura

Typically the patients who develop posttransfusion purpura are females. Thrombocytopenia usually develops 7–10 days following transfusion. Thrombocytopenia is usually severe, with platelet counts of less than $5000/\mu l$ not uncommon. The types of blood products that have been implicated include whole blood, packed red cell concentrates, and fresh frozen plasma. As many as 50% of patients experience severe transfusion reactions with blood product administration. Symptoms may include hypotension, hypertension, chills, bronchospasm, fever, and chills. The duration of thrombocytopenia may range from 4 to 40 days, although it is unclear if those patients with longer durations of thrombocytopenia may not have other clinical conditions leading to more prolonged duration of thrombocytopenia (25).

In patients known to be PI^{A1}-negative, the occurrence of posttransfusion purpura following transfusion is not predictable. Patients have been transfused blood several months after recovery to normal platelet counts without recurrent thrombocytopenia following a documented episode of posttransfusion purpura, whereas other patients have had a recurrent episode of posttransfusion purpura after transfusion.

Patient Management

Treatment of posttransfusion purpura should be individualized (1,26). If the patient is not bleeding and is not at risk for bleeding because of invasive procedures, observation may be all that is required. In postoperative patients or patients with bleeding, aggressive therapy may be indicated. Previously plasma exchange has been used. In general, this approach leads to an increase in the platelet count after one to two plasma exchanges. Patients may relapse and repeat exchanges are required. Platelet transfusions from PI^{A1} are not effective.

In many cases plasma exchange therapy may not be readily available or venous access may be limited. For these reasons, IVIG has been used. There are no controlled studies, and it is difficult to assess the relative effectiveness of a therapy where the natural history of the illness is to improve spontaneously (24,27,28). Nonetheless, it appears that the temporal high-dose intravenous gammaglobulin may promptly correct the thrombocytopenia. Platelet transfusions, even if found negative for the immunizing platelet specific antigen, usually are not effective.

Intravenous Immunoglobulin in Posttransfusion Purpura

The largest experience in the treatment of posttransfusion purpura with immunoglobulin comes from Kroll and co-workers (25). They studied 34 cases of posttransfusion purpura. All patients were female, with a mean age of 60.8 years (35–78 years, n = 32). The interval between transfusion and onset of purpura ranged form 2 to 14 days, with a clear maximum at 7 and 8 days. Hemorrhagic symptoms lasted 9.4 days (3–37 days, n = 16). The mean minimal platelet count was $7.1 \times 10^3/\mu l$ [$(0–28) \times 10^3/\mu l$, n = 29]. The platelet count rose to over $50 \times 10^3/\mu l$ after 13.9 days (2–61 days, n = 26), over $100 \times 10^3/\mu l$ after 17.0 days (3–75 days, n = 22). In one patient, posttransfusion purpura led to death due to intracranial hemorrhage. Twenty-two patients were treated with corticosteroids, 20 patients with intravenous immunoglobulins, and 17 patients both. Therapy with IVIG was successful in 14/19 patients. In general, platelet counts increase within 48–72 h. After discontinuation of the IVIG, platelet counts may decrease but generally do not reach the lowest levels seen before the initiation of therapy.

REFERENCES

1. Shulman NR, Marder V, Hiller M, Collier EM. Platelet and leucocyte isoantigens and their antibodies: clinical, physiologic and clinical studies. Prog Hematol 1964; 4:222.
2. Kunicki TJ. Biochemistry of platelet associated isoantigens and alloantigens. In: Kunicki TJ, JN George, eds. Platelet Immunobiology. Philadelphia: J. B. Lippincott, 1989:99.
3. Kunicki TJ, Newman PJ. The molecular immunology of human platelet proteins. Blood 1992; 80:1386–1404.
4. Kickler TS. The challenge of platelet alloimmunization: management and prevention. Transfusion Med Rev 1990; 4:8–18.

5. Kickler TS. Platelet immunology. In: Anderson KL, Ness PM, eds. Scientific Basis of Transfus Medicine. Philadelphia: W.B. Saunders, 194:304–315.
6. Mueller-Eckhardt C, Kiefel V, Santoso S. Review and update of platelet alloantigen systems. Transfus Med Rev 1990; 4:98–109.
7. Schiffer CA, Hogge DE, Aisner J, Dutcher JP, Lee EJ, Papenberg D. High dose intravenous gammagobulin in alloimmunized platelet transfusion recipients. Blood 1984; 64:937–944.
8. Lee EJ, Norris D, Schiffer CA. Intravenous immune globulin for patients alloimmunized to random donor platelet transfusions. Transfusion 1987; 27:245–250.
9. Ziegler ZR. Shadduck RK. Rosenfeld CS, et al. Intravenous gamma globulin decreases platelet-associated IgG and improves transfusion responses in platelet refractory states. Am J Hematol 1991; 38(1):15–23.
10. Ziegler Z, Shaddduck R, Rosenfeld CS. High dose intravenous gammaglobulin improves response to single donor platelets in patients refractory to platelet transfusion. Blood 1987; 70:1433–1439.
11. Kickler TS, Braine HG, Piantadosi S, Ness PM, Herman J, Rothko K. A randomized placebo controlled trial of intravenous gammaglobulin in alloimmunized thrombocytopenic patients. Blood 1990; 75:313–316.
12. Pearson HA, Shulman NR, Marder VJ, Cone TE. Isoimmune neonatal thrombocytopenic purpura. Clinical and therapeutic considerations. Blood 1964; 23:154–176.
13. Blanchette VS, Petere MA, Pegg-Feige K. Alloimmune thrombocytopenia. Review from a neonatal intensive care unit. Curr Stud Hematol Blood Transfus 1986; 52:87–96.
14. Blanchette VS, Chen L, de Friedberg ZS, et al. Alloimmunization to the PI[A1] platelet antigen: results of a prospective study. Br J Haematol 1990; 74:209–215.
15. Herman JH, Jumbelic MI, Ancona RJ, Kickler TS. In utero cerebral hemorrhage in alloimmune thrombocytopenia. Am J Pediatr Hematol Oncol 1986; 8:312–317.
16. Bussel JB, McFarland JG, Berkowitz RL. Antenatal management of fetal alloimmune and autoimmune thrombocytopenia. Transfus Med Rev 1990; 4:149–162.
17. Kaplan C, Daffos F, Forestier F, et al. Management of alloimmune thrombocytopenia: antenatal diagnosis and in utero transfusion of maternal platelets. Blood 1988; 72:340–343.
18. Derycke M, Dreyfus M, Ropert JC, Tchernia G. Intravenous immunoglobulin for neonatal isoimmune thrombocytopenia. Arch Dis Child 1985; 60–667–669.
19. Suarez CR, Anderson C. High-dose intravenous gammaglobulin (IVG) in neonatal immune thrombocytopenia. Am J Hematol 1987; 26:247–253.
20. Bussel JB, Berkowitz RL, McFarland JG, Lynch L, Chitkara U. Antenatal treatment of neonatal alloimmune thrombocytopenia. N Engl J Med 1988; 319:1374–1378.
21. Lynch L, Bussel JB, McFarland JG, Chitkara U, Berkowitz RL. Antenatal treatment of alloimmune thrombocytopenia. Obstet Gynecol 1992; 80:67–71.
22. Kroll H, Kiefel V, Giers G, et al. Failure of antenatal intravenous immunoglobulin to prevent intracranial hemorrhage. Transfus Med 1994; 4:293–296.
23. Murphy MF, Waters AH, Doughty HA, et al. Antenatal management of fetomaternal alloimmune thrombocytopenia—report of 15 affected pregnancies. Transfus Med 1994; 4:281–292.
24. Weiner E, Zasmer N, Bajoria R, et al. Direct fetal administration of immunoglobulins—another disappointing therapy in alloimmune thrombocytopenia. Fetal Diagn Ther 1994; 9:159–164.
25. Vogelsang G, Kickler TS, Bell WR. Post-transfusion purpura. Am J Hematol 1986; 21:259–267.
26. Kroll H, Kiefel V, Mueller-Eckhardt C. Clinical and serologic studies in 34 patients with post-transfusion purpura. Infusionsther Transfusionsmed 1993; 20(5):198–204.

27. Mueller-Eckhardt C, Kiefel V, Grubert A. High-dose treatment for neonatal alloimmune thrombocytopenia. Blut 1989; 59:145–146.
28. Berney SI, Metcalfe P, Wathen NC, Waters AH. Post-transfusion purpura responding to high-dose intravenous IgG: further observation on pathogenesis. Br J Haematol 1985; 61:627.

26

Guillain-Barré Syndrome

Frans G.A. van der Meché and Pieter A. van Doorn
University Hospital Rotterdam, Rotterdam, The Netherlands

INTRODUCTION

In this chapter the treatment of the Guillain-Barré syndrome (GBS) with intravenous immunoglobulin (IVIG) is discussed. The diagnosis of Guillain-Barré syndrome is essentially a clinical one. Therefore, first the spectrum and the pathogenesis of GBS and its clinical variants will be described.

The treatment of GBS with IVIG has been evaluated in two major trials compared to plasma exchange (PE). For that reason it is essential to consider the efficacy of PE in comparison to the natural course of the disease before the effect of IVIG can be discussed. After the discussion of PE, attention will be given to the results of the Dutch immunoglobulin trial in GBS in which IVIG was compared with PE in a so-called conservative trial—i.e., a trial aiming for equal efficacy. Preliminary data are now also available from an international study with a similar design, in which the results of the Dutch study were confirmed—namely, that IVIG is as effective as PE.

Despite the clear results in different trials it is not always easy to treat the individual patient. Questions arise when patients continue to deteriorate during treatment or when they initially improve and subsequently deteriorate. These questions will be handled later in this discussion. The chapter will finish with some ideas on further development of the treatment of GBS.

CLINICAL SPECTRUM AND PATHOGENESIS

GBS is clinically characterized by subacute symmetrical weakness and loss of myotactic reflexes. The cerebrospinal fluid shows, usually from the second week onward, an elevated total protein content without a rise in cell count. Very importantly, there is no other known cause for the polyneuropathy. GBS is primarily distinguished from chronic inflammatory demyelinating polyneuropathy (CIDP) by a different time course. By definition, the nadir of GBS is reached within 4 weeks, but in the majority of patients within 2 weeks. For CIDP, in contrast, a duration of progressive weakness of at least 2 months has been suggested as a criterion (1). More recently, a group of patients have been described with an intermediate time course (2). In fact, a large series showed that there is a continuum with a sharp peak of patients who have their nadir in the first few weeks and a long trail of patients who have a much longer and usually less fulminant course (3,4).

In 1978, diagnostic criteria for GBS were developed (5). These criteria were based on the assumption that GBS is essentially a demyelinating disorder of peripheral nerves in the extremities, although several variants were described. Further clinical studies in the Western world, and additionally in northern China, have revealed that axonal forms exist in patients with an otherwise typical clinical course of GBS. Furthermore, pathogenetic studies have shown that variants as diverse as the classical ascending form and the Miller-Fisher syndrome, characterized by ocular motor weakness, ataxia, and areflexia and often a descending paralysis, share to a large extent similar pathogenic phenomena. For those reasons, it is now acceptable to define GBS clinically, as described above, and thereby to include all variants within the syndrome as long as the weakness is symmetrical, either ascending from the legs or starting in the cranial nerves with a characteristic time course (6,7).

Although in the last 10 years more clinical and pathogenetic information has become available, there has been a tendency in the literature to split up GBS into different syndromes, such as primary axonal GBS, GBS related to *Campylobacter jejuni* or anti-ganglioside antibodies, and other categorizations. Since GBS is now primarily clinically defined, a whole set of characteristics may be added to describe the individual patient in more detail (Table 1) (7). The justification of this approach comes also from pathogenetic studies, showing that different clinical syndromes may share very similar mechanisms. In classical ascending GBS, evidence for molecular mimicry has been put forward between certain *C. jejuni* strains and the ganglioside GM1, whereas in the Miller-Fischer syndrome between certain *C. jejuni* strains and the ganglioside GQ1b (7–9). Table 2 summarizes the major associations of clinical patterns and pathogenetic findings. By analyzing large groups of patients in relation to detailed clinical and electrophysiological information, it may be that in the future specific clusters or subgroups can be distinguished that need specific therapy. Such suggestions come from our studies, in which we showed that in a group of patients with pure motor GBS, who frequently have prior *C. jejuni* infections and high-titer anti-GM1-IgG antibodies, there was a better response to immunoglobulin therapy than to plasma exchange (10,11).

TREATMENT

General Aspects

Although at present specific treatment is available, general care is still of utmost importance for the GBS patient. A comprehensive review has been given by Ropper et al. (12). Progressive weakness of the respiratory muscles and muscles involved in swallowing especially should be monitored with great care. Aspiration in a patient with respiratory weakness may result in acute respiratory distress. Patients at risk should therefore be monitored in an intensive care unit and intubated in a timely fashion. Decreasing respiratory force is paralleled by a decreasing vital capability. Elective intubation is indicated in patients who still are deteriorating if the vital capacity is about 15 ml/kg or just above 1 L in a 70-kg person. In addition to the vital capacity, an increasing respiratory rate and subjective increased effort in breathing are indicators of impending respiratory failure. Blood gas analysis may not be very informative; PCO_2 and PO_2 may be within normal limits until respiratory failure occurs. If atelectasis or

Table 1 Further Characterization of
Clinically Defined GBS

Neurological examination
  Classically ascending
    sensorimotor
    pure motor
    severe sensory
    hyperacute with severe prognosis
  Cranial nerve variant
    Miller-Fisher syndrome
    lower bulbar variant
Epidemiology
  late summer outbreak in children in China
Laboratory studies
  Electrodiagnostic studies
    demyelination vs. axonal
Pathological studies
  demyelination vs. axonal
  inflammatory characteristics
Microbiological studies
  Campylobacter jejuni
  CMV, EBV, HIV
  Mycoplasma pneumoniae
Immunological studies
  activation markers
  antiganglioside antibodies

respiratory infection occurs, however, this may result in shunting and lowering of the PO_2 with increased respiratory effort. By monitoring the vital capacity, respiratory rate, and subjective breathing load, however, severe complications may be prevented by physical therapy and elective intubation. Cardiovascular dysautonomia should be treated only when necessary, since the response to medication may be unpredictable. Hypotension may best be treated by an increase in fluid infusions. Serious arrhythmias may be anticipated in patients requiring ventilation and developing wide fluctuations of pulse or blood pressure and transient asystole following tracheal suction or just after exturbation (13).

Table 2 Clinical Pattern and Laboratory Characteristics

Clinical variant	Associated infection	Associated antigen
Miller-Fisher	*C. jejuni*	GQ1b
Pure motor	*C. jejuni*	GM1
Motor-sensory with severe sensory involvement	CMV	GM2
Primary axonal (AMAN[a])	*C. jejuni*	GM1

[a]Acute motor axonal neuropathy.

Plasma Exchange

Specific treatment has been sought over the years, since morbidity is high in the acute phase of the disease; about 25% of patients need artificial ventilation, and about 5% will die. In addition, about 25% of the patients included in the major trials were not able to walk independently after 6 months.

The first randomized controlled trial appeared in 1984 (14). In that study, 14 patients received plasma exchange (PE) and 15 served as controls. No sham pheresis was applied in the control group, since this was believed unethical in these cardiovascular, often unstable patients. (For this reason, in subsequent trials, treatment was open-label.) Five exchanges of 55 ml plasma/kg body weight per exchange were performed in 10 days. Patients were included if they fulfilled the GBS criteria and were entered within 30 days after disease onset. No overall beneficial effect was seen in this study. Analyzing the effect in a subgroup of 20 patients randomized within 14 days after disease onset resulted in a clear positive trend. The control patients deteriorated 0.27 points on a 7-point functional scale, whereas the treated group had an average improvement of 0.44 points ($P = .07$). This was important, since in the later large North American study it was demonstrated that treatment started 2 weeks or more from onset was not effective (15). In retrospect, this study demonstrated similar results to later, much larger trials.

A second study was published in 1984 (16). In this trial performed in four centers, 38 patients were included with a mean disease duration of just less than 1 week. They were, however, not randomized but treated in an alternate order, and dropouts were replaced by the next patient. Patients not willing or not able to be fully exchanged were considered to be dropouts as well. Thus, this study can be regarded as preliminary and explanatory. In total, at least 10 kg of plasma had to be removed in at least three sessions and within 8 days. In this study, a beneficial effect was noted in the PE group. Treated patients were able to walk independently 40 days earlier than the nontreated group; the median stay in hospital was 30 days for the PE group and 78 for the control group.

In 1985, the first large-scale randomized trial involving 245 patients was published (15). This study was analyzed both according to the intention-to-treat paradigm and in an explanatory fashion. A total of 200 to 250 cc/kg body weight was exchanged in 7–14 days. The primary outcome measure, the proportion of patients with functional improvement 4 weeks after randomization, favored PE, as did all secondary outcome measures. Clinically, most interesting are the following statistically significant findings: the median time on the respirator—7 days for the PE group and 23 days for the control group; time until independent locomotion—53 days for the PE group and 85 days in the control group: and outcome at 6 months—18% treated with PE were not able to walk independently versus 29% in the control group. It was also confirmed in this study that an effect could be seen only in the group of patients randomized within 2 weeks after disease onset. Apparently, as may have been expected, PE has, as an immune modulatory treatment, an effect only in that phase of the disease in which an active immune attack occurs.

In general, albumin has been used as a replacement fluid in these plasma exchange studies. The use of fresh frozen plasma was a subject of study in the French plasma exchange trial (17). In that trial, 220 patients were randomized with a mean disease duration of less than 1 week. One hundred nine patients were exchanged of whom 52 received fresh frozen plasma instead of albumin (based on random assignment). This study confirmed the effect of plasma exchange. In the exchange group, 21% of the patients went on the respirator after entry, in contrast to 43% in the control group. The median time to regain independent locomotion was 70 days in the treatment group and 111 days in the control group. Six-month data were available for the outcome "walking with support" but not for "walking independently"; the former did not show a significant difference. Comparing albumin and fresh frozen plasma as replacement fluids, it was found that a trend but no consistent difference in outcome was obtained in favor of fresh frozen plasma. Since the complication rate of fresh frozen plasma was higher, including viral hepatitis, the authors recommended abandoning fresh frozen plasma as a replacement fluid.

It may be concluded from these studies that PE reduces acute morbidity considerably, whereas the largest study also showed improvement of long-term outcome at 6 months. In addition, after 6 months some further improvement may occur, but only very slowly and incompletely, as may be extrapolated from the survival curves of the outcome measures in all major trials discussed. Since 1985, PE has been the mainstay as specific treatment in GBS. It has even been calculated that it is cost-effective in all stages of the disease (18).

However, PE has major drawbacks. It is contraindicated in cardiovascular instability. For that reason, 25 of the 325 patients evaluated for entry in the French GBS trial had to be excluded. Furthermore, complications of PE have been described, and this has led to withdrawal of 10% of the PE-treated patients in the North American GBS trial and to discontinuation of one or more sessions in 18% of the patients in the French GBS trial. In the latter study, at least one adverse incident was observed in 76% of the PE-treated patients (19). Moreover, PE facilities are not available everywhere or immediately available in acute situations. For those reasons, an alternative for PE was desirable. In 1988, the first open study with high-dose immunoglobulin was published (20). Further studies with immunoglobulin have aimed for equal efficacy compared to PE; an equally effective alternative with a better risk profile and which is easier to employ would be preferred.

Immunoglobulin Treatment

The first randomized clinical trial comparing IVIG with PE appeared in 1992 (21). This study strictly followed a conservative design. This included a clinical judgment of equal efficacy based on confidence limits and power calculations to determine the suitable number of patients. In addition, an early stopping rule was developed along these lines, although there were no general rules for this within the statistical literature. After 150 patients were randomized, the study was halted since significantly more patients in the IVIG group fulfilled the major outcome criterion compared to the PE group. Based on the conservative design, it was concluded that IVIG was a least as good as PE but not superior to it. Although that latter might be the case, an additional study aiming to demonstrate such a difference would be required.

In the Dutch Guillain-Barré study 150 patients were randomized. Three patients were incorrectly randomized and excluded, leaving 147 patients: 74 in the IVIG group and 73 in the PE group. No patients were lost to follow-up. Patients were eligible if they fulfilled the clinical criteria for GBS, were within 2 weeks of onset of weakness, and were so severely afflicted that independent locomotion was no longer possible.

Patients were scored according to a 7-point functional scale for which 0 denoted healthy, 1 = having minor symptoms and signs but fully capable of manual work, 2 = able to walk at least 10 m without assistance, 3 = able to walk at least 10 m with a walker or support, 4 = bedridden or chairbound, 5 = requiring assisted ventilation for a least part of the day, and 6 = dead. The main outcome criterion based on this scale was improvement by one or more grades 4 weeks after randomization. Important secondary outcome criteria were time until one grade improvement, time until independent locomotion, need for assisted ventilation, and complication rate. In fact, the study was designed to make possible a direct comparison with earlier PE trials. Also, PE treatment was given according to the former North American trial protocol: exchange 200–250 ml plasma/kg body weight in five sessions within 7–14 days. Albumin was used as the replacement fluid. PE was started as soon as possible after randomization (median delay 1 day) and always under optimal conditions, to avoid complications as much as possible. IVIG treatment also was started as soon as possible and, due to its easier application, started, in general, at the day of randomization. The dose was 0.4 g IVIG/kg body weight/day for 5 consecutive days (Gammagard, Baxter Healthcare, Glendale, CA). Patients were followed for 6 months according to a rigid scheme. Since it was an open study, because of the PE procedure, bias was controlled during the follow-up period. All patients were seen at least once by one of the study coordinators, who were blinded to the treatment modality. Their score was compared with the score of the unblinded investigator in the center. By using this method, no evidence of bias was observed. The proportion of patients fulfilling the primary outcome criterion—i.e., functional improvement with one or more grades—was 34% in the PE group and 53% in the IVIG group (95% confidence interval of 3–34%; $P = .024$).

In addition, the secondary outcome criteria were in favor of IVIG: time until functional improvement ($P = .05$), the proportion of patients with multiple complications ($P < .01$), and the proportion of patients needing artificial ventilation in the second week ($P < .05$). Time until independent locomotion ($P = .07$) and the proportion of patients able to walk independently at 6 months ($P = .16$) also showed a difference in favor of IVIG, but did not reach significance. Based on the main aim of this conservative trial, we concluded that IVIG was at least as effective as PE but may be superior.

In some comments following the publication of this study, the PE arms of the North American, French, and Dutch GBS trials were compared and some concern expressed about the differences (12). In the North American GBS trial, improvement in the PE group started somewhat earlier. In the French and Dutch PE arms, the time until independent locomotion was 70 and 69 days, respectively. In the North American PE arm this was 53 days. The difference between the two European GBS trials and the North American study may be due to differences in referral pattern and the method of analysis. In the French and Dutch GBS studies, the duration of the disease until entry was about 6 days; in the North American GBS study it was just over 11 days. Comparison of the main outcome criteria in the North American and Dutch PE groups using similar methodology (intention-to-treat analysis) and correcting for a difference of over 5 days of disease duration yielded a similar proportion of patients with functional improvement at the same number of days from onset of disease: 49% in the Dutch PE group, and 52% in the North American PE group (22). These comparisons further substantiate the efficacy of IVIG in GBS.

A multicenter study coordinated from London has recently been completed, but the results have only been communicated in meetings and are not yet available in print. In this study, 383 patients were randomized to three treatment arms. In two arms the equal efficacy of plasma exchange and immune globulins was evaluated, and in a third arm the administration of IVIG after completing a course of PE was considered. The preliminary results of this study substantiate the similar effectiveness of IVIG and PE. The combination of the two treatments did not improve the outcome significantly. It is important to note that IVIG used in this study was manufactured from a different donor population by another manufacturer. This implies that the clinical effect of IVIG in GBS may not be brand-specific, despite the fact that smaller differences in efficacy may exist due to the biological nature of the product. It is expected that after publication of these results, IVIG will become the primary choice of treatment in GBS in even more centers than at present.

Cost-effectiveness has been proven for PE (18). IVIG may have a similar cost to PE depending on the local circumstances (21); in the Dutch GBS study, IVIG reduced hospital costs by shortening the duration of artificial ventilation by an average of 7 days and hospital stay by 2 weeks, as estimated from the time until independent locomotion (21). Thus, based on cost, IVIG seems a well-balanced choice.

Treating the Individual Patient

The clinical trials discussed show that in large groups in GBS patients IVIG and PE are effective therapies. Large studies were necessary to prove efficacy due to the variability of the disease in individual patients. In clinical practice, however, we must manage individual patients, and other questions may therefore come up. When and how should one treat individual patients, and what should one do if a patient further deteriorates during or even after treatment? Since GBS has only a short phase of active disease in which immune-modulating therapy may be effective, treatment should not start too late. In the North American GBS study, it was shown that PE starting in the third week was not effective (15). Treatment therefore should start as soon as possible, at least before the end of the second week after diagnosis. An exception to this rule may be the patient who is still progressive in the third or fourth week of the disease, indicating an ongoing immune attack. In the Dutch GBS study, about 15% reached their nadir beyond 2 weeks; a possible effect in such a small subgroup may have been lost in the North American trial.

Should a GBS patient be treated who is as yet only mildly affected? Final outcome is strongly related to age and severity of the disease in the early phase (21,23,24); therefore, mildly affected patients carry a limited risk for residual deficit. Recently, however, it has been shown in a large study from France that mildly affected patients who were still able to walk independently benefited from half the intensity of PE used in more severe GBS patients (25). Whether a lower dose of IVIG is sufficient under these circumstances is not yet known, but is the subject of a planned study in France.

Do children or patients with variants like the Miller-Fisher syndrome benefit from treatment? No large trials have been performed in children alone, but small studies indicate similar improvement as in adults with PE (26) or IVIG (27,28). In the Miller-Fischer syndrome, case histories indicate that PE (29) or IVIG (30,31) may be of help. At present no pathogenic differences between childhood and adult GBS are known, and classical GBS and variants will likely share disease mechanisms. Because of these similarities and since large-scale clinical trials are unlikely to be performed in these subgroups, it may be practical to treat children, at least if they are more severely affected, according to the results obtained in the large studies with predominantly adults with classical GBS.

During treatment, the individual GBS patient may improve, stabilize, or further deteriorate. If a patient improves, it is impossible to determine whether the therapy actually caused improvement or improvement was achieved spontaneously. On the other hand, a patient who will continue to deteriorate may have had a more severe course without therapy; i.e., treatment may have been effective in reducing the deterioration. In fact, it may be impossible to judge the efficacy of any treatment in one individual patient. Despite this, the treating neurologist may feel in conflict if a patient deteriorated during PE or IVIG. Thus, one may struggle with whether a patient should be switched to the alternative treatment. It is therefore important to know what to expect from the clinical course after starting IVIG or PE. From studies in CIDP it is known that the effect of IVIG or PE may sometimes be seen almost immediately, but usually within a week after the start of IVIG treatment (32). If the immune attack is more fulminant as in GBS, one should anticipate that it may take even longer to reach recovery phase.

To know more quantitatively what may be expected in the first 2 weeks after the onset of the treatment, the clinical course in the first 2 weeks for the patients involved in the Dutch IVIG PE trial has been analyzed (7). It was shown that in a considerable proportion of patients, the clinical condition deteriorated during the first 2 weeks after the onset of treatment. On the functional scale, a quarter of the patients in the IVIG group demonstrated deterioration, compared to a third in the PE group. Therefore, we concluded that further deterioration during either IVIG or PE treatment occurs frequently and a management strategy must be developed based on this knowledge. It may be tempting to change therapy in a patient showing further deterioration. On the other hand, it is clear that improvement starts in over one-third of the patients in the second week; therefore, one should wait at least until the second week after the onset of treatment. It was further observed that after one course of IVIG, rapid and full improvement may start even in the third week in a patient who initially deteriorated rapidly from walking with support to being bedridden and on artificial respiration. If such a patient had been treated with the alternative treatment, one certainly might have ascribed the improvement to that and not to the initial therapy. If one plans to switch to another treatment 2 weeks after the first, the majority of patients will be at the end of the third week of the disease, and any treatment is then very unlikely to be of benefit (15). We therefore use as a pragmatic treatment rule that GBS patients should only be given one full treatment as long as we lack knowledge of factors that predict the efficacy of either IVIG or PE. Only in a special situation will there be a clear indication of the effect of treatment: about 10% of GBS patients treated either with IVIG or PE initially improve and subsequently deteriorate again. Such treatment-related clinical fluctuations do respond to a further course of the same treatment (33). Recent small, open studies showed variable effects during or after IVIG treatment that may be explained by the selection of either fast- or late-improving patients. Some patients worsened during or after IVIG treatment (34,35), whereas others showed a very favorable response (27,36,37). Overall it is difficult to draw conclusions from these small studies (38), but, taken together, they fit the pattern of wide variation in the clinical course of the disease seen in the large clinical trials.

FUTURE DEVELOPMENTS

Future developments in the treatment of Guillain-Barré syndrome should focus on clear predictive factors for a guided treatment choice in the individual patient and on new treatment strategies in general. High-dose methylprednisolone (MP) at a dose of 500 mg for 5 days has received renewed interest. The GBS steroid trial group reported a lack of effect (39). However, in this study PE was permitted if required, and the increased application of PE in the placebo group may have masked some positive effect of MP treatment. In idiopathic thrombocytopenic purpura, it has been suggested from case histories that IVIG in combination with MP may show a synergistic effect (40). The Dutch GBS Study Group demonstrated in a pilot study in 25 GBS patients that the combined treatment of 0.4 g IVIG/kg and 0.5 g methylprednisolone for 5 consecutive days caused a significant improvement in the clinical course compared to a historical control group of 74 patients treated with IVIG alone who were evaluated with an identical follow-up scheme (41). A multicenter study has been designed and is running with patients randomly assigned to either IVIG and placebo or IVIG and methylprednisolone treatment.

REFERENCES

1. Cornblath DR, Asbury AK, Albers JW, et al. Research criteria for diagnosis of chronic inflammatory demyelinating polyneuropathy (CIDP). Neurology 1991; 41:617–618.
2. Hughes RAC, Sanders E, Hall S, et al. Subacute idiopathic demyelinating polyradiculoneuropathy. Arch Neurol 1992; 49:612–616.
3. Ropper AH, Wijdicks EFM, Truax BT. Guillain-Barré Syndrome. Contemporary Neurology Series. Philadelphia: F. A. Davis Company, 1991.
4. Gibbels, Giebisch U. Natural course of acute and chronic monophasic inflammatory demyelinating polyneuropathies (IDP). Acta Neurol Scand 1991; 85:282–291.
5. Asbury AK, Arnason BG, Karp HR, McFarlin DE. Criteria for diagnosis of Guillain-Barré syndrome. Ann Neurol 1978; 3:565–566.
6. WHO-AIREN meeting on the differential diagnosis of acute onset flaccid paralysis: comparison of poliomyelitis, the Guilliain-Barré syndrome and related conditions. Geneva: WHO, 1993.
7. Van der Meché FGA, van Doorn PA. Guillain-Barré syndrome and chronic inflammatory demyelinating polyneuropathy: immune mechanisms and update on current therapies. Ann Neurol 1995; 37(suppl 1):S14–S31.
8. Oomes PG, Jacobs BC, Hazenberg MHP, Bänffer JRJ, van der Meché FGA. Anti-GM1 IgG antibodies and *Campylobacter* bacteria in Guillain-Barré syndrome: evidence of molecular mimicry. Ann Neurol 1995; 38:170–175.
9. Jacobs BC, Endtz HPh, van der Meché FGA, Hazenberg MP, Achtereekte HAM, van Doorn PA. Serum anti-GQ1b IgG antibodies recognize surface epitopes on *Campylobacter jejuni* from patients with Miller-Fisher syndrome. Ann Neurol 1995; 37:260–264.
10. Visser LH, van der Meché FGA, van Doorn PA, et al. Guillain-Barré syndrome without

sensory loss (acute motor neuropathy): a subgroup with specific clinical, electrodiagnostic and laboratory features. Brain 1995; 118:841–847.

11. Jacobs BC, van Doorn PA, Schmitz PIM, et al. Clinical, prognostic and therapeutic significance of *Campylobacter jejuni* infections and anti-GM1 antibodies in patients with Guillain-Barré syndrome. Ann Neurol 1996; 40(2):181–187.

12. Ropper AH. The Guillain-Barré syndrome. N Engl J Med 1992; 326:1130–1136.

13. Winer JB, Hughes AC. Identification of patients at risk of arrhythmia in the Guillain-Barré syndrome. Q J Med N Ser 1988; 68:735–739.

14. Greenwood RJ, Hughes RAC, Bowden AN, et al. Controlled trial of plasma exchange in acute inflammatory polyradiculoneuropathy. Lancet 1984; 1:877–879.

15. Guillain-Barré Syndrome Study Group. Plasmapheresis and acute Guillain-Barré syndrome. Neurology 1985; 35:1096–1104.

16. Osterman PG, Lundemo G, Pirskanen R, et al. Beneficial effects of plasma exchange in acute inflammatory polyradiculoneuropathy. Lancet 1984; 2:1296–1299.

17. French Cooperative Group on Plasma Exchange in Guillain-Barré Syndrome. Efficiency of plasma exchange in Guillain-Barré syndrome: role of replacement fluids. Ann Neurol 1987; 22:753–761.

18. Audet AM, Eckman M. Plasmapheresis in the treatment of Guillain-Barré syndrome: a cost-effective analysis. Med Decis Making 1989; 9:324.

19. Bouget J, Chevret S, Chastang C, et al. Plasma exchange morbidity in Guillain-Barré syndrome: results from the French prospective, double-blind, randomized, multicenter study. Crit Care Med 1993; 21:651–658.

20. Kleyweg RP, van der Meché FGA, Meulstee J. Treatment of Guillain-Barré syndrome with high dose gammaglobulin. Neurology 1988; 38:1639–1642.

21. Van der Meché FGA, Schmitz PIM, Dutch Guillain-Barré Study Group. A randomized trial comparing intravenous immune globulin and plasma exchange in Guillain-Barré syndrome. N Engl J Med 1992; 326:1123–1129.

22. Van der Meché FGA. The Guillain-Barré syndrome. In: McLeod JG, ed. Inflammatory Neuropathies. Baillière's Clin Neurol 1994; 3:73–94.

23. McKhann GM, Griffin JW, Cornblath DR, et al. Plasmapheresis and Guillain-Barré syndrome: analysis of prognostic factors and the effect of plasmapheresis. Ann Neurol 1988; 23:347–353.

24. Winer JB, Hughes RAC, Osmond C. A prospective study of acute idiopathic neuropathy. 1. Clinical features and their prognostic value. J Neurol Neurosurg Psychiatry 1988; 51:605–612.

25. Raphael JC, Chevret S, Chastang CL, et al. Détermination du nombre optimal d'échanges plasmatiques dans le syndrome de Guillain-Barré selon la gravité. Résultats d'une étude multicentrique randomisée. Société de Réanimation de Langue Française, Paris, 20–22 Jan 1994. Rean Urg 1993; 2:704.

26. Lamont PJ, Johnston HM, Berdoukas VA. Plasmapheresis in children with Guillain-Barré syndrome. Neurology 1991; 41:1928–1931.

27. Suri M, Suri ML, Shahani BT. Intravenous gammaglobulin (IVGG) therapy in children with severe acute inflammatory demyelinating polyneuropathy (AIDP). Neurology 1993; 43:A347.

28. Vallée L. Dulac O, Nuyts J, et al. Intravenous immune globulin is also an efficient therapy of acute Guillain-Barré syndrome in afflicted children. Neuropediatrics 1993; 24:235–236.

29. Irvine AT, Tibbles J. Treatment of Fischer's variant of Guillain-Barré syndrome by exchange transfusion. Can J Neurol Sci 1981; 8:49–50.

30. Zifko U, Drlicek M, Senautka G, et al. High dose immunoglobulin therapy is effective in the Miller-Fisher syndrome. J Neurol 1994; 241:178–179.

31. Arakawa Y, Yoshimura M, Kobayashi S, et al. The use of intravenous immunoglobulin in Miller-Fisher syndrome. Brain Dev 1993; 15:231–233.

32. Van Doorn PA, Vermeulen M, Brand A, et al. Intravenous immunoglobulin treatment in

patients with chronic inflammatory demyelinating polyneuropathy. Clinical and laboratory characteristics associated with improvement. Arch Neurol 1991; 48:217–220.

33. Kleyweg RP, van der Meché FGA. Treatment related fluctuations in Guillain-Barré syndrome after high-dose immunoglobulins or plasma exchange. J Neurol Neurosurg Psychiatry 1991; 54:957–960.

34. Castro LHM, Ropper AH. Human immune globulin infusion in Guillain-Barré syndrome: worsening during and after treatment. Neurology 1993; 43:1034–1036.

35. Irani DN, Carnblath DR, Chaudhry V, et al. Relapse in Guillain-Barré syndrome after treatment with human immune globulin. Neurology 1993; 43:872–875.

36. Jackson MC, Godwin-Austen RB, Whitely AM. High-dose intravenous immunoglobulin in the treatment of Guillain-Barré syndrome: a preliminary open study. J Neurol 1993; 240:51–53.

37. Kamei T, Nakagawa H, Uchiyama F, et al. Treatment of Guillain-Barré syndrome with high-dose intravenous immunoglobulins—a comparison with plasma exchange. Risho Shinkeigaku 1993; 33:660–662.

38. Van der Meché FGA, van Doorn PA, Schmitz PIM. Intravenous immunoglobulin versus plasma exchange in Guillain-Barré syndrome. Neurology 1993; 43:2730.

39. Guillain-Barré Syndrome Steroid Trial Group. Double-blind trial of intravenous methylprednisolone in Guillain-Barré syndrome. Lancet 1993; 341:586–590.

40. Duncombe AS, Kesteven PJ, Savidge GF. Combination of steroids and immunoglobulin in chronic refractory idiopathic thrombocytopenic purpura (ITP) enabling renal stone fragmentation by lithotripsy. Clin Lab Haematol 1986; 8:315–319.

41. Dutch Guillain-Barré Study Group. Treatment of Guillain-Barré syndrome with high-dose immune globulins combined with methylprednisolone: a pilot study. Ann Neurol 1994; 35:749–752.

27

Chronic Inflammatory Demyelinating Polyneuropathy

Pieter A. van Doorn and Frans G. A. van der Meché
University Hospital Rotterdam, Rotterdam, The Netherlands

INTRODUCTION

Chronic inflammatory demyelinating polyneuropathy (CIDP) is considered to be the chronic variety of the Guillain-Barré syndrome (GBS)—an acute, generally severe, immune-mediated polyneuropathy (1).

CIDP and GBS differ mainly in onset, course, and prognosis. GBS patients have progressive weakness of less than 4 weeks (2). In order to make a clear separation between CIDP and GBS, criteria for CIDP require a progressive phase of 2 months at least (3). In fact, these neuropathies are at the poles of a spectrum, ranging from the very acute variety of GBS on one side to a very slowly progressive CIDP on the other side. The group of patients with a progressive phase exceeding 4 weeks but less than 8 weeks is sometimes named "subacute" idiopathic demyelinating polyneuropathy (4). Not only from a scientific point of view, but certainly also from the clinical, it is relevant to make a distinction between GBS and CIDP. GBS has a monophasic course that very infrequently relapses; treatment has to be administered for a short period of time within the first weeks after the onset of progressive weakness. Patients with CIDP, on the other hand, can have a course characterized by relapses and remissions (Fig. 1). Additionally, there is no rapid progression of weakness, and most patients need to be treated for a long period of time.

Patients with CIDP have symmetrical distal and proximal weakness which generally predominates over sensory loss; areflexia is common. Cerebrospinal fluid generally shows an increased protein content without a cellular reaction. Electrophysiological criteria for CIDP have been proposed and include evidence for demyelination with features such as conduction blocks, dispersion of the compound muscle action potential, increased distal latencies, or slowed conduction velocities (3) (Table 1).

Prior to making the diagnosis of CIDP, it is essential to rule out other causes of chronic polyneuropathies. Disease such as hereditary neuropathies, vasculitis, cryoglobulinemia, multiple myeloma, and many others have to be excluded. The clinical diagnosis of CIDP in principle can only be made in the absence of systemic disease (5).

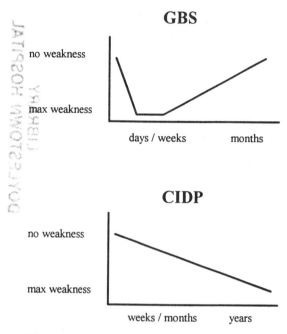

Figure 1   Clinical course of GBS and chronic progressive CIDP.

However, it seems that CIDP can also occur in the setting of some concurrent diseases (6,7). At present it is still a matter of debate whether the diagnosis of CIDP can be made when a monoclonal protein of undetermined significance (MGUS) is present. Several studies have excluded patients with a clinical diagnosis of CIDP who also have a MGUS, from the final diagnosis of CIDP (5,8); others have included patients who had a MGUS of the IgG isotype (6,9).

IMMUNE MECHANISMS

Immune mechanisms involved in CIDP have recently been reviewed (10). Many parallels may be drawn with GBS, but there are differences. Information on these mecha-

Table 1   Chronic Inflammatory Demyelinating
Polyneuropathy Clinical and Laboratory
Features

Progressive weakness ≥ 8 weeks
Motor ≥ sensory symptoms
Symmetric weakness in arms and legs
Hypo- or areflexia
Cerebrospinal fluid : protein increased, no cells
EMG : demyelination
No other cause of polyneuropathy

nisms can be obtained from the pathology, the occurrence of antecedent infections, and the results from various immunological and therapeutic studies.

In nerve biopsies or autopsy material, frank inflammatory infiltration is generally less obvious than in GBS patients, probably reflecting the more smoldering course of the disease. If inflammatory cells are present, they are usually within the endoneurium. Perivascular infiltrates, if present, are mainly located in the epineurium. As in nerve biopsies in GBS, T cells and macrophages disrupting the myelin sheath may be present in the biopsy material, but B cells are rarely seen (1). Immunoglobulin deposits on the external Schwann cell membrane have been demonstrated in some but not all studies (11,12). Whether macrophages, activated T cells, cytokines, adhesion molecules, or antibodies play an active role in the initial events leading to the disruption of myelin is not certain. Circulating antibodies against neural tissue have been demonstrated in patients with CIDP by many authors using different techniques (1,10). Antibodies against various glycolipids such as GM1, GD1b, GD1a, GT1b, GM2, and LM1 have been demonstrated in patients with a CIDP, but mostly in a rather low percentage (13). Lundkvist et al. found antibodies presumably directed against a neutral glycolipid present on a neuroblastoma cell line in almost half of the patients with a CIDP (14). The exact molecular structure of the putative antigen is unknown (Lundkvist, unpublished). In parallel with GBS, it may well be that different antigens are related to more or less specific clinical subgroups of CIDP.

Studies on T cell activation by measuring soluble interleukin (IL) or IL-receptor levels have also been performed in CIDP. Serum levels of IL-2 and soluble IL-2 receptors were increased in some CIDP patients, but did not show a correlation with disease activity (15,16). These and other studies suggest that CIDP, like GBS, is, at least partially, a T-cell–mediated disorder. A failure to pick up measurable concentrations of cytokines in serum or CSF does not preclude the local production of cytokines, since it is known that at least some of these cytokines are not stable over longer periods of time. Further studies on interleukin production, if possible at the RNA level, might be more meaningful in patients with signs of an active process of disease.

Initial studies on a genetic predisposition to CIDP initially suggested an association with certain HLA antigens (17–19). It was not possible, however, to demonstrate a significant relationship with any of the HLA-A, B, C, DR, or DQ antigens in a large group of CIDP patients (20). Additionally, we could not demonstrate a significant HLA association between the group of CIDP patients who improved after IVIG and those who did not improve (20). Thus, the results from HLA typing do not support the idea that CIDP has a genetic predisposition.

Antecedent infections are not as frequent as reported in GBS. The passage of time before neurological evaluation may in part reflect a failure to recall a preceding infection. However, Prineas et al. reported various infections within a month before onset of neurological symptoms in 15 of 23 (65%) CIDP patients in whom upper respiratory tract infections were the most frequent (21). Some evidence for a CMV infection was found in 19 of 39 (49%) CIDP patients (8). Studies on antecedent *Campylobacter jejuni* infections in CIDP have not, to the best of our knowledge, been published. We have found evidence for an increased titer of antibodies against *C. jejuni* in 47% of 36 CIDP patients, compared to 14% in normal controls, when tested by counter immunoelectrophoresis (10). Whether these observations suggest an active infection or represent a prior infection needs reevaluation.

TREATMENT

Many uncontrolled studies and only a few controlled trials have been performed in CIDP. Controlled studies and the largest series evaluating the effect of steroids and PE will be discussed shortly. Trials and some other studies on the initial and long-term effect of IVIG and a recent study comparing the effect of PE and IVIG will be discussed in more detail.

Steroids

Steroids are considered to be effective in patients with CIDP. It is, however, reported that improvement after prednisone was often not apparent over protracted periods (5). A controlled trial in 28 patients treated with 120 mg prednisone every other day tapered in 3 months versus no treatment showed that prednisone caused a small but significant improvement (22). The two largest retrospective studies reported improvement after corticosteroids in 49 of 76 (65%) (8) and in 56 of 59 (95%) CIDP patients (6). The time lapse between initiation of prednisone treatment until onset of clinical improvement varied from 1 or 2 weeks up to 3.5 months (23). Barohn et al. reported that the mean time to the first signs of improvement was 1.9 months and that maximal improvement was reached not earlier than 6.6 months (6). Although it was concluded that the majority of patients initially improved, relapses occurred in 70% of the patients after discontinuation of steroids (6). Long-term treatment with corticosteroids can cause serious side effects, but the incidence and severity are not well known and need further evaluation (24).

Plasma Exchange

Two PE trials in CIDP have been performed. In the first study, 15 patients were treated with PE and 14 patients received a sham exchange (25). After 3 weeks, the reflexes and nerve conduction velocities were improved in favor of the PE group. Improvement in the neurological disability score in five patients treated with PE exceeded the largest improvement attained by any patient receiving sham exchange. Improvement was observed both in patients with slowly progressive disease and in those with a remitting course. Improvement after PE was transient, since it began to fade 10–14 days after finishing the course of PE. Hahn et al. recently published a double-blind, sham-controlled, crossover study showing that PE is effective in newly diagnosed, previously untreated CIDP patients (26). Eighteen previously untreated patientsof whom six patients had a chronic progressive course, and 12 a relapsing course received PE for 4 weeks. After a washout period of 5 weeks, the patients were crossed over. In total, three patients did not complete the trial, leaving 15 patients to be analyzed. Twelve of these 15 patients (80%) had a major response to PE. Improvement was found in the neurological disability score as a whole, and the clinical grade, grip strength, and distal amplitude ($P < .007$). Seven of the 12 patients (58%) relapsed 7–14 days after the last PE, but stabilized with subsequent PE plus immunosuppressive drug therapy.

There is no study available that focuses on long-term treatment with PE, which seems to be inevitable in most patients with a CIDP. PE is expensive and requires special equipment and good vascular access. It therefore appears not to be an attractive treatment for patients needing long-term treatment.

IVIG Treatment

In the early 1980s, when the results of the corticosteroid and PE trials in patients with CIDP were not available, fresh-frozen plasma (FFP) and later on IVIG were administered at our department to a 15-year-old patient with severe CIDP who did not respond to steroids. This patient clearly responded to regularly performed PE, but this procedure became increasingly difficult because of problems with vascular access. The results of IVIG treatment in this patient and in 16 other CIDP patients were published in 1985 (27). These results were the basis for further studies on IVIG in patients with inflammatory neuropathies.

Initial Effect of IVIG

Uncontrolled studies. In the first study on IVIG treatment of CIDP, it was observed that improvement after IVIG occurred in 13/17 patients (70%); furthermore, it appeared that improvement started within a week after the onset of therapy. Most of the patients needed intermittent treatment, and none of them became refractory to IVIG treatment (27). Since then, several uncontrolled studies claimed that 20–100% of CIDP patients improved after IVIG treatment (9,27–33) (for a review see Ref. 34). The results of the studies involving more than two CIDP patients treated with IVIG are shown in Table 2. Since some patients with CIDP can improve spontaneously (27) and most

Table 2 Studies in Patients with CIDP Treated with IVIG

Study	Type of study	IVIG dose g/kg/day × number of days	Improvement After IVIG Proportion of patients	%
Vermeulen (35)	double-blind	0.4 × 5	4/15	27
		placebo	3/13	
Van Doorn (36)	double-blind crossover	0.4 × 5	7/7	100
		placebo	0/7	
Hahn (37)	double-blind crossover	0.4 × 5	19/30	63
		placebo	5/30	
Vermeulen (27)	open	0.1 1 FFP/kg or 0.4 × 5	12/17	70
Curro Dossi (28)	open	0.4 × 5	4/4	100
Faed (29)	open	0.4 × 3	9/9	100
Vedanarayanan (30)	open	0.4 × 5	4/4	100
Cornblath (31)	open	0.3–0.4 × 4–5	3/15	20
Van Doorn (9)	open	0.4 × 5	32/52[a]	62
Azulay (32)	open	0.4 × 5	4/8	50
Nemni (33)	open	0.4 × 5	7/9[b]	78

FFP = fresh frozen plasma.
[a]32/52 improved; 2/32 only shortlasting; 9/32 one course followed by clinical remission; 21/32 intermittent treatment necessary.
[b]1/7 became refractory for IVIG.

of these studies report on patients who were selected for IVIG treatment, these percentages are difficult to interpret.

In a retrospective study involving 52 CIDP patients, it was found that 32 patients (62%) improved after IVIG. Twenty-one patients (40%) needed intermittent IVIG infusions to maintain clinical improvement, suggesting that, at least in these patients, the effect was due to treatment (9). In two of the 32 patients there was a short-lasting improvement, and subsequent IVIG infusions had no effect.

In a retrospective study, the following variables were significantly associated with a high chance for improvement after IVIG treatment: disease duration of less than 1 year; progression of weakness until treatment; absence of discrepancy in weakness between arms and legs; areflexia of the arms; and decreased motor nerve conduction velocity of the median nerve (9). It was calculated that the chance of improvement after IVIG treatment was over 90% if these five factors were present. Patients with CIDP who had active disease with weakness both in arms and legs had the highest chance of improvement after IVIG.

Controlled trials.   The observations in the open studies of IVIG treatment were supported by the results of a double-blind, placebo-controlled, crossover trial in patients with CIDP who were judged to have responded to IVIG treatment and who needed repeated IVIG infusions to maintain their improved condition (36). In this crossover study all patients deteriorated after discontinuation of regular IVIG treatment. Thereafter, the patients were randomized to IVIG (0.4 g/kg) or placebo (albumin) treatment for 5 consecutive days. All patients responded after IVIG; none of the patients responded after placebo treatment. Improvement after IVIG was always observed within 1 week after the start of treatment. The time lapse from the end of trial treatment to deterioration was significantly longer after treatment with IVIG (mean 6.4 weeks) than after placebo treatment (mean 1.3 weeks). Therefore, it was surprising that it was not possible to demonstrate the efficacy of IVIG treatment in a double-blind, placebo-controlled study in 28 patients with a clinical diagnosis of CIDP who were not treated with IVIG previously (35). Furthermore, three patients with a slowly progressive deterioration before the start of trial treatment had a rapid and dramatic clinical improvement within days after the start of placebo treatment. Another explanation for the results of this study may be the skewed deviation of CIDP patients within the treatment groups; as many as 10 of 13 patients in the placebo group and only six of 15 patients in the IVIG treatment group fulfilled the five criteria that were associated with improvement after IVIG treatment (9). These observations indicate that only a subgroup of patients with a CIDP seem to respond to IVIG treatment. These prognostic factors, however, need to be evaluated in a properly designed prospective study.

Recently Hahn et al. examined 30 CIDP in a double-blind, placebo-controlled, crossover trial. Seventeen patients had a chronic progressive and 13 had a chronic relapsing course of disease. After IVIG, 10 of the 17 chronic progressive patients (60%) and nine of the 13 chronic relapsing patients (69%) improved in the neurological disability score, clinical grade, and grip strength ($P < .002$). Improvement after placebo was seen in five patients; two of these five patients improved more while on IVIG treatment. The patients improving after IVIG were stabilized either with a single treatment course or with repeated IVIG treatment sometimes with additional small doses of immunosuppressive drugs (37). No trial is available at present that evaluates the effect IVIG over a long period of time.

Long-Term Treatment

Since IVIG treatment of patients with CIDP started in our department in the early 1980s, we have been able to follow these patients for a significant period of time. We analyzed 53 such CIDP patients who were treated with IVIG (38). None of the patients were on other treatments when IVIG was started. Clinical improvement was defined as improvement of at least 1 grade of the modified Rankin disability scale (39). Of the 53 patients treated with 0.4 g IVIG/kg for 5 consecutive days, 41 (77%) improved. Improvement was observed within 1–9 days (median 3.8 days) from onset of IVIG.

Since improvement could also be due to the natural course of the disease, we had a closer look at the 30 patients (73%) who needed intermittent IVIG treatment for at least 6 months. In this group of patients, it was strongly suggested that improvement was due to the effect of IVIG. The patients were followed for a median duration of 4.7 years (range 0.5–14 years). During this period we regularly tried to reduce the IVIG dosage. In the most extreme patient, intermittent treatment was needed for a period of 12 years in order to prevent relapses. After 6 months of treatment, two factors were associated with the necessity to maintain intermittent IVIG treatment for an additional period of at least 2 years. These factors were a low MRC sum score ($<50/60$) before onset of IVIG treatment (indicating profound muscular weakness), and lack of full clinical recovery (Rankin 0–1) within 6 months after the initiation of treatment. If these two factors are present at 6 months, the chance to stop IVIG within 2 years is about 30%; if these factors were not present, the chance to stop IVIG within 2 years was over 80%. This observation may have important implications for decision making, since intermittent IVIG treatment is very expensive. One may consider additional treatment or a change of treatment when there is a very high chance that IVIG will have to be continued for a long period of time. Serious side effects have not been observed in the patients, even in individuals who required intermittent IVIG treatment for up to 14 years.

Comparison Between Treatment with Steroids, PE, and IVIG

Several uncontrolled studies have included CIDP patients who were treated with PE, steroids, or other immunosuppressive treatments prior to IVIG treatment, or alternatively, after a failure of IVIG treatment. These studies show that some CIDP patients may improve after immunosuppressive treatment, PE, or IVIG, while other patients improve only after one particular treatment (9,33,34). This is also strikingly shown in a recent study by Nemni et al., who administered IVIG to nine CIDP patients who previously failed to improve after prednisone and/or PE. Six of these patients showed obvious clinical improvement after IVIG (33). This suggests that it is generally worthwhile to try another treatment modality in an individual patient if prednisone, PE, or IVIG fails. Figure 2 gives a schematic impression of the response to different treatments; the actual overlap between the responders to these various treatments appears to be greater.

There is only one controlled study comparing PE with IVIG (40). In this crossover study, 20 patients were randomized to receive either of the two treatments for 6 weeks, followed by a washout period before they received the other treatment. The treatment schedule was two PE sessions during the first 3 weeks followed by one exchange for the following 3 weeks, or 0.4 g IVIG/kg in weeks 1–3 and 0.2 g/kg in weeks 4–6. Of 20 patients, only 13 received both treatments, whereas four did not worsen

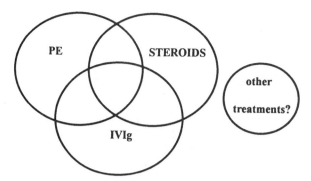

Figure 2 Response to various treatments in CIDP. Schematic impression of the response to different treatments; the actual overlap between the responders to these various the treatments appears to be greater.

sufficiently to receive the second treatment; 3 patients left the study for various reasons. With both treatment schedules, statistically significant improvement occurred compared to baseline for the following end points: overall neurological disability score, muscle weakness, and compound muscle action potentials (CMAP) of various muscles ($P < .001–.006$). Improvement after IVIG was comparable to the effect of PE. Furthermore, the treatment schedules were chosen in such a way that the costs were comparable. Subsequently, the patients were able to enter an open trial; as expected, the duration of improvement was transient in most patients, and the maintenance frequency and IVIG dosage varied greatly among patients. The authors suggested that IVIG may be the preferable initial treatment in many patients.

The cost of treatment is important. IVIG and PE are both expensive treatments. To compare the costs of IVIG and PE, one has to take into account the costs for PE personnel, equipment, and other logistics. Not only in our country (The Netherlands), but also in the United States, the cost of five PE sessions or an IVIG course totaling 2 g/kg seems to be more or less equal (41). Corticosteroids, on the other hand, are cheap, but the complications can be severe and expensive to treat as well. Because of the potentially serious side effects of prednisone, especially in children, we start treatment with IVIG as soon as the patient has reached a degree of muscular weakness that significantly interferes with lifestyle or prevents an independent existence. The effectiveness and the advantages and disadvantages of PE, steroids, and IVIG treatment are summarized in Table 3.

Treatment Schedule

The best IVIG dosage schedule in CIDP patients is not known. Initially most patients are treated with 0.4 g IVIG/kg/day for 5 consecutive days. With this dosage no major complications are observed. One may treat a CIDP patient with 1.0 g IVIG/kg/day for 2 days or even the double dosage in a single day; it was shown in Kawasaki disease that such a rapidly administered total dosage appeared to be even more effective (42). However, especially in older patients, one has to beware of possible fluid dysbalance and increased plasma viscosity due to an overhead of IVIG (43) resulting in vascular

Table 3 Comparison Between Various Treatments for CIDP

Treatment	Effective	Estimated % responders	Major side effects	Availability/ logistics	Cost
Prednisone	+	80	yes	+	low
Plasma exchange	+	80	no	±	high
IVIG	+	70[a]	no	+	high

[a]Depending on selection of patients (9).

problems (44). We usually treat CIDP patients with 0.4 g IVIG/kg/day for 5 days, and no major complications have been observed in more than 65 patients of which many needed repeated treatment. If a patient improves after IVIG treatment, we wait and observe. When secondary deterioration follows, a 0.4 g IVIG/kg course for 1 day is recommended. We then put the patient on a regular treatment scheme of 1 treatment day every 3–4 weeks depending on the severity and rate of deterioration. If this is insufficient, the treatment frequency is increased to 1 day every other week. If the patient reaches a stable condition, we gradually reduce the dosage instead of increasing the interval between the administered IVIG dosages. Figure 3 shows the IVIG treatment schedule we generally use.

IVIG MECHANISM OF ACTION

It is known from studies of various autoimmune diseases that IVIG can interfere with the regulation of the immune network, either by stimulation, blockage, or down-regulation. Overviews on the clinical use of IVIG and the various mechanisms of immunomodulation by IVIG have been published (45,46) and are also discussed elsewhere in this book. Studies on the mechanism of IVIG in CIDP are limited. In vitro studies have shown that IVIG contains anti-idiotypic antibodies that recognize a cross-reactive idiotype on antineuroblastoma (NBL) cell line antibodies present in roughly 50% of patients with GBS or CIDP. F(ab)$_2$ antibodies present in serum from recovered GBS patients can inhibit anti-NBL antibody activity in serum from patients with CIDP or with active GBS (14,47–49). These inhibitory antibodies, which develop during recovery from GBS, are also present in IVIG. Affinity chromatography revealed that these anti-idiotypic antibodies constitute less than 1% of the total IgG antibodies present in IVIG (49). It is not proven, however, that these various antibodies, including anti-NBL antibodies, have a direct pathogenic role in the process of disease. Whether a large pool of donors is essential for improvement of GBS or CIDP is questionable, since it was observed that improvement from CIDP can also occur after intermittent infusion of fresh frozen plasma (FFP) obtained from a limited number (20–28) of donors (27). A recent case report suggested that the mechanism of IVIG in CIDP is not primarily mediated by a specific Fc interaction (50). The mechanism of action of IVIG in patients with GBS or CIDP is far from clear, but there are arguments obtained from in vitro studies that a V region–dependent interaction plays a role in the regulation of GBS and CIDP.

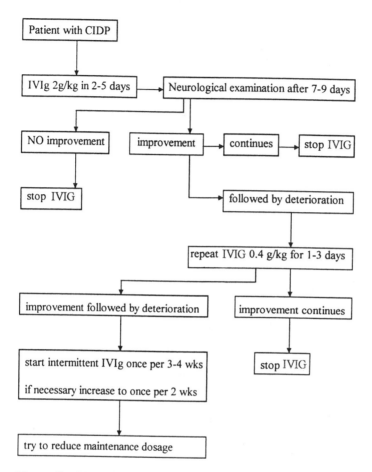

Figure 3   IVIG treatment schedule.

CONCLUSION AND FUTURE DIRECTIONS

Intravenous immunoglobulin treatment is effective in patients with a chronic inflammatory demyelinating polyneuropathy (CIDP). The proportion of patients that improve after IVIG treatment depends on the selection of patients. Patients with active disease and clear involvement of both arms and legs appear to have the highest chance to improve after IVIG treatment, but additional or prospective studies are needed to verify these criteria. One trial showed that IVIG is as effective as PE. All controlled studies have focused on the initial effect of treatment. Since CIDP is a chronic disease and most patients need treatment for a longer period of time, studies that focus on the long-term effect of treatment are now essential. We retrospectively followed such a group of patients for a long period of time. Over 50% needed intermittent treatment for at least

6 months. It appeared that most patients finally reached clinical remission after discontinuation of regular IVIG treatment. Even after years of intermittent IVIG treatment, no serious side effects occurred. We conclude that IVIG is effective and safe in CIDP even after a long duration of treatment (51). New studies are under way to compare IVIG with different steroid regimens. Further studies on the mechanism of IVIG in CIDP may reveal important features that can help to unravel the pathogenesis of the inflammatory demyelinating polyneuropathies.

REFERENCES

1. Dyck PJ, Prineas J, Pollard JD. Chronic inflammatory demyelinating polyneuropathy. In: Dyck, Thomas, eds. Peripheral Neuropathy. Philadelphia: Saunders, 3rd ed. 1993:1498–1518.
2. Asbury AK, Cornblath DR. Assessment of current diagnostic criteria for Guillain-Barré syndrome. Ann Neurol 1990; 27(suppl):S21–S24.
3. Cornblath DR, Asbury AK, Albers JW, et al. Research criteria for diagnosis of chronic inflammatory demyelinating polyneuropathy (CIDP). Neurology 1991; 617–618.
4. Hughes RAC, Sanders E, Hall S, Atkinson P, Colchester A, Payan P. Subacute idiopathic demyelinating polyradiculoneuropathy. Arch Neurol 1992; 49:612–616.
5. Dyck PJ, Lais AC, Ohta M, et al. Chronic inflammatory polyradiculoneuropathy, Mayo Clin Proc 1975; 50:621–637.
6. Barohn RJ, Kissel JT, Warmolts, et al. Chronic inflammatory demyelinating polyradiculoneuropathy, clinical characteristics, course and recommendations for diagnostic criteria. Arch Neurol 1989; 14: 878–884.
7. Steck AJ. Inflammatory neuropathy: pathogenesis and clinical features. Curr Opin Neurol Neurosurg 1992; 5:633–637.
8. McCombe PA, Pollard JD, McLeod JG. Chronic inflammatory demyelinating polyradiculoneuropathy. A clinical and electrophysiological study of 92 cases. Brain 1987; 110:1617–1630.
9. Van Doorn PA, Vermeulen M, Brand A, et al. Intravenous immunoglobulin treatment in patients with chronic inflammatory demyelinating polyneuropathy. Clinical and laboratory characteristics associated with improvement. Arch Neurol 1991; 48:217–220.
10. Van der Meché FGA, Van Doorn PA. Guillain-Barré syndrome and chronic inflammatory demyelinating polyneuropathy: immune mechanisms and update on current therapies. Ann Neurol 1995; 37(S1):S14–S31.
11. Dalakas MC, Engel WK. Immunoglobulin and complement deposits in peripheral nerves of patients with chronic relapsing polyneuropathy. Arch Neurol 1980; 37:637–640.
12. Liebert UG, Seitz RJ, Weber T, et al. Immunocytochemical studies of serum proteins and immunoglobulins in human sural nerve biopsies. Acta Neuropathol 1985; 68:39–47.
13. Ilyas AA, Mithen FA, Dalakas MC, et al. Antibodies to acidic glycolipids in Guillain-Barré syndrome and chronic inflammatory demyelinating polyneuropathy. J Neurol Sci 1992; 107:111–121.
14. Lundkvist I, Van Doorn PA, Vermeulen M, et al. Regulation of Autoantibodies in inflammatory demyelinating polyneuropathy: spontaneous and therapeutic. Immunol Rev 1989; 110:105–117.
15. Hartung HP, Hughes RAC, Taylor WA, et al. T cell activation in Guillain-Barré syndrome and in MS. Elevated serum levels of soluble IL-2 receptors. Neurology 1990; 40:215–218.
16. Hartung HP, Reiners K, Schmidt B, et al. Serum interleukin-2 concentrations in Guillain-Barré syndrome and chronic inflammatory demyelinating polyradiculoneuropathy: comparison

with other neurological diseases of presumed immunopathogenesis. Ann Neurol 1991; 30:48–53.

17. Stewart GJ, Pollard JD, McLeod JG, et al. HLA antigens in the Landry-Guillain-Barré syndrome and chronic relapsing polyneuritis. Ann Neurol 1978; 4:285–289.

18. Adams D, Festenstein H, Gibson JD, et al. HLA antigens in chronic relapsing idiopathic inflammatory polyneuropathy. J Neurol Neurosurg Psychiatry 1979; 42:184–186.

19. Feeney DJ, Pollard JD, McLeod JG, et al. HLA antigens in chronic inflammatory demyelinating polyneuropathy. J Neurol Neurosurg Psychiatry 1990; 53:170–172.

20. Van Doorn PA, Schreuder GMT, Vermeulen M, et al. HLA antigens in patients with chronic inflammatory demyelinating polyneuropathy. J Neuroimmunol 1991; 32:133–139.

21. Prineas JW, McLeod JG. Chronic relapsing polyneuritis. J Neurol Sci 1976; 27:427–458.

22. Dyck PJ, O'Brien PC, Oviatt KF, et al. Prednisone improves chronic inflammatory demyelinating polyradiculoneuropathy more than no treatment. Ann Neurol 1982; 11:136–141.

23. De Vivo DC, Engel WK. Remarkable recovery of a steroid-responsive recurrent polyneuropathy. J Neurol Neurosurg Psychiatry 1970; 33:62–69.

24. Dyck PJ. Intravenous immunoglobulin in chronic inflammatory demyelinating polyradiculoneuropathy and in neuropathy associated with IgM monoclonal gammopathy of unknown significance. Neurology 1990; 40:327–328.

25. Dyck PJ, Daube J, O'Brien, et al. Plasma exchange in chronic inflammatory demyelinating polyradiculoneuropathy. N Engl J Med 1986; 314:461–465.

26. Hahn AF, Bolton CF, Pilay N, et al. Plasma-exchange therapy in chronic inflammatory demyelinating polyneuropathy (CIDP): a double-blind, sham-controlled cross-over study. Brain 1996; 119:1055–1066.

27. Vermeulen M, van der Meché FGA, Speelman JD, et al. Plasma and gamma-globulin infusion in chronic inflammatory demyelinating polyneuropathy. J Neurol Sci 1985; 70:317–326.

28. Curro Dossi B, Tezzon F. High-dose intravenous gammaglobulin for chronic inflammatory demyelinating polyneuropathy. Ital J Neurol Sci 1987; 8:321–326.

29. Faed JM, Day B, Pollock M, et al. High-dose intravenous human immunoglobulin in chronic inflammatory demyelinating polyneuropathy. Neurology 1989; 39:422–425.

30. Vedanarayanan VV, Kandt RS, Lewis DV, et al. Chronic inflammatory demyelinating polyradiculoneuropathy of childhood. Treatment with high-dose intravenous immunoglobulin. Neurology 1991; 41:828–830.

31. Cornblath DR, Chaudry V, Griffin JW. Treatment of chronic inflammatory demyelinating polyneuropathy with intravenous immunoglobulin. Ann Neurol 1991; 30:104–106.

32. Azulay JPh, Pouget J, Pellissier JF, et al. Polyradiculonevrites chroniques. Rev Neurol (Paris) 1992; 148:752–761.

33. Nemni R, Amadio S, Fazio R, et al. Intravenous immunoglobulin treatment in patients with chronic inflammatory demyelinating neuropathy not responsive to other treatments. J Neurol Neurosurg Psychiatry 1994; 57(suppl):43–45.

34. Van Doorn PA. Intravenous immunoglobulin treatment in patients with chronic inflammatory demyelinating polyneuropathy. J Neurol Neurosurg Psychiatry 1994; 57(suppl):38–42.

35. Vermeulen M, Van Doorn PA, Brand A, et al. Intravenous immunoglobulin treatment in patients with chronic inflammatory demyelinating polyneuropathy: a double-blind, placebo-controlled study. J Neurol Neurosurg Psychiatry 1993; 56:36–39.

36. Van Doorn PA, Brand A, Strengers PFW, et al. High-dose intravenous immunoglobulin treatment in chronic inflammatory demyelinating polyneuropathy. A double-blind placebo-controlled cross-over study. Neurology 1990; 40:209–212.

37. Hahn AF, Bolton CF, Zochodne D, et al. Intravenous immunoglobulin treatment in chronic inflammatory demyelinating polyneuropathy. A double-blind, placebo-controled, cross-over study. Brain 1996; 199:1067–1077.

38. Van Doorn PA, Van Burken MMG, Vermeulen M, et al. Longterm I. V. immunoglobulin

(IVIg) treatment in patients with chronic inflammatory demyelinating polyneuropathy (CIDP). Annual Meeting of the Peripheral Nerve Society, Antalya, Turkey, Oct 6–9, 1995.

39. Van Swieten JC, Koudstaal PK, Visser MC, et al. Interobserver agreement for assessment of handicap in stroke patients. Stroke 1988; 19:604–607.

40. Dyck PJ, Litchy WJ, Kratz KM, et al. A plasma exchange versus immune globulin infusion trial in chronic inflammatory demyelinating polyradiculoneuropathy. Ann Neurol 1994; 36:838–845.

41. Thornton CA, Griggs RC. Plasma exchange and intravenous immunoglobulin treatment of neuromuscular disease. Ann Neurol 1994; 35:260–268.

42. Newberger JW, Takahashi M, Beiser AS, et al. A single intravenous infusion of gamma-globulin as compared with four infusions in the treatment of Kawasaki syndrome. N Engl J Med 1991; 324:1633–1639.

43. Reinhart WH, Berchtold PE. Effect of high-dose intravenous immunoglobulin therapy on blood rheology. Lancet 1992; 339:662–664.

44. Woodruff RK, Grigg AP, Firkin FC, et al. Fatal thrombotic events during treatment of autoimmune thrombocytopenia with intravenous immunoglobulin in elderly patients. Lancet 1986; ii:217–218.

45. Dwyer JM. Manipulating the immune system with immune globulin. N Engl J Med 1992; 326:107–116.

46. Hurez V, Kaveri SV, Kazatchkine MD. Normal polyspecific immunoglobulin G (IVIg) in the treatment of autoimmune diseases. J Autoimmun 1993; 6:675–681.

47. Van Doorn PA, Brand A, Vermeulen M. Anti-neuroblastoma cell line antibodies in inflammatory demyelinating polyneuropathy: inhibition in vitro and in vivo by IV immunoglobulin. Neurology 1988; 38:1592–1595.

48. Van Doorn PA, Rossi F, Brand A, et al. On the mechanism of high-dose intravenous immunoglobulin treatment of patients with chronic inflammatory demyelinating polyneuropathy. J Neuroimmunol 1990; 29:57–64.

49. Lundkvist I, Van Doorn PA, Veermeulen M, et al. Spontaneous recovery from the Guillain-Barré syndrome is associated with anti-idiotypic antibodies recognizing a cross-reactive idiotype on anti-neuroblastoma cell line antibodies. Clin Immunol Immunopathol 1993; 67:192–198.

50. Vermeulen M, Van Schaik IN. Anti-D immunoglobulin treatment in chronic inflammatory demyelinating polyneuropathy. J Neurol Neurosurg Psychiatry 1995; 58:383–384.

51. Van de Meché FGA, Van Doorn PA. The current place of high-dose immunoglobulins in the treatment of neuromuscular disorders. Muscle Nerve 1997: 20:136–147.

28

Intravenous Immunoglobulin in the Management of Myasthenia Gravis

David Grob

*Maimonides Medical Center and State University of New York
Health Science Center, Brooklyn, New York*

MANIFESTATIONS OF MYASTHENIA GRAVIS

Symptoms and Course

Myasthenia gravis (MG) is a chronic disease characterized by weakness and abnormal fatigability of any or all of the skeletal muscles. In 14% of patients the disease remains clinically limited to the extraocular muscles and orbiculares oculi, with ptosis and/or diplopia, while in 86% it becomes generalized—in 87% of these within a year after onset, and in 94% within 3 years (1). In patients with generalized MG, weakness and fatigability of muscles of the eyes, face, neck, trunk, and limbs occur, and in nearly half the patients there are episodes of difficulty swallowing, chewing, speaking, coughing, and, less often, breathing.

The course of the disease is variable. In most patients, there is gradual extension of the affected areas and fluctuating increase in severity of weakness during the first 1–3 years after onset. The maximal level of weakness is reached during the first year in 55%, the first 3 years in 70%, and the first 5 years in 85%. Most patients improve after the first 1–3 years, 11% have a complete remission, 33% remain unchanged; only 4% become worse after the first 1–3 years, and less than 4% die of the disease, usually during the first 3 years (2). Exacerbation of the disease may occur during upper respiratory tract infection, other infectious illness, emotional tension, or inadequate or excessive anticholinesterase medication, or may occur without obvious cause.

Serological Changes in MG

Elevated serum level of antibody to acetylcholine receptor of skeletal muscle, a glycoprotein located at the postsynaptic membrane of the neuromuscular junction, occurs in 90% of patients with generalized myasthenia gravis and 50% of patients with localized ocular myasthenia gravis (3). Most patients with myasthenia gravis also have elevated serum levels of other autoantibodies, most commonly skeletal muscle antibody and antithyroglobulin antibody, less often anti–single-strand DNA antibody, antinuclear antibody and antimicrosomal antibody, and, even less frequently anti–double-strand DNA antibody, antiparietal cell antibody, anticardiolipin antibody, Sjögren's antibody, anti-SM antibody, anti-RNP antibody, anti-JO-1 antibody, and antimitochondrial anti-body, among others. Hyperglobulinemia occasionally occurs (4,5), and hypogamma-globulinemia, especially decreased serum IgA, occasionally occurs, usually associated with thymoma or, less often, an extrathymic neoplasm (6-8).

Association of MG with Other Autoimmune Diseases

Other autoimmune diseases occur in 10% of female and 5% of male MG patients, and in 13% and 8% of patients with and without thymoma, respectively (9). In 3% of MG patients the associated autoimmune disease is thyroid (Graves' disease, Hashimoto's thyroiditis, or hypothyroidism), and in each of less than 1% psoriasis, pemphigus, au-toimmune leukopenia, thrombocytopenia and/or aplastic anemia, polymyositis, rheuma-toid arthritis, glomerulonephritis, systemic lupus erythematosus, ulcerative colitis, Crohn's disease, diabetes mellitus, or multiple sclerosis. Some of these diseases may, like MG, improve temporarily after administration of intravenous immunoglobulin (IVIG).

Mechanism of Weakness in MG

The weakness and fatigability of MG have been attributed to circulating antibodies to the acetylcholine receptor (3,10-12), although serum levels correlate poorly with the severity and clinical course of MG, except for the gradual decline in antibody level and severity of disease that occur after the initial 1-3 years after onset (2), and although the manifestations of antibody-negative disease are generally the same as of antibody-positive disease. These polyclonal antibodies decrease the number of acetylcholine re-ceptors at the neuromuscular junction and/or act to block their reactivity to the trans-mitter acetylcholine. With complement, they may lyse the postsynaptic membrane at the neuromuscular junction (11).

It is not clear which component of the acetylcholine receptor antibodies or which of these mechanisms is most important in the underlying pathogenesis of the disease. Immunization of animals with animal or human acetylcholine receptor induces antibodies to this protein and results in neuromuscular block resembling MG, a model for MG (12). Neuromuscular block can be passively transferred to animals using serum, im-munoglobulin, or acetylcholine receptor antibody from MG patients (13) or from ani-mals immunized with acetylcholine receptor (10). Immunoglobulin from MG patients degraded acetylcholine receptors at normal neuromuscular junctions more rapidly than immunoglobulin from normal subjects, at a rate that was correlated with severity of disease but not with serum levels of acetylcholine receptor antibody (14). The compo-nents of serum immunoglobulin and of the polyclonal acetylcholine receptor antibod-ies responsible for neuromuscular block in antibody-positive and antibody-negative MG patients have not been identified.

MANAGEMENT OF MG

Anticholinesterase Compounds

The weakness of MG is almost always ameliorated, although to a variable and usually limited degree, by anticholinesterase compounds, which delay the hydrolysis of ace-tylcholine by cholinesterase enzymes and thereby increase and prolong its action on the receptors. This response serves as the basis for diagnosis and symptomatic management of the disease in almost all patients. Oral pyridostigmine (Mestinon) parenteral neostigmine (Prostigmin) or pyridostigmine is administered in the lowest doses that have optimal effect on strength, especially of swallowing, cough, and respiration. During exacerbation of the disease, the patient becomes weaker and less responsive to anticholinesterase medication, presumably because more receptors have become unavailable or unresponsive to acetylcholine (2,15).

Other Therapeutic Measures

In patients in whom anticholinesterase medication does not provide sufficient symptomatic relief, corticosteroid and/or cytotoxic immunosuppressant medications are prescribed. In patients with generalized disease plasmapheresis or immunoadsorption and/ or IVIG may be administered and thymectomy performed (15). These measures are believed to produce improvement by altering the immunological parameters of the disease, although the mechanisms remain unclear. Any or all of these measures may be employed, in any order. In severely weak patients, especially those with respiratory failure, the more rapidly acting measures, such as corticosteroid, plasmapheresis, immunoadsorption, and/or intravenous immunoglobulin, are employed first.

Assisted Ventilation

During severe exacerbation of MG, dysphagia, weakness of respiration, cough, and obstruction of the upper airway often develop. Endotracheal intubation, suction, and mechanical ventilation are employed at any time when needed to maintain respiration and remove secretions. The approach of the emergency is recognized by weakening cough and aspiration of saliva, and by decreasing vital capacity, which can be measured if the orbicularis oris is strong enough to hold the mouthpiece. When vital capacity approaches the tidal volume, intubation and mechanical ventilation are usually needed. Adequate fluid intake is maintained to prevent dehydration and inspissation of mucus in the bronchioles. Atropine is employed only if necessary to diminish excessive secretions, and then used in small doses to avoid overatropinization, which causes drying of mucus in the respiratory tract, difficulty in suctioning, and atelectasis. Electrolyte balance is maintained by intravenous administration of sodium chloride and potassium chloride daily. A nasogastric tube is inserted, and feeding is begun to maintain an adequate nutritional state and for the enteral administration of pyridostigmine if desired. Antacid and ramotidine (Pepcid) or ranitidine (Zantac) are given to prevent peptic ulceration induced by anoxia, stress, anticholinesterase compounds, or corticosteroid administration. Because the dysphagia and impairment of cough and respiration that precede institution of mechanical ventilation predispose to atelectasis and pneumonia, a high index of suspicion must be maintained for pneumonia, which must be vigorously treated with intravenous antibiotics.

EFFECT OF IVIG IN MG

Effect on Strength and Vital Capacity

Pooled immunoglobulin was administered intramuscularly in small weekly doses to patients with MG in the 1970s, with reported benefit, but no detailed studies were carried out (16). In 1982, 20 g IVIG was administered three times a week for 2 weeks for treatment of idiopathic thrombocytopenic purpura (ITP) to a patient who also had MG; improvement was noted in both diseases (17). Since then, several studies have reported improvement in MG after IVIG (18–30). These studies have been open, nonblinded, and mostly on small numbers of patients. Arsura (28) reviewed eight studies of 60 patients, Edan and Landgraf (30) reviewed three more studies of 57 additional patients, and Ferreri et al. described 15 patients (24). Of these 132 patients, 110 received one or more courses of 0.4 g/kg IVIG daily for 5 days, 16 patients received 0.6–0.9 g/kg for 5 days (21), and six patients received 10 g daily for 5 days (22). The IVIG was usually administered as 3–6% solution in normal saline, or, less often, 9–12% in normal saline or distilled water. In some studies Sandoglobulin (Sandoz, Minneapolis, MN) was administered (18,25–27), and in some Intraglobulin (Biotest, Frankfurt, Germany) (17), Venoglobulin I (Alpha Therapeutic, Los Angeles, CA, and Institut Merceux, France) (21), Gamimmune N (Miles, West Haven, CT), Gammagard (Baxter, Glendale, CA), Gammar IV (Armour Pharmaceutical, Collegeville, PA), and Polygam (Baxter, American Red Cross, Washington, D.C.) (31). A large majority of patients had severe myasthenia gravis. Most had previously had thymectomy, and several had a thymoma or had been thymomectomized. About half received IVIG during acute exacerbation of MG, usually during respiratory failure, while about half received IVIG during a period of weakness that had been fairly static for 2–6 months. Nearly all patients were being treated with anticholinesterase medication, and most with corticosteroid or azathioprine or both, but doses of medication were kept fairly constant before, during, and after IVIG administration. In three studies of 21, 15, and 10 patients, no medication except anticholinesterase drugs were being administered (21,24,30).

Improvement in MG occurred in 74% of 132 patients (24,28,30) and in 50–100% ($73 \pm 30\%$) of each reported group, with the exception of one group of six patients who received only 10 g IVIG daily for 5 days, with no improvement (22). There was no significant difference between the rate of improvement in patients who received IVIG during acute exacerbation of MG and those treated during a period of static weakness: over 70% of patients in each group improved. Improvement in strength began within 1–20 days after the onset of IVIG, usually within the first week; reached a peak usually during the second week; and lasted 30–120 days. A decrease in strength, usually mild, occurred in 25% of MG patients after about two infusions of IVIG and lasted about 2 days.

In the more detailed studies of Arsura et al. (25,26), 14 patients with severe exacerbation of generalized MG were administered 31 courses of 3–6% IVIG (Sandoglobulin) 0.4 g/kg in normal saline, on each of 5 consecutive days. All other medications were kept constant. Improvement in muscle strength, including vital capacity, occurred after 22 of 31 courses (71%) in 11 of 14 patients (79%). Three patients had no improvement after each of two courses, while 11 patients improved after 22 of 25 courses. Improvement began a mean of 4.3 ± 1.2 days after the start of each course, peaked at 8.2 ± 2 days, and lasted a mean of 63 ± 56 days after a single course, 144 ± 73 days after two courses, 110 ± 38 days after the three courses, and 107 ± 49 days after the courses all patients received. Severity of disease improved from a mean Osserman class (25) 4.0 ± 0.5 (generalized moderately severe weakness) to 1.4 ± 0.5 (mild limb girdle weakness) (Fig. 1), and functional status (25) improved from a mean of 4.3 ± 0.7 to 1.4 ± 0.5. Vital capacity improved from a mean of 1944 ± 641 cc to 3028 ± 880 cc ($P < .01$) after a single course, 1261 ± 598 cc to 2558 ± 769 cc

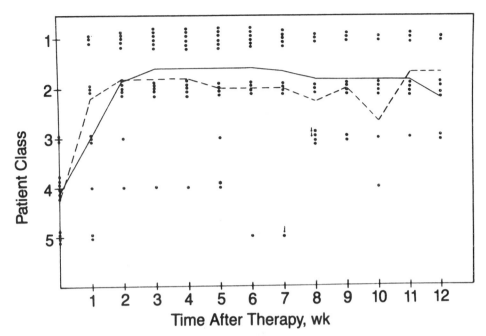

Figure 1 Effect of a 5-day course of daily IVIG on severity and distribution of weakness in 12 patients with class 4 or 5 moderately severe to very severe generalized myasthenia gravis (solid line), five of whom also received a second 5-day course of IVIG (broken line) after relapsing a mean of 36 days after the first course. (From Arsura et al., 25.) Class 1: oculofacial weakness; class 2: oculofacial and mild limb girdle weakness; class 3: oculofacial, mild limb girdle, and pharyngeal weakness; class 4: moderately severe generalized weakness, symptomatic at rest and restricted in daily activity; class 5: very severe generalized weakness, completely dependent for care.

($P < .05$) after two courses, 983 ± 165 cc to 2800 ± 1088 cc after three courses ($P < .05$), and 1845 ± 459 to 2844 ± 762 cc ($P < .01$) after the courses all patients received (Figs. 2, 3). Patients who were receiving corticosteroid were twice as likely to improve after IVIG as those who were not receiving corticosteroid, and had longer duration of improvement after IVIG—64 ± 63 days compared to 34 ± 31 days (28). In patients who were receiving prednisone, the daily dose could be reduced after IVIG from a mean of 60 ± 41 mg to 25 ± 13 mg without recurrence of weakness. In four of 14 patients, strength decreased transiently, beginning a mean of 1.8 ± 1.2 days after starting IVIG and lasting 2.3 ± 2.2 days, to a mild degree in three patients and severely in one patient on the second day.

Effect on Course of MG

IVIG administered three times a week for 2 weeks produced improvement lasting a mean of 34 days, occasionally up to 120 days, and the duration of improvement was prolonged to a mean of 64 days by the administration of corticosteroid (28). Since the course of MG improves after the first 1–3 years in the majority of patients (2), and since improvement is accelerated in varying degrees by corticosteroid, cytotoxic immunosup-

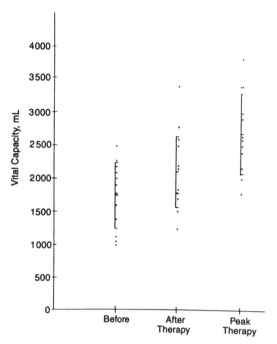

Figure 2 Vital capacity of 12 patients with moderately severe to very severe generalized myasthenia gravis before and after five daily infusions of IVIG and at peak vital capacity 8.6 ± 4.6 days after initiation of IVIG. (From Ref. 25.)

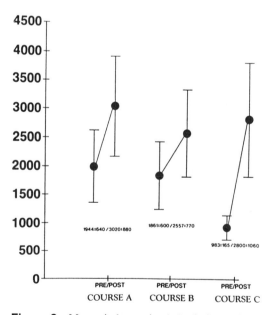

Figure 3 Mean vital capacity (cc) of nine patients with moderately severe to very severe myasthenia gravis who received 23 5-day courses of daily IVIG. The average vital capacity before and after all courses was 1845 ± 459 cc and 2844 ± 762 cc. (From Ref. 26.)

pressant drugs, and thymectomy, which are usually employed at some time, it is difficult to measure the effect of IVIG on the course of MG. Most studies have indicated that repeated courses of IVIG can each improve the disease for about a month, or for about 2 or more months if corticosteroid or cytotoxic immunosuppressant medication is also administered, but the long-term course of the disease is probably not altered (25,26,28,30).

ADVERSE EFFECTS OF IVIG

Less Serious Adverse Effects

Headache and Aseptic Meningitis

The most common adverse effect of IVIG has been diffuse, throbbing headache, which has occurred in 10% (32) to 56% (33) of patients, usually beginning after the last two infusions of a course of five, particularly after larger doses and more rapid infusion of any of the IVIG preparations. The headache was sometimes severe, but abated within hours to up to 3–5 days, especially after administration of an analgesic or narcotic. Severe headache has been attributed to aseptic meningitis, which has been demonstrated after the administration of IVIG in 1% (32) to 11% (33) of patients with MG (34,35) or other diseases, especially those with a history of migraine. Headache, meningismus, photophobia, nausea and sometimes vomiting, and fever began within 24 h after IVIG and lasted 3–5 days. The spinal fluid showed pleocytosis and increased concentration of protein and immunoglobulin. The cause of aseptic meningitis is not known (33).

Vasomotor Reactions

In about 5% of patients, IVIG infusion has been followed by fever, chills, myalgia, vasomotor, cardiovascular, and hypersensitivity reactions thought to be immune-mediated reactions to immunoglobulins, or secondary to bioactive substances such as prekallikrein activator or kallikrein (31). In the past, IVIG preparations produced allergic anaphylactoid reactions in 25% of patients, especially those with immunoglobulin deficiency, but removal of aggregated immunoglobulin from current preparations has rendered such reactions much less common. Immune complexes have been found in the serum of some patients after allergic reaction to IVIG (9).

Less that 5% of patients developed mild pedal edema or shortness of breath after IVIG, attributable to volume expansion (28). Less often, asthma has been precipitated or has recurred.

Serious Adverse Effects

These have been rare and have included thromboembolic events, hepatitis C transmission, and acute renal failure.

Thromboembolic Events

Thromboembolic events have been the most serious complication of IVIG, but have been rare. IVIG increases viscosity of the serum by 0.1–1 centripoise (mean 0.55), which can impair blood flow and trigger a thromboembolic event, especially in patients with preexisting vascular disease, high lipoproteins, or cryoglobulinemia (36). Fatal pulmonary embolus in one patient, and spinal cord infarction in another, occurring 2 and 7 days after the second IVIG infusion were described. A case of aseptic meningitis followed by bilateral cerebral thrombosis was reported in a 27-year-old woman with myasthenia gravis after 0.4 g/kg IVIG (Sandoglobulin) daily for 5 days (37). The patient developed severe, throbbing headache, nausea, vomiting, and fever after the fourth IVIG infusion. The spinal fluid contained 41 white blood cells/mm^3, with 32% neutrophils, 27% lymphocytes, 41% monocytes-histiocytes, 28 mg/dl protein and 49 mg/dl glucose (serum glucose 171 mg/dl). Ten days after completion of IVIG, while still having headaches, the patient developed a right homonomous hemianopia, right hemiparesis, and a hemisensory defect involving the face, arms, and leg. MRI of the brain showed ischemic infarctions in both frontal lobes and the left parietal and occipital lobes.

Rapid rise of platelet count after IVIG with thrombosis has occurred rarely in elderly atherosclerotic patients, or in neonates, who developed enterocolitis (36,37). Elderly patients and neonates have also been at risk for fluid overload, hypernatremia, hyperglycemia, increased proteinuria, and increased serum creatinine.

Hepatitis C

Hepatitis C virus (HCV) was transmitted before 1995 by certain preparations of IVIG, including Gammagard (Hyland Divsiion of Baxter Healthcare Corporation, Glendale, CA), Polygram (Baxter from American Red Cross plasma), and Gammonativ (Kabivitram, Stockholm, Sweden) (38–46). The risk of transmission of HCV was higher in patients with hypogammaglobulinemia. IVIG prepared after May 1994 is available and is considered to have a high degree of safety with respect to HCV contamination. Most manufacturers now use only anti-HCV-negative plasma donors, and include solvent-detergent treatment (Gammagard-SD, Polygam, and Venoglobulin S [Alpha Therapeutic]), enzyme treatments (Sandoglobulin [Sandoz] and Iveegam [Immuno-U.S.]), or incubation at room temperature (Gamimmune N [Miles]), procedures that inactivate viruses. Additional viral inactivation measures are being developed, such as exposure to ultraviolet light or heat pasteurization, and IVIG preparations currently produced are considered to be safe, though no process can guarantee absence of all viruses, including those still unknown. There has been no transmission of human immunodeficiency virus (HIV) by any preparation of IVIG, though reverse transcriptase was found in the serum of two recipients in 1986 (47).

Acute Renal Failure

At least 39 adult patients, half of whom had preexisting renal disease, have been reported to have developed reversible acute renal failure during IVIG therapy with 0.35–1 g/kg/day (48–52). Increase in serum creatinine was noted after 1–6 days of IVIG administration (48,49). Oliguria or anuria developed in one-third of the patients, with dialysis becoming necessary in one-fourth. Creatinine returned to baseline within 2–60 days after discontinuation of IVIG, in 84% within 14 days. Although the concentration of IVIG solution and the rate of administration have seldom been reported, it is believed that more rapid administration of higher concentrations of IVIG may be more likely to cause renal injury. In one patient, IVIG was successfully readministered when the daily dose was decreased by 50% and the infusion rate was reduced by half (50). Almost all commercially available IVIG preparations have on rare occasions produced acute renal failure, especially in patients with renal insufficiency or fluid depletion (51). The cause is not known, but the biopsy finding of markedly swollen and vacuolated proximal tubular cells with preservation of the brush borders suggests that it may be due to uptake by these cells of sucrose, maltose, or sorbitol, which are employed in 5–10% concentration as stabilizing agents in the immunoglobulin solutions employed (49,52).

EFFECT OF IVIG ON BLOOD

Effect of IVIG on Serum Level of Acetylcholine Receptor Antibody

In most studies IVIG produced no consistent change in the serum level of AChR antibody (Fig. 4) (19,22,25–28). In some of the smaller trials, a decline in level during (17,20,21) or 1–10 days after IVIG (24) was reported, followed in one of these trials by a return to the initial level 25 days after IVIG (21). A correlation was reported between the decline in antibody level and improvement in strength, but these reports have not been confirmed.

Effect of IVIG on Other Components of Blood

IVIG affects many of the components of blood, but the relation of these changes to the therapeutic actions of IVIG is not clear. Administration of IVIG increases the plasma

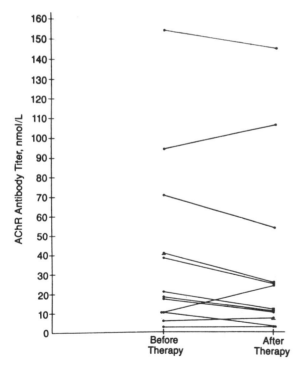

Figure 4 Serum level of acetylcholine receptor antibody of 12 patients with moderately severe to very severe myasthenia gravis before and after a 5-day course of daily IVIG. The mean serum level was 40.7 ± 35.7 nmol/L before IVIG, 35.7 ± 45.5 nmol/L after the fifth day infusion, and 39.2 ± 50.9 nmol/L 1 month later. (From Ref. 25.)

concentration of immunoglobulin to about 200% of baseline value for several days (24), and decreases production and increases the rate of disappearance of immunoglobulin from the plasma; hypoglobulinemia has the opposite effect (54). A small decrease in white blood count, attributed to decrease in both polymorphonuclear leukocytes and lymphocytes, has been reported (17,25–28), with return to baseline within a week (26). Occasionally more severe leukopenia has occurred. Immunoglobulin-positive cells rose from 13% to 26% after the fifth day of IVIG, attributed to passive acquisition of IgG by a subset of lymphocytes (25). An increase in CD8 and NK T cells and a decrease in CD4 T cells, with a decrease in the ratio of helper to suppressor cells, has been reported (19,25), but another study found no change in the number of any of these cells (22). Complement components (17,25–28), and immune complexes measured by C1q binding, did not change (23), but the binding of C3 and C4 to antibody sensitized cells was inhibited (55), and release of interleukin-1 and tumor necrosis factor (TNF) was reduced.

MECHANISM BY WHICH IVIG IMPROVES MG

IVIG has many effects on immunological functions (56), but its mechanism of action in MG is not known, though there are several possibilities. The immunoglobulin in the serum of MG patients degrades acetylcholine receptors in the neuromuscular junction at a rate correlated with severity of disease, but not with the level of acetylcholine receptor antibodies (14), resulting in neuromuscular block (10,13). IVIG might reduce the neuromuscular block by competitively blocking this action of immunoglobulin of the MG patient on the acetylcholine receptors or on the postsynaptic membrane, similar to the blockade of the Fc receptors of the reticuloendothelial system produced by IVIG in patients with idiopathic thrombocytopenic purpura (55,56), but such a mechanism has not yet been demonstrated in MG.

Administered IVIG has been reported to react with acetylcholine receptor antibodies (24,53,57) and immune complexes (58) in the serum of MG patients. While IVIG did not significantly alter the total reactivity of polyclonal acetylcholine receptor antibodies in the serum of MG patients, the effect of IVIG on the monoclonal antibodies, or on the as yet unidentified component of immunoglobulin that causes neuromuscular block, or on the reactivity of this component with acetylcholine receptors or postsynaptic membrane, is not known.

IVIG administration floods the recipient with a diverse array of antibody molecules, some of which are anti-idiotypic antibodies which bind to the variable region of other antibodies, including autoantibodies. ("Idiotype" refers to an antigenic marker located within variable regions of the immunoglobulin molecule.) Anti-idiotypic antibodies in IVIG have been reported to neutralize acetylcholine receptor antibodies in the serum of MG patients and to delay synthesis of antibody (24,53), similar to the effect of anti-idiotypic antibodies in IVIG on the binding of antithyroglobulin, anti-DNA, anti-intrinsic factor, and anti–factor VIII antibodies to their autoantigens in vitro (59), and perhaps on the synthesis of these antibodies.

IVIG inhibits the binding of activated complement to some target cells (55,60) and might inhibit the complement-mediated damage to neuromuscular junctional folds that occurs in MG (11), similar to the inhibition by IVIG of other complement-mediated immune damage (55). Such inhibition has not, however, been demonstrated in MG.

It has been reported that IVIG downregulates the activity of CD4 T cells (25,61). While this has not been associated with a decrease in total polyclonal acetylcholine receptor antibodies in MG serum, it is not known if there are any changes in production of monoclonal antibodies or in the component of immunoglobulin responsible for neuromuscular block. IVIG has also been reported to downregulate production and activity of some cytokines, such as interleukin-1 and TNF (61), but the role of this in MG is not known. Most IVIG preparations contain small amounts of HLA class I and class II antigens, certain cytokines, and soluble CD4 and CD8, which could interfere with antigen presentation through inhibition of the interaction between HLA class II and membrane-bound CD4, which is important for T cell activation (61). This could be a mechanism for immunosuppression.

It has been suggested that IVIG might block and internalize Fc receptors on phagocytic or effector cells, similar to the removal of antibody-coated platelets by reticuloendothelial cells of the spleen and liver in autoimmune thrombocytopenia (61,62), but such a mechanism has not been shown in MG.

COMPARISON OF IVIG WITH OTHER THERAPEUTIC MEASURES FOR MG

Corticosteroids

In patients whose weakness interferes with normal activity, especially swallowing, speech, cough, or respiration, despite anticholinesterase medication, the next step in therapy is usually administration of corticosteroid, 30–60 mg of prednisone or 2–4.5 mg of dexamethasone daily. A decrease in strength occurs in most patients beginning within 3 days and reaching maximum within 5–10 days, of moderate to severe degree in some, occasionally requiring intubation and assisted ventilation (63). Improvement above the initial level of strength occurs in 90% of patients, beginning between days 4 and 15 and reaching maximum between days 10 and 20, of moderate to marked degree in 50%. Larger doses of corticosteroid produce more rapid improvement, and very high dose "pulses"—e.g., 2 g methylprednisolone or 400 mg dexamethasone intravenously every 3–5 days for three doses—produce less severe exacerbation of weakness (64). Increase in weakness occurs on days 1–2 after each infusion, and increase in strength above the original level begins on days 2–4 after each infusion and reaches maximum between days 3 and 15 after the third infusion. Small doses of corticosteroid that are slowly increased over many weeks also produce less frequent and less marked exacerbation, but improvement is of slower onset and sometimes of lesser degree.

Maintenance of improvement requires continued administration of corticosteroid, which usually sustains improvement indefinitely except for intermittent exacerbations of weakness, which may occur at any time, especially during respiratory infections, and may require increase of maintenance dose. The maintenance dose of corticosteroid is gradually reduced to the lowest level compatible with adequate strength, and the corticosteroid is discontinued whenever possible, because high doses of prolonged administration may produce peptic ulcer, glucose intolerance, hypertension, weight gain, mood changes, cataracts, osteoporosis, vertebral compression, aseptic necrosis of the femoral heads, steroid myopathy, and increased susceptibility to infection.

The improvement in strength that occurs in 90% of patients within 1–2 weeks after starting corticosteroid is more consistent and generally of greater degree than that produced by IVIG, plasmapheresis or immunoadsorption, or cytotoxic immunosuppressant drugs, and of much more rapid onset than that produced by cytotoxic drugs or thymectomy. Corticosteroid is therefore usually the initial measure added to anticholinesterase medication when exacerbation of the disease occurs. In the minority of patients who do not improve on corticosteroid or who require maintenance doses that produce serious side effects, IVIG and/or plasmapheresis or immunoadsorption can be added to or substituted for corticosteroid, though the duration of improvement after these measures (1–2 months) is usually of much shorter duration than that of maintenance corticosteroid. The side effects of IVIG and decrease in strength during the first few days of administration are much less frequent and less severe than after corticosteroid.

Plasmapheresis

A series of exchanges of plasma for an equal volume of saline and 5% albumin (usually 2 L three times a week) resulted in excellent to good improvement in 68%, fair in 15%, and poor in 15% of 328 reported MG patients (65). Improvement usually began about 48 h after the first exchange (occasionally as early as 3–7 h), reached a peak after the fourth exchange (occasionally up to 14 exchanges), and lasted 1–2 months (occasionally 3–6 months) or longer if supplemented by the administration of corticosteroid or cytotoxic immunosuppressant drug. Improvement in strength has been attributed to reduction in the serum concentration of acetylcholine receptor antibody to a mean of 32% of the original level, with return to or above the original level within 2–3 weeks, though improvement usually began days after the fall in serum concentration, lasted weeks after return to the original level, and was the same in seronegative as in seropositive patients. Adverse effects of plasma exchange occurred in about one-fourth to one-half the exchanges in one-half the patients, were due mainly to the removal of blood or plasma more rapidly then replacement by 5% albumin and saline, and consisted of hypotension, lightheadedness, nausea, and, less often, vomiting, headache, chilliness, or abdominal cramps. Less often, citrate used as an anticoagulant caused bleeding and paresthesias or tetany due to hypocalcemia, and least often hypofibrinogenemia caused bleeding. More severe hypotension occurred in 2% of exchanges in 5–19% of patients. Death occurred in 0.03–0.6% of exchanges in 0.1–3% of patients and was attributed to cardiac arrest, pulmonary embolus, sepsis, bleeding, or anaphylaxis.

Although plasma exchange and IVIG administration have opposite effects on serum concentration of immunoglobulin and acetylcholine receptor antibody, the incidence, time course, and duration of improvement in MG have been about the same after each procedure. The two procedures have been used sequentially in MG patients, with additive effects on strength (66). A high degree of improvement has been more frequent after plasma exchange, and there has been a report of four patients whose MG crisis improved after plasma exchange following failure to respond to 3–5 days of 0.2–0.4 g/kg IVIG daily, and in three of the four to corticosteroids as well (67). Minor adverse effects are common, and major adverse effects uncommon, after plasma exchange or IVIG, and may be less common after IVIG. If equipment and trained personnel are available, plasma exchange is usually performed prior to IVIG administration in more severely weak MG patients, especially those in respiratory failure, because it is likely to be more effective. IVIG administration is usually performed first in less severely weak patients, since it is easier to administer, requires no special equipment, and has less frequent side effects.

Immunoadsorption

Perfusion of 2500 ml of plasma through a polyvinyl alcohol resin on each of four alternate days resulted in about the same incidence, time course, degree and duration of improvement, and fall in serum concentration of acetylcholine receptor antibody in 14 studied and 83 reported MG patients, as did plasma exchange in 328 reported patients (65). Adverse effects of immunoadsorption were attributable to withdrawal of blood more rapidly than it was returned, and were almost completely prevented or ameliorated by infusing sufficient isotonic saline intravenously before or during the procedure. While the incidence of mild hypotensive symtpoms was the same as during plasma exchange, the incidence of more severe adverse effects was much lower. Immunoadsorption has the advantage over plasma exchange of less severe side effects and no need for protein replacement, and has the advantage over IVIG of a higher incidence of more marked improvement and a lower incidence of adverse effects, but it requires equipment that is not yet generally available in the United States.

Cytotoxic Immunosuppressant Drugs

The drugs so far available do not begin to produce improvement until after 2–12 months of administration; maximal improvement occurs in twice this time, so that their efficacy is difficult to evaluate in a disease that usually improves spontaneously after 1–3 years. Nevertheless, azathioprine (Imuran), 150–200 mg (2–3 mg/kg) daily by mouth, the most widely used immunosuppressant, is recommended for patients with moderate to severe disease who do not have adequate strength on doses of corticosteroid small enough to avoid significant side effects (15). Because azathioprine or other immunosuppressants may produced leukopenia, and less often thrombocytopenia or anemia, dose- and duration-related, the blood count should be monitored every week or 2. Because leukopenia may develop suddenly and be first indicated by infection, especially tonsillitis, the white blood cell count should be repeated as soon as a bacterial infection is suspected. Cyclophosphamide (Cytoxan) is similar in dose, effect, and complications but may also cause hemorrhagic cystitis. Methotrexate, 2.5–5 mg daily by mouth, has also been used. Cyclosporine (Sandimmune) (3–5 mg/kg/day by mouth) is a more potent immunosuppressant, but its nephrotoxicity needs to be monitored. None of the cytotoxic immunosuppressant drugs acts rapidly or effectively enough to be substituted for corticosteroid, plasmapheresis, immunoadsorption, or IVIG in the management of exacerbations of MG. They may be of help as maintenance therapy, particularly to reduce the maintenance dose of corticosteroid.

Thymectomy

Sixty percent of patients with MG have a hyperplastic thymus containing germinal centers; 25% have a thymus that is normal or, in the elderly, normally involuted or undetectable; and 15%, mainly those over the age of 40 years and with generalized disease, have a thymoma. Although the natural course of the disease is usually one of gradual improvement after the first 1–3 years and no prospective trial of thymectomy has been performed, most patients who have undergone removal of a hyperplastic thymus do appear to improve more than matched controls (30% during the first year and over 50% within 5 years) (2). The best results usually occur in younger patients, in those with disease of recent onset, in females, and in patients who have a "total" thymectomy with removal of all detected or suspected thymic tissue after splitting the sternum. While some patients, especially young females with recent onset of MG and high serum level of acetylcholine receptor, improve within days or weeks after thymectomy, the procedure does not substitute for more rapidly acting measures such as corticosteroids, plasmapheresis or immunoadsorption, or IVIG.

Thymectomy will also remove small, unsuspected thymomas or prevent their later development. Thymomas must be detected by x-ray, CT, or MRI and removed as early as possible, before local invasion has occurred. Thirty percent of patients with thymoma have or develop myasthenia gravis, 20% nonthymic cancer, and 5% one of the other diseases of autoimmunity, especially red cell or bone marrow aplasia (68). The associated disease usually determines the prognosis. Myasthenia gravis in patients with thymoma tends to be more severe and to carry double the mortality rate of MG in patients without thymoma. Removal of thymoma, even in toto, does not usually affect the course of MG or of other associated disease.

ROLE OF IVIG IN THE MANAGEMENT OF MG

While IVIG administration improves strength in most patients with severe MG, very few clinical trials have been carried out to ascertain optimal dose or duration of treatment, comparison with other therapeutic measures, or administration with or sequential to other therapeutic measures. The most commonly employed dosage schedule (one or more courses of 0.4 g/kg/day for 5 days) is the same as was employed in the first therapeutic trial of IVIG in immune thrombocytopenia 15 years ago. Half this daily dose was ineffective in each of six MG patients (22). Additional controlled studies are needed before the optimal dose and role of IVIG in the management of MG can be accurately assessed.

Each course of IVIG, usually about 5 days, improves MG for about a month, or about 2 months if supplemented by corticosteroid. Continued administration of IVIG for more than 5 days, or sequential administration of several courses, prolongs improvement, but there is no good evidence that it affects the long-range course of the disease. Less serious adverse effects of IVIG are common, and major adverse effects are rare. However, major adverse effects such as thromboemboli, acute renal failure, and transmission of hepatitis C are sufficiently serious that IVIG should be reserved for treatment of severe MG that is not being adequately managed by anticholinesterase medication and doses of corticosteroid that are not producing serious side effects.

The time of onset of improvement of severe MG treated by IVIG, corticosteroid, plasma exchange, and immunoadsorption is about the same, beginning during the first week of treatment and increasing during the second week, while improvement produced by cytotoxic immunosuppressant drugs or thymectomy usually begins after several months.

The incidence and degree of improvement of severe MG are greatest after corticosteroid, and duration of improvement is usually maintained by continued administration of corticosteroid, though it is necessary to reduce the dose to avoid serious side effects. The incidence and degree of improvement of severe MG after plasma exchange or immunoadsorption appear to be somewhat greater than after IVIG, while the duration of improvement appears to be about the same.

Both minor and major adverse effects of high doses of corticosteroid are more frequent than those of the other therapies, but can usually be lessened by reducing the dose. Minor adverse effects are common after IVIG or plasma exchange, but major adverse effects are uncommon. While major adverse effects after IVIG or plasma exchange are rare, they may be serious, so that these therapies are reserved for patients with severe MG who cannot be adequately managed with anticholinesterase compounds and doses of corticosteroid that are not producing serious side effects.

In the management of severe MG not adequately controlled by anticholinesterase medication, the first step is to assist ventilation if this is impaired. The next measure is usually corticosteroid administration. If the patient does not respond adequately, the next measure is usually plasma exchange or immunoadsorption if equipment is available, or IVIG if equipment is unavailable. If the patient responds inadequately to plasma exchange or immunoadsorption, IVIG is usually then administered. If the weakness is not very severe, IVIG is sometimes administered in lieu of plasma exchange or immunoadsorption, because of greater ease of administration and lesser, though still high, expense. The purchase cost of immunoglobulin for intravenous administration is about $25 per gram, or $3000 for 5 days' infusion of 24 g/day to a 60-kg patient. Regardless of which measure is initially employed, other measures may be added simultaneously or sequentially, depending on need. Cytotoxic immunosuppressant medication may be begun at any time and thymectomy performed, preferably early in the course of MG, usually after an attempt has been made to improve ventilation.

While IVIG increases the serum concentration of immunoglobulin and does not affect the level of acetylcholine receptor antibody, and plasma exchange (or immunoadsorption) decreases the serum concentration of both, these measures have similar effects in improving strength of MG patients and can be employed sequentially in the management of MG (66). If plasma exchange is carried out after IVIG administration, it removes some of the infused IVIG. If used sequentially, it would seem preferable to administer IVIG after completing a course of plasma exchange, as has been done in the treatment of refractory autoimmune thrombocytopenia (62), but this is still to be evaluated in MG.

REFERENCES

1. Grob D. Myasthenia gravis: a review of pathogenesis and treatment. Arch Intern Med 1961; 108:615–638.
2. Grob D, Arsura EL, Brunner NG, Namba T. The course of myasthenia gravis and therapies affecting outcome. Ann NY Acad Sci 1987; 505:472–499.
3. Lindstrom JM, Seybold ME, Lennon VA, Whittingham S, Duane DD. Antibody to acetylcholine receptor in myasthenia gravis: prevalence, clinical correlates, and diagnostic value. Neurology 1976; 26:1054–1059.
4. Oosterhuis HJGH, Vander Geld H, Feltkamp TEW, Peetom F. Myasthenia gravis with hypergammaglobulinemia and antibodies. J Neurol Neurosurg Psychiatry 1964; 27:345.

5. Rowland LP, Osserman EF, Scharfman WB, Balsam RF, Ball S. Myasthenia gravis with myeloma-type gamma-G (IgG) immunoglobulin abnormality. Am J Med 1969; 46:599–605.

6. TeVelde K, Huber J, Vander Slikke LB. Primary acquired hypogammaglobulinemia, myasthenia and thymoma. Ann Intern Med 1966; 65:554.

7. Behan PO, Simpson JA, Behan WMH. Decreased serum-IgA in myasthenia gravis. Lancet 1976; 1:593–594. Letter.

8. Brahms J, Shane C, Papatestis AE, Genkins G, Aufses AH Jr. Serum IgA in myasthenia gravis. Lancet 1976; 1:1243–1244. Letter.

9. Palmisani MT, Evoli A, Batocchi AP, Bertoccioni E, Tonali P. Myasthenia gravis and associated autoimmune diseases. Muscle Nerve 1994; 17:1234–1235. Letter.

10. Lindstrom JM, Engel AG, Seybold ME, Lennon VA, Lambert EH. Pathological mechanisms in experimental myasthenia gravis. II. Passive transfer of experimental autoimmune myasthenia gravis in rats with antiacetylcholine receptor antibodies. J Exp Med 1976; 144:739–753.

11. Nakano S, Engel AG. Myasthenia gravis: quantitative immunochemical analysis of inflammatory cells and detection of complement membrane attack complex at the end plate. Neurology 1993; 43:1167–1172.

12. Patrick J, Lindstrom J. Autoimmune response to acetylcholine receptor. Science 1973; 180:871–872.

13. Howard JF, Sanders OB. Passive transfer of human myasthenia gravis to rats. 1. Electrophysiology of the developing neuromuscular block. Neurology 1980; 30:760–764.

14. Takeo G, Masakatsu M, Matsuo H, et al. Effect of myasthenia IgG on degradation of junctional acetylcholine receptor. Muscle Nerve 1993; 16:840–848.

15. Grob D. Myasthenia gravis. In: Rakel RE, ed. Conn's Current Therapy. 1992:864–872.

16. Genkins G, Papatestas AE, Kornfeld P, Horowitz SH. Studies in myasthenia gravis: staging and gammaglobulin. In: Dau P, ed. Plasmapheresis and the Immunobiology of Myasthenia Gravis. Boston: Houghton Mifflin, 1979:144–149.

17. Fateh-Moghadam A, Besinger U, Guersen RG. Ein kliniches Modell zur Regulation der Humoralen. Immunantwort: Infusion therapie. Beitr Infusionther. Klin Ernahr 1982; 9:69–79.

18. Devathason G, Kueh YK, Chong PN. High-dose intravenous gammaglobulin for myasthenia gravis. Lancet 1984; 2:809–810.

19. Ippoliti G, Cosi V, Piccolo G, Lombardi M, Mantegaz R. High-dose intravenous gammaglobulin for myastghenia gravis. Lancet 1984; 2:809.

20. Besinger UA, Fateh-Moghadam A, Knorr-Helds, Wick M, Kissel H, Albiez M. Immunomodulation in myasthenia gravis by high-dose intravenous 7-S immunoglobulins. Ann NY Acad Sci 1987; 505:828–831.

21. Gadjos PH, Outin HD, Morel E, Raphael JC, Goulon M. High-dose intravenous gammaglobulin for myasthenia gravis: an alternative to plasma exchange? Ann NY Acad Sci 1987; 505:842–844.

22. Uchiyama M, Yukinovu I, Takaya N, Moriuchi J, Shimizu H, Arimori S. High-dose gammaglobulin therapy of generalized myasthenia gravis. Ann NY Acad Sci 1987; 505:868–871.

23. Ibars Bonaventura I, Ponseti J, Espanol T, Guiu-Matias J, Codina-Puiggros A. High-dose intravenous gamma-globulin therapy for myasthenia gravis. J Neurol 1987; 234:363.

24. Ferrero B, Durelli L, Cavallo R, et al. The mechanism of action of high-dose immunoglobulin G. Ann NY Acad Sci 1993; 681:563–566.

25. Arsura EL, Bick A, Brunner NG, Namba T, Grob D. High-dose intravenous immunoglobulin in the management of myasthenia gravis. Arch Intern Med 1986; 146:1365–1368.

26. Arsura EL, Bick A, Brunner NG, Grob D. Effects of repeated doses of intravenous immunoglobulin in myasthenia gravis. Am J Med Sci 1988; 295:438–443.

27. Cook L, Howard JF, Folds TD. Immediate effects of intravenous IgG administration on peripheral blood band T cells and polymorphonuclear cells in patients with myasthenia gravis. J Clin Immunol 1988; 8:23–31.

28. Arsura EL. Experience with intravenous immunoglobulin in myasthenia gravis. Clin Immunol Immunopathol 1989; 53:S170–S179.

29. Evoli A, Bartoccioni E, Palmisani MT, Provenzano C, Tonali P. IgG therapy in myasthenia gravis patients. J Autoimmun 1991; 4(6):XXXI.

30. Edan G, Landgraf F. Experience with intravenous immunoglobulin in myasthenia gravis: a review. J Neurol Neurosurg Psychiatry 1994; 57:55–56.

31. Weisman L. The safety of intravenous immunoglobulin preparations. Isr J Med Sci 1994; 30:459–463.

32. Scribner CL, Kapit RM, Phillips ET, Rickles NM. Aseptic meningitis and intravenous immunoglobulin therapy. Ann Intern Med 1994; 121:305–306.

33. Sekul EA, Cupler EJ, Dalakas MC. Aseptic meningitis associated with high-dose intravenous immunoglobulin therapy: frequency and risk factors. Ann Intern Med 1994; 121:259–262.

34. Meiner Z, Ben-Hur T, River Y, Reches, A. Aseptic meningitis as complication of intravenous immunoglobulin therapy for myasthenia gravis. J Neurol Neurosurg Psychiatry 1993; 56:(7)830–831. Letter.

35. Ellis RJ, Swenson MR, Bajorek J. Aseptic meningitis as a complication of intravenous immunoglobulin therapy for myasthenia gravis. Muscle Nerve 1994; 17:683–684.

36. Dalakas MC. High-dose intravenous immunoglobulin and serum viscosity: risk of precipitating thromboembolic events. Neurology 1994; 30:459–463.

37. Steg RE, Lefkowitz DM. Cerebral infarction following intravenous immunoglobulin therapy for myasthenia gravis. Neurology 1994; 44:1180–1181.

38. Lever AM, Webster AD, Brown D, Thomas HC. Non-A, non-B hepatitis occurrence in agammaglobulinemic patients after intravenous immunoglobulin. Lancet 1984; 2:1062–1064.

39. Ochs HD, Fischer SH, Virant FS, Lee ML, Kingdom HS, Wedgewood RI. Non-A, non-B hepatitis and intravenous immunoglobulin. Lancet 1985; 1:404–405.

40. Schiff RI. Transmission of viral infections through intravenous immune globulins. N Engl J Med 1994; 33:1649–1650. Editorial.

41. Centers for Disease Control and Prevention. Outbreak of hepatitis C associated with intravenous immunoglobulin administration—United States, Oct 1993–June 1994. JAMA 1994; 272:424–425.

42. Bjoro K, Froland SS, Zhibing Y, Samdal HH, Haaland T. Hepatitis C infection in patients with primary hypogammaglobulinemia after treatment with contaminated immune globulin. N Engl J Med 1994; 331:1607–1611.

43. Gomperts ED. HCV and Gammagard in France. Lancet 1994; 344:201. Letter.

44. Nixon RR, Smith SA, Johnson RL, Pillers DA. Misleading hepatitis C serology following administration of intravenous immunoglobulin. Am J Clin Pathol 1994; 101:327–328.

45. Douglas SD, Slade HB. Hepatitis C and immune globulin. N Engl J Med 1995; 332:1235–1236. Letter.

46. Schiano TD, Black M. Possible transmission of hepatitis C virus infection with intravenous immunoglobulin. Ann Intern Med 1995; 122:802–803. Letter.

47. Webster ADB, Dalgleish AG, Malkovsky M, et al. Isolation of retroviruses from two patients with "common variable" hypogammaglobulinemia. Lancet 1986; 1:581–583.

48. Pasatiempo AMG, Kroser JA, Rudnick M, Hoffman BI. Acute renal failure after intravenous immunoglobulin therapy. J Rheumatol 1994; 21:347–349.

49. Cantu TG, Hoehn-Savic EW, Burgess KM, Racusen L, Scheel PJ. Acute renal failure associated with immunoglobulin therapy. Am J Kidney Dis 1995; 25:228–233.

50. Tan E, Hajinazarian M, Bay W, Neff J, Mendell JR. Acute renal failure resulting from intravenous immunoglobulin therapy. Arch Neurol 1993; 50:137–139.
51. NIH Concensus Conference: Intravenous immunoglobulin. Precaution and treatment of disease. JAMA 1990; 264:3189–3193.
52. Ahsan N, Palmer BF, Wheeler D, Greenlee RG Jr, Toto RD. Intravenous immunoglobulin-induced osmotic nephrosis. Arch Intern Med 1994; 154:1985–1987.
53. Durelli L, Ferrero B, Aimo G, Cavallo R, Beramamaco B, Bergamini L. Anti-idiotypic (ID) mechanisms of high dose gamma globulin (HIG) in myasthenia gravis (MG). Neurology 1992; 42 (Suppl 3):307.
54. Thornton CA, Griggs RC. Plasma exchange and intravenous immunoglobulin treatment of neuromuscular disease. Ann Neurol 1994; 35:260–268.
55. Basta M, Kirshborn P, Frank MM, Fries LF. Mechanism of therapeutic effects of high dose intravenous immunoglobulin: Alteration of acute, complement-dependent immune damage in a guinea pig model. J Clin Invest 1989; 84:1974–1981.
56. Rondo N, Hurez Z, Kazarchkine MD. Intravenous immunoglobulin therapy of autoimmune and systemic inflammatory diseases. Vox Sang 1993; 64:65–72.
57. Liblau R, Gajdos PH, Bustarret FA, El Habib R, Buch IF, Morel E. Intravenous gamma-globulin in myasthenia gravis: interaction with anti-acetylcholine receptor antibodies. J Clin Immunol 1991; 11:128–131.
58. Bartoloni C, Guidi L, Scopetta C, Tonali P, Bartoccioni E, Flamini G, Gambacci G, Terranova T. Circulating immune complexes in myasthenia gravis. A study in relation to thymectomy. Clinical severity and thymic histology. J Neurol Neurosurg Psychiatry 1981; 44:901–905.
59. Rossi F, Kazarchkine MD. Antiidiotypes against autoantibodies in pooled human polyspecific IG. J Immunol 1989; 143:4104–4109.
60. Basta M, Fries FL, Frank MM. High doses of intravenous Ig inhibit in vitro uptake of C4 fragments onto sensitized erythrocytes. Blood 1991; 77:376–380.
61. Ballow M. Mechanisms of action of intravenous imune serum globulin therapy. Pediatr Infect Dis J 1994; 13:806–811.
62. Bussel JP, Saal S, Gordon B. Combined plasma exchange and intravenous gammaglobulin in the treatment of patients with refractory immune thrombocytopenic purpura. Transfusion 1988; 28:38–41.
63. Brunner NG, Namba T, Grob D. Corticosteroids in management of severe, generalized myasthenia gravis and comparison with corticotroprin therapy. Neurology 1972; 22:603–610.
64. Arsura E, Brunner NG, Namba T, Grob D. High dose intravenous methylprednisolone in myasthenia gravis. Arch Neurol 1985; 42:1149–1153.
65. Grob D, Simpson D, Mitsumoto H, Hoch B, Mokhtarian F, Bender A, Greenberg M, Koo A, Nakayama S. Treatment of myasthenia gravis by immunoadsorption of plasma. Neurology 1995; 45:338–344.
66. Dau PC. Immune globulin intravenous replacement after plasma exchange. J Clin Apheresis 1983; 1:104–108.
67. Stricker RB, Kwiatkowska BJ, Habis JA, Kiprov DD. Myasthenic crisis: Response to plasmapheresis following failure of intravenous gamma-globulin. Arch Neurol 1993; 50:837–840.
68. Namba T, Brunner NG, Grob D. Myasthenia gravis in patients with thymoma, with particular reference to onset after thymectomy. Medicine 1978; 57:411–433.

29

Multiple Sclerosis

Anat Achiron

Multiple Sclerosis Center, Sheba Medical Center, Tel-Hashomer, Israel

INTRODUCTION

Multiple sclerosis (MS) is the most common demyelinating disease of the central nervous system (CNS) that affects young to middle-aged adults and the third leading cause of significant disability in this age group, after trauma and arthritis. The disease first appears between the ages of 20 and 40 years, with an excess incidence among females (1). The clinical course of MS typically appears as either relapsing-remitting or chronic-progressive. In the relapsing-remitting course, new neurological symptoms appear, usually over a period of several days and lasting for 6–8 weeks, then gradually resolve. The annual relapse rate in these patients is the main factor affecting neurological disability, since with additional consecutive relapses the possibility of complete clinical remission decreases (2). In the chronic-progressive course symptoms progress over the years with different rates of progression among patients; even for the same patient the rate of progression can differ over various spans (3). Scattered inflammatory and demyelinating CNS lesions produce varying combinations of motor, sensory, coordination, visual, and cognitive impairments, as well as symptoms of fatigue and urinary tract dysfunction. The prognosis is unpredictable, ranging from occasional mild relapses over an entire lifetime to severe neurological disability within a few months (4,5).

The target for the inflammatory response in MS is the CNS myelin, which serves as a cable to insulate axons, thereby enhancing nerve conduction. Myelin is thick and lipid-rich, thus of high resistance and low capacitance, and therefore well-designed to permit rapid, saltatory axonal transmission of nerve impulses. Neurological dysfunction results primarily from partial, complete, or intermittent block of nerve conduction through demyelinated areas.

The classic lesions of MS—the demyelinating plaques—are microscopically characterized by myelin fragmentation followed by the appearance of activated microglia and macrophages that scavenge the myelin debris. Ultrastructural studies of ongoing myelin breakdown at the edges of expanding plaques show that myelin destruction is mediated by macrophages, which physically remove myelin, while in the surrounding white matter, the process of gliosis commences and perivascular cuffs of lymphocytes, plasma cells, and lipid-laden macrophages become increasingly prominent (6). This inflammatory process was the first indication of immune system involvement in the pathogenesis of MS.

Several factors, such as a viral infection during adolescence, genetic susceptibility (e.g., race, recurrence risks in relatives of affected individuals, concordance rates in twins), are believed to contribute to disease pathogenesis. The initiation and continuation of the disease process are attributed to immunological processes involving T cell–mediated mechanisms that cause selective injury to the CNS myelin (7).

The premise that MS may represent an autoimmune disorder where the immune system recognizes components of myelin as non-self, thus disrupting self-tolerance, is supported by:

1. The pathology of MS lesions in the CNS including the presence of interleukins, interferons, TNF, and various T cell subsets in MS plaques along with MHC class II expression on astrocytes, macrophages, and microglial cells in the lesions.
2. Increased production of IgG within the CNS with the appearance of oligoclonal bands.
3. Expression of immunological activation markers (e.g., specific T cell antigens, cytokines) in the peripheral blood of MS patients during acute relapse or progression.
4. The association of disease frequency with specific MHC class II alleles (DRw15, DQwr).
5. The animal model of experimental autoimmune encephalomyelitis (EAE), a prototype autoimmune disease mediated by CD4+ T cells, with clinical and pathological characteristics that resemble MS (8–11).

THERAPEUTIC TRIALS IN MS

Clinical trials in MS are aimed mainly at the following therapeutic objectives: induction of remission, maintenance of remission, and improvement of neurological disability. Current treatments are based on the concept that MS is a disease of immune regulation with complex genetic predisposing factors, triggered by as yet undetermined infectious agent(s). To alter the course of the disease and ultimately to arrest progression, immune regulatory drugs are being widely explored. In recent years, several controlled clinical trials were conducted using treatments aimed at removing or suppressing antigen-specific autoreactive cells. These various regimens included immunosuppressive therapy with cyclophosphamide (12,13), azathioprine (14), total lymphoid irradiation (15), and cyclosporine (16,17). These trials have shown controversial and inconclusive clinical effects. Moreover, such therapeutic modalities often produced serious side effects, which curtailed their long-term use. A recent multicenter, placebo-controlled, double-blind trial using subcutaneous injections of interferon-β-1b on alternate days, showed reduction in the frequency and severity of acute exacerbations, and slowed progression of brain lesions by magnetic resonance imaging (MRI) (18,19). Other interferons—both β and α—and the synthetic compound copolymer-I, have also been proved to be effective in relapsing-remitting MS.

RATIONALE FOR IVIG TREATMENT IN MS

Since immune mechanisms have been implicated in the pathogenesis of MS, treatment with immunoglobulins as nonspecific modulators of the immune response might be used as a strategy to alter the grievous course of this disease.

Intravenous immunoglobulin (IVIG) has been shown to be beneficial in the treatment of other immune regulation disorders such as idiopathic thrombocytopenic purpura (ITP), autoimmune hemolytic anemia, immune neutropenia, aplastic anemia, rheumatoid artritis, systemic lupus erythematosus (20–22), and various immune neurological diseases such as Guillain-Barré syndrome (23), chronic inflammatory demyelinating polyneuropathy (24), stiff-man syndrome (25), inflammatory myopathies (26), multifocal motor neuropathy (27), and myasthenia gravis (28,29).

IVIG Treatment in MS: Clinical Trials

In early uncontrolled studies IVIG was administered to reduce acute exacerbations and to arrest disease progression. Rotherfelder et al. (30) treated 20 relapsing-remitting MS patients with IVIG, 5 g once every 2 months for 1 year, and reported reduction in exacerbation rate compared with the rate during the year before IVIG treatment. Schuller and Govaerts (31) treated 31 MS patients with intramuscular injections of immunoglobulin (5 g, three times a week) for at least 1 year, and later continued the treatment with IVIG (5 g per week) for a mean period of 4 years. Overall, one-third improved, one-third were stable, and one-third deteriorated. Soukop and Tschabitscher (32) treated 22 relapsing-remitting and five primary-progressive MS patients with IVIG (50 mg/kg) during an acute exacerbation or progression, for a period of 2–3 weeks. Sixteen (62%) patients improved within 24 h.

Achiron et al. (33) conducted an open, controlled trial in 10 relapsing-remitting MS patients treated with IVIG at a dose of 0.4 g/kg/day for 5 consecutive days, with booster doses administered once every 2 months for the next 12 months. Ten untreated relapsing-remitting MS patients, matched for age, disease duration, and number of attacks per year, served as controls. IVIG treatment was well tolerated with no side effects. The exacerbation rate decreased from 3.7 ± 1.2 exacerbations per year before treatment, to 1.0 ± 0.7 exacerbations per year during treatment in the IVIG-treated patients ($P < .001$), and remained unaltered in the controls. Neurological disability evaluated by the Kurtzke Expanded Disability Status Scale (EDSS) (34) decreased from a mean of 4.45 at study onset to 4.15 after 1 year, whereas in control MS patients mean EDSS scores increased from 3.55 to 3.75. These results suggested that IVIG suppressed the ongoing pathological process in MS and prompted continuation of the treatment for a period of 3 years (35).

Effect of IVIG on Frequency of Acute Exacerbations

The mean annual exacerbation rate (AER) decreased during the second and third years of the study; IVIG-treated MS patients had significantly fewer exacerbations than untreated patients. The mean AER in the IVIG group after the second year was 0.8 ± 0.8, compared to 2.1 ± 1, in the controls ($P = .005$). The mean AER in the IVIG group after the third year of treatment was 0.5 ± 0.5, and 1.7 ± 0.7 in the control patients ($P < .001$). AER correlated inversely with duration of IVIG treatment and neurological disability after 3 years. The severity of acute exacerbations was also influenced by IVIG treatment. The majority of exacerbations in the IVIG-treated patients were mild to moderate, while in untreated controls most of the acute exacerbations were moderate to severe (35).

Effect of IVIG Treatment on Neurological Disability

The mean change in neurological disability evaluated by the EDSS (ΔEDSS) showed a trend of reduced disability in the IVIG group at the 1-year end point (ΔEDSS $= -0.3$

± 0.58), compared with the control group (ΔEDSS = 0.2 ± 1.0; P = .182). At the 3-year end point the ΔEDSS became significant between the two groups; in the IVIG group ΔEDSS was 0.35 ± 0.58, compared with 1.7 ± 0.98 in the control patients (P = .001).

Cook et al. (36), in an attempt to prevent disease progression, administered IVIG (0.5 – 2 g/kg) with methylprednisolone monthly to 14 patients with progressive MS for a mean period of 7.8 months. Although the treatment was safe, with the dosage used the authors failed to show that IVIG plus methylprednisolone prevented further clinical attacks in steroid-dependent patients with progressive MS. Van Engelen et al. (37) reported that IVIG treatment may be followed by recovery of visual function in patients with chronic optic neuritis who failed to respond to steroids.

Noseworthy et al. (38) treated 10 MS patients with recently acquired muscle weakness with IVIG, and found improvement in isometric muscle testing in five of six patients available for analysis after a period of 6 months.

Effect of IVIG Treatment on Brain MRI

The most specific and characteristic pathological change in MS is that of demyelination. MRI can provide an accurate and sensitive assessment of the appearance and extent of MS lesions, and thus may also measure disease activity (39). Regular MRI follow-up serves as a measure of therapeutic effect in clinical trials (19).

To evaluate the impact of IVIG treatment on the disease process we scored the total lesional area of demyelinated brain plaques in IVIG-treated relapsing-remitting MS patients at baseline and after 3 years, in comparison with the untreated, control patients (40). In IVIG-treated patients, the MRI score improved in five; two showed no change; and in three the lesion area increased. In the untreated MS patients, the score remained unchanged in one, whereas in nine patients the MRI score increased. The mean MRI score in IVIG-treated patients decreased from 2.89 at baseline to 2.7 after 3 years; this decrease did not reach statistical significance. In the control group, the mean MRI score increased significantly from 2.13 at baseline to 3.33 after 3 years (P < .05), suggesting disease progression. The change in the MRI score (ΔMRI score) between the groups suggested that IVIG treatment arrested disease progression. Thus, the beneficial effect of the drug in reducing the frequency of relapses and neurological disability was confirmed by the neuroradiological findings. Despite the small number of patients investigated, the change in the brain MRI lesion score between groups demonstrated progression in untreated patients and decrease in progression over time in IVIG-treated patients.

Sorensen (41) reported the design of a randomized, placebo-controlled, crossover study in 22 relapsing-remitting or progressive-relapsing MS patients who will be treated with IVIG, 1 g/kg/d for 2 consecutive days, at intervals of 4 weeks over a period of 6 months, using serial MRI for evaluation of efficacy.

In an effort to extend these findings, we have designed a randomized, double-blind, placebo-controlled trial to further evaluate the efficacy of IVIG treatment in relapsing-remitting patients (age 20–55) with definite MS (42), disease duration of 2–10 years, and an exacerbation frequency of of 1–3/year during the 2 years prior to the study. Patients were examined monthly and brain MRI studies done at entry and after the first and second years of the trial. The results of this trial confirmed the benefits of IVIG in reducing the frequency of acute relapses and arresting disease progression, as was shown in the open-controlled trial. Moreover, the side effects of IVIG are minimal, the drug is given intravenously once every 2 months, and is safe during pregnancy. IVIG may serve as an important alternative to β-interferon, which is given by injections on alternate days and has prominent side effects.

Effect of IVIG Treatment on the Prevention of Childbirth-Associated Acute Exacerbations in MS

Many patients with MS develop the disease during the reproductive period; it is well documented that the postpartum period is associated with increased frequency of exacerbations (43,44). No therapeutic trials have been implemented to try to prevent exacerbations in the postpartum period. We conducted a pilot study using IVIG treatment (45) in an attempt to reduce the number of childbirth-associated acute exacerbations. Nine MS patients with a history of 12 childbirth-associated acute exacerbations which had occurred 2–9 weeks following previous deliveries were treated with IVIG at a dose of 0.4 g/kg/day for 5 consecutive days during the first week after childbirth, and at 6 and 12 weeks thereafter. None of the treated patients relapsed during the 6-month period after delivery. Three patients had a remote relapse; two at 8 months and one at 10 months postpartum, probably representing the natural course of disease and unrelated to childbirth. This important indication for IVIG treatment needs further investigation in a larger population to confirm efficacy.

Effect of IVIG on EAE

EAE can be induced by active immunization with myelin basic protein (MBP) or its peptide fragments as well as by the adoptive transfer of MBP-specific T cell lines and clones, following in vitro stimulation with MBP (46,47). EAE is characterized by invasion of T lymphocytes into the CNS, resulting in demyelination and acute, chronic, or chronic-relapsing paralysis. This model has provided the opportunity to investigate mechanisms that play a role in the inflammatory processes in the CNS which leads to demyelination, as well as evaluation of the effects of various drugs on the immune mechanisms associated with the disease. To evaluate the effect of IVIG on EAE, Lewis rats were immunized with MBP or by adoptive transfer of MBP-specific CD4+ T cells. Treatment with IVIG efficiently suppressed active EAE (48). In the adoptive transfer model of EAE, as well as in control animals treated either with protein or 10% maltose, IVIG did not alter the disease course. The different results obtained in actively induced versus adoptive-transfer EAE suggest that IVIG may act predominantly on the induction phase of the immune process.

IVIG in MS: Possible Mechanisms of Action

Fc Receptor Blockade

IVIG has been shown to block Fc receptors (FcR) in ITP (Fig. 1), leading to FcR internalization and thus decreasing the ability of effector cells to phagocyte and remove platelets (21). A similar mechanism was suggested in myasthenia gravis, where IVIG treatment was thought to inhibit acetylcholine receptor antibodies binding through the FcR (49). The possibility that IVIG bind to other FcR-bearing cells may also play a role in their immunomodulatory effects in MS, since FcRs were detected on activated

T cells from MS patients. When different subsets of T cells were assessed for FcR expression in the resting state and in response to activation, two distinct patterns were found: activation through the T cell receptor (TCR), which induced de novo expression of multiple classes of FcR on T cells (CD4+/TH2 cells and some subpopulations of γδ TCR+ cells) (50,51) and the constitutive expression of FcR (52). This pattern may be of importance in MS, where FcR modulation by IVIG can affect immunoregulatory activity.

In the CNS, FcγRs have been demonstrated on cells in the choroid plexus, arachnoid granulation, perivascular macrophages, microglia, and endothelial cells (53,54). The FcγR in the choroid plexus and arachnoid granulations may be involved in the transcellular transport of IgG from blood to cerebrospinal fluid, while FcγR expression on microglia, which has been shown to be upregulated within active MS lesions, probably plays a role in myelin breakdown and also contributes to immune-mediated phagocytosis (55,56). Binding of IgG to FcγF could also block these inflammatory and cytotoxic effects within the CNS, thereby explaining the beneficial effects of treatment as seen by MRI.

Major Histocompatibility Class II Blockade

Susceptibility of animals immunized against MBP to develop EAE is linked to MHC, and MS is linked to certain HLA molecules (DR15, DQw6) (57). In addition to activated T cells and macrophages, microglial cells also express MHC class I and II antigens and function simultaneously as antigen-presenting cells and scavengers of myelin

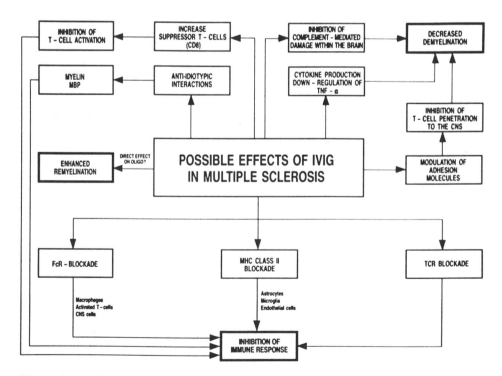

Figure 1   Possible mechanisms of action of IVIG in MS.

(58), thereby amplifying the inflammatory demyelinating process. Thus, it is theoretically possible to treat MS using antibodies against certain regions of MHC molecules. MHC blockade was demonstrated to prevent EAE induction using modified peptides of the encephalitogenic determinant MBP (59–61).

An important effect of IVIG may be its ability to prevent the immune response by masking the recognition of class II MHC (D/DR) that is frequently expressed in autoimmune disorders (62). It is thus possible that IVIG can suppress autoimmune reactivity in MS by interfering with the antigen presentation either systemically (activated T cells and macrophages) or within the CNS (microglia).

T Cell Receptor Blockade

Normally, T cells involved in an autoimmune response contain a diverse TCR repertoire. However, analysis of T cells in EAE and MS have shown that they use a restricted number of TCRs (63). The possibility that IgG binds to the TCR may be of significance in MS; specific T cell clones associated with disease activation may thus be eliminated.

The TCR has many structural similarities to immunoglobulins, which could promote physical interaction between homologous and heterologous domains of the TCR and IgG peptides. The injection of monoclonal antibodies specific for a predominant TCR Vβ8 chain can reduce the incidence of EAE in mice (63). Thus, it can be postulated that IgG, either by direct interaction with specific epitopes of the TCR or by competing with peptide fragments of the pathogenic autoantigen, may block antigen presentation by T cells and thereby prevent an immune response.

Moreover, as TCR blockade is restricted by specific MHC molecules, it is possible that IVIG has a dual effect, interrupting both MHC presentation of the antigen and its TCR recognition.

Induction of Antigen-Specific Suppressor Cells

In MS, reduction in the number of CD8+ suppressor T cells and a selective defect in suppressor cell function occur, especially during periods of disease activity in both the relapsing-remitting and chronic-progressive forms of the disease (64–66). Similar alterations in suppressor cell activity have also been demonstrated in EAE.

Several studies have examined the effect of IVIG on lymphocyte subsets. Amran et al. (67) studied the effects of IVIG on in vitro proliferation of human T cells. They found that IVIG inhibited anti-CD3-stimulated T cell proliferation. This inhibition was reversed by the addition of IL-2 or IL-4, implying that the effect of IVIG is mediated through interference with cytokine-dependent T cell proliferation. Achiron et al. (48) showed that the T cell proliferative responses to Con-A, ovalbumin, and BSA, 10 days after active induction of EAE, were not affected by IVIG treatment. However, antigen-specific proliferative responses to BP and the 71–90 encephalitogenic peptide were increased in EAE rats treated with IVIG, compared with untreated controls. Thus, the mechanism by which IVIG alters the natural course of the disease may be associated with a strong T cell response to the target encephalitogenic peptides.

In ITP during IVIG treatment, a reduction in the CD4/CD8 ratio with an increase in the relative number of CD8+ cells correlated with clinical response (68,69). In myasthenia gravis, IVIG was reported to increase the number of T suppressor cells, an effect that may also be important in MS (70). An attractive hypothesis is that the defect in suppressor function in MS, which lowers the threshold for T cell activation, can be prevented by IVIG treatment, thus establishing a new immunological equilibrium. This hypothesis is further supported by studies in EAE showing that long-term resistance to reinduction of the disease is mediated by a population of CD4 suppressor lymphocytes. Moreover, the amino acid residues 21–49 of the first extracellular domain of human CD4 bind immunoglobulin (71). Together these findings suggest that surface CD4 may cooperate with FcR in handling aggregated immunoglobulins.

Modulation of Cytokine Production

Cytokines secreted by activated T cells and macrophages play a major role in enhancing or suppressing the immune response at multiple levels of the lymphocytic cellular network. During acute EAE, the first cytokines to appear in the CNS are lymphotoxin and IL-12. This coincides with the first appearance of immunohistochemically detectable inflammatory cells in the brain, shortly before onset of clinical signs (72). Later, during the acute phase of the disease, IFN-γ and TNF-α appear, and their level of expression parallels the severity of clinical signs and degree of inflammatory cell infiltration. TGF-β peaks shortly before onset of recovery, while IL-10 increases dramatically in the recovery phase (72,73). In MS, both TNF-α and TNF-β were identified in acute and chronically active lesions, but were absent from chronically silent lesions (74,75). TNF-α was also demonstrated in cerebrospinal fluid of patients with active MS (76). In another study TNF-α levels in cerebrospinal fluid correlated with signs of blood-brain barrier (BBB) damage (77). These studies support the role of cytokines in promoting MS lesions. Less is known about putatively disease downregulatory cytokines. Among these, TGF-β and IL-10 are key candidates as evident from experimental models. MS patients with severe disease showed less RNA message for TGF-β than those with no or only slight disability (78). Taken together, these findings strongly support the role of cytokine-promoting and cytokine-suppressing mechanisms that are involved in both the experimental and human disease processes.

The possible effects of IgG on the inflammatory cascade is as yet unknown as the effects of cytokines are time-, site-, and dose-dependent. For example, treatment of EAE rats with anti-IFN-γ antibodies at the time of immunization manifests completely different effects compared with treatment shortly before onset of disease (79). We can thus hypothesize that during the disease process the effects of IgG will either be to decrease production of disease-promoting cytokines such as TNF-α and IFN-γ, and/or to increase disease-suppressing cytokines such as TGF-β and IL-10. Abe et al. (80) and Andersson et al. (81) studied the anticytokine nature of human immunoglobulin and its modulation of cytokine production. They found that IgG preparations significantly inhibited production of IL-2, IFN-γ, TNF-β, TNF-α, and IL-10 in anti-CD3 monoclonal antibody–stimulated cultures. Similarly, we reported that IVIG treatment downregulated TNF-α secretion by autoreactive T cells, while suppressing the clinical signs of EAE (48). As TNF-α induces selective destruction of oligodendrocytes in cultures (82), monoclonal antibody to TNF-α can prevent EAE, TNF-α is localized in MS plaques (74), and increased levels of TNF-α in the CSF of MS patients were reported to be associated with activation of the disease (76), the effects of IVIG on its level are of significance to the immune process in MS.

Adhesion Molecules

Adhesion molecules play a major role in the traffic of activated T cells across the BBB and initiation of the immune response within the normally sequestered CNS. During inflammation, leukocyte-endothelial interaction and regulation of leukocyte migration are regulated by adhesion molecules and cytokines (83). Expression of vascular cell adhesion molecule (VCAM-1), which is upregulated by the proinflammatory cytokines IL-1 and TNF-α, plays an important role in the recruitment of T cells and monocytes to sites of inflammation (84). Increased serum concentrations of soluble ICAM-1 were reported in MS patients during exacerbation of the disease (85).

Successful amelioration of EAE has been accomplished using monoclonal antibodies against the integrin very late antigen 4 (VLA-4), which mediates the adhesion and penetration of T cells and monocytes into the CNS (86). The counterreceptor of VLA-4 found on endothelial cell membrane is the (VCAM-1). In fact, enhancement of VCAM-1 expression is associated with lymphocyte infiltration (87), and serum levels of soluble VCAM-1 are elevated in patients with active MS (85).

Accordingly, the effect of IVIG on adhesion molecules might be related to restoration of proinflammatory homeostasis through binding to their ligands and inhibiting the effector phase of the immune response.

Idiotypic Network Interactions

Healthy humans can produce antibodies against variable region-defined recognition structures termed idiotypes, as well as against constant region structures, and the levels of these can increase markedly in autoimmune diseases. Immune responses to self antigens are interconnected within a network of idiotypic interactions involving antibodies and lymphocytes (88,89). Thus, the emergence of pathological autoimmunity may result from an unregulated expansion of autoreactive clones associated with decreased or defective connectivity (90,91). Although the contribution of the idiotype network to the pathogenesis of MS is unknown, this mechanism may underlie the therapeutic benefit of IVIG. Previous studies (92–94) demonstrating anti-idiotypes against autoantibodies in the serum of patients who spontaneously recovered from autoimmune diseases and of anti-idiotypes against autoantibodies in normal human polyspecific immunoglobulins, support the role for idiotypic interactions in the prevention of expression of autoimmune diseases in healthy individuals as well as in the exacerbating-remitting forms of many autoimmune diseases. Moreover, these data also suggest that the beneficial effect of IVIG prepared from large pools of normal donors in autoimmune diseases may depend on increased or reestablished feedback inhibition. IVIG contain a high number of antibodies capable of interacting with a variety of antigens as well as other antibodies (95). For instance, autoantibodies directed against variable and constant region markers of the α/β TCR were reported in healthy individuals (96). Modification of EAE has been successfully carried out by immunization with synthetic peptides corresponding to the CDR2 and Fr3/CDR3 segments, and immunization of humans with synthetic vβ CDR2 segments may prove helpful in MS. IVIG may bind to the antibody combining site of monoclonal and oligoclonal polyspecific IgM autoantibodies secreted by Epstein-Barr virus–transformed B cells from normal donors (97). These observations may be of potential relevance to the immunomanipulation of autoimmune disease, since they imply the possibility that IVIG can influence antigen-specific TCR and, through this, influence the regulation of autoimmunity.

Several lines of evidence demonstrate that inhibition of autoantibody activity by IVIG is dependent on idiotypic–anti-idiotypic interactions between idiotypes on autoantibodies and anti-idiotypes in IVIG. Olsson et al. (98) described cells producing IgG antibodies against myelin and MBP in the cerebrospinal fluid of MS patients. Antibodies generated against myelin components, such as myelin glycoprotein or glycolipids, may exert a direct myelinotoxic effect. Warren and Catz (99) stress the importance of a MBP antibody cascade in the mechanism of MS. The mechanism of action of IVIG would extend beyond the mere input of a restricted panel of anti-idiotypes recognizing idiotypic determinants of autoantibodies by providing, in addition to these anti-idiotypes, a set of interconnected antibodies. Through physiological antibody interactions IVIG could shift the connectivity equilibrium that characterizes the immune system of patients with autoimmune diseases to a more "normal" steady state in which selection of the expressed repertoire by anti-idiotypic interactions maintains "free" autoantibodies at very low levels (100). Pooled immunoglobulins in IVIG may express anti-idiotypic specificities that are not present or are only poorly represented in plasma from individual donors. It is also conceivable that even though specific activity may be diluted in the pool, some individuals may be higher "contributors of anti-idiotypes" to the pool than others. Thus, individuals who recovered or are in remission from an autoimmune disease may represent a privileged source of anti-idiotypes.

Complement-Mediated Tissue Damage

There is evidence that humoral mechanisms are involved in myelin injury; mediators may be introduced into the CNS or synthesized locally following T cell damage to the BBB. Induction of the EAE model by synergistic use of MBP sensitized T cells, together with a monoclonal antibody directed against myelin oligodendrocyte glycoprotein (101), results in a widespread loss of myelin that involves complement activation. Complement activation also occurs in MS patients, and C4 and C9 CSF levels were reported to be reduced, compared with controls (102,103). The role of complement in mediating myelin injury may be modulated by IVIG treatment. Though this mode of action has not been evaluated in MS, Basta and Dalakas (104), reported that in dermatomyositis IVIG treatment modulated complement-dependent tissue damage by blocking endomysial deposition of activated complement fragments.

Effect of IVIG on Remyelination

Oligodendrocytes synthesize myelin by the repetitive wrapping of their plasma membranes around axons. Unlike astrocytes, which are acknowledged as being capable of division, oligodendrocytes have been regarded as fully differentiated cells, which, like neurons, are incapable of division and therefore cannot be regenerated from precursor cells. However, in recent years it has become evident that oligodendrocytes are capable of mitosis and are involved in the remyelination process in areas of demyelination induced using JHM virus and cuprizone models (105,106). Further studies have demonstrated that oligodendrocytes attached to myelin sheathes can synthesize DNA preparatory to division, and there is presumptive evidence that they do proceed to divide (107,108). Current evidence based on the size of lesions that remyelinate effectively suggests that there is a limit to the distance that these cells can travel to remyelinate areas depleted of oligodendrocytes; the maximal distance of migration is a few millimeters (109,110).

Enhancing remyelination seems, therefore, a major direction in therapeutic strategies for MS in order to reverse long-term neurological disability. Rodriguez and Lennon (111) and Rodriguez (112) used the Theiler's virus model of chronic progressive demyelination to examine the possible effects of IgG treatment to enhance remyelination. They reported that remyelination of CNS axons was extensively promoted by systemic injection of serum IgG. The polyclonal mouse IgG used in their experiments was commercially prepared from nonsyngeneic donor mice and therefore analogous to human IgG preparation used in clinical trials. These findings raise the possibility that IVIG may also influence myelin repair and may account for our results showing reduction of demyelination by MRI in IVIG-treated MS patients. The mechanism by which IVIG promotes remyelination may at present involve unknown effects of IgG on intracellular transcriptional processes leading to oligodendrocyte proliferation and new myelin formation.

IgG and the Blood-Brain Barrier

The effective seal produced by the tight junctions of the brain capillaries usually inhibits transudation of IgG into the CNS. During the active process of demyelination the BBB is damaged. In EAE clinical signs appear shortly after the onset of BBB damage (113). In active MS, breakdown of the BBB is readily demonstrated with the appearance of enhanced lesions on MRI after gadolinium injection. Although raising the IgG serum concentration from the average value of 10 g/L to 30 g/L will only increase the CSF concentration from approximately 25 mg/L to 65 mg/L when the BBB is intact, (114), during BBB breakdown increased amounts of IgG can penetrate. In addition, the presence of FcR on the choroid plexus cells may enhance the active transport of IgG to the brain (53). The ability of IVIG to penetrate the BBB is of major potential benefit in MS, since the main inflammatory response is within the white matter of the CNS. Interferons that have been shown to be beneficial in MS do not cross the BBB, and their action is mostly focused on the periphery (115).

SIDE EFFECTS

Immunoglobulin has proved to be a very safe product, tens of millions of grams have been infused worldwide without serious problems. We have gained an extensive experience using the IVIG preparation by Bayer-Miles (GamimuneN). The Cohn fractionation process removes hepatitis B and human immunodeficiency virus, and incubation at room temperature during manufacturing inactivates hepatitis C virus. None of our MS patients treated with IVIG for a period of 3 years had elevations of liver enzymes. Side effects seen during IVIG treatment occurred in a minority of patients. These adverse reactions were mild and self-limited; they included drug eruption for several hours to 2 days, headaches, and low-grade fever. Side effects did not correlate with the duration of treatment and did not recur with subsequent infusions.

SUMMARY

IVIG treatment appears to orchestrate several immunoregulatory mechanisms involved in the pathogenesis of MS. Modulation of the disease control by IVIG is achieved through both limitation of the inflammatory process and enhancement of remyelination.

At present, clinical evidence of the effects of IVIG in MS is based on the results of small open trials, some of which have been encouraging and clearly support a role for IVIG in the treatment of MS. Confirmation of a beneficial effect of IVIG must await the results of placebo-controlled, double-blind trials.

Further studies integrating clinical and experimental data are needed to define specific mechanisms by which IVIG may affect the pathogenic processes underlying MS.

To conclude I will use an old American-Indian parable: An old Indian chieftain decided to test his heir. He captured a small bird and held it tightly in his fist. Turning to the future leader he inquired: "Is the bird alive or dead?" Planning to obstruct any possible answer, the old chief had decided beforehand that if the answer would be "alive," he would crush the bird to death, and if "dead," he would release it to fly away—thus disallowing a true solution. The young heir thought long and hard. Finally he bowed before his elder and said: "Honorable father, the answer is in your hand. . . ."

At this important crossroad of MS research, future therapy is in our hands to provide educated and skillful integrative pharmacotherapy.

REFERENCES

1. Martyn C. Epidemiology. In: Matthews WB, Compston A, V Allen I, Martyn, CN, eds. McAlpine's Multiple Sclerosis. 2nd ed. London: Churchill Livingstone, 1991:3–40.
2. McAlpine D. The benign form of multiple sclerosis: a study based on 241 cases seen within three years of onset and followed up until the tenth year or more of the disease. Brain 1961; 84:186–203.
3. Patzold U, Pocklington PR. Course of multiple sclerosis. First results of a prospective study carried out on 102 MS patients from 1976–80. Acta Neurol Scand 1982; 65:248–266.
4. Shepherd DI. Clinical features of multiple sclerosis in north-east Scotland. Acta Neurol Scand 1979; 60:218–230.
5. Poser S, Wikstrom J, Bauer HJ. Clinical data and identification of special forms of multiple sclerosis with a standardized documentation system. J Neurol Sci 1979; 40:159–168.
6. Prineas JW. Multiple sclerosis: pathology of the early lesion. In: Herndon RM, Seil FJ, eds. Multiple Sclerosis. Current Status of Research and Treatment. New York: Demos Publications, 1991:113–130.
7. Dijkstra CD, Polman CH, Berkenbosch F. Multiple sclerosis: some possible therapeutic opportunities. TiPS 1993; 14:124–129.
8. Antel JP, Freedman MS, Brodovsky S, et al. Activated suppressor cell function in severely disabled patients with multiple sclerosis. Ann Neurol 1989; 25:204–207.
9. Adachi K, Kumamoto T, Araki S. Interleukin-2 receptor levels indicating relapse in multiple sclerosis. Lancet 1989; 1:559–560.
10. Trotler JL, Cliford DB, McHinis JE, et al. Correlation of immunological studies and disease progression in chronic progressive multiple sclerosis. Ann Neurol 1989; 25:172–178.
11. Brosnan CF, Cannella B, Battistini L, Raine CS. Cytokine localization in multiple sclerosis lesions: correlation with adhesion molecule expression and reactive nitrogen species. Neurology 1995; 45(suppl 6):16–21.
12. Carter JL, Hafler DA, Dawson DM, et al. Immunosuppression with high-dose IV cyclophosphamide and ACTH in progressive multiple sclerosis: cumulative 6-year experience in 164 patients. Neurology 1988; 38(suppl 2):9–14.
13. Likosky WH. Experience with cyclophosphamide in multiple sclerosis: the cons. Neurology 1988; 38(suppl 2):14–18.
14. British and Dutch Multiple Sclerosis Azathioprine Trial Group. Double masked trial of azathioprine in multiple sclerosis. Lancet 1988; II:180–183.
15. Cook SD, Devereux C, Tvoiano R, et al. Effect of total lymphocyte irradiation in chronic progressive multiple sclerosis. Lancet 1986; 1:1405–1409.

16. Dommasch D. Comparative clinical trial of cyclosporine in multiple sclerosis: the pros. Neurology 1988; 38(suppl 2):28–29.

17. Rudge P. Cyclosporine and multiple sclerosis: the cons. Neurology 1988; 38(suppl 2):29–30.

18. IFNB Multiple Sclerosis Study Group. Interferon beta-1b is effective in relapsing-remitting multiple sclerosis. I. Clinical results of a multicenter, randomized, double-blind, placebo-controlled trial. Neurology 1993; 43:655–661.

19. Paty DW, Li DKB, UBC MS/MRI Study Group, IFNB Multiple Sclerosis Study Group. Interferon beta-1b is effective in relapsing-remitting multiple sclerosis. II. MRI analysis results of a multicenter, randomized, double-blind, placebo-controlled trial. Neurology 1993; 43:662–667.

20. Berkman SA, Lee ML, Gale RP. Clinical uses of intravenous immunoglobulins. Semin Hematol 1988; 25:140–158.

21. Bussell J, Hilgartner MW. Usage of intravenous gammaglobulins in the treatment of chronic idiopathic thrombocytopenic purpura. In: Morell A, Nydegger UE, eds. Clinical Uses of Intravenous Immunoglobulins. Orlando, FL: Academic, 1986:217–221.

22. Francioni C, Galeazzi M, Fioravanti A, et al. Long-term IVIG treatment in systemic lupus erythematosus. Clin Exp Rheumatol 1994; 12:163–168.

23. Van der Meche FGA. The Guillain-Barre syndrome: plasma exchange or immunoglobulins intravenously. J Neurol Neurosurg Psychiatry 1994; 57(suppl):33–34.

24. Van Doorn PA. Intravenous immunoglobulin treatment in patients with chronic inflammatory demyelinating polyneuropathy. J Neurol Neurosurg Psychiatry 1994; 57(suppl):38–42.

25. Amato AA, Cornman EW, Kissel JT. Treatment of stiff-man syndrome with intravenous immunoglobulin. Neurology 1994; 44:1652–1654.

26. Cherin P, Herson S. Indications for intravenous gammaglobulin in inflammatory myopathies. J Neurol Neurosurg Psychiatry 1994; 57(suppl):50–54.

27. Dalakas MC, Stein DP, Otero C, et al. Effect of high-dose intravenous immunoglobulin on amyotrophic lateral sclerosis and multifocal motor neuropathy. Arch Neurol 1994; 51:861–864.

28. Edan G, Landgraf F. Experience with intravenous immunoglobulin in myasthenia gravis: a review. J Neurol Neurosurg Psychiatry 1994; 57(suppl):55–56.

29. Arsura EL, Bick A, Brunner NG, Grob B. Effects of repeated doses of intravenous immunoglobulin in myasthenia gravis. Am J Med Sci 1988; 295:438–443.

30. Rotherfelder U, Neu I, Pelka R. Therapy for multiple sclerosis with immunoglobulin G. Munch Med Wochenschr 1982; 124:74–78.

31. Schuller E, Govaerts A. First results of immunotherapy with immunoglobulin G in multiple sclerosis patients. Eur Neurol 1983; 22:205–212.

32. Soukop W, Tschabitscher H. Gamma globulin therapy in multiple sclerosis. Theoretical considerations and initial clinical experience with 7S immunoglobulins in MS therapy. Wien Med Wochenschr 1986; 136:477–480.

33. Achiron A, Pras E, Gilad R, et al. Open controlled therapeutic trial of high-dose intravenous immunoglobulins in relapsing-remitting multiple sclerosis. Arch Neurol 1992; 49:1233–1236.

34. Kurtzke JF. Rating neurologic impairment in multiple sclerosis: an expanded disability status scale (EDSS). Neurology 1983; 33:1444–1452.

35. Achiron A, Gilad R, Margalit R, et al. Intravenous gammaglobulin treatment in multiple sclerosis and experimental autoimmune diseases: delineation of usage and mode of action. J Neurol Neurosurg Psychiatry 1994; 57(suppl):57–61.

36. Cook SD, Troiano R, Rohowsky-Kochin C, et al. Intravenous gamma globulin in progressive MS. Acta Neurol 1992; 86:171–175.

37. van Engelen BG, Hommes OR, Pinckers A, et al. Improved vision after intravenous immunoglobulin in stable demyelinating optic neuritis. Ann Neurol 1992; 32:834–835.

38. Noseworthy JH, Rodriguez M, An KN, et al. IVIG treatment in multiple sclerosis: Pilot study rsults and design of placebo-controlled, double-blind clinical trial. Ann Neurol (abstr) 1994; A:325(P266).

39. Gass A, Barker GJ, Kidd D, et al. Correlation of magnetization transfer ratio with clinical disability in multiple sclerosis. Ann Neurol 1994; 36:62–67.

40. Achiron A, Barak Y, Goren M, et al. Intravenous immunoglobulin in multiple sclerosis: clinical and neuroradiologic results and implications for possible mechanisms of action. Clin Exp Immunol 1996; 104(suppl 1):67–70.

41. Sorensen PS. Treatment of multiple sclerosis with IVIG: potential effects and methodology of clinical trials. J Neurol Neurosurg Psychiatry 1994; 57(suppl):62–64.

42. Poser CM, Paty DW, Scheinberg L, et al. New diagnostic criteria for multiple sclerosis: guidelines for research protocols. Ann Neurol 1983; 13:227–231.

43. Korn-Lubetzki I, Kahana E, Cooper G, Abramsky O. Activity of multiple sclerosis during pregnancy and puerperium. Ann Neurol 1984; 16:228–231.

44. Birk K, Ford C, Smeltzer S, Ryan D, Miller R, Rudick RA. The clinical course of multiple sclerosis during pregnancy and the puerperium. Arch Neurol 1990; 47:738–742.

45. Achiron A, Rotstein Z, Noy S, et al. Intravenous immunoglobulin treatment in the prevention of childbirth-associated acute exacerbations in multiple sclerosis—a pilot study. J Neurol 1996; 243:25–28.

46. Mokhatarian VF, McFarlin DE, Raine CS. Adoptive transfer of myelin basic protein-synthesized T cells produce chronic relapsing demyelinating disease in mice. Nature 1984; 309:356–358.

47. Lemire JM, Weigle WO. Myelin basic protein-specific T cell clones and experimental allergic encephalomyelitis. Pathol Immunopathol Res 1986; 5:248–252.

48. Achiron A, Margalit R, Hershkoviz R, et al. Intravenous immunoglobulin treatment of experimental T-cell mediated autoimmune diseases: up-regulation of T cell proliferation and down-regulation of TNF-α secretion. J Clin Invest 1994; 93:600–605.

49. Zweiman B. Theoretical mechanisms by which immunoglobulin therapy might benefit myasthenia gravis. Clin Immunol Immunopathol 1989; 53:583–591.

50. Sandor M, Gajewski T, Thorson J, et al. CD4+ murine T cell clones that express high levels of immunoglobulin binding belong to the interleukin-4-producing T helper cell type 2 subset. J Exp Med 1990; 171:2171–2176.

51. Sandor M, Houlden BW, Bluestone JA, et al. In vitro and in vivo activation of murine γ/δ T cells induce the expression of IgA, IgM, and IgG Fc receptors. J Immunol 1992; 148:2363–2369.

52. Sandor M, Daeron M, Ibraghimov A, Lynch RG. Fc receptor expression on murine epidermal T cells. FASEB J 1991; A1464:6339.

53. Nyland H, Nilsen R. Localization of Fcγ receptors in the human central nervous system. Acta Pathol Microbiol Immunol Scand 1982; 90:217–221.

54. Ulvetad E, Williams K, Vedeler C, et al. Reactive microglia in multiple sclerosis lesions have an increased expression of receptors for the Fc part of IgG. J Neurol Sci 1994; 121:125–131.

55. Ulvetad E, Williams K, Matre R, et al. Fc receptors for IgG on cultured human microglia mediate cytotoxicity and phagocytosis of antibody coated targets. J Neuropathol Exp Neurol 1994; 53:27–36.

56. Vedeler C, Ulvetad E, Nyland H, et al. Receptors for gammaglobulin in the central and peripheral nervous system. J Neurol Neurosurg Psychiatry 1994; 57(suppl):9–10.

57. Bansil S, Cook SD, Rohowsky-Kochan C. Multiple sclerosis: immune mechanism and update on current therapies. Ann Neurol 1995; 37(S1):S87–S101.

58. Maynier M, Cosso B, Brochier J, Clot J. Identification of class II HLA alloantibodies in placenta-eluted gamma globulin used for treating rheumatoid arthritis. Arthritis Rheumatism 1987; 30:375–381.

59. Sakai K, Zamvil SS, Mitchell DJ, et al. Prevention of experimental allergic encephalomyelitis with peptides that block interaction of T cells with major histocompatibility complex proteins. Proc Natl Acad Sci USA 1989; 86:9470–9474.

60. Lamont G, Sette A, Fujinami R, et al. Inhibition of experimental autoimmune encephalomyelitis induction in SJL/J mice by using a peptide with high affinity for IA molecules. J Immunol 1990; 145:1687–1693.

61. Guatam M, Glynn P. Competition between foreign and self proteins in antigen presentation: ovalbumin can inhibit activation of myelin basic protein-specific T-cells. J Immunol 1990; 144:1177–1180.

62. Hayes GM, Woodroofe MN, Cuzner ML. Microglia are the major cell type expressing MHC class II in human white matter. J Neurol Sci 1987; 80:25.

63. Acha-Orbea H, Mitchell DJ, Timmermann L, et al. Limited heterogeneity of T cell receptors from T lymphocytes mediating autoimmune encephalomyelitis allows specific immune intervention. Cell 1988; 54:263–273.

64. Rose LM, Ginsberg AH, Rothstein TL, et al. Selective loss of a subset of T helper cells in active multiple sclerosis. Proc Natl Acad Sci USA 1985; 82:7389–7393.

65. Morimoto C, Hafler DA, Weiner HL, et al. Selective loss of the suppressor-inducer T-cell subset in progressive multiple sclerosis. N Engl J Med 1987; 316:67–72.

66. Reinherz EL, Weiner HL, Hauser SL, et al. Loss of suppressor T cells in active multiple sclerosis. N Engl J Med 1980; 303:125–129.

67. Amran D, Renz H, Lack G, et al. Suppression of cytokine-dependent human T-cell proliferation by intravenous immunoglobulin. Clin Immunol Immunopathol 1994; 73:180–186.

68. Tsubakio T, Kurato Y, Katageri S, et al. Alteration in T cell subsets and immunoglobulin synthesis in vitro during high dose gammaglobulin therapy in patients with idiopathic thrombocytopenic purpura. Clin Exp Immunol 1983; 53:697–702.

69. Macey MG, Newland AC. Modulation of T and B cell subpopulations during high dose intravenous immunoglobulin therapy. Plasma Ther Transfus Technol 1988; 9:139–147.

70. Arsura EL, Bick A, Brunner NG, Grob B. Effects of repeated doses of intravenous immunoglobulin in myasthenia gravis. Am J Med Sci 1988; 295:438–443.

71. Metha RL, Lenert P, Zanetti M. Synthetic peptides of human CD4 enhance binding of immunoglobulins to monocyte/macrophage cells. II. Mechanisms of enhancement. Cell Immunol 1994; 156:146–54.

72. Olsson T. Cytokine-producing cells in experimental autoimmune encephalomyelitis and multiple sclerosis. Neurology 1995; 45(suppl 6):S11–S15.

73. Renno T, Lin JY, Piccirillo C, et al. Cytokine production by cells in cerebrospinal fluid during experimental allergic encephalomyelitis in SJL/J mice. J Neuroimmunol 1994; 49:1–7.

74. Selmaj KW, Raine CS, Cannella B, Brosnan CF. Identification of lymphotoxin and tumor necrosis factor in multiple sclerosis lesions. J Clin Invest 1991; 87:949–954.

75. Cannella B, Raine CS. The adhesion molecule/cytokine profile of multiple sclerosis lesions. Ann Neurol 1995; 37:424.

76. Sharief MK, Hentges R. Association between tumor necrosis factor-α and disease progression in patients with multiple sclerosis. N Engl J Med 1991; 325:467–472.

77. Sharief MK, Thompson EJ. In vivo relationship of tumor necrosis factor-α to blood-brain barrier damage in patients with active multiple sclerosis. J Neuroimmunol 1992; 38:27–33.

78. Link J, Soderstrom, M, Olsson T, et al. Increased TGF-β, IL-4 and IFN-γ in multiple sclerosis. Ann Neurol 1994; 35:197–203.

79. Strigard K, Holmdahl R, van der Meide P, et al. In vivo treatment for rats with monoclonal antibodies against gamma interferon: effects on experimental allergic neuritis. Acta Neurol Scand 1989; 80:201–207.

80. Abe Y, Horiuchi A, Miyake M, Kimura S. Anti-cytokine nature of natural human im-

munoglobulin: one possible mechanism of the clinical effect of intravenous immunoglobulin therapy. Immunol Rev 1994; 139:5-19.

81. Andersson U, Bjork L, Skansen-Saphir U, Andersson J. Pooled human IgG modulates cytokine production in lymphocytes and monocytes. Immunol Rev 1994; 139:21-42.

82. Selmaj KW, Raine CS. Tumor necrosis factor mediates myelin and oligodendrocyte damage in vitro. Ann Neurol 1988; 23:339-346.

83. Albelda SM, Smith CW, Ward PA. Adhesion molecules and inflammatory injury. FASEB J 1994; 8:504-512.

84. Pober JS, Cotran RS. What can be learned from the expression of endothelial adhesion molecules in tissues? Lab Invest 1991; 64:301-305.

85. Hartung HP, Archelos JJ, Zielasek J, et al. Circulating adhesion molecules and inflammatory mediators in demyelination: a review. Neurology 1995; 45(suppl 6):S22-S32.

86. Yednock TA, Cannon C, Fritz LC, Sanchez-Madrid F, Steinman L, Karin N. Prevention of experimental autoimmune encephalomyelitis by antibodies against $\alpha4\beta1$ integrin. Nature 1992; 356:63-66.

87. Damle NK, Khissman K, Linsley PS, Aruff A. Differential costimulatory effects of adhesion molecules B7, ICAM-1, LFA-3, and VCAM-1 on resting and antigen-primed CD4+ T lymphocytes. J Immunol 1992; 148:1985-1992.

88. Zanetti M. Idiotypic regulation of autoantibody production. CRC Crit Rev Immunol 1986; 6:151-183.

89. Martinez AC, Pereira P, Toribio ML, et al. The participation of B cells and antibodies in the selection and maintenance of T cell repertoires. Immunol Rev 1988; 101:191-215.

90. Roitt IM, Cooke A. Idiotypes and autoimmunity. In: Cinader B, Miller RG, eds. Progress in immunology VI. London: Academic Press, 1986:512.

91. Kazatchkine MD, Dietrich G, Hurez V, et al. V region–mediated selection of autoreactive repertoires by intravenous immunoglobulin. Immunol Rev 1994; 139:79-107.

92. Geha RS. Idiotypic interactions in the treatment of human diseases. Adv Immunol 1986; 39:255-297.

93. Burdette S, Schwartz RS. Idiotypes and idiotypic networks. N Engl J Med 1987; 317:219-224.

94. Rossi F, Dietrich G, Kazatchkine MD. Anti-idiotypes against autoantibodies in normal immunoglobulins: evidence for network regulation of human autoimmune responses. Immunol Rev 1989; 110:135-149.

95. Tankersley DL, Preston MS, Finlayson JS. Immunoglobulin G dimer: an idiotype–anti-idiotype complex. Mol Immunol 1988; 25:41-48.

96. Marchalonis JJ, Schluter SF, Wang E, et al. Synthetic autoantigens of immunoglobulins and T-cell receptors: their recognition in aging, infection, and autoimmunity. Proc Soc Exp Biol Med 1994; 207:129-147.

97. Seigneurin MJ, Guilbert B, Bourgeat MJ, Avrameas S. Polyspecific natural antibodies and autoantibodies secreted by human lymphocytes immortalized with Epstein-Barr virus. Blood 1988; 71:581-585.

98. Olsson T, Baig S, Hofeberg B, Link H. Antimyelin basic protein and anti myelin-producing cells in multiple sclerosis. Ann Neurol 1990; 27:132-136.

99. Warren KG, Catz I. A myelin basic protein antibody cascade in purified IgG from cerebrospinal fluid of multiple sclerosis patients. J Neurol Sci 1990; 96:19-27.

100. Jerne NK. Idiotypic networks and other preconceived ideas. Immunol Rev 1984; 79:5-24.

101. Linington C, Bradl M, Lassmann H, et al. Augmentation of demyelination in rat acute allergic encephalomyelitis by circulating mouse monoclonal antibodies directed against a myelin oligodendrocyte glycoprotein. Am J Pathol 1988; 130:443-454.

102. Jans H, Heltberg A, Zeeberg I, et al. Immune complexes and the complement factor C4 and C3 in cerebrospinal fluid and serum from patients with chronic progressive multiple sclerosis. Acta Neurol Scand 1984; 69:34-38.

103. Hartung HP, Heininger K. Non-specific mechanisms of inflammation and tissue damage in MS. Ann Inst Pasteur 1989; 140:226–233.
104. Basta M, Dalakas MC. High dose intravenous immunoglobulin exerts its beneficial effect in patients with dermatomyositis by blocking endomysial deposition of activated complement fragments. J Clin Invest 1994; 94:1729–1735.
105. Ludwin SK. An autoradiographic study of cellular proliferation in remyelination of the central nervous system. Ann J Pathol 1979; 95:683–696.
106. Arenella L, Herndon RM. Mature oligodendrocytes: division following experimental demyelination in adult animals. Arch Neurol 1984; 41:1162–1165.
107. Ludwin SK. Proliferation of mature oligodendrocytes after trauma to the central nervous system. Nature 1984; 308:274–275.
108. Ludwin SK, Bakker DA. Can oligodendrocytes attached to myelin proliferate? J Neurosci 1988; 8:1239–1244.
109. Baulac M, Lachapelle F, Gout O, et al. Transplantation of oligodendrocytes in the newborn mouse brain: extension of myelination by transplanted cells. Anatomical study. Brain Res 1987; 420:39–47.
110. Gansmuller A, Lachappele F, Baron–Van Evercooren A, et al. Transplantation of newborn CNS fragments into the brain of shiverer mutant mice: extensive myelination by transplanted oligodendrocytes. II. Electron microscopic study. Dev Neurosci 1986; 8:197–207.
111. Rodriguez M, Lennon VA. Immunoglobulins promote remyelination in the central nervous system. Ann Neurol 1990; 27:12–17.
112. Rodriguez M. Immunoglobulins stimulate central nervous system remyelination: electron microscopic and morphometric analysis of proliferating cells. Lab Invest 1991; 64:358–370.
113. Hirano A, Dembitzer HM, Becker NH, et al. Fine structural alterations of the blood brain barrier in experimental allergic encephalomyelitis. J Neuropathol Exp Neurol 1970; 29:432–440.
114. Wurster U, Haas J. Passage of intravenous immunoglobulin and interaction with the CNS. J Neurol Neurosurg Psychiatry 1994; 57(suppl):21–35.
115. Dalakas MC. Basic aspects of neuroimmunology as they relate to immunotherapeutic targets: present and future prospects. Ann Neurol 1995; 37(S1):2–13.

30

Polymyositis/Dermatomyositis

Lori B. Tucker
New England Medical Center, Boston, Massachusetts

Earl D. Silverman
The Hospital for Sick Children, University of Toronto, Toronto, Ontario, Canada

INTRODUCTION

Polymyositis (PM) and dermatomyositis (DMS) are disorders of muscle inflammation with unknown etiology (1–6). These disorders belong to the group of inflammatory myopathies that also includes the less common entity of inclusion-body myositis. These disorders are rare. The incidence of PM/DMS has been reported to be 0.2–0.55 new cases per 100,000, or roughly 10 new cases per million persons per year (7,8). Recent data from a collaborative pediatric rheumatology database in northeastern United States show the mean annual incidence of juvenile DMS to be 0.4 new cases per 100,000 children (9). PM is more commonly seen in adults and rarely in childhood, whereas DMS is seen in children and adults.

PM and DMS are quite different diseases in clinical presentation, although they share the central clinical finding of proximal muscle weakness (6). The onset of PM is generally more insidious, with the gradual development of muscle weakness. DMS may be more easily clinically identifiable because patients develop a typical rash consisting of red-purple discoloration (called a "heliotrope") of the eyelids, and scaley, red raised patches over the extensor surfaces of the fingers, knees, and elbows (Figs. 1 and 2). Patients may present with the gradual appearance of muscle weakness or the sudden, rapid deterioration of functional abilities. Involvement of the pharyngeal muscles may result in difficulty swallowing, and the risk of aspiration, or weakness of respiratory muscles, can result in respiratory insufficiency. Vasculitis involving the gastrointestinal tract can result in perforation; this was a frequent precipitant of death in the pretreatment era. Clinical findings of muscle weakness in PM/DMS are accompanied by elevations of serum muscle enzymes such as creatine kinase, aldolase, aspartate aminotransferase, alanine aminotransferase, lactate dehydrogenase, and typical abnormalities on electromyographic testing.

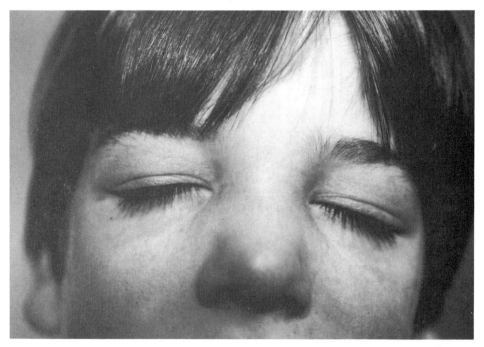

Figure 1   DMS heliotrape of the eyelids.

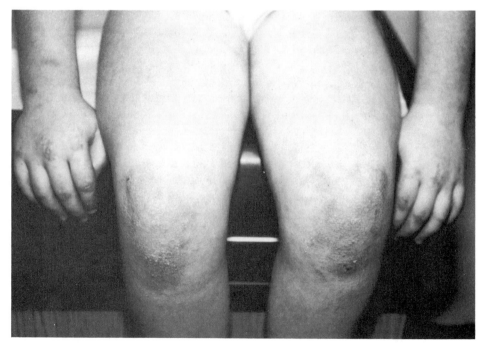

Figure 2   DMS red scaled patches on the knees.

HISTOLOGY

The histological findings differ in PM and DMS, suggesting a different disease pathogenesis. In DMS, there is endothelial cell damage, with B lymphocytes, CD4+ T lymphocytes, and immunoglobulin deposition seen in the perivascular regions of the muscles (10). There is activation of complement membrane attack complex (C5b–C9) on vascular endothelium of intramuscular capillaries, suggesting humorally mediated destruction of the microvasculature resulting in ischemia of muscle cells and the characteristic histological findings of perifasicular atrophy (11). In PM, however, there is an increase in CD8+ T lymphocytes and macrophages in endomysial regions, with activated CD8+ T cells infiltrating muscle fibers. The muscle fibers themselves have an increase in Class I antigen expression (8).

ETIOLOGY AND PROGNOSIS

Although the etiology and pathogenic mechanisms of PM and DMS are unknown, evidence for both humoral and cellular immune system participation in development of disease can be found (6,12,13). Recent work in adults has shown that 60–80% of patients with inflammatory myositis have the presence of specific myositis-related autoantibodies directed against intracellular antigens, such as aminoacyl synthetases or signal recognition particles (14). The presence of particular autoantibodies is associated with specific clinical findings (8,15).

The prognosis of PM and DMS prior to effective treatments with immunosuppressant agents was poor. For patients with DMS, one-third died from their disease, one-third were left with significant disability, and one-third recovered completely (16,17). Wedgwood et al. were among the first to recognize the utility of cortisone therapy in children with DMS (18). Steroid therapy is now the recommended treatment of choice for patients with PM and DMS, prescribed in high doses given either orally or intravenously, to achieve disease control (13,16,19). Slow tapering of the steroid over months to several years is undertaken once disease activity is controlled, with careful attention for any signs of disease flare.

STEROID THERAPY AND IVIG

Although many patients will have an excellent response to high-dose steroid therapy alone, some patients do not. Many patients will develop a flare of disease while the steroid dose is being tapered. Some patients have disease recalcitrant to high-dose prednisone therapy and continue to exhibit smouldering muscle weakness and abnormal serum muscle enzymes. Other patients may develop unacceptable side effects of steroid therapy such as steroid myopathy, diabetes, avascular necrosis, cataracts, or hypertension. In these situations, alternative or adjunctive immunosuppressant therapy may be necessary.

Immunosuppressant medications and treatments such as azathioprine, methotrexate, cyclosporine, and plasmapheresis have been reported to be useful for adjunctive therapy in PM and DMS, although the reports are from small-scale open trials or case reports (20–24). No large-scale randomized trials have been carried out to determine the effectiveness of these treatments for myositis. These drugs all have significant toxicities, which may limit their benefit. Thus, an alternative agent for the effective therapy of PM/DMS would be of benefit to patients.

Based on the need for new alternative therapies in PM/DMS and the variety of immune mechanisms involved in disease pathogenesis, intravenous immunoglobulin (IVIG) has been tried by a number of investigators, mostly in small trials, with promising results (25–31). Tables 1 and 2 outline the published experience of IVIG in the treatment of inflammatory myositis.

DISCUSSION

Roifman and colleagues first reported the successful use of IVIG in treating a patient with PM who was resistant to steroid therapy (30). In 1991, Cherin et al. treated 20 adult patients with refractory DMS or PM with IVIG, with good results (26). All patients had been treated with daily oral steroids, and the majority had failed treatment with adjunctive immunosuppressants. Significant improvement in muscle strength was noted in 15/20 patients; only one patient had worsening of clinical strength. Steroid doses were able to be tapered in 13/16 patients as well.

Lang et al. published a small series of five children with JDMS treated with IVIG after failure to improve with high-dose steroids and adjunctive immunosuppressants or development of significant steroid side effects. The rash of DMS showed dramatic improvement within 2–4 months of IVIG treatment (29). Muscle strength improved in all patients, and corticosteroid doses were able to be tapered and, in two cases, discontinued completely.

Two additional small open studies using IVIG in JDMS have substantiated the initial positive report. Collet et al. treated two children with IVIG after only 2 months of treatment with high-dose oral steroid (27). They reported excellent clinical response and were able to taper the children's steroids within 6 months of starting IVIG. Sansome and Dubowitz reviewed the course of nine children with JDMS treated with IVIG for a variety of indications including disease relapse during treatment with steroids and immunosuppressants, persistent weakness despite therapy, or steroid dependency (31). The IVIG administration schedule in this study differed significantly from all other published reports, with a 2 g/kg dose given divided over 5 days; all other studies administered this dose over 2 days. Despite this difference, all patients showed some degree of improvement and were able to have their steroid doses either maintained or tapered considerably.

Although the bulk of published reports show efficacy of IVIG in treating recalcitrant patients with inflammatory myositis, there is one brief report which documents two cases where patients developed clinical signs of disease flare, with elevations of muscle enzymes and muscle weakness, during a treatment course of monthly IVIG (32). These cases are a reminder that the total number of patients treated to date with IVIG is quite small. Further investigation may help to determine which patients are likely to respond or not respond to this form of treatment.

The use of IVIG as a first-line therapeutic choice for PM/DMS was investigated by Cherin and colleagues in a small open study with 11 adult patients (33). The patients were given IVIG monthly for an average of 4 months prior to treatment with steroids or other agents. Although serum creatine kinase levels dropped in 8/11 patients

Table 1 Reports of Treatment of PM/DMS with IVIG: Patient Characteristics, Dosing, and Side Effects

Reference	No. of patients	Diagnosis	Age (years)	Previous treatments	Dose of IVIG	No. of cycles	Side effects
Roifman (30)	1	PM	15	pred + cyto[a]	1/g/kg/d × 2 q mo	6	none
Lang (29)	5	DM	2.5-15	2—prednisone 3—prednisone + cyto	1 g/kg/d × 2 q mo	9	none
Cherin (26)	20	14 PM 6 DM	21-83 mean 43	prednisone + cyto; pharesis; TLI[b]	1 g/kg/d × 2 or 0.5 g/kg/d × 5	3-12 mean 4	4—headache, fever 1—delirium
Collet (27)	2	DM	7 and 12	prednisone	1 g/kg/d × 2 q mo	9	none
Dalakas (28)	15	DM	18-55 mean 36	prednisone + cytoto	1 g/kg/d × 2 q mo	3	none
Cherin (33)	11	5 PM 6 DM	mean 55.6	none	1 g/kg/d × 2 q mo	3-6 mean 4	1—fever and chills
Reimold (32)	2	DM	47 and 52	prednisone + cyto	1 g/kg/d × 2 q mo	6	none
Sansome (31)	9	DM	mean 10.6	prednisone + cyto	2 g/kg over 5 days q mo	1-6 mean 4	4—headache 2—diarrhea 1—fever

[a]Cytotoxic drugs, which include methotrexate, azathioprine, cyclosporine, hydroxychloroquine, and chlorambucil.
[b]Total lymphoid irradiation in one patient.

Table 2 Reports of Treatment of PM/DMS with IVIG: Efficacy

Reference	Muscle strength improved	Rash improved	Serum muscle enzymes[a]	Able to taper steroid
Roifman (30)	100%	NA	75%	100%
Lang (29)	80%[b]	100%	50%	100%
Cherin (26)	75%	NR	90%	81%
Collet (27)	100%	100%	100%	100%
Dalakas (28)	92%	100%	100%	NR
Cherin (33)	27%	NR	72%	NA
Reimold (32)	0[c]	NR	0[c]	0[c]
Samsone (31)	80%	NR	NR	25%

NA = not applicable in the study.
NR = not recorded.
[a]Muscle enzymes normalized or improved > 50%.
[b]One patient was too young to assess accurately.
[c]The two patients in this study had an initial positive response to IVIG, but developed increasing muscle enzymes and weakness while undergoing monthly therapy.

during the infusion treatment period, only 3/11 patients showed improved clinical muscle strength during the treatment period. Of interest, one of the responders was a patient who developed PM coincident to acute infection with Coxsackie B virus, and one was a patient who developed DMS during treatment with penicillamine therapy for rheumatoid arthritis. Although these results do not support the routine use of IVIG for first-line treatment of PM/DMS, there may be a particular indication for its use in patients with a clear viral trigger to their disease.

A carefully designed placebo-controlled trial of the utility of IVIG in DMS was carried out by Dalakas et al. with 15 patients who had treatment-resistant disease (28). Outcome was measured using a clinical muscle strength testing, a neuromuscular symptom score, changes in skin rash, and histological changes in repeated muscle biopsies. Significant improvements in muscle strength and symptoms were seen in all eight patients receiving IVIG after three treatments, with some patients manifesting remarkable improvement. Of the placebo-treated patients, 3/7 worsened, 2/7 had mild improvement, and 2 showed no change. Patients receiving IVIG during the first part of the trial either worsened or did not change when crossed over to placebo treatment. The clinical improvements were accompanied by decrease in the serum CPK and improvement in skin rash. Muscle biopsies, done before and after IVIG treatment, showed changes strongly suggesting that IVIG interferes with the pathogenic process of the disease. Membrane attack complex, seen on capillary endothelium during active disease, became undetectable, with resolution of overexpression of MHC Class I. There was regeneration of capillaries in posttreatment specimens, as well as reduction in number of regenerating muscle fibers and inflammatory cell infiltrates. This study is the first to link clinical improvement to histological and immunological changes in the muscles, and provides valuable data suggesting possible mechanisms of IVIG in resolving inflammatory myositis.

The exact mechanism of IVIG in treating autoimmune disorders is largely unknown. Proposed theories of IVIG effects in treating PM/DM include:

1. Providing a source of neutralizing antibody to an as yet unknown causative infectious agent.
2. Acting as a source of anti-idiotypic antibody to suppress autoantibody formation.
3. Blocking IgG Fc receptors on phagocytic cells.
4. Suppression of immunoglobulin and T cell proliferation.
5. Interference with complement system.
6. Blocking of cytokine activation or action.

Basta and Dalakas (34) have provided strong evidence for the role of IVIG in modulation of complement-dependent immunopathology in patients with DMS. Their elegant studies showed suppression of in vitro C3 uptake onto sensitized human erythrocytes after treatment with IVIG, which correlated with clinical improvement. Treatment with IVIG was associated with a decrease to normal of circulating late complement cascade complexes (C5b–9) in serum; membrane attack complexes, present on endothelial cells and muscle fibers in active disease, were no longer detected.

CONCLUSION

In summary, IVIG has been shown in a small number of studies to be an effective adjunctive therapy in patients with recalcitrant PM/DMS. Despite the high cost of this mode of therapy, there has been a low rate of side effects and toxicity compared to other currently accepted therapies. Early data do not support the use of IVIG as sole first-line therapy for PM/DMS, although further studies should be done. Although the exact mechanism of action is not known, data point to immunomodulation of an activated complement system as a key component in treatment efficacy.

REFERENCES

1. Banker BQ, Victor M. Dermatomyositis (systemic angiopathy) of childhood. Medicine 1966; 45:261–289.
2. Bitnum S, Daeschner CW, Travis LB, Dodge HC. Dermatomyositis. J Pediatr 1964; 64:101–131.
3. Bohan A, Peter JB. Polymyositis and dermatomyositis. Part 1. N Engl J Med 1975; 292:344–347.
4. Bohan A, Peter JB. Polymyositis and dermatomyositis. Part 2. N Engl J Med 1975; 292:403–407.
5. Sullivan DB, Cassidy JT, Petty RE. Dermatomyositis in the pediatric patient. Arthritis Rheum 1977; 20:327–331.
6. Pearson CM. Polymyositis and dermatomyositis. Bull Rheum Dis 1962; 12:269–272.
7. Oddis CV, Conte CG, Steen VD, Medsger TA. Incidence of polymyositis dermatomyositis: A 20 year study of hospital diagnosed cases in Allegheny County, PA, 1963–1982. J Rheum 1990; 17:1329–1334.
8. Plotz PH, Rider LG, Targoff IN, Raben N, O'Hanlon TP, Miller FW. Myositis: immunologic contributions to understanding cause, pathogenesis, and therapy. Ann Intern Med 1995; 122:715–724.

9. Denardo BA, Tucker LB, Miller LM, Szer IS, Schaller JG. Demography of a regional pediatric rheumatology patient population. J Rheum 1994; 21:1553–1561.

10. Whitaker JN, Engel WK. Vascular deposits of immunoglobulins and complement in idiopathic inflammatory myopathy. N Engl J Med 1972; 286:333–338.

11. Kissel JT, Mendell JR, Rammohan KW. Microvascular deposition of complement membrane attack complex in dermatomyositis. N Engl J Med 1986; 314:329–334.

12. Currie S, Saunders M, Knowles M, Brown AE. Immunological aspects of polymyositis. Q J Med 1971; 40:63–84.

13. Dalakas MC. Clinical, immunopathologic, and therapeutic considerations of inflammatory myopathies. Clin Neuropharm 1992; 15:327–351.

14. Targoff IN. Autoantibodies in polymyositis. Rheum Dis Clin North Am 1992; 18:455–482.

15. Love LA, Leff RL, Fraser DD, et al. A new approach to the classification of idiopathic inflammatory myopathy: myositis-specific autoantibodies define useful homogeneous patient groups. Medicine 1991; 70:360–374.

16. Jacobs JCJ. Treatment of dermatomyositis. Arthritis Rheum 1977; 20:338–341.

17. Sullivan DB, Cassidy JT, Petty RE, Burt MT. Prognosis in childhood dermatomyositis. J Pediatr 1972; 80:555–563.

18. Wedgwood RJ, Cook CD, Cohen J. Dermatomyositis: report of 26 cases in children with a discussion of endocrine therapy in 13. Pediatrics 1953; 12:447–466.

19. Dubowitz V. Treatment of dermatomyositis in childhood. Arch Dis Child 1976; 51:494–500.

20. Heckmatt J, Saunders C, Peters AM, et al. Cyclosporin in juvenile dermatomyositis. Lancet 1989; i:1063–1066.

21. Lueck CJ, Trend P, Swash M. Cyclosporin in the management of polymyositis and dermatomyositis. J Neurol 1991; 54:1007–1008.

22. Miller LC, Sisson BA, Tucker LB, DeNardo BA, Schaller JG. Methotrexate treatment of recalcitrant childhood dermatomyositis. Arthritis Rheum 1992; 35:1143–1149.

23. Miller FW, Leitman SF, Cronin ME, et al. Controlled trial of plasma exchange and leukpaheresis in polymyositis and dermatomyositis. N Engl J Med 1992; 326:1380–1384.

24. Olson NY, Lindsley CB. Adjunctive use of hydroxychloroquine in childhood dermatomyositis. J Rheumatol 1989; 16:1545–1547.

25. Sussman GL, Pruzanski W. The role of intravenous infusions of gamma globulin in the therapy of polymyositis and dermatomyositis. J Rheum 1994; 21:990–992.

26. Cherin P, Herson S, Wechsler B, et al. Efficacy of intravenous gammaglobulin therapy in chronic refractory polymyositis and dermatomyositis: an open study with 20 adult patients. Am J Med 1991; 91:162–168.

27. Collet E, Dalac S, Maerens B, Courtois JM, Izac M, Lambert D. Juvenile dermatomyositis: treatment with intravenous gammaglobulin. Br J Dermatol 1994; 130:231–234.

28. Dalakas MC, Illa I, Dambrosia JM, et al. A controlled trial of high-dose intravenous immune globulin infusions as treatment for dermatomyositis. N Engl J Med 1993; 329:1993–2000.

29. Lang BA, Laxer RM, Murphy G, Silverman ED, Roifman CM. Treatment of dermatomyositis with intravenous gammaglobulin. Am J Med 1991; 91:169–172.

30. Roifman CM, Schaffer FM, Wachsmuth SE, Murphy G, Gelfand EW. Reversal of chronic polymyositis following intravenous immune serum globulin therapy. JAMA 1987; 258:513–515.

31. Sansome A, Dubowitz V. Intravenous immunoglobulin in juvenile dermatomyositis—four year review of nine cases. Arch Dis Child 1995; 72:25–28.

32. Reimold AM, Weinblatt ME. Tachyphylaxis of intravenous immunoglobulin in refractory inflammatory myopathy. J Rheum 1994; 21:1144–1146.

33. Cherin P, Piette JC, Wechsler B, et al. Intravenous gamma globulin as first line therapy in

polymyositis and dermatomyositis: an open study in 11 adult patients. J Rheum 1994; 21:1092–1097.

34. Basta M, Dalakas MC. High-dose intravenous immunoglobulin exerts its beneficial effect in patients with dermatomyositis by blocking endomysial deposition of activated complement fragments. J Clin Invest 1994; 94:1729–1735.

31

Use of Intravenous Immunoglobulin in Therapy of Rheumatoid Arthritis

David E. Yocum
Arizona Arthritis Center, Arizona Health Sciences Center, University of Arizona, Tucson, Arizona

INTRODUCTION

Rheumatoid arthritis (RA) is a chronic inflammatory disease of unknown etiology characterized clinically by morning stiffness associated with swelling and pain of involved joints. In its worse stages, cartilage and boney erosions occur with marked destruction and disability (1). The proposed immunological mechanisms include abnormal cellular immune function, primarily involving T helper cells, humoral immune mechanisms, with involvement of rheumatoid factor; and other cellular mechanisms, including macrophage and synovial fibroblast release of cytokines and growth factors associated with the release of neutral proteases and other destructive enzymes.

The hypothesized mechanisms of action of intravenous immunoglobulin (IVIG) in RA include direct antibacterial activity, Fc-mediated blockade of reticuloendothelial cells, interference with immune complex binding, acting as a sump for complement activation products, suppression of monocyte and macrophage function, enhanced secretion of anti-inflammatory cytokines, anti-idiotypic regulatory antibodies, and immunoregulatory anti–T cell receptor antibodies (2–11). While only a few uncontrolled clinical trials have been performed in rheumatoid arthritis, all have demonstrated efficacy with minimal side effects (12–16). This is not surprising considering the immunological pathogenesis of RA and the hypothesized mechanisms of action of IVIG.

CLINICAL TRIALS

While used by many physicians as a "last-ditch" effort to control severe rheumatoid arthritis, there have been a few reported clinical trials using IVIG (Table 1). All trials to date have either been anecdotal or uncontrolled and prospective. There has also been variation in the source of the immunoglobulin as well as the dosage regimen used. However, all reported trials have been promising except in the treatment of immune-mediated neutropenia secondary to Felty's syndrome.

Table 1 Efficacy of IVIG in Rheumatoid Arthritis

Investigators	Trial Type	Dose	Response	N	Reference
Savery (12)	Case report	40 mg/kg/wk then 40 mg/kg/mo after 4–15 weeks	3/3 (subjective)	3	12
Tumiati et al. (13,16)	Prospective, open, uncontrolled	400 mg/kg/day × 5 days then 400 mg/kg/day q mo × 6 mos	9/10 (objective and subjective)	10	13
Combe et al. (15)	Prospective, open uncontrolled	1500 mg/day × 7 days q 1–1.5 mos and 3500 mg/day × 3 days	17/31 with > 50% response	31	15
Becker et al. (14)	Prospective, open uncontrolled	10 g/day × 3 days q month	6/10 with ≥ 30% ↓ in activity index	11	14

In a report using placenta-eluted gammaglobulin, Combe et al. noted a 50% improvement in 60% of patients with rheumatoid arthritis (15). Improvement included decreased activity indices as well as morning stiffness and walking time. Of the 22 patients treated with 1500 mg/day for 7 days, every 30–45 days, 14 (64%) had a >50% decrease in disease activity, with six patients achieving a full remission. While 750 mg/day for 7 days each month was not effective, 3500 mg/day for 3 days resulted in one of four patients achieving a >50% response. Similar doses of serum-derived immunoglobulin were not efficacious. Immunologically, there was a significant increase in E-rosetting (T) cells and a decrease in EA-rosetting (Fc binding) cells along with an enhanced peripheral blood monocuclear cell response to PHA. However, these responses could not be correlated with the clinical response. Patients with shorter disease duration appeared to do better.

At about the same time, Breedveld et al. reported on the use of IVIG in the treatment of immune-mediated Felty's syndrome (17). Five patients with sustained leukopenia of less than 2000 white blood cells and splenomegaly were treated with 400 mg/kg daily for 5 days. None of the patients experienced increases in their white blood cell count either during or subsequent to the treatment. There were no reports of what happened to the patients' arthritis in this trial. Similarly, Yocum (personal communication) treated two patients with Felty's syndrome with 500 mg/kg/day of immunoglobulin for 5 days. Neither patient experienced increases in their leukocyte count or improvement in their rheumatoid arthritis.

Three patients with the onset of rheumatoid arthritis (?JRA) between the ages of 12 and 16 were treated with IVIG later in their disease (12). These patients were not characterized as being seropositive or having definite or classical rheumatoid arthritis. In addition, the dosages were quite different from those previously used (40 mg/kg on a weekly basis). All three patients noted significant improvement subjectively, and two of the three continued on the same dose given on a monthly basis. No further data were given on these patients.

Becker et al. treated 11 RA patients with 10 g/day IVIG for 3 days, each month for up to 18 months (14). One patient was discontinued due to noncompliance, and of the remaining 10, six noted efficacy at 3 months, five at 5 months, and three at 7 months. The response was most evident during the 2 weeks immediately following infusion. Immunological and laboratory data demonstrated significant decreases in the number of circulating lymphocytes, the percentage of CD4+ lymphocytes, and the CD4/CD8 ratio, which was associated with an increase in the percentage of CD8+ lymphocytes. While there was no change in the titer of rheumatoid factor or ANA, the percentage of B cells, anti-u stimulation of B cells, and the levels of circulating immune complexes decreased significantly.

In a prospective, unblinded trial reported by Tumiati et al., 10 patients with active rheumatoid arthritis unresponsive to first- and second-line agents were administered intravenous gammaglobulin over a 6-month period (13). The dosage of gammaglobulin was 400 mg/kg/day for 5 days for the first week of the first month and then 400 mg/kg/month for 6 months. Of the 10 patients, one dropped out due to noncompliance, and of the remaining nine, all eight demonstrated objective and subjective improvement in disease activity. Overall, there was significant improvement by week 4 in the articular index, the number of swollen joints, and the visual pain analog scale. Morning stiffness decreased by 50%, and six of seven patients were able either to discontinue or to decrease their steroid dosage. However, there is no significant change in the grip strength. While clinical improvement was sustained for 8 months, 2 months after discontinuation of therapy, all except one of the patients demonstrated loss of efficacy. There were no significant side effects except for mild dizziness, nausea, and hypotension in two patients. Immunologically, there were significant decreases in the C-reactive protein level beginning at week 4 but no significant changes in the sedimentation rate. There were no changes in the rheumatoid factor, antinuclear antibody titers, or complement levels. In addition, overall immunoglobulin levels remained unchanged during the treatment. Further immunological data looking at cell surface receptors demonstrated a significant reduction in the number of T lymphocytes, especially those of the CD4+ CD45RA+ cell population. This latter population represents the naive T cells; this has been reported to be low in rheumatoid arthritis. There were no significant changes in activation markers or the number of circulating B lymphocytes. The increase in CD45RA+ CD4+ cells demonstrates a strict correlation with clinical improvement. Discontinuation of therapy and flare of disease were associated with a decrease in this population to pretreatment levels.

DISCUSSION

The proposed mechanism of action of IVIG strongly suggests efficacy in rheumatoid arthritis. The mechanisms that would appear to be most important would be the effects on Fc binding in the reticuloendothelial system, regulation of monocyte and macrophage function, anti-idiotypic regulation of cellular immunity, enhancement of anti-inflammatory cytokines, and regulation of cellular immune function through anti–T cell receptor antibodies. In recent studies, Marchalonis et al. have demonstrated that all individuals who contain antibodies to T cell receptors as demonstrated by an in vitro assay using synthetic putative T cell receptor peptides (10,11). Interestingly, these apparent autoantibodies, which are probably immunoregulatory, are increased in rheumatoid arthritis, most significantly in the IgM class. This would suggest that these antibodies, somewhat similar to rheumatoid factor, may be an attempt by the patient to regulate their immune response. Interestingly, patients with systemic lupus have similar elevations of anti–T cell receptor antibodies, but these are primarily of the IgG class. At present, these researchers are attempting to isolate B cell clones to further identify the potential actions of these anti–T cell receptor antibodies. Such data may be very important, not only therapeutically but also in understanding the pathogenesis of RA.

The reported efficacy of intravenous gammaglobulin in rheumatoid arthritis, while limited by uncontrolled trials, appears as effective as clinical trials using anti-CD4 and anti-CD5 monoclonal antibodies. Certainly, the side effects are significantly less and not associated with significant T cell suppression or infectious complications. In fact, intravenous gammaglobulin is protective against infectious complications.

The prolonged benefit of up to 2 months postdiscontinuation of therapy of IVIG would suggest a regulatory mechanism with more sustained activity than Fc receptor binding in the reticuloendothelial system. It suggests the induction of certain T cell suppressor lines or, as suggested by Tumiati et al., a shift in the memory and naive T cell populations. The shift toward naive T cell populations would suggest mechanisms of decreasing activated arthritis specified T cells, even though CD25+ CD4+ cells were apparently not affected.

Potentially as important would be the induction of immunosuppressive cytokines which, if enhanced over a 6-month period, may result in a prolonged antiarthritic effect. Attempts through other mechanisms at induction of anti-inflammatory cytokines have not been successful.

SUMMARY

While preliminary data would suggest a promising role for the use of IVIG in therapy of rheumatoid arthritis, no prospective, double-blind controlled trials have been done. All preliminary trials to date have demonstrated efficacy using dosages from 40 to 400 mg/kg/day on a weekly or monthly basis. Efficacy has been sustained up to 3 months postcompletion of therapy, and positive laboratory parameters have been observed in at least two trials. The proposed mechanism of action of this form of therapy is extremely exciting and associated with low adverse experiences. Unfortunately, this mode of therapy is limited by cost and inconvenience, although if a monthly injection would work, this may not be the case. Recent research into mechanisms of action including anti-T cell receptor antibodies is very exciting. Controlled, double-blind trials using intravenous gammaglobulin in RA are warranted.

REFERENCES

1. Harris ED Jr. Rheumatoid arthritis: pathophysiology and implications for therapy. N Engl J Med 1990; 322:1277–1289.
2. Kimberly RP, Salmon JE, Bussel JB, Crown MK, Hilgartner MW. Modulation of mononuclear phagocyte function by intravenous gammaglobulin. J Immunol 1984; 132:745.
3. Kurlander RJ, Hall J. Comparison of intravenous gammaglobulin and a monoclonal anti-Fc receptor antibody as inhibitors of immune complexes in vivo in mice. J Clin Invest 1986; 77:2010–2018.
4. Mannhalter JW, Ahmad R, Wolf HM, Eibl M. Effect of polymer IgG on human monocyte functions. Int Arch Allergy Appl Immunol 1987; 82:159–167.
5. Shimozato TF, Iwata M, Kawada H, Tamura N. Human immunoglobulin preparation of intravenous use induces elevation of cellular cyclic adenosine 3' 5'-monophosphate levels, resulting in suppression of tumor necrosis factor alpha and interleukin 1 production. Immunology 1991; 72:497–501.
6. Kaveri SV, Dietrich G, Hurez V, Kazatchkine MD. Intravenous immunoglobulins (IVIg) in the treatment of autoimmune disease. Clin Exp Immunol 1991; 86:192–199.
7. Stohl W, Mayer L. Inhibition of T cell–dependent human B cell proliferation and B cell differentiation by poly-specific monomeric IgG. Clin Exp Immunol 1987; 70:649–659.
8. Basta M, Kirshbom P, Frank MM, Fries LF. Mechanisms of therapeutic effect of high-dose intravenous immunoglobulin. Attenuation of acute, complement-dependent immune damage in a guinea pig model. J Clin Invest 1989; 84:1974–1981.
9. Roux RH, Tankersley DL. A view of the human idiotypic repertoire. Electron microscopic and immunologic analysis of spontaneous idiotype–anti-idiotype dimers in pooled IgG. J Immunol 1990; 144:1387–1395.
10. Marchalonis JJ, Schluter SF, Wang E, et al. Synthetic autoantigens of immunoglobulins and T-cell receptors: their recognition in aging, infection and autoimmunity. Proc Soc Exp Biol Med 1994; 207:129–147.

11. Marchalonis JJ, Kaymaz H, Schluter SF, Yocum DE. Human autoantibodies to a synthetic putative T-cell receptor-chain regulatory idiotype: expression in autoimmunity and aging. Exp Clin Immunogenet 1993; 10:1–15.

12. Savery F. Intravenous immunoglobulin treatment of rheumatoid arthritis–associated immunodeficiency. Clin Ther 1988; 10:527–529.

13. Tumiati B, Cusoli P, Veneziani M, Rinaldi G. High-dose immunoglobulin therapy as an immunomodulatory treatment of rheumatoid arthritis. Arthritis Rheum 1992; 35:1126–1133.

14. Becker H, Mitropoulou G, Helmke K. Immunomodulatory therapy of rheumatoid arthritis by high-dose intravenous immunoglobulin. Klin Wochenschr 1989; 67:286–290.

15. Combe B, Cosso B, Clot J, Bonneau M, Sany J. Human placenta-eluted gammaglobulin in immunomodulating treatment of rheumatoid arthritis. Am J Med 1985; 78:920–928.

16. Tumiati B, Bellelli A, Veneziani M, Castellini G. Use of high-dose immunoglobulin in rheumatoid arthritis. Prog Rheumatol 1990; 4:39–45.

17. Breedveld FC, Brand A, Aken WG. High dose intravenous gammaglobulin for Felty's syndrome. J Rheumatol 1985; 12:700–702.

32

Treatment of Systemic Lupus Erythematosus with Pooled Human Intravenous Immunoglobulin

Stanley C. Jordan

Cedars-Sinai Medical Center, Los Angeles, California

INTRODUCTION

Systemic lupus erythematosus (SLE) is a multisystem disease in which dysfunctional immune regulation results in autoantibody production, immune complex formation, and activation of inflammatory cytokine pathways with subsequent tissue injury and disease manifestations. Although the etiology of SLE remains enigmatic, it is likely that antibodies to DNA are an integral component of the disease process (1).

Since the report of Ballow in 1991 (2) detailing the use of pooled human intravenous immunoglobulin (IVIG) in SLE and autoimmune disorders, new reports regarding the effectiveness of IVIG in autoimmune diseases and vasculitic disorders have appeared. This chapter will summarize those reports, focus on the rationale for the use of IVIG in SLE, and address some of the complications of IVIG therapy. To begin with, I would like to discuss the pathological regulation of autoantibody production in SLE and how this might be modified by IVIG.

ETIOLOGY OF ANTI-DNA ANTIBODIES IN SLE

The presence of anti-DNA antibodies in the sera of SLE patients has long been considered a marker of, and pathogenic factor responsible for, renal disease and other systemic manifestations of the disease (1,3,4). Normal human sera contain antibodies which are reactive with numerous autoantigens, including DNA (5–7). These natural autoantibodies in normal human sera are usually of the IgM isotype and are encoded by V region genes in a germ line configuration (5,8–10). Normal human sera also contain IgG anti-DNA antibodies. The role of these natural autoantibodies is unclear, but has been proposed to be maintenance of homeostasis and competence of the immune system in normal healthy individuals (11). Recent data (12,13) suggest that polyclonal activation of autoantibody-producing B cells may be responsible, at least in part, for disease manifestations of SLE. Isenberg et al. (14) suggest that this observed polyclonal activation in human SLE might best be described as a limited and focused response. This may be related to the expansion of preactivated B cells with autoimmune potential (i.e., anti-DNA–producing B cells) in genetically predisposed individuals.

Recent data by Mayet et al. (15) lend credence to this hypothesis. These investigators showed that human B cells from patients with autoimmune diseases such as Wegener's granulomatosis and SLE could be transformed by Epstein-Barr virus (EBV) in vitro with subsequent production of large quantities of disease-specific autoantibodies (C-ANCA in Wegener's and anti-DNA in SLE). We have recently observed two patients (one Wegener's and one SLE) in whom high levels of EBV DNA was measured in peripheral blood mononuclear cells (PBMCs) by virus-specific PCR during disease relapse. Each relapse was associated with a marked increase in C-ANCA and anti-DNA antibody levels and clinical disease manifestations. EBV DNA was not detected when these patients were in remission.

It is also known that many other viruses have the capacity to induce polyclonal activation of B cells and could be important activators of autoimmune diseases (16). It would thus appear that the clinical expression of autoimmune diseases such as SLE depends on the exposure of a genetically autoimmune-prone individual to environmental factors (most commonly infectious) that polyclonally activate B cells to produce autoantibodies that result in a prolonged and dysfunctional immune response to self (i.e., DNA).

IVIG IN THE TREATMENT OF SLE

Numerous immunological abnormalities have been identified in SLE that could be amendable to the immunoregulatory actions of IVIG. The most characteristic abnormality is generalized polyclonal B cell activation, resulting in autoantibody production and immune complex formation. SLE is considered an immune complex disorder in which tissue injury (skin, CNS, kidney, etc.) occurs as a direct result of immune complex–mediated injury through complement activation. IVIG may inhibit autoantibody production through anti-idiotypic networks; but are there other possible mechanisms through which IVIG might work in a disease like SLE (Table 1)? Since complement activation can be an important mechanism for tissue injury in SLE, one possible protective effect of very high concentrations of IVIG may be the uptake of biologically active complement components. Basta et al. (17) were the first to show that very high levels of IVIG in fluid phase compete directly for nascent C4 fragments, thereby preventing C4 binding to target cells with subsequent inhibition of tissue injury and destruction. IVIG may also solubilize immune complexes, reducing their size and subsequent ability to activate complement and to produce tissue injury. Tomino et al. (18) were the first to report in vitro solubilization of tissue immune deposits in renal biopsy cortex tissue of patients with membranous nephropathy.

Immune complexes also possess strong proinflammatory effects by virtue of their ability to induce, in a wide variety of cell types, cytokine mRNA synthesis and subsequent release. We have shown that aggregated human gammaglobulin (AHG), an in vitro surrogate for circulating immune complexes, has the capacity to induce cytokine release from normal human peripheral blood mononuclear cells (PBMCs). We have also shown that TNF-α and IL-6 mRNA synthesis is stimulated in human PBMCs by ag-

Table 1 Intravenous Immunoglobulin Therapy for Patients with Systemic Lupus Erythematosus

Investigator	Res/Total	Improvements	Detrimental effects
Ballow and Park	1/3	Steroid sparing, cutaneous vasculitis	None
Gaedicke et al.	1/2	Cutaneous vasculitis	None
Lin and Racis	3/6	Reduced immune complexes (5/6), cutaneous vasculitis, thrombocytopenia	Proteinuria (2)
Akashi et al. (41)	2/2	Pancytopenia, proteinuria	None
Corvette et al.	2/3	Encephalitis, pancytopenia	Renal function
Jordan (37)	1/6	Encephalitis, pancytopenia	Proteinuria

gregated immunoglobulin. These immune complex aggregates are > 19S in size, which is critical for their ability to activate complement and cytokine release from mononuclear cells (19).

Could IVIG mediate its immunoregulatory effects by inhibition of cytokine synthesis and/or release by immune complex–stimulated mononuclear cells? Data to support this contention come from investigations into the beneficial effects of IVIG in Kawasaki disease. In this childhood vasculitis (Table 2), IVIG is known to exert beneficial anti-inflammatory and immunoregulatory effects which reduce the morbidity from coronary artery vasculitis. We and others (20,21) have detected high levels of cytokines (TNF-α, γ-IFN, and IL-1) in the sera of Kawasaki disease patients. Leung et al. (21) showed that IVIG can inhibit the expression of endothelial cell activation markers such as endothelial leukocyte adhesion molecule-1 (ELAM-1) and intercellular adhesion molecule-1 (ICAM-1) in Kawasaki disease patients through inhibition of IL-1. Other investigators suggest that IVIG acts through the production of IL-1 receptor antagonist (IL-1RA) in mononuclear cells, thereby blocking IL-1 activity (22,23). Our group has shown that sera from active SLE patients activates resting human umbilical vein endothelial cells (HUVECs) to express MHC class 1 molecules, apparently secondary to the presence of α-IFN and TNF-α in the sera of active SLE patients as monoclonal antibodies to these (but not other) cytokines remove this activity from SLE sera (24).

IL-6 is a pleiotropic cytokine which enhances B-cell immunoglobulin production, stimulates mesangial cell proliferation, and mediates mesangial-proliferative glomerulonephritis in animal models. It appears to be very important for immunoglobulin and autoantibody production in polyclonally activated B cells (25). Dysfunctional IL-6 production has been associated with autoimmune phenomena in humans, including mesangial proliferative glomerulonephritis. Data from our group (26) have shown overexpression of IL-6 mRNA and protein levels in patients with active SLE when compared with normals and patients with inactive SLE. High IL-6 levels appear to correlate well with high levels of polyclonal B cell activation and autoantibody produc-

Table 2 Classification of Systemic Immune-Mediated Vasculitides

Pathogenic mechanism	Clinical syndrome
Immune complex–mediated	
Immune	Leukocytoclastic angiitis (2nd serum sickness)
	PAN (2nd HBV)
	Leukocytoclastic angiitis (2nd cyroglob)
Autoimmune	Leukocytoclastic angiitis (2nd SLE)
Direct antibody attack	
Antibasement membrane	PRS (Goodpasture's)
Antiendothelia cell	Kawasaki disease
	PAN
	SLE
	IgA nephropathy
	Allograft rej. vascular
ANCA-associated	Wegener's vasculitis
	PAN
	PRS with capillaritis
	Churg-Strauss synd.
	HSP? (IgA-ANCA)
Cell-mediated	
	Giant cell arteritis
	Allograft rejection vascular

Modified from Jennette et al. (43).

tion in SLE patients (26). We have recently reported that IVIG is a potent inhibitor of pokeweed mitogen (PWM)-stimulated Ig (IgG, IgM, IgA) production in PBMCs (19,27,28), which is mediated, in part, by a potent inhibitory efect on PWM-stimulated IL-6 production. The potent and consistent inhibition of PWM-stimulated Ig production by IVIG occurs early after incubation and is Fc-dependent. IVIG strongly inhibited IL-6, γ-IFN, IL-2, and IgG mRNA production at time points when maximal amounts of mRNA were produced, and showed a marked inhibitory effect on PWM-stimulated IL-6 and γ-IFN protein levels (19,28). Andersson et al. (29,30) have recently shown that IVIG has potent effects on cytokine-producing cell generation. These investigators have used multiple mechanisms to stimulate T cells, including anti-CD3 stimulation. In this model, IVIG is a potent inhibitor of anti-CD3–stimulated cytokine release, as well as IL-2 receptor expression. These investigators also noted that IL-1RA was upregulated in resting PBMCs incubated with IVIG alone. We feel that the inhibitory effects on Ig production are mediated primarily through inhibition of cytokine(s) important for the generation of Ig-secreting B cells. Since IL-6 and other proinflammatory cytokines are important in SLE, it is not unreasonable to expect that IVIG might exert at least some of its beneficial effects through inhibition of key immunoregulatory and proinflammatory cytokines, or stimulation of anti-inflammatory cytokines such as IL-1RA.

There are ample experimental data to suggest a role for IVIG in the treatment of the immune abnormalities encountered in SLE and other similar autoimmune disorders (Table 3). However, the real proof of efficacy comes from data generated in clinical trials. As of now, no controlled clinical trials have occurred. The available reported data on the efficacy of IVIG in the treatment of SLE are anecdotal and is summarized are follows: Ballow (2) reported that IVIG showed beneficial effects in the treatment of SLE and primary Sjögren's syndrome. This group also reported that IVIG had good effects on the cutaneous manifestations of SLE, and exerted a steroid-sparing effect.

Others have reported beneficial effects of IVIG therapy in the treatment of various cytopenias associated with SLE and with encephalitis. Francioni et al. (31) treated 12 SLE patients with IVIG in doses of 400 mg/kg/day for 5 consecutive days, monthly for 6–24 months. Patients were chosen because of unresponsiveness to or complications from standard immunosuppressive therapies. Progressive clinical improvement was seen in 11 of 12 patients. Improvement was defined as increased hemoglobin, total serum hemolytic complement activity, C3 and C4 levels, and improved platelet counts in two thrombocytopenic patients. A marked improvement in serum urea nitrogen and creatinine clearance was also observed. The authors conclude that IVIG therapy was very promising but that further controlled trials were necessary to prove efficacy.

Silvestris et al. (32) reported that IVIG contains anti-idiotypic antibodies which inhibit the activity of pathogenic anti-DNA antibodies expressed in active SLE patients.

Table 3 Intravenous Immunoglobulin as Therapy for Autoimmune Disorders

Immune cytopenias
    ITP[a]
    Autoimmune hemolytic anemia
    Immune neutropenia
Autoimmune coagulopathies
    Antihemophilic factor VIIIc inhibitor
    Antiphospholipid antibody syndrome
Vasculitic disorders
    ANCA (+) vasculitides
    Kawasaki disease
Collagen vascular disorders
    SLE[b]
    Rheumatoid arthritis
    Polymyositis
Autoimmune neurological disorders
    Myasthenia gravis
    Chronic inflammatory polyneuropathy
    Guillain-Barré syndrome
    Intractable childhood seizures
Inflammatory bowel disease
    Crohn's disease
    Ulcerative colitis
Organ-specific autoimmune disease
    Insulin-dependent diabetes

[a]ITP: idiopathic thrombocytopenic purpura.
[b]SLE: systemic lupus erythematosis.

The authors conclude that the variable results seen in treatment of SLE with IVIG may result from the differing levels of blocking anti-idiotypes to these pathogenic anti-DNA antibodies in various lots of IVIG preparations.

Ronda et al. (33) also showed that IVIG preparations contain antibodies with V regions capable of binding anti–endothelial cell antibodies (AECA) from SLE patients. The authors conclude that their findings are relevant to the understanding of the mechanisms that control the expression of natural autoantibody and how this may be applied to dysfunctional autoantibody expression in autoimmune disease.

Aharon et al. (34) reported that IVIG was an excellent alternative to cytotoxic drug therapy in the treatment of elderly men with SLE. Two male patients >65 years of age were described. One patient was treated with traditional steroid and cytotoxic drug therapy and developed multiple complications. A second patient received only IVIG and developed a remission. The authors conclude that IVIG may be a successful alternative therapy for elderly patients with SLE.

Winder et al. (35) reported two patients with life-threatening manifestations of SLE who were treated with high-dose IVIG. Following IVIG therapy, lupus pneumonitis and encephalitis in the first patient and SLE nephritis in the second resolved. Continued treatment with IVIG monthly for up to 20 months resulted in prolonged clinical and laboratory remission. These authors also stopped treatment with cytotoxic agents and lowered corticosteroids. The second patient had an exacerbation of SLE 10 months after initiation of IVIG therapy.

Pirner et al. (36) described six patients who were treated with IVIG (400 mg/kg for 5 days). One patient had a 6-month remission, one a 36-month remission; however, three patients experienced deterioration in renal function within 1 month of IVIG administration. Several authors including our group (36–38) have reported a worsening of proteinuria and renal function in SLE patients treated with IVIG. Migliaresi et al. (39) reported four patients treated with IVIG who responded well to IVIG without complications. Horng et al. (40) reported an infant born to a mother with SLE who had neonatal pancytopenia and evidence for neonatal SLE (transmitted by active transport of pathogenic autoantibodies across the placenta). The child was treated with IVIG and showed a dramatic response. These data suggest that pathogenic autoantibodies which are actively transported across the placenta can produce disease in the neonate and are susceptible to V region inhibition by anti-idiotypic antibodies in the IVIG.

Barron et al. (38) reported that IVIG effectively treated three patients with SLE, but resulted in an exacerbation of renal disease in three others. Since our last report (19), we have tested a total of seven patients who developed severe SLE with IVIG. All but two showed no discernible beneficial effect, and in fact, two showed increased proteinuria. The patients who showed a beneficial effect had primary CNS involvement and cytopenia. The other patients were severely ill from their SLE, and had failed standard pulse cytoxan protocols. All also had significant nephrotic syndrome with renal failure and evidence for CNS involvement as well. So these patients were given IVIG as a "last-ditch" therapy where other, more standard therapies had failed. Indeed, this may not be the best way to assess the efficacy of IVIG therapy in SLE patients.

Other colleagues have reported anecdotal cases where IVIG has been beneficial in controlling the glomerulonephritis and CNS symptoms associated with SLE. In fact, one pediatric nephrologist reports he uses monthly IVIG therapy to replace cytoxan pulses in young female SLE patients (total eight) who refuse cytoxan therapy. Others report that IVIG has been less effective. It is very important to realize that these are anecdotal reports. Dosages and disease status at the time of IVIG therapy vary greatly and may affect any potential benefit. My feeling, at the present time, is that IVIG should not be considered as a primary therapy for SLE, and in fact may cause deleterious side effects such as increased proteinuria in patients with significant renal involvement. Despite this, there are SLE patients who clearly appear to benefit from IVIG therapy.

The report by Akashi et al. (41) showed that IVIG therapy in two drug-resistant SLE patients actually reduced proteinuria and improved other clinical parameters dramatically. It is also important to consider why IVIG might not be effective in certain subsets of SLE patients. First, my own experience has been with SLE patients with severe nephrotic syndrome. This is a condition in which all serum proteins are low, including immunoglobulins. These may be lost in the urine, but are primarily low due to inhibited production and hypercatabolism of proteins.

It is possible that IVIG therapy given to such individuals has no effect because it is so rapidly lost from the body either through urinary loss or through catabolism. This would not explain why patients would get worse after IVIG therapy, however. I do not fully understand this, but it is possible that deleterious autoantibodies, especially those directed at IgG, may result in pathogenic immune complex formation and result in renal inflammation and injury as the immune complexes are trapped in the glomerular capillary bed.

We were called to see one patient with Henoch-Schonlein purpura who was treated with IVIG. The patient exhibited minimal urinary findings prior to IVIG, but developed a full-blown acute glomerulonephritis with hematuria and proteinuria immediately after IVIG administration. The hematuria and proteinuria resolved spontaneously when no further IVIG was given. The timing of this reaction strongly suggests that IVIG was responsible for the acute glomerulonephritis. It is of interest to note in this regard that patients with Henoch-Scholein purpura often have IgA–anti-IgG (IgA–rheumatoid factor) antibodies. It is possible that the presence of anti-IgG antibodies in a permissive level could result in phlogistic immune complex formation with development of acute glomerulonephritis. However, recent data (42) suggest that high-dose IVIG improves the outcome of severe IgA nephropathy and Henoch-Schonlein purpura nephritis, reducing proteinuria and improving serum creatinine levels. A blinded controlled trial of IVIG therapy in active SLE patients would help sort out many of these problems.

REFERENCES

1. Worrall J, Snaith ML, Batchelor R, Isenberg DA. Systemic lupus erythematosus: a rheumatological view. Q J Med 1990; 275:319–330.
2. Ballow M. Mechanisms of action of intravenous immunoglobulin therapy and potential use in autoimmune and connective tissue diseases. Cancer 1991; 68:1430–1436.
3. Andres GA, Accinni L, Beiser SM, et al. Localization of fluorescein labeled anti-nucleoside antibodies in glomeruli of patients with systemic lupus erythematosus. J Clin Invest 1970; 49:2106–2118.
4. Koffler D, Agnello V, Kunkel HG. Polynucleotide immune complexes in serum and glomeruli of patients with systemic lupus erythematosus. Am J Pathol 1974; 74:109–124.
5. Mouthon L, Haury M, Sebastien L-D, Barreau C, Coutinho A, Kazatchkine M. Analysis of the normal human IgG antibody repertoire: evidence that IgG autoantibodies of healthy adults recognize a limited and conserved set of protein antigens in homologous tissues. J Immunol 1995; 154:5769–5778.

6. Ronda N, Haury M, Nobrega A, Kaveri S, Coutinho A, Kazatchkine M. Analysis of natural and disease-associated autoantibody repertoires: anti-endothelial cell autoantibody activity in the serum of healthy individuals and patients with systemic lupus erythematosus. Int Immunol 1994; 11:1651.

7. Pfueller SL, Logan D, Tran T, Bilston R. Naturally occurring human IgG antibodies to intracellular and cytoskeletal components of human platelets. Clin Exp Immunol 1990; 79:367.

8. Avrameas S, Dighiero G, Lymberi P, Guilbert B. Studies of natural antibodies and autoantibodies. Ann Immunol 1983; 134D:103.

9. Dighiero G, Lymberi P, Holmberg D, Lundquist I, Coutinho A, Avrameas S. High frequency of natural autoantibodies in normal newborn mice. J Immunol 1985; 134:765.

10. Cairns E, Kwong P, Misener V, Ip P, Bell A, Siminovitch KA. Analysis of variable region genes encoding a human anti-DNA antibody of normal origin: implications for the molecular basis of human autoimmune responses. J Immunol 1989; 143:685.

11. Varela F, Coutinho A. Second generation immune networks. Immunol Today 1991; 12:159.

12. Dar O, Salaman MR, Seifert NH, Isenberg DA. Spontaneous antibody-secreting cells against DNA and common environmental antigens in SLE. J Autoimmun 1990; 3:523–530.

13. Dar O, Salaman MR, Seifert NH, Isenberg DA. Does mitogen-induced antibody production by normal blood cells mimic spontaneous production in lupus? Autoimmunity 1992; 13:285–290.

14. Isenberg D, Ehrenstein M, Longhurst C, Kalsi J. The origin, sequence, structure, and consequences of developing anti-DNA antibodies. Arthritis Rheum 1994; 37:169–180.

15. Mayet W, Hermann E, Kiefer B, et al. In vitro production of anti-neutrophilcytoplasm antibodies (ANCA) by Epstein-Barr virus–transformed B-cell lines in Wegener's granulomatosis. Autoimmunity 1991; 11:13–19.

16. Ahmed R, Oldstone MBA. Mechanisms and biological implications of virus-induced polyclonal B-cell activation. In: Notkins AL, Oldstone MBA, eds. Concepts in Viral Pathogenesis. New York: Springer-Verlag, 1984:231.

17. Basta M, Fries LF, Frank MM. High dose intravenous immunoglobulin inhibit in vitro uptake of C4 fragments onto sensitized erythrocytes. Blood 1991; 77:376–380.

18. Tomino Y, Sakai H, Takaya M, et al. Solubilization of intraglomerular deposits of IgG immune complexes by human sera or gamma globulin in patients with SLE. Clin Exp Immunol 1984; 58:42–48.

19. Jordan SC, Toyoda M. Treatment of autoimmune and systemic vasculitis with pooled human IVIG. Clin Exp Immunol 1994; 97:31–38.

20. Jordan SC, Toyoda M, Mason E, Takahashio M. Serum cytokine levels in Kawasaki disease. Relationship to IVIG therapy. Third International Kawasaki Disease Symposium, Tokyo, Japan. Nov. 29–Dec. 3, 1988. Abstract.

21. Leung DYM, Kurt-Jones E, Newburger JW, et al. Endothelial cell activation and high interleukin-1 secretion in the pathogenesis of acute Kawasaki disease. Lancet 1989; 2:1298–1302.

22. Arend WP, Smith MF Jr, Janson RW, Joslin FG. IL-1 receptor antagonist and IL-1 beta production are regulated differently. J Immunol 1991; 147:1530–1536.

23. Aukrust P, Froland P, Liabakk N-B et al. Release of cytokines, soluble cytokine receptors, and interleukin-1 receptor antagonist after IVIG administration in vivo. Blood 1994; 84:2136–2143.

24. Yap HK, Ng SC, Lee BW, et al. Modulation of MHC expression on human endothelial cells by sera from patients with SLE. Clin Immunol Immunopathol 1993; 68:321–326.

25. Van Snick J. Interleukin-6: an overview. Annu Rev Immunol 1990; 8:253–278.

26. Linker-Israeli M, Deans RJ, Wallace DJ, Prehn J, Ozeri-Chen T, Klinenberg J. Elevated levels of endogenous IL-6 in SLE. J Immunol 1991; 147:117–123.

27. Toyoda M, Jordan SC. Intravenous immunologlobulin inhibits immunoglobulin production and cytokine mRNA production in human PBMCs. Kawasaki Dis 1993; 4:423–430.

28. Toyoda M, Zhang Z-M, Petrosian A, Galera O, Wang S-J, Jordan SC. Modulation of immunoglobulin production and cytokine mRNA expression in peripheral blood mononuclear cells by IVIG. J Clin Immunol 1994; 14:178–189.
29. Andersson JP, Andersson UG. Human intravenous immunoglobulin modulates monokine production in vitro. Immunology 1990; 71:372–376.
30. Andersson J, Skansen-Saphir U, Andersson U. Intravenous immunoglobulin has effects on cytokine production in T-lymphocytes and monocytes/macrophages. Clin & Exp Immunol. 1996; 104(suppl.) 1:10–20.
31. Francioni C, Galeazzi M, Fioravanti A, Gelli R, Marcolongo R. Long-term IVIG treatment in systemic lupus erythematosus. Clin Exp Rheum 1994; 12:163–168.
32. Silvestris F, Cafforio P, Dammacco F. Pathogenic anti-DNA idiotype-reactive IgG in IVIG preparations. Clin Exp Immunol 1994; 97:19–25.
33. Ronda N, Haury M, Nobrega A, Coutinho A, Kazatchkine M. Selectivity of recognition of variable (V) regions of autoantibodies by IVIG. Clin Immunol Immunopathol 1994; 70:124–128.
34. Aharon A, Zandman-Goddard G, Shoenfeld Y. Autoimmune multiorgan involvement in elderly men. Is it SLE? Clin Rheum 1994; 13:631–634.
35. Winder A, Molad Y, Ostfeld I, Kenet G, Pinhas J, Sidi Y. Treatment of SLE by prolonged admininstration of high-dose IVIG: report of 2 cases. J Rheum 1993; 20:495–498.
36. Pirner K, Rubbert A, Burmester GR, Kalden JR, Manger B. Intravenous administration of IVIG in SLE: review of the literature and initial clinical experiences. Infusionsther Transfusionsmed 1993; 20(Suppl 1):131–135.
37. Jordan SC. Intravenous gamma globulin therapy in systemic lupus erythematosus and immune complex disease. Clin Immunol Immunopathol 1989; 53:S164–S169.
38. Barron KS, Sher M, Silverman E. IVIG: magic or black magic. J Rheum 1992; 33:94–97.
39. Migliaresi S, Gallo M, Tirri G. Treatment of SLE with IVIG: preliminary study. Clin Ther 1992; 141:83–84.
40. Horng YC, Chou YH, Tsou-Yau KI. Neonatal lupus erythematosus with negative anti-Ro and anti-La antibodies: report of one case. Acta Paediatr Sin 1992; 33:372–375.
41. Akashi K, Nagasawa K, Mayuri T, et al. Successful treatment of refractory SLE with IVIG. J Rheum 1990; 17:375–379.
42. Rostoker G, Desvaux-Belghiti D, Yannick P, et al. High-dose immunoglobulin therapy for severe IgA nephropathy and Henoch-Schonlein purpura. Ann Intern Med 1994; 120:476–484.
43. Jennette J et al. Autoimmune vasculitis. In: Rose N, MacKay R, eds. The Autoimmune Diseases. New York: Academic Press, 1992: 279–301.

33

Intravenous Immunoglobulin Therapy of Systemic Necrotizing Vasculitis

Leonard H. Calabrese
Cleveland Clinic Foundation, Cleveland, Ohio

INTRODUCTION

The systemic necrotizing vasculitides are a heterogeneous group of clinicopathological syndromes characterized by the presence of necrotizing inflammation of the blood vessels. Their clinical features are protean and depend on the nature and intensity of the inflammatory response and the distribution and degree of target organ damage. The vascular inflammation is believed to be immunologically mediated, but only rarely have causative agents been identified. Even in those rare instances, the immunopathological mechanisms of tissue destruction are incompletely understood.

The mainstays of therapy for these disorders include corticosteroids and cytotoxic drugs. The use of these agents has resulted in a high degree of disease control, but relapses unfortunately do occur and long-term remission is often elusive. More importantly, even when vasculitis is well controlled, an unacceptable number of patients experience significant disease and therapy-related morbidity (1). In view of these limitations there has been a continuing search for alternative therapies including the use of intravenous immunoglobulin (IVIG).

The enthusiasm for IVIG as a therapeutic modality for systemic vasculitis has been stimulated by two important observations: the established efficacy of IVIG in Kawasaki disease, and the identification of anti-idiotype antibodies reactive with antineutrophil cytoplasmic antibodies (ANCA) in pooled IVIG. Based on these observations, varying regimens of IVIG therapy have been applied to a variety of vasculitic conditions and reported mostly in the form of isolated case reports and several uncontrolled series. There are no randomized controlled trials of IVIG in any form of systemic vasculitis thus far reported.

CLINICAL STUDIES

ANCA-Associated Diseases

The largest reported clinical trial of IVIG is that of Jayne et al. (2), treating 26 patients with systemic vasculitis either unresponsive to therapy or previously untreated.

The study group consisted of 14 patients with Wegener's granulomatosis, 11 with microscopic polyarteritis nodosa, and one with rheumatoid vasculitis. Among the previously treated patients, immunosuppressive regimens were maintained on a stable dose for 8 weeks after IVIG. Monitoring of disease activity included a clinical score as well as a variety of adjunctive measures including serial ANCA, C-reactive protein, chest x-rays, and impaired [111]indium white cell scans. The therapeutic intervention consisted of Sandoglobulin (Sandoz) 400 mg/kg/day for 5 days.

The results of this open trial revealed that, clinically, 13 patients achieved remission by 8 weeks without change in immunosuppressive therapy. This was mirrored by falls in ANCA, CRP, and erythrocyte sedimentation rate. In addition, at least partial clearing of radiographic abnormalities on chest x-ray and paired white blood cell scanning were also noted. Transient exacerbations of constitutional symptoms were observed between 10 days and 4 weeks in six patients, but did not require a specific treatment. There were no exacerbations of renal dysfunction in the study group.

Of particular importance was the inclusion of nine patients who were previously untreated. All were reported to improve initially, and four entered full remission for 1 year; the remainder required some form of additional therapy.

After a mean follow-up of 12 months, 19 of their patients were in full remission, six were in partial remission, and one had succumbed to infectious complications. IVIG appeared to be associated with long-term clinical improvement in 18, with six relapses requiring further therapy. The mean dose of cyclophosphamide of the entire group fell from 55 to 16 mg/day while the mean dose of prednisone fell from 50 to 6 mg/day at 12 months of follow-up. Of some note was the paucity of progressive renal disease in this study group suggesting, that overall these patients had relatively mild disease. These investigators cautiously concluded that some or all of the therapeutic benefits from IVIG could be due to placebo or the effects of spontaneous fluctuations in disease activity, and they have strongly endorsed the need for a randomized controlled trial.

A smaller open trial of IVIG has recently been reported by Richter and colleagues (3) in 15 patients with ANCA-associated vasculitis described as poor responders to traditional therapy. The therapeutic intervention consisted of single or multiple doses of IVIG (30 g/day × 5 days). Clinical improvement was noted in six of 15, but was limited to a single organ system such as skin or upper respiratory tract. No improvement was noted in nephritis, pericarditis, or ocular disease. Even when multiple infusions were administered, there was no additional clinical benefit. Overall, 40% of the group appeared to benefit, but there were no complete remissions noted.

Henoch-Schonlein Purpura

IVIG has also been reported to be efficacious in the treatment of Henoch-Schonlein purpura (HSP) as well as for severe IgA-associated nephropathy. Rostoker et al. (4) have recently reported the results of an open prospective cohort study of 11 patients with severe IgA nephropathy including two who had HSP. Patients in this study were followed for 3–10 months before IVIG therapy to document the rate of renal decline. The subjects were given three monthly infusions of high-dose IVIG followed by biweekly intramuscular immunoglobulin. No other treatments were given. The results of this study demonstrated that proteinuria decreased significantly from a median of 5.2 to 2.5 g/day. Histological improvement and staining for IgA in renal biopsies improved as well. In the two patients with HSP, systemic symptoms were reported to clear following IVIG therapy. In addition to this open trial, a single successfully reported case was reported by Heldrich et al. (5). Last, Jordan reported a single case of HSP treated with IVIG that resulted in the onset of gross hematuria (6).

Other Diseases

In addition to the reports noted above, there are a number of isolated case reports of the therapeutic application of IVIG in other vasculitic syndromes including Churg-Strauss (7), Wegener's-like disease (8), and essential mixed cryoglobulinemia (9).

MECHANISM OF ACTION

The mechanism of action of IVIG and autoimmune disease in general (and systemic necrotizing vasculitis in particular) is unknown but is likely due to multiple effects. IVIG is known to perturb numerous Fc-dependent immune functions including phagocytic cell activities as well as certain B and T cell functions (10). In addition, there is also evidence that IVIG modulates the synthesis and release of inflammatory cytokines (11). In the treatment of ANCA-associated vasculitis, there is growing experimental support that IVIG may exert its beneficial effect via idiotypic regulation of the immune system.

A series of laboratory observations are in support of an idiotypic mechanism of IVIG. These have been reported in a series of investigations (12–14). These observations include:

1. F(ab')2 fragments of IVIG contain ANCA anti-idiotypic activity, and these can be enriched by affinity purification of these fragments over sepharose-bound F(ab')2 prepared from the sera of patients with Wegener's granulomatosis.

2. Anti-idiotypic antibodies directed against ANCA are found in the recovery, but not the acute, sera from patients with Wegener's. These anti-idiotypic antibodies recognize public determinants which react with ANCA from other patients.

3. Levels of ANCA anti-idiotypes fluctuate over time and bear an inverse relationship to ANCA titer.

4. Following IVIG therapy, ANCA titers have been observed to rise briefly and then fall to about 50% of pretreatment levels for several months, suggesting active and persistent immunomodulation.

In addition, if IVIG exerts its beneficial effect through an anti-idiotypic mechanism, this also may explain the variability of its therapeutic effectiveness. These same investigators have documented considerable variation in the inhibitory effects of individual IVIG preparations against different ANCA-containing sera. This has also been demonstrated against antiproteinase 3 and antimyeloperoxidase (MPO)-containing sera (14). Explanations for this variation may include the size of the donor pool, the proportion of dimers in the IVIG preparation, and the contribution of privileged donors who have previously developed the relevant autoantibody in the pool. Thus, some preparations of IVIG and even some lots of IVIG may be more or less effective in the treatment of ANCA-associated vasculitis and other diseases. While these data are intriguing, they are far from conclusive and do not supply a satisfying explanation for the effectiveness of IVIG in other (non-ANCA) forms of vasculitis. Further studies are clearly necessary.

TOXICITY

In general, in the majority of isolated case reports as well as several open clinical trials of IVIG reported thus far in systemic necrotizing vasculitis, toxicities have been minimal. Despite this paucity of reports, a significant degree of caution is warranted in the therapeutic application of IVIG in these settings. Potential toxicities include not only allergic and anaphylactic reactions and infections, but also hyperviscosity and thromboembolic events and exacerbations of preexisting renal disease (15). Acute renal failure has been reported from IVIG therapy, which may be particularly important in patients with vasculitis with renal involvement. A recent study, which included renal biopsies performed on two patients who developed acute renal failure following IVIG therapy, demonstrated prominent swelling and vacuolization of the proximal tubule cells similar to that associated with the use of mannitol (16). Of note is that in the series of Jayne et al. (2), the four patients with preexisting but stable renal disease did not experience exacerbations. In a single case report by Jordan and Toyoda (11) of IVIG therapy for HSP, gross hematuria followed the treatment. The cause for this was unknown. Jordan and Toyoda (11) have also reported worsening of proteinuria in patients with systemic lupus erythematosus treated with IVIG.

Other toxicities of importance in this group are IVIG-associated hyperviscosity and thromboembolic disease. Dalakas (17) has reported that IVIG can increase blood viscosity to clinically relevant ranges and can be associated with cerebrovascular thromboembolism. This may be particularly important in patients with underlying cardiovascular disease, in the elderly, and in patients with hypergammaglobulinemia or other hypercoagulable states. To date there are no reports of this complication in patients with vasculitis, though this complication may be underrecognized in such a severely ill population with multisystem disease.

SUMMARY

The efficacy of IVIG therapy for systemic necrotizing vasculitis is unproven. While several large uncontrolled trials have been reported, the data range from extremely promising to somewhat cautious. As always in the absence of randomized controlled trials, initial published studies are more likely to positive in their outcome. Given the lack of other highly effective and nontoxic therapies for these conditions, however, clinicians are likely to empirically use IVIG in the absence of conclusive data. Extreme caution should be applied when IVIG is utilized in such situations, particularly in patients who are critically ill with multisystem disease—especially in those with renal insufficiency.

REFERENCES

1. Hoffman GS, Kerr GS, Leavit RY, et al. Wegener's granulomatosis: an analysis of 158 patients. Ann Intern Med 1992; 116:488.
2. Jayne DRW, Esnault VLM, Lockwood CM. ANCA anti-idiotype antibodies and the treatment of systemic vasculitis with intravenous immunoglobulin. J Autoimmun 1993; 6:207–219.

3. Richter C, Schnabel E, Csernok E, et al. Treatment of ANCA-associated systemic vasculitis with high-dose intravenous immunoglobulin. Arthritis Rheum 1994; 37(9):S353.
4. Rostoker G, Behlgiti DD, Pilatte Y, et al. High dose immunoglobulin therapy for severe IgA nephropathy and Henoch Schonlein purpura. Ann Intern Med 1994; 120:476-484.
5. Heldrich F, Minkin S, Gatdula C. Intravenous immunoglobulin in Henoch Schonlein purpura: a case study. Maryland Med J 1993; 42:577-579.
6. Jordan S. Intravenous gamma globulin therapy in SLE and immune complex disease. Clin Immunol Immunopathol 1989; 53:S164-S169.
7. Hamilos D, Christensen J. Treatment of Churg-Strauss syndrome with high-dose intravenous immunoglobulin. J Allergy Clin Immunol 1991; 88:823-824.
8. Tuso P, Moudgil A, Hay J, et al. Treatment of antineutrophil cytoplasmic autoantibody-positive systemic vasculitis and glomerulonephritis with pooled intravenous gammaglobulin. Am J Kidney Dis 1992; 124:504-508.
9. Boom BW, Brand A, Bavink J, et al. Severe leukocytoclastic vasculitis of the skin in a patient with essential mixed cryoglobulinemia treated with high dose gamma globulin. Arch Dermatol 1988; 124:1550-1554.
10. Dwyer JM. Manipulating the immune system with immune globulin. N Engl J Med 1992; 326:107-116.
11. Jordan SC, Toyoda M. Treatment of autoimmune diseases and systemic vasculitis with pooled human intravenous immune globulin. Clin Exp Immunol 1994; 97(suppl 1):31-38.
12. Jayne D, Esnault V, Lockwood C. ANCA anti-idiotype antibodies and the treatment of systemic vasculitis with intravenous immunoglobulin. J Autoimmun 1993; 6:207-219.
13. Rossi F, Jayne D, Lockwood C, Kazatchkine M. Anti-idiotypes against anti-neutrophil cytoplasmic antigen autoantibodies in normal human polyspecific IgG for therapeutic use and in the remission sera of patients with systemic vasculitis. Clin Exp Immunol 1991; 83:298-203.
14. Pall AA, Varagunam V, Adu D, et al. Anti-idiotypic activity against anti-myeloperoxidase antibodies in pooled human immunoglobulin. Clin Exp Immunol 1994; 95:257-262.
15. Misbah SA, Chapel HM. Adverse effects of intravenous immunoglobulin. Drug Safety 1993; 9(4):254-262.
16. Tan E, Hajinazarian M, Bay W, Neff J, Mandell JR. Acute renal failure resulting from intravenous immunoglobulin therapy. Arch Neurol 1933; 50:137-139.
17. Dalakas MC. High-dose intravenous immunoglobulin and serum viscosity: risk of precipitating thromboembolic events. Neurology 1994; 44:223-226.

34

Lambert-Eaton Myasthenic Syndrome

John Newsom-Davis
University of Oxford, Oxford, England

INTRODUCTION

Intravenous immunoglobulin (IVIG) infusion is being used increasingly to treat a range of neuromuscular disorders that are believed to be autoimmune in origin, as other chapters in this text document. How immunoglobulin exerts its beneficial effects, however, remains uncertain (1). The primary pathological process in most of these disorders involves humoral factors, likely to be autoantibodies. Evidence for this at the clinical level is the short-term improvement observed in these patients following plasma exchange [as, e.g., in myasthenia gravis (2)] and the sustained response that immunosuppressive drugs can engender.

The effector mechanism in some of these autoimmune disorders is a direct antibody-mediated interference with target function (by modulation, complement-dependent destruction, or pharmacological block), while in others it is probably immune complex–mediated, e.g., dermatomyositis. But understanding in greater depth the mode of action of IVIG therapy is hampered in most of these conditions by the specificities of the causative autoantibodies being unknown, so that one cannot investigate what influence, if any, the IVIG exerts on them. Where the causative autoantibodies are indeed known, as is the case in myasthenia gravis, there appear to be no reports of the effects of IVIG therapy in the setting of a placebo-controlled crossover trial.

The Lambert-Eaton myasthenic syndrome (LEMS) is an autoantibody-mediated disorder of neuromuscular transmission causing muscle weakness and autonomic disturbances (3). It can occur as a paraneoplastic disorder (in association with lung cancer) or arise apparently spontaneously (4). Because the antigenic target is known to be voltage-gated calcium channels (VGCCs) and the IgG autoantibodies can be measured in a sensitive radioimmunoassay, it presents an opportunity to investigate the clinical and concurrent serological effects of IVIG therapy. This chapter briefly outlines the clinical features and immunopathogenesis of the disorder, documents single case reports of the effects of IVIG therapy, and describes the results of a randomized, placebo-controlled crossover trial that we have recently completed.

CLINICAL FEATURES

Proximal weakness of the legs is typically the earliest symptom, causing difficulty in walking and a characteristic rolling gait (4). Weakness is often also present at the shoulders and, in more severe cases, may affect all limb muscles as well as respiratory and bulbar muscles. Ptosis can be present, and intermittent double vision may occur. One can usually detect characteristic augmentation of muscle strength during the first few seconds of a maximal voluntary effort, and the depressed tendon reflexes will often be increased following 10-s maximum voluntary activation of the muscle being tested. Patients also experience autonomic symptoms, notably dry mouth, constipation and sexual impotence, which can sometimes precede the motor symptoms.

LEMS is associated with small-cell lung cancer (C-LEMS) in about 60% of cases (4). The neurological symptoms typically precede radiological evidence of the tumor by 2 years and occasionally by up to 5 years. The prevalence of LEMS in small-cell lung cancer in a recent prospective study was 3%, implying approximately 250 new cases of LEMS in this population in the United Kingdom (5). However, the neurological diagnosis is often overlooked in these lung cancer patients. LEMS is also weakly associated with lymphoproliferative disorders (3).

The clinical phenotype in those without cancer (NC-LEMS), who are usually nonsmokers, cannot be distinguished from those with C-LEMS. Such patients have been followed for >10 years without developing a neoplasm.

LEMS also shows an increased association with other autoimmune diseases including vitiligo and thyroid disease. It occasionally associates with myasthenia gravis. Additionally, there is an increased association with certain immune response genes, notably HLA-B8 and -DR3 and with certain Ig heavy chain markers.

DIAGNOSIS

The diagnosis of LEMS has until recently depended on the clinical features and the electromyographic (EMG) findings. The latter are characterized by a greatly reduced amplitude of the compound muscle action potential (CMAP), recorded with surface electrodes over a small muscle of the hand, for example, which greatly increases (>100%) following 10–15 s maximum voluntary contraction of the muscle. There may also be an increased decrement in the CMAP amplitude at low rates of stimulation, e.g., 3 Hz, and increased jitter on single fiber EMG, but these changes are not specific for LEMS, being also found in myasthema gravis.

The diagnosis of LEMS can now also be substantiated by detection of serum anti-VGCC antibodies (see below).

IMMUNOPATHOLOGY

The antibody-mediated nature of LEMS, first suggested by the response to plasma exchange, has been established by experimental studies in which injection of patients' IgG has passively transferred to mice the pathophysiological (6–8) and morphological features of the disease (9,10). The causative autoantibodies interfere with the quantal release of acetylcholine from motor nerve terminals at the neuromuscular junction, leading to the characteristic impairment of transmission. There is strong evidence that the primary targets for these autoantibodies are the VGCCs at the nerve terminal on which neurotransmitter (acetylcholine) release depends. The autoantibodies cause a decrease in the number of functional VGCCs by crosslinking adjacent channels, resulting in an increased rate of internalization. Complement does not appear to contribute, since complement-deficient mice are as susceptible to passive transfer of LEMS IgG as normal mice (3).

Several different subtypes of VGCCs are present in neurons. They can be distinguished by their electrophysiological properties and by the actions of neurotoxins specific for particular subtypes (Table 1). Current evidence suggests that the VGCC subtype subserving transmitter release at the neuromuscular junction is the P/Q-type VGCC (11).

A radioimmunoassay based on the cone snail (*Conus geographus*) toxin GVIA (CgTx GVIA) detets serum antibodies to N-type VGCCs in 40-80% of LEMS cases (12,13). However, the toxin of a different cone snail *Conus magus* (CmTx MVIIC), which labels P/Q-type VGCCs, is positive in 85–95% of patients (11,14). Although the antibody titer does not correlate with disease severity across individuals (likely to be explained by antibody heterogeneity), there is a broad correlation within an individual. Leys et al. (13) showed, using the CgTx GVIA assay, that the serum titer of anti-VGCC antibodies was inversely related to an EMG index of disease severity. A similar relationship exists using the ^{125}I-CmTx MVIIC assay (unpublished observations). Such a relationship is consistent with a pathogenic action of these autoantibodies, and provides a means of monitoring within individuals the effectiveness of therapy.

LAMBERT-EATON SYNDROME AS A PARANEOPLASTIC DISORDER

Small-cell lung carcinoma, which associates not only with LEMS but also with several other neurological disorders (subacute sensory neuropathy, cerebellar degeneration, encephalomyelitis) is neuroectodermal in origin. The tumor cells express VGCCs, and LEMS IgG blocks K^+-stimulated (voltage-gated) $^{45}Ca^{2+}$ flux into these cells in culture (15). Inhibition of flux correlates with disease severity (16), and specific tumor therapy

Table 1 Voltage-Gated Calcium Channels

	Type			
	L	N	P	Q
Distribution				
Neurons	+	+	+	+
Skeletal muscle	+	–	–	–
Smooth/cardiac muscle	+	–	–	–
Ligands				
Dihydropyridines	+	–	–	–
Conus geographus (ω-CgTx-GVIA)	–	+	–	–
A. aperta (ω-Aga-IVA)	–	–	+	–
Conus magus (ω-CmTx-MVIIC)	–	–	+/–	+

is often followed by improvement or even full recovery of the neurological disorder (17). Thus, tumor VGCCs appear to trigger the autoantibody response in these patients. The provoking factor in NC-LEMS is unknown.

EXISTING TREATMENT

Most patients benefit from 3,4-diaminopyridine (18), a compound that blocks voltage-gated potassium channels. This action lengthens the period of depolarization at the nerve terminal, prolonging the opening of voltage-gated calcium channels and thereby increasing Ca^{2+} influx and neurotransmitter release.

As mentioned above, symptoms of C-LEMS may improve or resolve after specific tumor therapy. In C-LEMS and NC-LEMS, patients often improve following prednisolone treatment. In NC-LEMS, azathioprine is a valuable addition to prednisolone therapy (19).

Plasma exchange helped to established the antibody-mediated nature of LEMS (6,19), and it is useful as short-term treatment. Typically, improvement peaks at about 10 days after a 5-day course of plasma exchange, but the beneficial effects largely disappear by 6 weeks.

IVIG TREATMENT

LEMS Case Reports

There have been two recent case reports of IVIG treatment in LEMS. Bird (20) reported a 68-year-old woman with a 6-month history of fatigable muscle weakness and typical electromyographic changes of the Lambert-Eaton syndrome. There was no evidence of an underlying malignancy. Anti-VGCC antibody titers were not reported. She received azathioprine treatment and also underwent repeated courses of plasma exchange, improving initially following each course, but then relapsing in a characteristic manner. A 5-day course of IVIG (0.4 g/kg/day) was followed by clear-cut clinical and electromyographic improvement, and 14 days posttreatment limb strength was observed to be normal. Repeated treatment courses every 10–12 weeks was followed by similar improvements.

The subject of the second case report (21) was a 68-year-old man with biopsy-proven small-cell lung cancer, typical electromyographic changes of LEMS, and a raised titer of anti-N-type VGCC antibodies. He received repeated courses of chemotherapy for his cancer at approximately 4-week intervals, during which time he also underwent two 2-day courses of plasma exchange. Three weeks later he received a single course of IVIG therapy (0.4 g/kg × 5 days). This treatment schedule was associated with a slow decline in anti-VGCC antibodies and by clinical and electromyographic improvement. However, because of the ongoing chemotherapy necessary for the malignancy, it is uncertain how far his improvement can be attributed to the IVIG treatment.

Randomized Crossover Trial of IVIG Infusion in LEMS

In order to try to substantiate whether IVIG was beneficial, and to investigate whether it had an influence on the serum level of the causative autoantibodies, we (22) undertook a randomized, double-blind, placebo-controlled crossover trial of IVIG treatment in nine patients with NC-LEMS. Existing immunosuppressive treatment (prednisolone and azathioprine) was continued unchanged. Patients were followed for 8 weeks after receiving an infusion on 2 consecutive days of IVIG at 1 g/kg/day (total dose 2.0 g/kg) or an equivalent volume of placebo (0.3% albumin). They then crossed over to the alternative preparation (placebo or IVIG) and were similarly followed for 8 weeks. Serial indices of limb, respiratory and bulbar muscle strength, and the serum titers of P/Q-type VGCC antibodies were compared over the 8-week periods in the two limbs of the trial, using the area-under-the-curve approach.

IVIG infusion was followed by significant improvements in the three strength measures ($P = .017 - .038$) that peaked at 2–4 weeks, and were declining by 8 weeks. The serum titers of anti-VGCC antibodies were unchanged at 1 week (strength was not measured at that time), but thereafter declined significantly ($P = .028$), showing a clear inverse relationship with muscle strength.

To look for a direct anti-idiotypic effect on anti-VGCC antibodies by the IVIG preparation, patients' pretreatment serum was preincubated with the IVIG (or with albumin) before carrying out the binding assay in the usual way (22). No significant effect was observed in the resulting antibody titers. This observation, together with the unchanged serum value of anti-VGCC antibodies at 1 week following IVIG infusion, suggests that direct anti-idiotypic neutralization of anti-VGCC antibodies is not the explanation for the late fall in the antibody titer and the associated improvement in strength. A delayed anti-idiotypic action cannot be excluded, however. It seems very likely that it is the ability of the IVIG infusion to induce the decline in serum pathogenic autoantibodies in LEMS that underlies the observed clinical improvement. Other autoantibody-mediated disorders that improve following IVIG treatment may similarly be associated with a decrease in pathogenic antibodies.

IVIG TREATMENT IN PARANEOPLASTIC NEUROLOGICAL DISORDERS

Although this study was confined to those with NC-LEMS, there seems no reason to suppose that patients with C-LEMS will not also similarly benefit. Other paraneoplastic neurological disorders have been reported to improve in single case reports. A 44-year-old woman with bilateral breast adenocarcinoma showed a striking recovery in her severe ataxia following early treatment with chemotherapy, plasma exchange, and a 5-day course (0.4 g/kg) of IVIG (23). As the authors point out, however, improvement cannot be confidently attributed to the IVIG treatment itself.

A 57-year-old man with LEMS, subacute cerebellar degeneration, seropositivity for antineuronal nuclear antibodies, and an associated small-cell lung cancer showed improvement in his ataxia and nystagmus within 1 week of starting a similar course of IVIG (24). In both of these cases, early treatment will have been important, because autopsies in established cases show very extensive Purkinje cell destruction that will be irreversible.

Opsoclonus-myoclonus associated with a nonresectable ganglioneuroblastoma in an 18-month-old girl responded to IVIG infusion (2 g/kg), and remission was obtained following chemotherapy and repeated IVIG infusions (1 g/kg) over a period of about a year (25).

SUMMARY

LEMS is an autoimmune disorder causing proximal muscle weakness and autonomic symptoms, and is mediated by IgG anti-P/Q-type VGCC antibodies. A randomized crossover trial of IVIG therapy substantiated the single case reports of its short-term clinical benefits and showed an inverse relationship between improvement in strength measures and decline in anti-VGCC antibodies. No anti-idiotypic neutralization of the specific antibodies could be demonstrated. IVIG treatment can help to control symptoms in the short term; its place in the long-term management of LEMS remains to be determined.

REFERENCES

1. Dwyer JM. Manipulating the immune system with immune globulin. N Engl J Med 1992; 326:107–116.
2. Pinching AJ, Peters DK, Newsom-Davis J. Remission of myasthenia gravis following plasma exchange. Lancet 1976; ii:1373–1376.
3. Lang B, Newsom-Davis J. Immunopathology of the Lambert-Eaton myasthenic syndrome. Springer Semin Immunopathol 1995; 17:3–15.
4. O'Neill JH, Murray NM, Newsom-Davis J. The Lambert-Eaton myasthenic syndrome. A review of 50 cases. Brain 1988; 111:577–596.
5. Elrington GM, Murray NMF, Spiro SG, Newsom-Davis J. Neurological paraneoplastic syndromes in patients with small cell lung cancer: a prospective survey of 150 patients. J Neurol Neurosurg Psychiatry 1991; 54:764–767.
6. Lang B, Newsom-Davis J, Wray D, Vincent A, Murray NMF. Autoimmune aetiology for myasthenic (Eaton-Lambert) syndrome. Lancet 1981; ii:224–226.
7. Lang B, Newsom-Davis J, Prior C, Wray D. Antibodies to motor nerve terminals: an electrophysiological study of a human myasthenic syndrome transferred to mouse. J Physiol (Lond) 1983; 344:335–345.
8. Lang B, Newsom-Davis J, Peers C, Prior C, Wray DW. The effect of myasthenic syndrome antibody on presynaptic calcium channels in the mouse. J Physiol (Lond) 1987; 390:257–270.
9. Fukunaga H, Engel AG, Osame M, Lambert EH. Paucity and disorganisation of presynaptic membrane active zones in the Lambert-Eaton myasthenic syndrome. Muscle Nerve 1982; 5:686–697.
10. Fukunaga H, Engel AG, Lang B, Newsom-Davis J, Vincent A. Passive transfer of Lambert-Eaton myasthenic syndrome with IgG from man to mouse depletes the presynaptic membrane active zones. Proc Natl Acad Sci USA 1983; 80:7636–7640.
11. Motomura M, Johnston I, Lang B, Vincent A, Newsom-Davis J. An improved diagnostic assay for Lambert-Eaton myasthenic syndrome. J Neurol Neurosurg Psychiatry 1995; 58:85–87.
12. Sher E, Canal N, Piccolo G, et al. Specificity of calcium channel autoantibodies in Lambert-Eaton myasthenic syndrome. Lancet 1989; ii:640–643.
13. Leys K, Lang B, Johnston I, Newsom-Davis J. Calcium channel autoantibodies in the Lambert-Eaton myasthenic syndrome. Ann Neurol 1991; 29:307–314.
14. Lennon VA, Kryzer TJ, Griesmann GE, et al. Calcium-channel antibodies in the Lambert-Eaton syndrome and other paraneoplastic syndromes. N Engl J Med 1995; 332:1467–1474.
15. Roberts A, Perera S, Lang B, Vincent A, Newsom-Davis J. Paraneoplastic myasthenic syndrome IgG inhibits $^{45}Ca^{2+}$ flux in a human small cell carcinoma line. Nature 1985; 317:737–739.

16. Lang B, Vincent A, Murray NM, Newsom-Davis J. Lambert-Eaton myasthenic syndrome: immunoglobulin G inhibition of Ca^{2+} flux in tumor cells correlates with disease severity. Ann Neurol 1989; 25:265–271.

17. Chalk CH, Murray NM, Newsom-Davis J, O'Neill JH, Spiro SG. Response of the Lambert-Eaton myasthenic syndrome to treatment of associated small-cell lung carcinoma. Neurology 1990; 40:1552–1556.

18. McEvoy KM, Winderbank AJ, Daube JR, Low PA. 3,4-Diaminopyridine in the treatment of Lambert-Eaton myasthenic syndrome. N Engl J Med 1989; 321:1567–1571.

19. Newsom-Davis J, Murray NM. Plasma exchange and immunosuppressive drug treatment in the Lambert-Eaton myasthenic syndrome. Neurology 1984; 34:480–485.

20. Bird SJ. Clinical and electrophysiologic improvement in Lambert-Eaton syndrome with intravenous immunoglobulin therapy. Neurology 1992; 42:1422–1423.

21. Takano H, Tanaka M, Koike R, Nagai H, Arakawa M, Tsuji S. Effect of intravenous immunoglobulin in Lambert-Eaton myasthenic syndrome with small-cell lung cancer: correlation with the titer of anti–voltage-gated calcium channel antibody. Muscle Nerve 1994; 17:1073–1075.

22. Bain PG, Motomura M, Newsom-Davis J, et al. Effects of intravenous immunoglobulin on muscle weakness and calcium-channel autoantibodies in the Lambert-Eaton myasthenic syndrome. Neurology. 1996; 47:678–683.

23. Moll JWB, Henzen-Logmans SC, Van der Meché FGA, Vecht CH. Early diagnosis and intravenous immune globulin therapy in paraneoplastic cerebellar degeneration. J Neurol Neurosurg Psychiatry 1993; 56:112. Letter.

24. Counsell CE, McLeod M, Grant R. Reversal of subacute paraneoplastic cerebellar syndrome with intravenous immunoglobulin. Neurology 1994; 44:1184–1185.

25. Petruzzi MJ, de Alarcon PA. Neuroblastoma-associated opsoclonus-myoclonus treated with intravenously administered immune globulin G. J Pediatr 1995; 127:328–329.

35

Intravenous Gammaglobulin in the Treatment of Recurrent Pregnancy Loss

Ann L. Parke

University of Connecticut Health Center, Farmington, Connecticut

INTRODUCTION

Although the precise mechanism of action of intravenous gammaglobulin (IVIG) in the treatment of autoimmune diseases is unknown, there is now considerable proof that this therapy is very useful in the management of a variety of immune-mediated diseases including cytopenias, Kawasaki disease, dermatomyositis (1–3) and, most recently, recurrent pregnancy loss, as it has become clear that certain maternal autoantibodies are associated with a predisposition to recurrent fetal loss. One example of this disease process is the phospholipid antibody (aPL) syndrome (4). This review will address the role of IVIG in the management of recurrent fetal loss in patients with phospholipid antibodies and in the treatment of other autoimmune diseases which result in fetal wastage and congenital abnormalities.

ANTIPHOSPHOLIPID SYNDROME

The association of (aPL) with recurrent fetal wastage was first described in the early 1970s (5) and followed by additional reports in the 1980s (6,7). Recent animal studies have suggested that it is the antibodies themselves that are responsible for the fetal wastage rather than some associated epiphenomenon (8,9). These antibodies are also associated with a predisposition to recurrent thrombosis, both arterial and venous (10,11). Although it has been suggested that the placental insufficiency that leads to fetal wastage is a consequence of recurrent thrombosis in the placental bed leading to placental infarction and placental death (12,13), not all studies have confirmed these findings (14). Our studies demonstrated multiple infarcts in the placentas of some patients with aPL syndrome, whereas other patients displayed definite placental inflammation as a major pathology (15). The most impressive finding in our studies was recurrences of the same pathology in mothers studied in recurrent pregnancies, thereby explaining the recurrent nature of pregnancy losses in some women.

Once the potential for the pregnancy loss in patients with aPL syndrome was recognized, it was suggested that fetal wastage could be prevented by treatments designed to suppress antibody production and to prevent recurrent thrombosis (7,16). Lubbe et al. reported that women who had never previously completed pregnancy could become mothers if treated with aspirin and prednisone (7). Multiple other reports followed leading to the conclusion that the appropriate treatment for pregnant women with the phospholipid syndrome was anticoagulation and corticosteroids (16,17), even though large, randomized controlled trials had never been performed. This resulted in many women with aPL receiving these treatments throughout pregnancy regardless of their previous medical or obstetric histories. Unfortunately, some patients developed significant maternal morbidity, including toxemia of pregnancy, gestational diabetes, aseptic necrosis of various joints, and even cataracts (18,19).

It is not always possible to suppress the production of aPL, now known to be a family of antibodies, some of which are easier to suppress than others (18,20,21). Because some women successfully complete pregnancy despite the presence of aPL antibodies (18,22), we have previously questioned their precise role in the pathogenesis of fetal wastage. Gleicher postulates that the autoimmune state itself predisposes to fetal wastage, as other autoimmune disease, including thyroid disease, are also associated with recurrent fetal loss and infertility (23).

Our study demonstrated that women with more than one aPL, measured as a lupus anticoagulant (LAC), a falsely positive VDRL for syphilis, or IgG or IgM cardiolipin antibodies, were more likely to experience recurrent fetal wastage than women without aPL (24). Ramsey-Goldman et al. demonstrated that women with aPL experiencing one unexplained loss are more likely to have additional fetal losses (25).

There is no question that some form of treatment for pregnant aPL patients is better than no therapy, as many of these patients who had previously failed to complete any pregnancy successfully produced live infants when treated with anticoagulants and/or corticosteroids, even though the pregnancies were not normal (6,18). As these women are pregnant, anticoagulation requires self-injection at least twice a day with heparin. Oral prednisone poses little threat to the fetus as only very small amounts cross the placenta (26), but problems for the mother are numerous. These concerns have resulted in the demand for a better understanding of the underlying pathological process, and more convenient and less toxic therapies.

In 1985 McVerry et al. demonstrated that IVIG suppressed production of a lupus anticoagulant in a patient with thrombocytopenia (27). At the same time interest developed in the role of IVIG in the management of other autoimmune diseases, including systemic lupus erythematosus (SLE) (28). This stimulated us and others to study the use of IVIG in patients with aPL with previous fetal losses. (29–33).

In 1988 Carreras et al. reported a patient with an LAC and VDRL who had failed to complete 13 previous pregnancies. When treated with IVIG this patient successfully delivered a live infant at week 34 (29). This report raised two important issues: IVIG appeared to suppress the production of the LAC as this disappeared immediately following infusion of IVIG; and the pregnancy still could not be considered to be normal as there were signs of intrauterine growth retardation (IUGR) from week 28 onward. Unfortunately this report did not comment on the state of the placenta, which may have offered additional information (29). Francois et al. reported a patient with aPL syndrome and recurrent episodes of venous thrombosis and pulmonary emboli, who had failed to complete three previous pregnancies despite treatment with prednisone, low-molecular-weight heparin, and aspirin. When treated with IVIG this patient successfully completed pregnancy (30).

Our first aPL patient treated with IVIG was enrolled in a study to determine the role of IVIG in treating mild connective tissue diseases. The IVIG initially appeared to suppress the levels of the LAC but had no effect on the cardiolipin antibodies which remained positive throughout the pregnancy. Nonetheless, this pregnancy developed normally as the patient did not develop pre-eclampsia, or IUGR and the placenta was normal (31). This was the patient's first normal pregnancy despite the fact that she had been pregnant six previous times (18).

Subsequent case reports have also suggested that IVIG may be useful in the treatment of patients with aPL who have experienced recurrent fetal wastage (32–36), although suppression of aPL was not found consistently, even in the same patient. Spinnato et al. describes five patients with the aPL syndrome with previously unsuccessful pregnancies who successfully completed pregnancy when treated with IVIG. Cardiolipin antibody levels were lowered in three of the five patients studied (36), and there were no signs of IUGR in the infants and the placentas were normal.

One interesting report describes the benefit of IVIG in preventing fetal resorption in experimentally induced phospholipid antibody syndrome in mice (37). These authors previously demonstrated induction of the clinical features of the aPL syndrome in animals either actively or passively immunized with phospholipid antibodies. The injected animals demonstrated an increase in fetal resorption (9). These same authors showed that increase in fetal resorption could be neutralized if the animals were injected with IVIG 2 days after induction of the experimentally induced phospholipid syndrome (37). These reports and those of Branch et al. (8) suggest that aPL are directly involved in the pathogenesis of the fetal wastage and that IVIG may prevent this fetal loss.

SLE

The incidence of fetal wastage and preterm birth are increased in patients with SLE (38–40) by many factors, including disease activity (38–40). The association of disease activity with poor pregnancy outcome is so strong that we advise our patients not to try to conceive until at least 6 months after the underlying disease has become inactive.

The use of IVIG in patients with SLE has not been well studied. Several small studies suggest this therapy may be useful (41,42), but well-controlled randomized trials with large numbers of patients have not been done. One concern that has emerged is the reported association of IVIG with acute renal failure (43).

The management of pregnant lupus patients is comparatively easy as large doses of prednisone can be taken without fear of toxicity to the fetus since only small amounts of prednisone cross the placenta (26). IVIG has been used to treat some specific manifestations of SLE (i.e., thrombocytopenia) as well as patients who have antibody to Ro antigen and who were considered to be at risk for the development of the neonatal lupus syndrome with primary congenital complete heart block in the fetus (44,45).

This syndrome appears to be a consequence of the transplacental passage of maternal antibody which damages the fetal conducting system, resulting in primary congenital complete heart block (46). Unlike the dermatological manifestations associated with this disease, the heart block is irreversible, with some of these infants dying and others requiring permanent pacemakers (47,48). The difficulty in interpreting the results of therapeutic trials in these patients is the fact that the same mother with the same antibody present can deliver an abnormal child in one pregnancy but a normal child in the next. It is clear that certain fetal determinants also dictate the expression of this syndrome (49).

FETAL WASTAGE IN THE ABSENCE OF THE aPL SYNDROME

The causes of recurrent fetal wastage are multiple. The immune tolerance that permits a mother to remain pregnant is still not well understood. It is now evident that local immunosuppression at the maternal/fetal interface is essential for the maintenance of pregnancy aided by decidua-associated suppressor cells and placental suppressor factors (50,51). The fetus is an allograft, and for a pregnancy to be maintained there must be maternal allogeneic recognition. This has been the basis for the use of allogeneic leukocyte immunization therapy in patients with recurrent fetal wastage. A success rate of more than 60% has been reported (52). It is theorized that this therapy permits the development of "blocking" antibodies that are essential for the immunosuppression which permits pregnancy to continue.

Mueller-Eckardt et al. suggested that administration of IVIG could provide these antibodies passively and could be useful in the treatment of women with recurrent fetal wastage (53). Initial results with >80% success rate were encouraging (53), and subsequent studies have been equally encouraging (54); however, a large, multicentered double-blinded trial comparing IVIG to albumin failed to reveal any statistically significant difference between IVIG and albumin infusions (55). Heine and Mueller-Eckhardt (56) remind us that the probability of a woman with three previous unexplained fetal losses successfully completing her next pregnancy is 60% even with no intervention. To accurately evaluate the benefits of IVIG in women with recurrent fetal wastage, randomized controlled studies must be performed. These are under way.

CONCLUSION

IVIG is a comparatively safe treatment for a variety of autoimmune disorders, and initial results for its use in disorders that can result in fetal wastage are encouraging. The successful abrogation of SLE and primary aPL in animal studies encourages the use of IVIG in humans (57). However, this is a very expensive treatment and, in these days of cost containment, it will become increasingly difficult to prescribe IVIG without randomized, well-controlled trials that clearly demonstrate the benefits of IVIG in patients with recurrent fetal wastage and autoimmune diseases.

REFERENCES

1. Stiehm ER, Ashida E, Kim KW, Winston DJ, Haas A, Gale RP. Intravenous immunoglobulins as therapeutic agents. Ann Intern Med 1987; 107:367–382.
2. Leung DYM. Immunomodulation by intravenous immune globulin in Kawasaki disease. J Allergy Clin Immunol 1989; 84:588–594.

3. Ballow M. Mechanisms of action of intravenous immunoglobulin therapy and potential use in autoimmune connective tissue diseases. Cancer 1991; 68:1430–1436.

4. Hughes GRV, Harris EN, Gharavi AE. The anticardiolipin syndrome. J Rheumatol 1986; 13:486–488.

5. Nilsson IM, Asbedt V, Hedner U, et al. Intrauterine deaths and circulating anticoagulants (antithromboplastin). Acta Med Scand 1975; 197:153.

6. Firkin BG, Howard MA, Radford N. Possible relationship between lupus inhibitor and recurrent abortion in young women. Lancet 1980; 2:366.

7. Lubbe WF, Butler WS, Palmer SJ, et al. Fetal survival after prednisone suppression of maternal lupus anticoagulant. Lancet 1983; i:1361–1363.

8. Branch WD, Dudley DJ, Mitchell MD. Immunoglobulin G fractions from patients with antiphospholipid syndrome cause fetal death in balb/c mice: a model for autoimmune fetal loss. Am J Obstet Gynecol 1990; 163:210–216.

9. Blank M, Cohen J, Toder V, Shoenfeld Y. Induction of antiphospholipid syndrome in naive mice with mouse lupus monoclonal and human polyclonal anticardiolipid antibodies. Proc Natl Acad Sci USA 1991; 88:3069–3073.

10. Boey ML, Colaco CB, Gharavi AE, et al. Thrombosis in systemic lupus erythematosus: striking association with the presence of circulating anticoagulant. Br Med J 1983; 287:1021–1023.

11. Harris EN, Chan JK, Asherson RA, Aber VR, Gharavi AE, Hughes GR. Thombosis, recurrent fetal loss, and thrombocytopenia. Arch Intern Med 1986; 146:2153–2156.

12. Abramowsky CR, Vegas ME, Swinehart G, Gyves MT. Decidual vasculopathy in the placenta in lupus erythematosus. N Engl J Med 1980; 303:668–672.

13. Out HJ, Bruinse HW, Christiaens GCML, et al. A prospective, controlled multicenter study on the obstetric risks of pregnant women with antiphospholipid antibodies. Am J Obstet Gynecol 1992; 167:26–32.

14. Lockshin MD, Qamar T, Druzin ML, Goei S. Antibody to cardiolipin, lupus anticoagulant, and fetal death. J Rheumatol 1987; 14:259–262.

15. Parke AL, Ernst L, Starzy, KA, Salafia CM. Placental pathology in the phospholipid antibody syndrome and systemic lupus erythematosus. In press.

16. Branch DW, Scott JR, Kochenour NK, et al. Obstetric complications associated with the lupus anticoaulant. N Engl J Med 1985; 313:1322–1327.

17. Branch WD, Silver RM, Blackwell JL, Reading JC, Scott JR. Outcome of treated pregnancies in women with antiphospholipid syndrome: an update of the Utah experience. Obstet Gynecol 1992; 80:614–620.

18. Parke A, Maier D, Hakim C, Randolph J, Andreoli J. Subclinical autoimmune disease and recurrent spontaneous abortion. J Rheumatol 1986; 13:1178–1180.

19. Cowchock FS, Reece EA, Balaban D, et al. Repeated fetal losses associated with antiphospholipid antibodies (a collaborative randomized trial comparing prednisone with low dose heparin treatment). Am J Obstet Gynecol 1992; 166:1318–1323.

20. Matsuura E, Igarashi V, Fujimoto M, et al. Heterogeneity of anticardiolipin antibodies defined by the anticardiolipin cofactor. J Immunol 1992; 148:3885–3891.

21. Derksen RHWM, Beisma D, Bouma BN. Discordant effects of prednisone on anticardiolipin antibodies and the lupus anticoagulant. Arthritis Rheum 1986; 20:1295–1296.

22. Stafford-Brady FJ, Gladman DD, Urowitz MB. Successful pregnancy in systemic lupus erythemaotsus with an untreated lupus anticoagulant. Arch Intern Med 1988; 148:1647–1648.

23. Gleicher N. Autoantibodies and pregnancy loss. Lancet 1994; 343:747–748.

24. Parke AL, Wilson D, Maier D. The prevalence of antiphospholipid antibodies in habitual aborters, normal women and in women who have never been pregnant. Arthritis Rheum 1991; 34:1231–1235.

25. Ramsey-Goldman R, Kutzer JE, Kuller LH, Guzick D, Medsger TA Jr. Previous pregnancy outcome is an important determinant of subsequent pregnancy outcome in women with sys-

temic lupus erythematosus. First Annual Rheumatic Diseases in Pregnancy Conference, Jerusalem, Israel, May 1992.

26. Briggs GG, Freeman K, Yaffe SJ. Drugs in Pregnancy and Lactation. 2nd ed. Baltimore: Williams and Wilkins, 1986.

27. McVerry BA, Spearing R, Smith A. SLE anticoagulant: transient inhibition by high dose immunoglobulin infusions. Br J Haematol 1985; 61:579–580.

28. Ballow M, Parke A. The uses of intravenous immune globulin in collagen vascular disorders. J Allergy Clin Immunol 1989; 84:608–612.

29. Carreras LO, Perez GN, Vega HR, Casavilla F. Lupus anticoagulant and recurrent fetal loss: successful treatment with gammaglobulin. Lancet 1988; ii:393–394.

30. Francois A, Freund M, Daffos F, Remy P, Aiach M, Jacquot C. Repeated fetal losses and the lupus anticoagulant. Ann Intern Med 1980; 993–994.

31. Parke A, Maier D, Wilson D, Andreoli J, Ballow M. Intravenous gamma-globulin, antiphospholipid antibodies, and pregnancy. Ann Intern Med 1989; 110:495–496.

32. Scott JR, Branch DW, Kochenour NK, Ward K. Intravenous immunoglobulin treatment of pregnant patients with recurrent pregnancy loss caused by antiphospholipid antibodies and Rh immunization. Am J Obstet Gynecol 1988; 159:1055–1056.

33. Wapner RJ, Cowchock FS, Shapiro SS. Successful treatment in two women with antiphospholipid antibodies and refractory pregnancy losses with intravenous immunoglobulin infusions. Am J Obstet Gynecol 1989; 161:1271–1272.

34. Kaaja R, Julkunen H, Ammala P, Palosuo T, Kurki P. Intravenous immunoglobulin treatment of pregnant patients with recurrent pregnancy losses associated with antiphospholipid antibodies. Acta Obstet Gynecol Scand 1993; 72:63–66.

35. Arnout J, Spitz B, Wittevrongel C, Vanrusselt M, Van Assche A, Vermylen J. High-dose intravenous immunoglobulin treatment of a pregnant patient with an antiphospholipid syndrome: immunological changes associated with a successful outcome. Thromb Haemostas 1994; 71:741–747.

36. Spinnato JA, Clark AL, Pierangeli SS, Harris EN. Intravenous immunoglobulin therapy for the antiphospholipid syndrome in pregnancy. Am J Obstet Gynecol 1995; 172:690–694.

37. Bakimer R, Guilbard B, Zurgil N, Shoenfeld Y. The effect of intravenous γ-globulin on the induction of experimental antiphospholipid syndrome. Clin Immunol Immunopathol 1993; 69(1):97–102.

38. Zurier RB, Argyros TG, Urman JD, et al. SLE management during pregnancy. Obstet Gynecol 1977; 51:178.

39. Gimovsky ML, Montoro M, Paul RH. Pregnancy outcome in women with systemic lupus erythematosus. Obstet Gynecol 1984; 63:686.

40. Mintz G, Niz J, Gutierrez G, et al. Prospective study of pregnancy in systemic lupus erythematosus: results of a multidisciplinary approach. J Rheumatol 1986; 13:732.

41. Francioni C, Galeazzi M, Fioravanti A, Gelli R, Megale F, Marcolongo R. Long term IVIG treatment in systemic lupus erythematosus. Clin Exp Rheumatol 1994; 12:163–168.

42. Winder A, Molad Y, Ostefeld I, Kenet G, Pinkhas J, Sidi Y. Treatment of systemic lupus erythematosus by prolonged administration of high dose intravenous immunoglobulin: Report of 2 cases. J Rheumatol 1993; 20;495–498.

43. Pasatiempo AMG, Kroser JA, Rudnick M, Hoffman BI. Acute renal failure after intravenous immunoglobulin therapy. J Rheumatol 1994; 21:347–349.

44. Kaaja R, Julkunen H, Ämmälä P, Teppo A-M, Kurki P. Congenital heart block: successful prophylactic treatment with intravenous gamma globulin and coritcosteroid therapy. Am J Obstet Gynecol 1991; 165:1333–1334.

45. Rider LG, Buyon JP, Rutledge J, Sherry DD. Treatment of neonatal lupus: case report and review of the literature. J Rheumatol 1993; 20:1208–1211.

46. Buyon JP, Ben-Chetrit E, Karp S, et al. Acquired congenital heart block: a pattern of maternal antibody resonse to biochemically defined antigens of the SSA/Ro–SSB/La system in neonatal lupus. J Clin Invest 1989; 84:627–634.

47. Lee LA. Maternal autoantibodies and pregnancy. II. The neonatal lupus syndrome. In: Parke AL, ed. *Pregnancy and the Rheumatic Diseases*. London: Bailliere Tindall, 1990; 4:69–84.

48. Watson RM, Lane AT, Bonnet NK, et al. Neonatal lupus erythematosus: a clinical serological and immunogenetic study with a review of the literature. Medicine 1984; 63:362.

49. Harley JB, Kane JL, Fox OF, et al. (SS/A) antibody and antigen in a patient with congenital complete heart block. Arthritis Rheum 1985; 28:1321.

50. Remacle-Bonnet MM, Rance RJ, Depieds RC. Non-specific immunoregulatory factors in the cytosol fraction of human trophoblast. J Reprod Immunol 1983; 5:123–134.

51. Menu E, Kinsky R, Hoffmann M, Chaouat G. Immunoreactive products of human placenta. IV. Immunoregulatory factors obtained from cultures of human placenta inhibit in vivo local and systemic allogeneic and graft versus host reactions in mice. J Reprod Immunol 1991; 20:195–204.

52. Unander AM. The role of immunization treatment in preventing recurrent abortions. Transfusion Med Rev 1992; 6:1–16.

53. Mueller-Eckardt G, Heine O, Neppert J, Künzel W, Mueller-Eckhardt C. Prevention of recurrent spontaneous abortion by intravenous immunoglobulin. Vox Sang 1989; 72:301–305.

54. Maruyama T, Makino T, Iwasaki K-I, et al. The influence of intravenous immunoglobulin treatment on maternal immunity in women with unexplained recurrent miscarriage. Am J Reprod Immunol 1994; 31:7–18.

55. German RSA/IVIG Group. Intravenous immunoglobulin in the prevention of recurrent miscarriage. Br J Obstet Gynecol 1994; 101:1072–1077.

56. Heine O, Mueller-Eckhardt G. Intravenous immune globulin in recurrent abortion. Clin Exp Immunol 1994; 97:39–42.

57. Krause I, Blank M, Kopolovic J, et al. Abrogation of experimental systemic lupus erythematosus and primary antiphospholipid syndrome with intravenous gamma globulin. J Rheumatol 1995; 22:1068–1074.

36

Intravenous Immunoglobulin and Other Autoimmune Diseases

Martin L. Lee
School of Public Health, University of California, Los Angeles, California

INTRODUCTION

Throughout the latter chapters of this book, there have been detailed discussions of the various uses of IVIG in autoimmune diseases. However, there are a number of other immune-mediated applications for which isolated reports are available. Typically, these involve a limited number of patients studied under anecdotal circumstances. As a result, we shall present here merely a listing of these applications with their reference numbers.

1. Factor VIII inhibitors (1–7)
2. Intractable childhood epilepsy (8–18)
3. Bullous pemphigoid (19)
4. Psychosis (secondary to SLE) (20)
5. von Willebrand's disease (21–24)
6. Amyotrophic lateral sclerosis (25,26)
7. Graves' ophthalmopathy (27,28)
8. Pure red cell or white cell aplasia (29–32)
9. Uveitis (33)
10. Epidermolysis bullosa acquisita (34)
11. Thrombotic thrombocytopenic purpura (35)

REFERENCES

1. Sultan Y, Kazatchkine MD, Malsonneuve P, Nydegger UE. Anti-idiotypic suppression of autoantibodies to factor VIII (antihemophilic factor) by high-dose intravenous gammaglobulin. Lancet 1984; 2:765–768.
2. Glanella-Borradori A, Hirt A, Luthy A, Wagner HP, Imbach P. Haemophilia due to factor VIII inhibitors in a patient suffering from an autoimmune disease: treatment with intravenous immunoglobulin. Blut 1984; 48:403–407.
3. Green D, Dwaan HC. An acquired factor VIII inhibitor responsive to high-dose gammaglobulin. Thromb Haemostas 1987; 58:1005–1007.

4. Zimmerman R, Kommerell B, Harenberg J, Elch W, Rother K, Schimpf K. Intravenous IgG for patients with spontaneous inhibitor to factor VIII. Lancet 1985; 1:273–274.

5. Heyman MR, Chakravarthy A, Edelman BB, Needleman SW, Schiffer CA. Failure of high-dose IV gammaglobulin in the treatment of spontaneously acquired factor VIII inhibitors. Am J Hematol 1988; 28:191–194.

6. Nilsson IM, Berntorp E, Zettervall O. Induction of immune tolerance in patients with hemophilia and antibodies to factor VIII by combined treatment with intravenous IgG, cyclophosphamide and factor VIII. N Engl J Med 1988; 315:947–950.

7. Nilsson IM, Berntorp E. Induction of immune tolerance in hemophiliacs with inhibitors, by combined treatment with IVIG, cyclophosphamide and factor VIII or IX—the Malmo model. In: Imbach P, ed. Immunotherapy with Intravenous Immunoglobulins. London: Academic Press, 1991:333–344.

8. Pechadre JC, De Villepin A, Sauvezi B, Gibert J. Gammaglobulines et epilepsie. Rev Med 1978; 34:1889–1901.

9. Laffont F, Esnault S, Gilbert A, Peytour MA, Cathola HP, Eygonnet JP. Effets des gammaglobulines sur des epiliepsies rebelles. Etude preliminaire. Ann Med Interne (Paris) 1979; 130:307–312.

10. Ariizumi M, Shiihara H, Hibio S, et al. High-dose gammaglobulin for intractable childhood epilepsy. Lancet 1993; 2:162–163.

11. Sandstedt P, Kostulas V, Larsson LE. Intravenous gammaglobulin for postencephalitic epilepsy. Lancet 1984; 2:1154–1155.

12. Bedini R, de Feo MR, Orano A, Rocchi L. Effects of gamma globulin therapy in severely epileptic children. Epilepsia 1985; 26:98–102.

13. Schwartz SA, Gordon KE, Johnston MN, Goldstein GW. Use of intravenous immune globulin in the treatment of seizure disorders. J Allergy Clin Immunol 1989; 84:603–607.

14. Duse M, Tibert S, Plebani M, et al. IgG2 deficiency and intractable epilepsy of childhood. Monogr Allergy 1986; 20:128–134.

15. Sterio M, Gebauer E, Vucicevic G, Zalisevskij G, Felle D, Kolarov N. Intravenous immunoglobulin in the treatment of malignant epilepsy in children. Wien Klin Wochensch 1990; 102:230–233.

16. Gross-Tsur V, Shalev RS, Kazir E, Engelhard D, Amir N. Intravenous high-dose gammaglobulins for intractable childhood epilepsy. Acta Neurol Scand 1993; 88:204–209.

17. Voit T. High-dose immunoglobulin treatment of epilepsy in children. Infusionsther Transfusionsmed 1993; 20(suppl 1):146–148.

18. Steriod M, Gebauer E, Felle D, Vucicevic G, Zalisevskij G. Malignant epilepsy in children: therapy with high doses of intravenous immunoglobulin. Medicinski Pregled 1992; 45:220–224.

19. Godard W, Roujeau JC, Guillot B, Andre C, Rifle G. Bullous pemphigoid and intravenous gammaglobulin. Ann Intern Med 1985; 103:965.

20. Tomer Y, Shoenfeld Y. Successful treatment of psychosis secondary to SLE with high dose intravenous immunoglobulin. Clin Exp Rheumatol 1992; 10:391–393.

21. Macik BG, Gabriel DA, White GC, High K, Roberts H. The use of high-dose intravenous gammaglobulin in acquired von Willebrand syndrome. Arch Pathol Lab Med 1988; 112:143–146.

22. Cataman G, Tosetto A, Rodeghiero F. Effectiveness of high-dose intravenous gammaglobulin in a case of acquired von Willebrand syndrome with chronic melena not responsive to desmopressin and factor VIII concentrate. Am J Hematol 1992; 41:132–136.

23. Delannoy AM, Saillez AC. High-dose intravenous gammaglobulin for acquired von Willebrand's disease. Br J Haematol 1988; 70:387.

24. van Genderen PJJ, Michiels JJ, Bakker JJ, van't Veer MB. Effectiveness of high-dose intravenous gamma globulin therapy in acquired von Willebrand's disease. Vox Sang 1994; 67:14–17.

25. Dalakas MC, Stern DP, Otero C, Sekul E, Cupler SE, McCrosky S. Effect of high-dose intravenous immunoglobulin (IVIG) on amyotrophic lateral sclerosis and multifocal motor neuropathy. Arch Neurol 1994; 51:861–864.

26. Savery F, Hang LM. Immunodeficiency associated with motor neuron disease treated with intravenous immunoglobulin. Clin Ther 1986; 8:700–702.

27. Antonell A, Saracino A, Alberti B, et al. High-dose intravenous immunoglobulins treatment in Graves' ophthalmopathy. Acta Endocrinol 1992; 126:13–23.

28. Dwyer JM, Benson EM, Currine JN, O'Day J. Intravenously administered IgG for the treatment of thyroid eye disease. In: Imbach P, ed. Immunotherapy with Intravenous Immunoglobulins. London: Academic Press, 1991:387–394.

29. Clauvell JP, Vainchenker W, Herrera A, et al. Treatment of pure red cell aplasia by high dose intravenous immunoglobulins. Br J Haematol 1983; 55:380–382.

30. McGuire WA, Yang HH, Bruno E, et al. Treatment of antibody-mediated pure red-cell aplasia with high dose intravenous immunoglobulin. N Engl J Med 1987; 317:1004–1008.

31. Ballester OF, Saba HI, Moscinski LC, Nelson R, Foulis P. Pure red cell aplasia: treatment with intravenous immunoglobulin concentrate. Semin Hematol 1992; 29(suppl 2):106–108.

32. Barbui T, Bassan R, Viero P, Minetti B, Comotti B, Buelli M. Pure white cell aplasia treated by high dose intravenous immunoglobulin. Br J Haematol 1984; 58:554–555.

33. Sunakawa M. High-dose intravenous gammaglobulin therapy for uveitis. Metab Pediatr Svs Ophthalmol 1989; 1293–1295.

34. Meiter F, Sonnichsen K, Schaumburg-Lever G, et al. Epidermolysis bullosa acquisita: efficacy of high-dose intravenous immunoglobulins. J Am Acad Dermatol 1993; 29:334–337.

35. Kolodziej M. Case report: high-dose intravenous immunoglobulin as therapy for thrombotic thrombocytopenic purpura. Am J Med 1993; 305:101–102.

37

Intravenous Immunoglobulin Therapy in Idiopathic Inflammatory Bowel Diseases

Douglas S. Levine
University of Washington, Seattle, Washington

INTRODUCTION

Crohn's disease and ulcerative colitis are the most common idiopathic inflammatory bowel diseases (IIBD) and affect about 2 million people in the United States. Crohn's disease involves any portion of the alimentary tract; ulcerative colitis is limited to the large intestine. These diseases most frequently affect adolescents and young adults and impact significantly upon lifestyles and productivity. The etiologies of IIBD are unknown, but ongoing research that includes clinical observations focused on patients who have received a wide variety of empirical therapies (1) is leading to a holistic concept of disease pathogenesis. At the present time, immune stimulation by intestinal luminal antigens, altered permeability of the intestinal mucosal barrier, disordered regulation of host gut mucosal and systemic immune systems, generation of various soluble proinflammatory mediators within intestinal mucosa, and other local gut physiological and anatomical factors are all suspected in the etiology and pathogenesis of IIBD in genetically predisposed individuals.

The type and severity of symptoms of IIBD relate to the intensity of inflammation in affected portions of the gut. These include gastrointestinal bleeding, abdominal pain, nausea, anorexia, vomiting, diarrhea, weight loss, malabsorption, growth failure, anemia, fevers, other constitutional symptoms, site-specific inflammatory complications such as fistulas and abscesses, secondary infections, the development of intestinal epithelial malignancies, and extraintestinal inflammatory disorders of other organs. Medical therapies for IIBD can suppress inflammation, improve symptoms, and induce temporary remissions of disease. Although medications do not provide a cure for these diseases, some can be used as maintenance therapy to prevent relapses. The commonly used drugs include aminosalicylates, corticosteroids, immunosuppressive agents, and antibiotics, which may be administered as oral, rectal, or parenteral formulations. Unfortunately, such therapies are incompletely effective in a substantial proportion of patients or cause side effects. Patients with ulcerative colitis can be essentially cured by surgical resection of the entire large intestine, but surgery is often not an acceptable option for some. Surgery in patients with Crohn's disease is quite appropriate for specific complications, but it is not curative and is frequently followed by disease recurrences.

Many factors are leading to an increased interest in drug development for patients with IIBD. The lack of effectiveness and the adverse-effect profiles of available drugs, and either the poor response to, or the lack of acceptance for, surgical intervention for these diseases, is stimulating more basic investigations of etiology and pathogenesis. The effects of this research activity are an improved understanding of the molecular and cell biological mechanisms of immune-mediated inflammatory damage to the alimentary tract that characterizes these diseases, and the development of new therapeutic strategies and better drug products that can prevent, inhibit, or otherwise interfere with immune reactions and thereby suppress inflammatory damage to the gastrointestinal tract with fewer adverse effects in patients. The available clinical data on the therapeutic use of intravenous immunoglobulins (IVIG) suggests that this treatment modality may prove to be effective in patients with IIBD.

IDIOPATHIC INFLAMMATORY BOWEL DISEASES

Clinical Description of IIBD

The two common forms of IIBD, Crohn's disease and ulcerative colitis, share many clinical, pathological, and epidemiological features, but there are sufficient differences to classify them as distinct clinical entities (2–5). When differentiation between them is not possible in some patients, a diagnosis of "indeterminate colitis" is applied. Other varieties of IIBD that are less common than Crohn's disease and ulcerative colitis include, for example, collagenous colitis, microscopic or lymphocytic colitis, diversion colitis, and eosinophilic gastroenteritis, among others. IIBD is differentiated from inflammatory bowel diseases resulting from known causes, such as host deficiency states, foods, infections, toxins, ischemia, diverticulitis, neoplasia, drugs, radiation, other physical agents, or graft-versus-host disease following allogeneic marrow transplantation.

What we diagnose as "Crohn's disease" or "ulcerative colitis" may be several different diseases that may become defined molecularly in the future (6). Ongoing investigations of IIBD may confirm observations suggesting that patients with these disorders seem to conform to a wide variety of subsets with different clinical presentations, pathological manifestations, medical or surgical treatment responses, and tendencies toward disease recurrence. Crohn's disease may affect any portion of the alimentary tract and may be transmural. Ulcerative colitis is generally limited to the relatively superficial mucosa of the large intestine. These diseases may vary both in inflammatory intensity and total surface area of involvement of the alimentary tract. Only a small portion of the ileum or rectum may be involved in limited forms. However, in severe forms a large portion of the small intestine or the entire colon is affected. Therefore, the spectrum of symptoms and clinical diagnostic abnormalities reflecting these varying pathological manifestations is diverse (2–5). In some patients inflammation may be so minimal it may only be detectable by endoscopic visualization and biopsy. In others, severe ulceration and hemorrhage are obvious, and inflammation may involve the entire bowel wall thickness and lead to formation of strictures or progression to perforation, fistulous tracts or sinuses, and abscesses with the potential for septicemia.

The clinical courses of patients with IIBD are highly variable and usually relate to the anatomical sites of gut involvement and the intensity of inflammation. Most patients give a history of periodic flares of disease interspersed with normal or near-normal health during time intervals that vary from months to a few years. In other patients, disease is chronic and unremitting with continuous bloody diarrhea, anemia, abdominal discomfort, and generalized or constitutional symptoms. Some have an initial acute attack followed by apparent good health for up to several years before they experience recurrent symptoms. Some develop small or large intestinal epithelial dysplasia and cancer independent of the inflammatory intensity and course of their disease.

The cardinal symptoms of Crohn's disease are abdominal pain and nonbloody diarrhea, reflecting a tendency to produce transmural inflammation, narrowing of the intestinal lumen, and partial obstruction. The most common symptoms of ulcerative colitis are tenesmus, hematochezia, and crampy abdominal pain due to involvement of the rectum and a variable extent of proximal colonic mucosa. Symptoms of IIBD are mild or moderate in the majority of patients, with some increase in the number of stools per day, insignificant gut blood loss, and tolerable levels of abdominal pain. For others, symptoms are severe with disabling diarrhea, anemia due to intestinal blood loss, abdominal pain, fevers, and extraintestinal manifestations. Fulminant disease occurs in the minority of patients who must be hospitalized for severe intestinal hemorrhage, vomiting, abdominal pain, fevers, malnutrition, dehydration, electrolyte imbalances, or infection. A subset of this group may develop toxic colitis with gross dilatation or perforation, and require emergent surgery to prevent peritonitis and sepsis.

Ulcerative colitis is diagnosed using sigmoidoscopy with mucosal biopsies. Other tests that provide imaging of the large intestine, such as air contrast barium enema or colonoscopy, are potentially hazardous and more uncomfortable in active disease. However, such exams may become necessary to differentiate ulcerative colitis from Crohn's disease or to assess the proximal extent and intensity of colitis as part of therapeutic planning and monitoring. These examinations also identify complications of colitis such as strictures, pseudopolyps, or adenocarcinoma. Diffuse, contiguous colonic mucosal involvement is characteristic of ulcerative colitis. Patients with active disease have loss of normal mucosal vascular detail, mucosal friability, erosions and/or ulcers, and the presence of inflammatory exudate composed of pus, mucus, and blood.

The diagnosis of Crohn's disease may be challenging insofar as symptoms and diagnostic results may mimic those of ulcerative colitis. Differentiating features may be suggested by findings on barium enema, and sigmoidoscopy or colonoscopy with mucosal biopsies, of focal or segmental colitis rather than contiguous colorectal disease. Evidence of disease involving other portions of the alimentary tract (which may be provided by upper endoscopy, or x-ray studies of the upper tract and small intestine) and the presence of fissures, fistulous tracts, mesenteric sinuses, or intra- or extra-abdominal abscesses also are more consistent with Crohn's disease.

The loss of mucosal integrity, as demonstrated endoscopically and histologically, is perhaps the most obvious feature of the inflamed intestinal mucosa in patients with IIBD. The differentiation between Crohn's disease and ulcerative colitis is difficult if Crohn's disease involvement is limited to the large intestine. However, radiological and endoscopic observations and certain histological features of mucosal biopsies may help differentiate these two disorders. Barium enema and total colonoscopy establish the presence of a diffuse, contiguous mucosal inflammatory process consistent with ulcerative colitis. Histological evaluation of colonic mucosal biopsies of patients with ulcerative colitis reveals diffuse inflammatory involvement with increased mucosal neutrophils, plasma cells, lymphocytes, and eosinophils. Crypt architecture is distorted, the epithelial surface loses its integrity and develops erosions, and crypt abscesses appear. In Crohn's disease of the colon, radiological and colonoscopic examination may reveal segmental disease, focal rather than diffuse inflammatory changes, and small aphthous or larger, irregularly shaped stellate, elliptical, and serpiginous ulcerations. Colonoscopic biopsies of patients with Crohn's colitis may share the same histological features of ulcerative colitis, but the presence of focal rather than diffuse inflammation or of noncaseating epithelioid granulomas is more consistent with a diagnosis of Crohn's disease.

Immunopathogenesis of IIBD

Current treatment strategies for patients with IIBD are empirical and based on hypotheses on the causes of these disorders. Two general theories are proposed for the causes of IIBD: the infectious hypothesis, and the immunological hypothesis. Infectious and immunoregulatory or autoimmune mechanisms are proposed (7–15), leading to the use of antibiotics, anti-inflammatory drugs, and immunosuppressive or immune-modulating agents in patients with these disorders (16–19). The infectious hypothesis proposes that a pathogen causes IIBD and the immune system responds appropriately to the infectious agent. However, extensive investigation has not led to the identification of any transmissible agent in patients with IIBD. The immunological hypothesis proposes that the immune system reacts abnormally or inappropriately against one or more antigens (e.g., intestinal bacterial, viral, dietary, or other environmental agents) to which everyone is commonly exposed. The manifestations of IIBD are postulated to result from immunological mechanisms based on intestinal pathological features, beneficial clinical responses to immunosuppressive drugs, systemic extraintestinal complications that are observed, and various laboratory observations of cell-mediated and humoral immune abnormalities, including circulating immune complexes (2–4, 8,10,14,20,21).

Multiple types of host immune system abnormalities are demonstrated in patients with IIBD. Whether or not these represent primary immunoregulatory abnormalities or secondary epiphenomena is vigorously debated. Nevertheless, altered immunoreactivity may be responsible for disease manifestations whether it is a primary etiological factor or a secondary manifestation that leads to intestinal tissue damage. These immune system abnormalities are probably interactive in susceptible patients, and may be broadly classified as follows: (1) stimulation by intestinal luminal antigens; (2) dysfunction of intestinal barrier epithelium; (3) defects in systemic and/or intestinal mucosal immunoregulation; (4) generation of mediators of intestinal inflammatory damage; and (5) other factors affecting immune-mediated intestinal inflammatory damage (1,2,4,22).

Stimulation by Intestinal Luminal Antigens

Any of a variety of alimentary tract luminal antigens may trigger an immune-mediated inflammatory response in the intestinal mucosa of susceptible individuals who develop IIBD (23). Such antigens include viral particles, cellular structural proteins or toxins from bacteria, dietary antigens, environmental agents, or proteins from sloughed intestinal epithelial cells. This hypothesis is suggested by several different investigations of the association of IIBD with exogenous agents that may trigger disease development, including: disease exacerbations following respiratory tract or enteric infections with bacterial or viral pathogens (24–27); geographic and seasonal patterns of disease incidence and prevalence that further suggest the possible influence of infections or other unknown environmental agents (28,29); and disease incidence related to smoking, diet, and drug ingestion habits (30–33).

Dysfunction of Intestinal Barrier Epithelium

An intact intestinal epithelium forms the most basic host defense mechanism against the large number of microbial populations and antigens that are present within the intestinal lumen (34,35). Primary abnormalities of intestinal epithelial permeability are detectable in patients with IIBD (36). In addition, intestinal epithelial destruction that is mediated by specific immune mechanisms or nonspecific inflammatory mediators leads to the secondary loss of integrity of the barrier epithelium. Such a breach of intestinal mucosal defense allows increased entry of microorganisms and luminal antigens into the mucosa, permitting propagation of immunostimulating and inflammatory processes.

Defects in Systemic and/or Intestinal Mucosal Immunoregulation

Abnormalities of TH1 and TH2 responses in patients with IIBD are demonstrable, examples of which include: identification of disease-specific autoantibodies (37–40); aberrations in B lymphocyte function and immunoglobulin secretion (41–47); abnormal T lymphocyte function (48–51); and elaboration of cytokines and cytokine receptors (52–59). The inflammatory distribution and microscopic pathology in the intestinal tract of patients with IIBD are similar to those in patients with other immunologically mediated diseases affecting the alimentary tract, such as intestinal graft-versus-host disease following allogeneic bone marrow transplantation (60,61). The pathogenesis of the mucosal necrosis, edema, and protein loss that is characteristic of intestinal graft-versus-host disease results from the activity of donor T lymphocytes leading to immune destruction of intestinal epithelial cells, local release of cytokines [particularly tumor necrosis factor (TNF), interleukin-1 (IL-1), and interferon-γ], breakdown of the intestinal barrier epithelium, massive intestinal wall edema, and secondary microbial invasion of the intestinal mucosa (62,63). Although the primary inciting events in IIBD are unknown, dysfunction of T lymphocytes, among other primary host immune abnormalities, is hypothesized (12,13,15), and the resulting cascade of inflammatory events leading to intestinal mucosal destruction is similar to that in intestinal graft-versus-host disease. Therefore, it is not surprising that the therapeutic approaches to intestinal graft-versus-host disease, Crohn's disease, and ulcerative colitis are similar, often involving the use of systemic immunosuppressive and anti-inflammatory medications, including IVIG.

Mediators of Intestinal Inflammatory Damage

In addition to possible primary intestinal epithelial damage caused by specific cell- or antibody-mediated immune mechanisms, epithelial cell destruction in IIBD also occurs via an innocent bystander reaction. Nonspecific inflammatory processes of IIBD are mediated by local generation of soluble mediators of inflammation in intestinal mucosa (23). Increased secretion of immunoglobulins can activate complement components (64) that attract macrophages and neutrophils to the intestinal mucosa, initiating release of injurious tissue proteases and free oxygen radicals. Activation of macrophages and neutrophils produces phospholipase-mediated release of arachidonic acid, which is the substrate for cyclo-oxygenase and lipoxygenase enzymatic pathways that lead to the production of prostaglandins and leukotrienes, respectively (65–67). Prostaglandins and leukotrienes are known mediators of the inflammatory response of the body; cause vasodilation, hyperemia, and edema, which are features of the mucosal inflammation of IIBD; and thus are important contributors to these inflammatory processes.

Other Factors Affecting Immune Intestinal Inflammatory Damage

Several other factors influence immune-mediated inflammatory damage to intestinal mucosa in IIBD. The access of immune effector cells to the intestinal mucosa is affected by local intestinal vascular and microcirculatory conditions, adhesion to vascular endothelium, and egress from the vascular compartment into the mucosal tissue. Intestinal mucosal immunoreactivity may be affected by a variety of neuropeptides and other molecules, the release of which may be initiated by psychological phenomena and the central nervous system. The contact of immunostimulating luminal microorganisms and other antigens with the intestinal mucosa may be influenced by disordered intestinal smooth muscle function and motility.

INTRAVENOUS IMMUNOGLOBULIN THERAPY IN IIBD

Rationale for IVIG in IIBD

As detailed elsewhere in this text, IVIG, as well as immune sera, is administered to individuals who are exposed and susceptible to a variety of infectious microorganisms, and to patients with primary or acquired immune deficiencies and immunoregulatory disorders such as autoimmune thrombocytopenic purpura, Kawasaki disease, and graft-versus-host disease following bone marrow transplantation (68–73), among others. The rationale for the use of immunoglobulins in patients with primary immunodeficiency diseases is to provide specific antibodies against pathogens (68–71). Other mechanisms of action for immunoglobulins have been demonstrated or hypothesized for immunoregulatory disorders, including decreasing autoantibody production by the infusion of anti-idiotypic antibodies that are present in the immunoglobulin preparations, altering B lymphocyte function, increasing natural killer and suppressor T lymphocyte activity, inhibiting cytokine release, enhancing clearance of antigen-antibody complexes, and interfering with Fc receptors on reticuloendothelial system cell membranes (68–79).

The immunoglobulins present in commercial preparations of IVIG have an extraordinary variety of idiotypic specificities; are of adequate mass and have sufficient half-life to produce measurable, lasting increases in serum immunoglobulin levels; and have distinct Fc receptor reactivities (77). In theory, these properties could produce ameliorative effects that are mediated by a variety of mechanisms in patients with IIBD, including neutralization of antigens, modification of gut luminal antigen processing in the mucosa, suppression of primary immunoregulatory effects, specific suppression or enhancement of T and B lymphocyte cellular functions, suppression of inflammation, and inhibition of egress of inflammatory cells from the vascular compartment into the gut mucosa. Further investigations of the modes of therapeutic action of exogenously administered IVIG to patients with IIBD could shed light on the etiology of these disorders.

The mechanisms of therapeutic action of IVIG in patients with IIBD may be similar to those in other diseases described throughout this text, and may involve direct or indirect systemic immunoregulatory activities. The demonstration of intestinal localization of technetium- or indium-labeled immunoglobulins in patients with IIBD, evaluated as part of efforts to improve noninvasive diagnostic imaging methods in Crohn's disease and ulcerative colitis (80–86), suggests that IVIG also may affect local intestinal mucosal immunoregulation. Potential mechanisms of action of immunoglobulins in patients with IIBD could include provision of specific antibodies that neutralize a pathogenic antigen, specific anti-CD4 or anti-interleukin receptor antibodies, immune modulation of anti-idiotypic antibodies, immune modulation of activated macrophages and T lymphocytes, and, ultimately, altered regulation of local intestinal mucosal generation of inflammatory mediators. Increased interleukin-1 is produced by activated intestinal lamina propria mononuclear cells obtained from patients with IIBD (87). Therefore, the finding that IVIG may interfere with the excess production and secretion of interleukin-1 in Kawasaki disease (88) also may be of relevance for IIBD.

Clinical Experience with IVIG in IIBD

Published Studies of Immune Sera and IVIG in IIBD

Exogenously administered immunoglobulins are reported to improve experimental inflammatory bowel disease in animal model systems. In a rat model of ulcerative colitis induced by administration of dextran sulfate, treatment of rats with immunoglobulin G ameliorated colitis while diminishing gut levels of TNF-α, IL-1, and IL-8 (89,90). The improvement in colitis and decrement in tissue cytokine levels were attributed to inhibition of activation of mucosal T cells (91). Intraperitoneal administration of gammaglobulin also improved experimental colitis in rats induced by trinitrobenzenesulfonic acid (92).

The available clinical literature on the use of immunoglobulin therapy in patients with IIBD is limited insofar as most publications are relatively brief case reports or summaries of case series published only in abstract form. This suggests that publication bias may exist because very few negative studies are published. Moreover, no blinded, randomized, controlled study on the use of IVIG is reported. However, a beneficial action of IVIG has been suggested by the available clinical observations on small numbers of patients with Crohn's disease or ulcerative colitis.

A controlled trial of antilymphocyte serum did not show any improved therapeutic efficacy compared to standard therapy for patients with ulcerative colitis (93).

In a review of immunoglobulin therapy, Cottier and Hassig allude to clinical improvements in seven patients with IIBD (five with ulcerative colitis and two with Crohn's disease) who received IVIG (94). Specific dosing regimens and clinical details are not provided for all patients in this report.

In a small case series of six patients (three with Crohn's disease and three with ulcerative colitis), Rohr *et al.* reported clinical improvement in all with a 7-day treatment course of IVIG 10 g/day (95). Remission of disease in the patients with ulcerative colitis was confirmed endoscopically, and improvement in those with Crohn's disease was documented with decrements in the Crohn's Disease Activity Index (CDAI).

A pilot, controlled trial of IgM-enriched immunoglobulin (Pentaglobin) was conducted in 10 patients with Crohn's disease in which the Pentaglobin was administered during a 4-day protocol (2.5 ml/kg/day) in addition to standard therapy (steroids, sulfasalazine, and elementary diet) (96). Control patients received the same standard therapy but no immunoglobulin. Those who received immunoglobulin had a marked reduction in the CDAI, C-reactive protein levels, erythrocyte sedimentation rate, and endotoxinemia compared to the control group.

Wolf *et al.* reported on a case of a 14-year-old child with Crohn's disease who was previously refractory to standard medical therapies but whose disease remitted with a course of IVIG (97). Two additional relapses of Crohn's disease also were successfully treated with IVIG.

An open-label study was carried out in corticosteroid-dependent Crohn's disease patients who received IVIG 400 mg/kg/day for 5 days, followed by injections every 3 weeks (98). An attempt was made to lower corticosteroid dosing, but this apparently failed because of an abridgement in the chronic dosing protocol necessitated by systemic side effects attributed to IVIG (headaches, shivers, fever). However, the disease course in patients appeared to stabilize for 1 year following IVIG treatment insofar as no further disease flares were observed, in contrast to the 1-year period preceding IVIG treatment, when frequent disease exacerbations were documented.

In an open-label pilot study, six patients with acutely active Crohn's disease were treated with IVIG 400 mg/kg/day for 5 days as a single agent without concomitant corticosteroid or sulfasalazine therapies (99,100). Three patients promptly relapsed within several days of completing IVIG therapy, but the other three enjoyed sustained clinical improvement for 6–12 months.

In an open-label study, 13 patients with active ulcerative colitis were administered IVIG 400 mg/kg/day for 5 days (101). Nine individuals responded clinically based on comparison colonoscopic evaluations conducted pretreatment and 2 weeks after treatment initiation. Serum immune complex levels, as well as C4 and C3 levels, were observed to decrease in responding patients.

A case series of 69 patients with IIBD treated with different formulations of immunoglobulin-containing antibodies to *E. coli* was reported (102). Among 29 patients with ulcerative colitis who received IVIG, 21 (72%) were reported to improve clinically. The remaining 40 patients (28 with ulcerative colitis, 12 with Crohn's disease) were administered complex immunoglobulin in suppositories, 50% of whom were reported to improve clinically. In a separate report, two individuals with pseudomembranous colitis secondary to *C. difficile* toxin, which was unresponsive to standard antibiotic therapy, were reported to improve following a single dose of IVIG 200 mg/kg (103). IVIG was analyzed and found to contain antibodies to *C. difficile* toxin.

Retention enemas containing immunoglobulin G were administered as part of an open-label trial to seven patients with distal ulcerative colitis (104). Of five individuals who completed the 2-week treatment trial, only one patient experienced clinical improvement. Whereas clinical improvement in IIBD has been noted with parenteral immunoglobulin administration, this study suggests that there is no apparent topical effect in ulcerative colitis. However, the bioavailability and biological action of immunoglobulin were not evaluated in this study.

The development of idiopathic inflammatory bowel disease was reported in a patient with agammaglobulinemia who received immunoglobulin replacement therapy but who had low serum immunoglobulin levels (105).

Ongoing investigations of the therapeutic potential of Fc fragments may have relevance for the therapy of IIBD because Fc fragments are reported to be 100–1000 times more effective than intact immunoglobulin molecules in inhibiting cellular immunity (106).

Seattle Study of IVIG in IIBD

At the time we were planning an independent therapeutic study, the available medical literature indicated that clinical improvement in small numbers of patients with IIBD was reported following treatment with IVIG. However, these observations may have reflected spontaneous remissions of IIBD, controls were not included, and the degree of refractoriness to standard medical therapies, the proximal extent of colonic disease, and the intensity of mucosal inflammatory change in the responders were not clearly described. To further assess its therapeutic potential in IIBD, we administered IVIG to patients with active and extensive idiopathic colitis who had not responded to standard medical therapies or who were dependent on systemic corticosteroids to remain in clinical remission. We monitored their responses to IVIG therapy clinically, as well as endoscopically and histologically in order to assess the results of treatment as objectively as possible (107–110).

To determine if IVIG produced demonstrable clinical improvement in patients with refractory idiopathic inflammatory bowel disease, a pilot, open-label, nonrandomized, safety and therapeutic efficacy study was carried out at the University of Washington, a tertiary care referral medical center. Twelve consecutive patients with refractory idiopathic colitis (nine with ulcerative colitis and three with Crohn's colitis) who were reluctant to receive immunosuppressive therapy or have surgical intervention were referred by physicians not participating as investigators in this study. Eleven patients were symptomatic for at least 6 months with endoscopically moderate or severe mucosal inflammation despite medical therapy, including systemic corticosteroids in all cases, and one patient was dependent on oral prednisone to remain in clinical remission. Ten patients had extensive colitis, six of whom had pancolitis and four of whom had colitis extending to the hepatic flexure or transverse colon. Nine patients required hospitalization for treatment of colitis. IVIG was administered in one or two induction phases (2 g/kg over 2 or 5 days) followed by a maintenance phase (200–500 mg/kg every 2 weeks for 12 or 24 weeks). Tapering of systemic corticosteroid therapy was attempted, whereas other medications for idiopathic colitis were continued. Treatment response was assessed clinically and by colonoscopy with multiple biopsies whenever possible.

IVIG therapy was well tolerated and did not produce any biochemical abnormalities. IgG subclass deficiencies were discovered in six patients before initiating IVIG therapy. Serum IgG levels increased significantly during IVIG therapy, 1076 $\pm$ 124 mg/dl to 3378 $\pm$ 183 mg/dl ($P <$ .001). In six patients who completed the treatment protocol, mean reductions $\pm$ SE were achieved in subjective symptoms as quantitated by a colitis activity score, 13.3 $\pm$ 1.2 to 4.7 $\pm$ 0.9 ($P <$ .001), and prednisone, 41.7 $\pm$ 8.0 to 1.9 $\pm$ 1.2 mg/day ($P <$ .001). For all 12 patients, statistically significant reductions were achieved in the colitis activity score and daily prednisone dose. Of five patients who completed the treatment protocol and improved clinically, four underwent posttreatment colonoscopic and biopsy evaluations and had unequivocal reductions in the intensity of colonic mucosal inflammation. Three patients who had objective improvement with IVIG experienced relapse of colitis after discontinuation of this therapy. Six patients did not complete the treatment protocol, two of whom required surgical intervention and four of whom withdrew to undergo colectomy electively.

CONCLUSIONS

Approaches to treatment of patients with IIBD have long included anti-inflammatory and immunomodulating agents. Many patients respond to intermittent or continued use of systemic corticosteroids and immunosuppressive agents such as azathioprine or 6-

mercaptopurine. More recently, other immunomodulating drugs have been found to be effective in subsets of patients with IIBD, including methotrexate and cyclosporine A. The ultimate immunosuppressive therapy, removal of lymphocytes by leukapheresis, is associated with considerable morbidity and is not practical as a long-term treatment strategy. Current clinical trials are assessing the therapeutic effects of other immune-modulating agents such as monoclonal antibodies against TNF and recombinant IL-10.

The results of the published pilot, open-label therapeutic trials of IVIG, although encouraging in some patients, must be considered preliminary. Collectively, these observations justify the undertaking of prospective, randomized controlled therapeutic investigations in patients who are carefully selected or stratified into different disease categories before IVIG can be recommended as a therapeutic option for patients with IIBD. The relationships between response to IVIG therapy and various factors that could be predictive of a beneficial therapeutic response require additional investigation, including: IIBD diagnosis (ulcerative colitis *vs.* Crohn's disease); colitis disease activity (proximal extent and intensity of mucosal inflammatory change); duration of disease; corticosteroid dosing; IgG subclass deficiencies; and perhaps other immunological markers. The possible need for extended treatment periods as well as increased dosages of IVIG must be evaluated because of the significant improvement in, but incomplete resolution of, colitis in many responders; the tendency for some responders to relapse following completion of maintenance courses of IVIG therapy; and the costs for such therapy.

IVIG therapy ultimately may be shown to produce long remissions of disease in selected patients or provide a satisfactory temporizing measure in severely ill patients who are destined for surgical intervention. Investigation of the mechanisms underlying the therapeutic response to IVIG could lead to the design of more practical, less expensive, and more effective immunomodulatory therapies. The devastating nature of IIBD and the evidence supporting the immunopathogenesis of these disorders justify continued investigation of immunomodulating therapeutic agents such as IVIG for affected patients.

REFERENCES

1. Levine DS. Immune modulating therapies for idiopathic inflammatory bowel diseases. Adv Pharmacol 1994; 25:171–234.
2. Levine DS. Inflammatory bowel diseases. In: Bierman CW, Pearlman DS, Shapiro GG, Busse WW, eds. Allergy, Asthma, and Immunology from Infancy to Adulthood. 3rd ed. Philadelphia: W. B. Saunders, 1996:687–702.
3. Levine DS. Clinical features and complications of Crohn's disease. In: Targan SR, Shanahan F, eds. Inflammatory Bowel Disease: From Bench to Bedside. Baltimore: Williams and Wilkins, 1994:296–316.
4. Levine DS. Ulcerative colitis. In: Rakel RE, ed. Conn's Current Therapy. Philadelphia: W. B. Saunders, 1996:468–473.
5. Targan SR, Shanahan F. Inflammatory Bowel Disease: From Bench to Bedside. Baltimore: Williams and Wilkins, 1994.
6. Yang H, Rotter JI, Toyoda H, et al. Ulcerative colitis: a genetically heterogeneous disorder defined by genetic (HLA class II) and subclinical (anti-neutrophilic cytoplasmic antibodies) markers. J Clin Invest 1993; 92:1080–1084.
7. Gibson PR, Jewell DP. Local immune mechanisms in inflammatory bowel disease and colorectal carcinoma. Gastroenterology 1986; 90:12–19.

8. Kirsner JB, Shorter RG, eds. Inflammatory Bowel Disease. Philadelphia: Lea and Febiger, 1988.

9. Elson CO. The immunology of inflammatory bowel disease. In: Kirsner JB, Shorter RG, eds. Inflammatory Bowel Disease. Philadelphia: Lea and Febiger, 1988:97–164.

10. MacDermott RP, Stenson WF. The immunology of inflammatory bowel disease. In: Kirsner JB, Shorter RG, eds. Diseases of the Colon, Rectum, and Anal Canal. Baltimore: Williams and Wilkins, 1988:295–315.

11. Jayanthi V, Probert CSJ, Sher KS, Mayberry JF. Current concepts of the etiopathogenesis of inflammatory bowel disease. Am J Gastroenterol 1991; 86:1566–1572.

12. Podolsky DK. Inflammatory bowel disease. N Engl J Med 1991; 325:928–937, 1008–1016.

13. Brandtzaeg P, Halstensen TS, Kett K. Immunopathology of inflammatory bowel disease. In: MacDermott RP, Stenson WF, eds. Inflammatory Bowel Disease. New York: Elsevier, 1992:95–136.

14. Rook GAW, Stanford JL. Slow bacterial infections or autoimmunity? Immunol Today 1992; 13:160–164.

15. Shanahan F, Targan SR. Mechanisms of tissue injury in inflammatory bowel disease. In: MacDermott RP, Stenson WF, eds. Inflammatory Bowel Disease. New York: Elsevier, 1992:77–93.

16. Hawthorne HA, Hawkey CJ. Immunosuppressive drugs in inflammatory bowel disease—a review of their mechanisms of efficacy and place in therapy. Drugs 1989; 38:267–288.

17. Sacher DB. Cyclopsorine treatment for inflammatory bowel disease: a step backward or a leap forward? N Engl J Med 1989; 321:894–896.

18. Peppercorn MA. Advances in drug therapy for inflammatory bowel disease. Ann Intern Med 1990; 112:50–60.

19. Geier DL, Miner PB Jr. New therapeutic agents in the treatment of inflammatory bowel disease. Am J Med 1992; 93:199–208.

20. Lowes JR, Jewell DP. The immunology of inflammatory bowel disease. Springer Semin Immunopathol 1990; 12:251–268.

21. Snook J. Are the inflammatory bowel disease autoimmune disorders? Gut 1990; 31:961–963.

22. Levine DS. Medical and surgical options for ulcerative colitis. Curr Opin Gastroenterol 1995; 11:29–35.

23. MacDermott RP, Stenson WF. Inflammatory bowel disease. In: Targan SR, Shanahan F, eds. Immunology and Immunopathology of the Liver and Gastrointestinal Tract. New York: Igaku Shoin, 1990:459–486.

24. Mee AS, Jewell DP. Factors inducing relapse in inflammatory bowel disease. Br Med J 1978; 2:801–802.

25. Goodman JM, Pearson KW, McGhie D, Dutt S. Deodhar SG. *Campylobacter* and *Giardia lamblia* causing exacerbation of inflammatory bowel disease. Lancet 1980; 2:1247.

26. Newman A, Lambert JR. *Campylobacter jejuni* causing flare-up of the inflammatory bowel disease. Lancet 1980; 2:919.

27. Kangro HO, Chong SKF, Hardiman A, Heath RB, Walker-Smith JA. A prospective study of viral and mycoplasma infections in chronic inflammatory bowel disease. Gastroenterology 1990; 98:549–553.

28. Ekbom A, Helmick C, Zack M, Adami HO. The epidemiology of inflammatory bowel disease: a large, population-based study in Sweden. Gastroenterology 1991; 100:350–358.

29. Sonnenberg A, McCarty DJ, Jacobsen SJ. Geographic variation of inflammatory bowel disease within the United States. Gastroenterology 1991; 100:143–149.

30. Boyko EJ, Koepsell TD, Perera DR, Inui TS. Risk of ulcerative colitis among former and current cigarette smokers. N Engl J Med 1987; 316:707–710.

31. Mayberry JF. Recent epidemiology of ulcerative colitis and Crohn's disease. Int J Colorectal Dis 1989; 4:59–66.

32. Sutherland LR, Ramcharan S, Bryant H, Fick G. Effects of cigarette smoking on recurrence of Crohn's disease. Gastroenterology 1990; 98:1123–1128.

33. Whelan G. Epidemiology of inflammatory bowel disease. Med Clin North Am 1990; 74:1–12.

34. Seidman E, Walker WA. Intestinal defenses. In: Kirsner JB, Shorter RG, eds. Inflammatory Bowel Disease. Philadelphia: Lea and Febiger, 1988:65–74.

35. Russell GJ, Walker WA. Role of the intestinal mucosal barrier and antigen uptake. In: Targan SR, Shanahan F, eds. Immunology and Immunopathology of the Liver and Gastrointestinal Tract. New York: Igaku Shoin, 1990:15–31.

36. Croitoru K, Beinenstock J, Ernst PB. Immunological alterations associated with inflammatory bowel disease. In: Freeman HJ, ed. Inflammatory Bowel Disease. Boca Raton, FL: CRC Press, 1989:39–58.

37. Fiocchi C, Roche JK, Michener WM. High prevalence of antibodies to intestinal epithelial antigens in patients with inflammatory bowel disease and their relatives. Ann Intern Med 1989; 110:786–794.

38. Saxon A, Shanahan F, Landers C, Ganz T, Targar S. A distinct subset of antineutrophil anticytoplasmic antibodies is associated with inflammatory bowel disease. J Allergy Clin Immunol 1990; 86:202–210.

39. Shanahan F, Landers C, Duerr R, Targan SR. Neutrophil autoantibodies as disease markers for ulcerative colitis. Immunol Res 1991; 10:479–484.

40. Shanahan F, Duerr RH, Rotter JI, et al. Neutrophil autoantibodies in ulcerative colitis: familial aggregation and genetic heterogeneity. Gastroenterology 1992; 103:456–461.

41. Stevens R, Oliver M, Brogan M, Heiserodt J, Targan S. Defective generation of tetanus-specific antibody-producing B cells after in vivo immunization of Crohn's disease and ulcerative colitis patients. Gastroenterology 1985; 88:1860–1866.

42. Kett K, Rognum TO, Brandtzaeg P. Mucosal subclass distribution of immunoglobulin G subclasses in patients with ulcerative colitis and Crohn's disease. Gastroenterology 1987; 93:919–924.

43. MacDermott RP, Nahm MH. Expression of human immunoglobulin G subclasses in inflammatory bowel disease. Gastroenterology 1987; 93:1127–1129.

44. Verspaget HW, Pena AS, Weterman IT, Lamers CBHW. Differences in the immunoglobulin synthesis by peripheral blood lymphocytes in Crohn's disease and ulcerative colitis. Digestion 1987; 38:245–253.

45. MacDermott RP, Nash GS, Auer IO, et al. Alterations in serum immunoglobulin G subclasses in patients with ulcerative colitis and Crohn's disease. Gastroenterology 1989; 96:764–768.

46. Wu KC, Mahida YR, Priddle JD, Jewell DP. Immunoglobulin production by isolated intestinal mononuclear cells from patients with ulcerative colitis and Crohn's disease. Clin Exp Immunol 1989; 78:37–41.

47. Wu KC, Mahida YR, Priddle JD, Jewell DP. Effect of human intestinal macrophages on immunoglobulin production by human intestinal mononuclear cells isolated from patients with inflammatory bowel disease. Clin Exp Immunol 1990; 79:35–40.

48. James SP, Neckers LM, Graeff AS, Cossman J, Balch CM, Strober W. Suppression of immunoglobulin synthesis by lymphocyte subpopulations in patients with Crohn's disease. Gastroenterology 1984; 86:1510–1518.

49. Raedler A, Fraenkel S, Klose G, Seyfarth K, Thiele HG. Involvement of the immune system in the pathogenesis of Crohn's disease: expression of the T9 antigen on peripheral immunocytes correlates with the severity of the disease. Gastroenterology 1985; 88:978–983.

50. Kramer JK, Depew WT, Szewczuk MR. T-cell immunoregulation in patients with inflammatory bowel disease. I. Differential helper T-cell function in ulcerative coltiis and Crohn's disease. J Clin Lab Immunol 1988; 25:9–17.

51. Kramer JK, Depew WT, Szewczuk MR. T-cell immunoregulation in patients with inflammatory bowel disease. II. Enhanced suppressor T-cell activity in ulcerative colitis. J Clin Lab Immunol 1988; 25:19–27.

52. Lieberman BY, Fiocchi C, Youngman KR, Sapatnekar WK, Profitt MR. Interferon gamma production by human intestinal mucosal mononuclear cells: decreased levels in inflammatory bowel disease. Dig Dis Sci 1988; 33:1297–1304.

53. Mahida YR, Gallagher A, Kurlak L, Hawkey CJ. Plasma and tissue interleukin-2 receptor levels in inflammatory bowel disease. Clin Exp Immunol 1990; 82:75–80.

54. Rubin LA, Nelson DL. The soluble interleukin-2 receptor: biology, function, and clinical application. Ann Intern Med 1990; 113:619–627.

55. Dinarello CA. Interleukin-1 and interleukin-1 antagonism. Blood 1991; 77:1627–1652.

56. Sartor RB. Pathogenetic and clinical relevance of cytokines in inflammatory bowel disease. Immunol Res 1991; 10:465–471.

57. Targan SR, Deem RL, Shanahan F. Role of mucosal T-cell–generated cytokines in epithelial cell injury. Immunol Res 1991; 10:472–478.

58. Braegger CP, Nicholls S, Murch SH, Stephens S, MacDonald TT. Tumour necrosis factor alpha in stool as a marker of intestinal inflammation. Lancet 1992; 339:89–91.

59. Dinarello CA, Wolff SM. The role of interleukin-1 in disease. N Engl J Med 1993; 328:106–113.

60. Snover DC. Biopsy interpretation in bone marrow transplantation. Pathol Annu 1989; 24:63–101.

61. Eigenbrodt ML, Eigenbrodt EH, Thiele DL. Histologic similarity of murine colonic graft-versus-host disease (GVHD) to human colonic GVHD and inflammatory bowel disease. Am J Pathol 1990; 137:1065–1076.

62. McDonald GB, Shulman HM, Sullivan KM, Spencer GD. Intestinal and hepatic complications of human bone marrow transplantation. Gastroenterology 1986; 90:460–477, 770–784.

63. Thiele DL, Eigenbrodt ML, Bryde SE, Eigenbrodt EH, Lipsky PE. Intestinal graft-versus-host disease initiated by donor T cells distinct from classic cytotoxic T lymphocytes. J Clin Invest 1989; 84:1947–1956.

64. Halstensen TS, Brandtzaeg P. Local complement activation in inflammatory bowel disease. Immunol Res 1991; 10:485–492.

65. Sharon P, Stenson WF. Enhanced synthesis of leukotriene B4 by colonic mucosa in inflammatory bowel disease. Gastroenterology 1984; 86:453–460.

66. Lauritsen K, Laursen LS, Bukhave K, Rask-Madsen J. Effects of topical 5-aminosalicylic acid and prednisolone on prostaglandin E2 and leukotriene B4 levels determined by equilibrium in vivo dialysis of rectum in relapsing ulcerative colitis. Gastroenterology 1986; 91:837–844.

67. Laursen LS, Naesdal J, Bukhave K, Lauritsen K, Rask-Madsen J. Selective 5-lipoxygenase inhibition in ulcerative colitis. Lancet 1990; 335:683–685.

68. Gordon DS, ed. Proceedings of a symposium: innovative uses of intravenous immunoglobulins in clinical hematology. Am J Med 1987; suppl 4A:1–56.

69. Berkman SA, Lee ML, Gale RP. Clinical uses of intravenous immunoglobulins. Ann Intern Med 1990; 112:278–292.

70. Sullivan KM, Kopecky KJ, Jocom J, et al. Immunomodulatory and antimicrobial efficacy of intravenous immunoglobulin in bone marrow transplantation. N Engl J Med 1990; 323:705–712.

71. Buckley RH, Schiff RI. The use of intravenous immune globulin in immunodeficiency disease. N Engl J Med 1991; 325:110–117.

72. Yocum MW, Kelso JM. Common variable immunodeficiency: the disorder and treatment. Mayo Clin Proc 1991; 66:83–96.

73. Dwyer JM. Manipulating the immune system with immune globulin. N Engl J Med 1992; 326:107–116.

74. Nydegger UE, Sultan Y, Kazatchkine MD. The concept of anti-idiotypic regulation of selected autoimmune diseases by intravenous immunoglobulin. Clin Immunol Immunopathol 1989; 53:S72–S82.

75. Dietrich G, Kazatchkine MD. Normal immunoglobulin G (IgG) for therapeutic use (intravenous Ig) contains antiidiotypic specificities against an immunodominant, disease-associated, cross-reactive idiotype of human antithyroglobulin autoantibodies. J Clin Invest 1990; 85:620–625.

76. Dietrich G, Rossi F, Sultan Y, Kaveri S, Nydegger UE, Kazatchkine MD. IVIG and regulation of autoimmunity through the idiotypic network. In: Imbach P, ed. Immunotherapy and Intravenous Immunoglobulins. San Diego: Academic Press, 1991:3–14.

77. Imbach P, ed. Immunotherapy and Intravenous Immunoglobulins. San Diego: Academic Press, 1991.

78. Newland AC, Macey MG, Veys PA. Intravenous immunoglobulin: mechanisms of action and their clinical application. In: Imbach P, ed. Immunotherapy and Intravenous Immunoglobulins. San Diego: Academic Press, 1991:15–25.

79. Nydegger UE. Hypothetic and established action mechanisms of therapy with immunoglobulin G. In: Imbach P, ed. Immunotherapy and Intravenous Immunoglobulins. San Diego: Academic Press, 1991:27–36.

80. Fischman AJ, Rubin RH, Khaw BA, et al. Detection of acute inflammation with ^{111}In-labeled nonspecific polyclonal IgG. Semin Nucl Med 1988; 18:335–344.

81. Buscombe JR, Lui D, Ensing G, de Jong R, Ell PJ. ^{99m}Tc-human immunoglobulin (HIG): first results of a new agent for the localization of infection and inflammation. Eur J Nucl Med 1990; 16:649–655.

82. Arndt JW, van der Sluys Veer A, Blok D, et al. A prospective comparison of ^{99m}Tc-labeled polyclonal human immunoglobulin and ^{111}In granulocytes of localization of inflammatory bowel disease. Acta Radiol 1992; 33:140–144.

83. Hebbard GS, Salehi N, Gibson PR, Lichtenstein M, Andrews JT. ^{99m}Tc-labelled IgG scanning does not predict the distribution of intestinal inflammation in patients with inflammatory bowel disease. Nucl Med Commun 1992; 13:336–341.

84. Naber AHJ, Oyen WJG, Claessens RAMJ, Jansen JB, van der Meer JWM, Corstens FHM. Three dimensional imaging of In-111 labelled human nonspecific immunoglobulin G (spect In-111-IgG scintigraphy) in the assessment of the localization of inflammatory bowel disease (IBD) activity. Gastroenterology 1992; 102:A669.

85. Rubin RH, Fischman AJ. The use of radiolabeled nonspecific immunoglobulin in the detection of focal inflammation. Semin Nucl Med 1994; 24:169–179.

86. Mairal L, de Lima PA, Martin-Comin J, et al. Simultaneous administration of ^{111}In-human immunoglobulin and ^{99m}Tc-HMPAO labelled leucocytes in inflammatory bowel disease. Eur J Nucl Med 1995; 22:664–670.

87. Fiocchi C. Lymphokines and the intestinal immune response: role in inflammatory bowel disease. Immunol Invest 1989; 18:91–102.

88. Leung DYM, Cotran RS, Kurt-Jones E, Burns JC, Newburger JW, Pober JS. Endothelial cell activation and high interleukin-1 secretion in the pathogenesis of acute Kawasaki disease. Lancet 1989; 2:1298–1302.

89. Nakajima T, Shintani N, Nagai M, et al. Effect of gammaglobulin in dextran sulfate-induced colitis in rats. Gastroenterology 1993; 104:A753.

90. Shintani N, Nakajima T, Nakakubo H, et al. Effect of gamma-immunoglobulin in experimental colitis induced by dextran sulfate. Nippon Shokakibyo Gakkai Zasshi 1994; 91:1936–1945.

91. Shintani N, Nakajima T, Nagai H, et al. Immunological effect of immunoglobulin on experimental colitis induced by dextran sulfate. Nippon Shokakibyo Gakkai Zasshi 1995; 92:1911–1921.

92. Kodama M, Tsukada H, Fukuda K, et al. The effects of an ultra-high dose of gamma-im-

munoglobulin on experimental colitis induced by trinitrobenzensulfonic acid. Gastroenterology 1996; 110:A939.

93. Heyworth MF, Truelove SC. A therapeutic trial of anti-lymphocytic globulin in acute ulcerative colitis. Digestion 1980; 20:221–224.

94. Cottier H, Hassig A. Immunoglobulin in chronic inflammatory diseases. Vox Sang 1986; 51(suppl 2):39–43.

95. Rohr G, Kusterer K, Schille M, et al. Treatment of Crohn's disease and ulcerative colitis with 7S-immunoglobulin. Lancet 1987; 1:170.

96. Raedler A, Ladehof E, Schug S, Schreiber S, Greten H. Therapy of Crohn's disease with IgM-enriched immunoglobulin. Gastroenterology 1988; 94:A363.

97. Wolf A, Gaedicke G, Leupold E, Kohne E. Behandlung von morbus Crohn mit intravenosem Immunoglobulin. Monatsschr Kinderheilkd 1988; 136:101–103.

98. Possoz P, Diaz D, Bories P, Michel H. May the administration of high dose intravenous gammaglobulin remove a long term steroid treatment in dependent Crohn's disease? Gastroenterology 1989; 96:A397.

99. Knoflach P, Muller C, Stetter M, Zielinski CC, Eibl MM. Treatment of Crohn's disease with high dose intravenous immunoglobulin. Gastroenterology 1989; 96:A261.

100. Knoflach P, Muller C, Eibl MM. Crohn disease and intravenous immunoglobulin G. Ann Intern Med 1990; 112:385–386.

101. Asakura H, Sasagawa T, Takizawa H, Bannai H, Yamaguchi M, Narisawa R. Clinical effectiveness and immunological changes in ulcerative colitis by massive immunoglobulin G treatment. Gastroenterology 1991; 100:A194.

102. Khalif IL, Kirkin BV, Gonsherenko SN. The use of immunoglobulin in the treatment of inflammatory bowel disease (IBD). Gastroenterology 1993; 104:A723.

103. Salcedo J, Keates S, Pothoulakis C, Castagliuolo I, LaMont JT, Kelly CP. Intravenous gammaglobulin, a novel treatment for severe unresponsive *Clostridium difficile* colitis. Gastroenterology 1996; 110:A1007.

104. Jarlov AE, Munkholm P, Schmidt PN, Langholz E, Vestergaard BF, Bech RM. Treatment of active distal ulcerative colitis with immunoglobulin G enemas. Aliment Pharmacol Ther 1993; 7:561–565.

105. Sorenson RU, Kallick MD. Clinical uses of intravenous immune globulin: immunoglobulin replacement therapy and treatment of autoimmune cytopenias. J Clin Apheresis 1988; 4:97–103.

106. Kawada K, Terasaki PI. Evidence for immunosuppression by high-dose gammaglobulin. Exp Hematol (Copenhagen) 1987; 15:133–136.

107. Fischer SH, Levine DS, Haggitt RC, Christie DL, Ochs HD. Immunoglobulin therapy for active and extensive idiopathic ulcerative and Crohn's colitis. Gastroenterology 1990; 98:A170.

108. Ochs HD, Fischer SH, Christie DL, Haggitt RC, Levine DS. Intravenous immunoglobulin in idiopathic inflammatory bowel disease: results of an open-label therapeutic trial. In: Imbach P, ed. Immunotherapy with Intravenous Immunoglobulins. San Diego: Academic Press, 1991:359–376.

109. Levine DS, Fischer SH, Christie DL, Haggitt RC, Ochs HD. Intravenous immunoglobulin therapy for active, extensive, and medically refractory idiopathic ulcerative or Crohn's colitis. Am J Gastroenterol 1992; 87:91–100.

110. Levine DS. Immunoglobulin therapy in inflammatory bowel disease. Can J Gastroenterol 1993; 7:187–195.

38

Development of Hyperimmune Immunoglobulins

William J. Landsperger and Roger Lundblad
Baxter Healthcare Corporation, Duarte, California

INTRODUCTION

Passive immunization arose as a concept in 1666 with Lower and King's early transfusion experiments described by Pepys as "mending of bad blood by borrowing from a better body," as related by Wedgwood and Riese (1). Beginning in the 19th century, many studies on the potential of immunoglobulins for use in the treatment of infectious diseases in humans were carried out for tetanus, diphtheria, scarlet fever, botulism, and snake venoms (2–7). During the early 20th century, antisera for prevention of tetanus infections in the U.S., meningococcus in Germany, and rubeola were investigated (3,6,8,9). However, the first large-scale demand for blood products that could be stored, transported, and administered quickly was created by World War II (10). Using procedures for large-scale separation of plasma productions and production of stabilized fractions by Cohn and co-workers (11–13), and with the discovery that antibodies were contained in the gammaglobulin fraction (14,15), the modern era of plasma fractionation and commercial immunoglobulin production began.

Early commercial human immunoglobulin preparations from normal plasma were developed as replacements for animal antisera and to provide passive immunization for diseases for which no effective vaccines or other treatments existed. They were suitable for intramuscular (IM) injection and given the general name immune serum globulins (ISG) or intramuscular immunoglobulins (IMIG). Today, standard ISG prepared from normal human plasma represents a pool of many thousands of plasma donors. Immune serum globulin has become a mainstay for propylactic use by travelers prior to travel to areas of endemic diseases, for both normal and HIV-infected persons with known or potential exposure to hepatitis and all patients exposed to measles when they were severely immunocompromised. However, ISG is contraindicated for persons who had been exposed to or received a measles vaccine. Antibody levels versus specific pathogens have not been precisely determined, and recommended doses of ISG vary. Lerman et al. (16) studied the effectiveness of 2 ml and 5 ml doses of standard ISG for preexposure prophylaxis against hepatitis A among Israel Defense Force troops serving in field units. At 4 months follow-up, the attack rates seen were similar for the two doses. Between 5 and 12 months postimmunization, attack rates were higher in the group given 2 ml doses. By 12 months postinfusion of ISG, the cumulative attack rate for hepatitis A was significantly different between the two groups ($P < .05$). Conclusions were that 2 ml doses were adequate for up to 4 months, while for 5–12 months the 5 ml dose was preferred. Current U.S. recommended dosages are 0.02 ml/kg for household/institutional contacts and less than 3 months of travel to 0.06 ml/kg for travel over 3 months.

Production of ISG formulations containing high titers of specific antibodies have been prepared and are available worldwide. These products were made from the plasma of donors immunized with appropriate vaccines or by screening of plasma donors for naturally occurring high antibody titers. These efforts have resulted in the availability of a large number of currently licensed ISG hyperimmune products for use in a variety of disease states. Varicella zoster virus (VZV) immunoglobulin (VZIG) is currently recommended for exposed susceptible adults (especially pregnant women), newborns (≥ 28 weeks' gestation) of susceptible mothers, and preterm infants (< 28 weeks or < 100 g). For both moderately and severely immunocompromised individuals, VZIG is recommended for both infants and adults following significant VZV exposure with doses ranging between 125 units (0–10 kg) and 625 units (> 40 kg). Protective levels of antibodies are unknown. Tetanus immunoglobulin (TIG) is recommended for those with serious wounds and all individuals having received less than three doses of tetanus toxoid. The usual prophylactic dose is 250–500 units, while 500–6000 units is indicated for therapy of tetanus infection.

Use of hepatitis B (HB) immunoglobulin (HBIG) is indicated for prophylaxis of infants born to HBsAg+ mothers and susceptible persons with percutaneous, sexual, or mucosal exposure to HB virus. Liver transplantation evolved as the therapy of choice in end-stage liver disease (17) and was associated with recurrence of viral hepatitis in the graft. For patients with active viral replication, liver transplantation should only be considered within the limits of predictable prevention of reinfection of the allograft. Protective equivalency has been shown for a single dose of HBIG given within 3 days of exposure followed by immediate vaccine administration or for vaccine alone over a 10-month period (18). Individual doses of HBIG for adults and children are in the range of a total of 3–5 ml. When persons not previously immunized against rabies are exposed to virus, the use of human rabies immunoglobulin (Imogam) is indicated. Usage is identical for all individuals regardless of immunological status. Doses are 0.13 ml/kg to be given as soon as possible postexposure. Vaccinia immunoglobulin (VIG) was previously indicated for passive, transient prevention of, or modification of, aberrant infections induced by vaccinia (smallpox) vaccine. Fortunately, the smallpox virus currently exists in only a few laboratories. For passive, transient protection against development of endogenous anti-Rh_0 or anti-D antibodies in nonsensitized Rh_0 or D antigen-negative persons who received Rh_0 or D antigen–positive blood, $Rh_0(D)$ immunoglobulin (RhIG) is indicated. Exposure could result in a number of ways, but prophylaxis is most common for prevention the alloimmunization of Rh_0-negative mothers by Rh_0-positive fetuses and for secondary prophylaxis of hemolytic disease of the fetus and newborn. WinRho is the latest and most potent of the $Rh_0(D)$ immunoglobulins. The armamentarium of specific immune globulin products that are available worldwide under a variety of names are listed on Table 1.

A novel IMIG product (bacterial polysaccharide immunoglobulin, BPIG) was conceptualized and produced at the Massachusetts Public State Biologics Laboratories

Table 1 U.S. and International Hyperimmune Intramuscular Immune Globulins

Hyperimmune IMIG	Dose/efficacy	Product names[a]
Varicella zoster	125 units (0–10 kg) to 625 units > 40 kg/ primary indication for immunodeficient children significantly reduces mortality	VZIG (generic U.S.) Haimazig, Varitect, Immunozig, Vacuman, Varicellon
Tetanus	250 units prophylaxis, 500–2000 units severe wound, up to 6000 units for therapy/high	Hyper-Tet, Humotet, Gammatet, Tetagam, Tetavenin, Tetuman
Rabies	0.133 ml/kg (29 IU/kg)/nearly 100%	Imogam, Hyperab, Berirab, Haimarab, Rabiabulin, Rabuman, Rabies-Gamma
Hepatitis B	0.06 ml/kg/75% sexual contact with HBsAg+ person, >98% in infants with combined vaccine usage	H-BIG, HyperHep, Aunativ, Hep-B-Gammagee, Haimabig, Uman-Big
Rh$_o$ (D) (anti-D)	Variable, 1–2 vials dependent on packed red cell volume/sensitization 1–2% postpartum, 0.1–0.7% antepartum	Gamulin Rh, Haima, Gammamen, WinRho S/D, Igrho, Rhega

[a]U.S. and international products.

by Siber et al. (19). Donors were immunized with a *H. influenzae* (Hib) capsular polysaccharide vaccine, a meningococcal vaccine against groups A, C, Y, and W-135 and a 23-valent *S. pneumoniae* vaccine. Prevention of Hib in high-risk Apache infants using BPIG was evaluated in a field trial (19). At doses of 0.5 ml/kg given at 2, 6, and 10 months of age, significant protection from invasive Hib disease was seen. Specific antibody levels reached 2–4 µg/ml at 72 h postinfusion, with a mean antibody half-life of 27 days. Another study tested BPIG in Alaskan native infants who, up to 1989, had the highest recorded Hib disease rate (2960/100,000) in children less than 13 months of age (20). Upon the introduction of the *H. influenzae* conjugate vaccine (PedvaxHIB), the clinical study protocol was modified to a passive-active strategy in which BPIG was given at birth and vaccine at 2, 4, and 12 months of age. Incidence of Hib was reduced from 2960 to 302:100,000 over the period of 1989 through 1992.

Prevention of acute otitis media (AOM) by BPIG was tested in a randomized, stratified, double-blind, placebo-controlled protocol (21). Children ≤24 months of age with one to three prior episodes of AOM received BIPG (0.5 ml/kg) or saline placebo at entry and 30 days later. Although the incidence of AOM due to all organisms during the 120-day study period was similar for both BPIG and placebo recipients, pneumococcal AOM was significantly less frequent in BPIG recipients (0.21 episodes per patient) than in placebo (0.45 episodes per patient, $P = .05$). At the time of this writing, BPIG has not been approved for licensure by regulatory agencies.

Despite worldwide availability of products (Table 1), there were major drawbacks in the usage of high-dose (volume) therapy of IMIG for passive immunization. Severe complement-mediated adverse reactions due to high anticomplementary activity were associated with early attempts at IV administration of ISG (22). When administered IM, varying amounts of antibody were degraded by proteolysis prior to reaching the circulation and 2 to 4 days was required before peak plasma levels of IgG could be reached (23). Pain and sterile abscesses sometimes developed at the site of injection, and the limitations on the amount of IMIG which could be infused provided a major impetus for development of IgG concentrates suitable for IV infusion.

The remainder of this chapter will review the rationale for the development of hyperimmune intravenous immunoglobulins (HYPERIVIG), their current availability, and new products under investigation. With a few exceptions, the emphasis will be placed on reports of recent clinical evaluations of polyclonal hyperimmune IVIGs in humans which are either licensed or in various stages of clinical development.

RATIONALE FOR HYPERIMMUNE IMMUNOGLOBULINS

Standard vs. Hyperimmune IVIG

Early preparations of IgG developed for IV usage used various enzymatic and chemical methods as part of the manufacturing process for the reduction of anticomplementary activity. Low pH treatments and/or the use of ion exchange chromatography were also evaluated. Both enzymatic and chemical modifications of IgG often resulted in adverse effects on antibody Fc function and variations in the concentrations of different IgG subclasses. Therefore, most products in use today have manufacturing processes to ensure that the IgG remains native and retains full functional activity. Standard intravenous immunoglobulins (IVIGs) are produced from donor pools of up to 30,000 donors. They have a number of disadvantages, such as limited and variable levels of antibodies for specific bacterial and viral organisms (24). In addition, large infusion volumes of 10–20 ml/kg body weight are required to obtain minimal protective antibody levels suitable for treatment of premature infants and neonates (25). Lastly, large doses of standard IVIGs increase both the risks of disease transmission and adverse reactions.

While normal individuals rarely contract serious infectious diseases, patient populations are at increased risk because of age and with those patients, with hematological malignancies and/or solid tumors having their lives extended by chemotherapy. There is an increased used of prosthetic heart valves, plastic shunts, and other foreign bodies which might be susceptible to contamination by bacterial biofilms. Individuals with primary and secondary immunodeficiencies remain most susceptible to nosocomial infections, and high morbidity and mortality are seen in spite of the best medical care and the use of antibiotics (26). If suitable HYPERIVIG preparations for passive immunotherapy were available, they would be useful in the treatment of a wide variety of nosocomial bacterial, viral, and, possibly, fungal infections in these patient populations. Potential advantages and increased benefits of HYPERIVIGs include significantly reduced volumes with possibly only 1–4 ml/kg being required. Increased amounts of specific and efficacious antibodies, i.e., those with opsonizing and protective activities, would be increased as a proportion of total IgG (high titers). Therefore, these preparations should provide an important adjunct and possibly synergistic therapy with antibiotics, thus providing significantly reduced morbidity and mortality.

Antibiotic Resistance

During a 3-day colloquium held at the 1993 American Society for Microbiology, Stuart Levy stated that "antibiotic resistance was becoming so commonplace that the 1990s were beginning to look like the "preantibiotic" era (27). The problem of resistance to antibiotics was global, with the situation rapidly becoming more serious. During the coming decade, physicians would increasingly be challenged with infections for which effective treatments are not available. Over the next 20 years, effective control of disease due to bacterial pathogens using new antibiotics would be limited, and new modes of treatment, such as organism-specific hyperimmune immunoglobulin products, were likely to be required. Recently, the U.S. public health system has been severely challenged by a myriad of newly identified pathogens and syndromes such as *Escherichia coli* 0157:H7, hepatitis C virus, human immunodeficiency virus, Legionnaires' disease, Lyme disease, and toxic shock syndrome (28). In addition, incidences of disease previously considered to be under control have also increased in many areas. Emerging infections place a disproportionate burden on immunocompromised persons, those in institutional settings (e.g., hospitals and child day care centers), and minority and underserved populations. Certain resistant strains of *Pneumococcus* and gram-positive organisms such as *S. epidermidis* can only be treated with vancomycin (to which resistance is increasing) and *S. pneumoniae* isolates resistant to most antibiotics are found virtually worldwide.

Recently, following organ transplantation, a number of young children suffered vancomycin-resistant *S. epidermidis* infections and could not be effectively treated (29). Even more significantly, a trend toward plasmid transmission of vancomycin resistance from *S. epidermidis* to *S. aureus* has been observed. At present, up to 50% of *S. aureus* nosocomial infections were due to vancoymcin antibiotic-resistant strains. Other clinically significant bacteria with demonstrated antibiotic resistance include *Pseudomonas, Klebsiella, Serratia, Proteus, Enterobacter*, and *E. coli* (one of the most important causes of community- and hospital-acquired infections). Each year up to 80,000 Americans die from hospital-acquired (nosocomial) infections (27), out of a total of over 2 million reported cases in the U.S. with 1–1.5 million cases reported from intensive care units alone (30).

Clinical Need

Gram-Positive Bacteria

Staphylococcus epidermidis and *Staphylococcus aureus*.   Disease due to gram-positive organisms represents one of infectious disease's major challenges. Both *S. epidermidis* and *S. aureus* were important causes of nosocomial infections and have become the most common cause of sepsis in premature infants (31). Impaired immunity in such infants is likely due to several factors, including diminished neutrophil function and low levels of both IgG and complement (32,33). As the major cause of opportunistic nosocomial infections, *S. epidermidis* was a major problem for patients undergoing continuous peritoneal dialysis (CAPD) as well as those with indwelling catheters and/or plastic implants. The role of antibody in immunity to *S. epidermidis* was incompletely understood, although low levels of opsonic antibody in neonatal sera suggested that neonatal susceptibility to *S. epidermidis* might be related to impaired opsonic activity (34). If opsonic antibodies were necessary for effective clearance of *S. epidermidis* and these antibodies were present in standard IVIG, they might be useful for prevention or treatment of these infections.

Three standard IVIG preparations (Gamimmune N, Sandoglobulin, and Gammagard) were compared in in vivo opsonophagocytic assays and in a staphylococcal suckling rat sepsis model. Opsonic titers varied greatly among preparations and among different lots of each product. Each preparation and different lots of each product were highly variable in antibody content. Only those with ≥90% opsonic activity promoted bacterial clearance from blood and significantly increased survival when compared with lots with ≤50% opsonic activity. Although these studies suggested that opsonic antibody may play an important role in immunocompromised patients, such as premature infants, standard IVIG was found to be unreliable in providing reliable therapy. Development of an appropriate HYPERIVIG for treatment of these diseases was highly desirable.

Group B Streptococcus.   Group B streptococci (GBS) were the leading cause of meningitis and sepsis in neonates in the United States (35), with an incidence of 1.8–3.2 cases per 1000 live births (36,37). GBS infections continue to cause significant morbidity and mortality among neonates and other immunocompromised hosts (38). It remains the most lethal organism in the neonatal ICU. Infections were divided into early-onset prenatally or perinatally acquired infections (≤7 days of age) and late-onset postnatally acquired infections (>7 days of age) (39). Host immunity to GBS depended on opsonization of the organisms by antibodies and complement, with subsequent killing by phagocytic leukocytes (40,41). Both opsonic and protective activities have been demonstrated for antibodies directed against the capsular polysaccharides. At least six capsular types have been associated with human disease and, except for potential cross-reactivity between types Ia and Ib and protective antibodies directed toward the individual capsular polysaccharides, are type-specific (35). GBS was important in both pregnant women and women of childbearing age and since these infections remain nonreportable in most states, previous levels of the frequency of disease have probably been underestimated.

Although immunoglobulin G (IgG) is acquired transplacentally by newborns (42), much of the IgG transference occurs during the third trimester of gestation. Premature infants (<32–34 weeks' gestation) are likely to have decreased levels of serum IgG (43). Since the specificities of transplacentally transferred antibodies are limited to the mother's previous exposure to specific pathogens, newborns (especially preterms) may have both qualitative and quantitative immunoglobulin deficiencies. In 1973, it was suggested that inadequate amounts of GBS antibody may play a role in human GBS infections (44). By 1976, the susceptibility of neonates to GBS infection due to a deficiency of maternal GBS antibody was established (45,46).

Risk factors for vertical transmission to neonates include the presence of GBS in the birth canal at time of birth, prematurity and low birth weight, prolonged interval between membrane rupture and birth, and lack of sufficient circulating maternal antibodies. In horizontal transmission, up to 40% of noninfected neonates become colonized in the hospital nursery; others, to a lesser extent, become infected in day care centers.

A vaccine composed of either purified bacterial polysaccharides alone or conjugated to tetanus toxoid was developed by Kasper for intended use in the immunization of women of child-bearing age (47). Unfortunately the antibody response in subjects or pregnant women immunized with the polysaccharide vaccine was reported to be unsatisfactory. Based on other vaccine experience (i.e., the Hib-conjugate vaccine), development of a polysaccharide carrier protein conjugate vaccine was begun. This preparation should be more immunogenic and suitable for donor immunization and production of a GBS HYPERIVIG (35).

Streptococcus pneumoniae. Infections with this organism continued to be a serious health problem, especially in children under 2, the immunoincompetent, the immunocompromised elderly, HIV-infected persons, those with chronic diseases, and certain bone-marrow transplant (BMT) patients. While for many years the infections caused by these bacteria were easily killed by low doses of penicillin, cases of pneumococcal disease resistant to penicillin (and even the newer antibiotics) were being reported at increased rates (49). *S. pneumoniae* caused potentially fatal infections, which reportedly strike ~3.5 million people per year with ~70% of infections occurring in individuals over the age of 45; and was the leading cause of year-round community-acquired pneumonia (30). On a global level, *Pneumococcus* is believed to be the most common bacterial cause of acute respiratory infections, which were estimated to result in more than 1 million childhood deaths each year (48). In HIV patients, it was the leading cause of nonmycobacterial bacteremia and was the primary infectious agent in patients surviving 6 months or longer following BMT. Physicians remain concerned owing to increasing resistance to antibiotics.

It has been known for decades that the pneumococcal capsular polysaccharides (PCP) of *Streptococcus pneumoniae* confer the antigenic specificity that defines different serotypes and that antibodies to these polysaccharides are type-specific and protective in humans (50). The currently licensed vaccine is composed of a cocktail of purified PCP representing 23 serotypes of *S. pneumoniae*. A recent study showed that these serotypes accounted for 93% of the isolates from 1054 invasive pneumococcal infections (51). However, the vaccine's efficacy was estimated to be only 61% in immunocompetent adults, and only about 10% of at-risk elderly persons are immunized. Children 2 years of age and under were unable to respond to the vaccine due to weak and short-lived responses to the T cell–independent PCP (52).

Specific serotypes associated with invasive disease varied in different geographies. For instance, types 1 and 5 were the most common in Israel, but were uncommon in Finland; type 19 was common in Finland but unknown in Israel (53,54). Previous U.S. studies showed regional and epidemiological differences between serotypes in children and adults. Generally, types 4, 6, 14, 18, 19, and 23 predominated in children (52,55,56), but unpredictable variations of serotypic prevalence occurred over time (57). Development of an *S. pneumoniae* hyperimmune IVIG (PN HYPERIVIG) prepared from the plasma of adults immunized with 23-valent vaccine may be a way to provide broad-spectrum prophylaxis and/or therapy.

Gram-Negative Bacteria

Pseudomonas aeruginosa. *Pseudomonas* continues to be a major nosocomial infectious disease. The relative frequency of infections has increased dramatically over the last 30 years for two primary reasons. First, advances in medical treatments and technologies have resulted in the prolonged survival of immunologically impaired hosts. Second, nosocomial infections have increased due to widespread antibiotic usage with the concomitant development of resistant strains (58–61). *Pseudomonas* has recently been noted to account for 11% of all nosocomial infections (62), and this frequency reflected an upward trend (63). Only 4–12% of healthy individuals were carriers of *P. aeruginosa*, whereas 40–50% of hospitalized patients were potential carriers (64). Patients with cancer who were neutropenic due to antineoplastic therapy were at high risk. Others at high risk were those with hematological malignancies, recipients of bone marrow, and those with solid tumors. In one group of 67 patients with underlying malignancies who developed *P. aeruginosa* bacteremia, 81% had a neutrophil count of $< 1000/mm^3$ (65). Two distinct phenotypes were associated with human infections: a nonmucoid, lipopolysaccharide (LPS)-smooth phenotype, mostly isolated from patients with nosocomial and community-acquired infections; and a mucoid LPS-rough phenotype, mostly isolated from cystic fibrosis (CF) patients with chronic respiratory infections (66). Immunity to these different variants was mediated by antibodies specific to O antigens and mucoid exopolysaccharide (alginate), respectively.

As far back as 1984, Collins and Roby demonstrated the protective activity of an IVIG (human) enriched in antibody against lipopolysaccharide antigens of *Pseudomonas aeruginosa* (PS HYPERIVIG), which was prepared by screening of plasma donors for high titers of antibodies to four serotypes of *Pseudomonas* (67). Evaluations of individual donors were done by ELISA to screen for Fisher-Devlin-Gnabasik immunotypes 1, 2, 4, and 6. Serum pools with titers to various immunotypes ranging between 1/1600 and 1/3200 were made. Using this high-titer product, Hunt and Purdue (68) evaluated 10 patients with *Pseudomonas* sepsis and eight with bacteremia. Doses of 500 mg/kg on 2 consecutive days were given. IgG levels rose after infusions and were maintained in the normal range throughout the septic course. *Pseudomonas* antibodies specific to each of the *Pseudomonas* immunotypes responsible for the bacteremias were represented in the hyperimmune globulin. Clinical improvement was seen, with 70%

of the patients surviving, including six of the seven with bacteremia. This benefit was correlated with a three- to 125-fold postinfusion in specific antibody titers.

Klebsiella pneumoniae. *Klebsiella* has been a frequently isolated nosocomial pathogen (69,70), and, despite the availability of potent antimicrobial agents, invasive *Klebsiella* infections were associated with a high mortality rate, ranging between 24% and 50% in bacteremic patients (69,71). Numerous studies had been reported regarding the immunogenicity of capsular polysaccharide antigens of the *Klebsiella* group (KCP) (72,73), but relatively little attention was given to the type O antigens. *Klebsiella* was shown to be the leading cause of epidemic extraintestinal infection in neonates, was second only to *P. aeruginosa* in case fatality rates, and was second only to *E. coli* as the cause of nosocomial infections (74,75).

Viruses

Respiratory Syncytial Virus.   Respiratory syncytial virus (RSV) was regarded worldwide as the most important pediatric pathogen of the lower respiratory tract. It caused annual epidemics between December and April in temperate zones of the northern hemisphere (76). Serological surveys worldwide had demonstrated that approximately half of the infants who lived through a single RSV epidemic were infected (77). RSV was the single most serious cause of respiratory disease in young children, the major cause of severe pneumonia and bronchiolitis, and the most common cause of acute lower respiratory tract diseases. Respiratory illness due to RSV was the most common cause for rehospitalization of preterm infants, both with and without bronchopulmonary dysplasia (78,79).

King et a. assessed the use of Ribavirin and standard IVIG combination therapy in cohorts of 83 infants born to HIV+ and 48 non-HIV-infected mothers (80). RSV shedding was prolonged in HIV+ children. One child, who shed RSV for 199 days, remained RSV-infected following this treatment regimen. Prolonged shedding of RSV in HIV+ children must be recognized and assessed during therapy.

Treatment of severe respiratory infection with specific immune globulin, either alone or in combination with antiviral drugs, was desirable. Ribavirin and amantadine ameliorated illness caused by RSV in children but were used infrequently due to lack of cost-effectiveness. Prevention of viral respiratory diseases was preferable to therapy because some lung damage occurred before the beginning of treatment, and damage resulting from the immune response could continue even after the virus was inhibited. Passive immunization with RSV immunoglobulin in infants and children has been shown to prevent or attenuate RSV in high-risk groups (81). In the absence of a safe and effective vaccine, passive immunization with an RSV HYPERIVIG remains the only proven means of protection against serious RSV illness (82,83).

Human Immunodeficiency Virus.   Development of vaccines for immunization against the HIV virus has been a long and frustrating road which yet seems elusive. Desirability of an HIV vaccine has been ranked No. 1 28 of 45 times as the single most urgently needed vaccine in the developing world, and No. 1 41 out of 50 times for the developed world (84). However, discussions of vaccine development were beyond the scope of this chapter. Efforts to develop hyperimmune globulins for the passive immunization of HIV infections were also being aggressively pursued and will be discussed in the following pages.

Passive hyperimmune therapy first emerged in an effort to delay the progression of a human immunodeficiency virus (HIV)-positive status to acquired immune deficiency syndrome (AIDS). An early report by Gao and co-workers (85) provided an overview of passive hyperimmune therapy, including benefits, adverse reactions, and other, similar therapies that were available. Nurses who cared for HIV-positive patients were shown to be a significant source of information for day-to-day patient responses to treatment.

Patients infected with HIV may eventually have both an antibody deficiency and a deficiency of cellular immunity. Restoration of antibody levels through IVIG administration benefited HIV-infected children and adults with recurrent bacterial infections. Platelet counts could also be raised to hemostatic levels at doses of IVIG of 200–400 mg/kg every 2–4 weeks in HIV-infected patients with idiopathic thrombocytopenic purpura (ITP) and life-threatening bleeding. Some retrospective evidence has suggested that IVIG is effective in prevention of *Pneumocystis carinii* pneumonia. Yap et al. (86) postulated that specific anti-HIV HYPERIVIG antibody preparations could have a therapeutic role, either as immunoglobulin concentrates or as immunoadhesions and immunotoxins. Further investigations were required to exclude effects of antibody enhancement of HIV infection by the Fc or complement receptor.

In 1991, a conference on the early diagnosis of HIV infection in infants was called to further encourage collaborative exchanges of information among researchers in the field (87). It was of special interest to determine if one or more subpopulations of anti-gp120/V3 loop-neutralizing antibodies could be associated with a reduction of vertical transmission of HIV infection. It was important to determine if those antibodies were truly protective or surrogate markers of a different mechanism(s). Some support for the first supposition was provided by finding HIV-specific antibodies in seropositive persons' saliva and breast milk, both of which had relatively low infectivity. However, the development and testing of specific HIV HYPERIVIG in controlled clinical trials were required to answer these questions.

Cytomegalovirus.   Infection by human cytomegalovirus (CMV) remains a major cause of morbidity and mortality after BMT (82). In infected patients, CMV is generally detected between 4 and 10 weeks following transplantation (88). Although the use of CMV-seronegative blood products was effective in the prevention of primary infection in seronegative patients with seronegative marrow donors, infection due to CMV-seropositive marrow donors continued to occur at the rate of about 40% (89,90). Up to 90% of patients with AIDS evidenced active CMV infection during their illness, as determined by autopsy and clinical studies, and up to 45% may experience life- or sight-threatening infections due to CMV (91–93). Historically, CMV disease developed in 30–49% of seropositive recipients with the predominant manifestation being interstitial pneumonitis, which was generally fatal (94). The most frequent cause of life-threatening opportunistic infections in patients with AIDS was CMV (95,96). CMV retinitis was the leading cause of blindness in HIV-infected patients, with disease progression occurring without early aggressive and appropriate antiviral therapy (97).

Standard IVIG has been evaluated extensively for use in the prevention of complications and disease due to CMV in transplant and immunocompromised clinical settings (98,99). Differences in IVIG preparations from various manufacturers, dosing regimens, donor and recipient CMV serology, prophylaxis of graft-versus-host disease (GvHD) and the use of white blood cell transfusions have greatly complicated interpretations of the prophylactic benefit. For CMV-negative transplant patients, IVIG decreased symptomatic CMV infection and interstitial pneumonia. For CMV-positive recipients, IVIG prevented interstitial pneumonia but not symptomatic CMV infection.

Siadak et al. suggested that the best currently established role for prophylactic use of standard IVIG in allogeneic BMT may be in the prevention of GvHD (98).

Research in the past decade had demonstrated that CMV antibody significantly modulated the expression of CMV disease (76). However, in spite of the availability of licensed CMV HYPERIVIG products, the incidence of CMV disease in seronegative recipients of seropositive allogenic bone marrow and solid organ transplants had not been eliminated, and the results have been variable (88). The benefits of IVIG (standard or hyperimmune) in transplant patients should be directly related to the pharmacokinetics of anti-CMV. In a study using Gammagard, anti-CMV half-life in bone marrow patients was ~ 6 days for both 250 mg/kg or 500 mg/kg doses, compared to a 22-day IgG half-life in normal subjects (100).

Perhaps an additional benefit could be derived from product with even higher antibody doses. North American Biologics Incorporated (NABI) is currently using a vaccine-stimulated HyperIVIG based on Biocine/Chiron's recombinant glycoprotein B vaccine. The HyperIVIG produced using vaccine-stimulated donor plasma was scheduled for clinical studies in 1996/1997.

Herpes Simplex Virus. Neonatal herpes simplex viral infections cause significant morbidity and mortality among infected babies despite the availability of antiviral therapy. The disease presents in one of three forms: skin, eye, and mouth involvement; encephalitis; or disseminated infection. More than 50% of infected babies with neonatal herpes fell into one of the two latter categories. Mortality and severe morbidity rates in these neonates exceeded 75%. Future therapeutic efforts must be directed toward improved disease outcome. One such effort was the evaluation of humanized monoclonal antibodies, human monoclonal antibodies and hyperimmune globulin as part of a concomitant approach for babies with encephalitis and disseminated infection (101). Since little transplacental maternal antibody was received at the time of birth, the combination of immunoglobulin and antiviral therapy could improve disease outcome.

HYPERIMMUNE INTRAVENOUS IMMUNOGLOBULINS

Preparation

HYPERIVIG can be prepared by screening and selecting high-titer donor pools or through the use of plasma donor pools from individuals who have been immunized with specific vaccines. However, distinct disadvantages of selecting screened donors were the limited availability of such plasma and the disqualification of those donors from use in preparation of normal IVIG. Ethical concerns over immunization of individuals for plasma donation continued to be important. Since normal individuals were at minimal risk for such infections as *P. aeruginosa* and CMV, immunization of these individuals may remain problematic. The advantages of donor immunization include the ability to establish donor pools with defined antibody titers. Product titers could be expected to be increased for immunized donors compared to screened donors; in addition, plasma availability should be extended.

The required development time for HYPERIVIG would be relatively short since methodologies and manufacturing techniques were already in place for production of standard IVIG. The lead time for a vaccine-based program was defined by the time required to produce a safe and immunogenic vaccine. HYPERIVIG production only required the replacement of normal plasma pools with high-titered plasma pools. Polyclonal antibodies with multiple specificities would aid in promotion of the rapid clearance of microorganisms and their virulence factors. Since the development of anti-idiotypic antibodies to human polyclonal antibodies was unlikely, these preparations could maintain a distinct advantage over humanized monoclonal antibodies (MAb). Finally, and perhaps most importantly, no organism was known to have developed resistance to high-titered polyclonal antibodies.

Properties

With few exceptions, attempts at intravenous usage of intramuscular immunoglobulin products in persons suffering from acute infections, usually children, had immediate and severe anaphylactic or anaphylactoid reactions (22,102,103). A primary cause for these severe adverse reactions was found by Barandun and colleagues to be due to the tendency for purified IgG molecules to aggregate. Both aggregated IgG and contaminating IgM were believed to be responsible for high anticomplement activity (104). While working in close cooperation with the Swiss Red Cross Laboratories, Barandun et al. first formulated IgG preparations at low pH (~4.0) isolated in the presence of trace amounts of pepsin in order to minimize reaggregation. They then listed the desired criteria for an optimal IVIG. Among these were: (1) maintenance of native structure and functional activities; (2) the entire spectrum of IgG antibodies present in a large representative blood donor population (i.e., large plasma pools); (3) all four IgG subclasses in physiological proportions; and (4) no infectious agents, aggregates, or other detrimental substances (105). Later, these properties were mandated for IVIG preparations by a World Health Organization (WHO) panel of experts (106). The foundation for immunoglobulin therapy was consequently laid, using the formulation developed by Barandun and colleagues. Since then, a large number of standard IVIG (and a limited number of HYPERIVIG) products have been accepted as standard therapy for a variety of therapeutic and/or prophylactic benefits including secondary immunodeficiencies and autoimmune diseases.

Licensed HYPERIVIGs

Anti-CMV HYPERIVIG

A number of commercially available high-titered CMV hyperimmune IVIG products (CMVIG) are produced for treatment of CMV infections (Table 2). In the United States, MedImmune has the only approved product; however, in Europe, several preparations are available. All currently available CMVIG products are based on the screening of plasma donors for selection of those with naturally acquired high titers of anti-CMV antibodies. Plasma donor selection was done by screening using a CMV enzyme-linked immunosorbent assay (ELISA). Recently, the major neutralizing epitopes of both "early" and "late" CMV antigens were identified (107). Improved ELISA assays based on recombinant antigens corresponding to immunodominant epitopes for the detection of CMV-specific antibodies were published. This methodology may lead to the production of a higher-titered and more effective hyperimmune CMV globulin.

Bone Marrow Transplantation.   A review by Zaia (94) supported the use of standard IVIG as general treatment in the allogenic bone marrow transplant recipient and

Table 2 Licensed Global Intravenous Hyperimmune Immunoglobulin Preparations

Disease	Manufacturer	Product name
Cytomegalovirus	MedImmune/Massachusetts Public Health Biologic Labs	CytoGam
	Bayer, Biotest	Cytoglobin®, Cytoglobin, Cytotect Polyglobin R
P. aeruginosa	Bayer, Germany	Psomaglobin N
Hepatitis B	Biotest, Europe	Hepatect IV
Rh$_o$ (D)	Berne, Switzerland	Rhesuman IV, Antirho D,
	Schiapparelli, Italy	Venogamma
Tetanus	Immuno, Italy	Tetaven IV
Varicella zoster	Schiapparelli, Italy	Var Zeta IV

CMV antibody-enriched immunoglobulin (hyperimmune CMVIG) for selected renal transplant recipients. For the treatment of CMV-associated pneumonitis, it was recommended that Ganciclovir and IVIG be used in combination for the bone marrow transplant recipient, and that Ganciclovir be used with or without IVIG in patients in other transplantation groups with high doses of CMVIG (1.0 g/kg once weekly for 120 days after transplant). He suggested that most CMV infections could be prevented, including CMV disease in CMV-seronegative allogeneic BMT recipients, even when the marrow donor was CMV-seropositive (108).

A Hungarian study evaluated the efficacy of standard IVIG versus anti-CMV HYPERIVIG (Cytotect) (109). Ten children who received bone marrow transplants received standard IVIG in doses of 100 mg/kg regularly 1 day before and 14, 28, 60, and 90 days following transplantation. Cytotect was given to 6 patients at the same 100 mg/kg doses. New CMV infections occurred in 3 of the 11 standard IVIG recipients, while in the group of six children given Cytotect prophylaxis, only one became infected from endogenous reactivation of CMV. The authors concluded that anti-CMV HYPERIVIG seemed to be more effective than standard IVIG in the prevention of CMV infection.

A study by Bowden et al. evaluated a CMV HYPERIVIG produced by Bayer (formerly Cutter Biologics) in a randomized controlled trial in CMV-seronegative marrow transplant patients receiving seropositive marrow for prevention of primary CMV infection during the first 100 days after transplant (110). Patients received 200 mg/kg CMVIG on days 8 and 6 before transplant, the day after transplant, weekly for the first month, and then every 2 weeks to complete 10 doses. Eligible patients were randomized into two groups, with each group receiving either total body irradiation (TBI) plus cyclophosphamide or other conditioning regimens such as busulfan and cyclophosphamide, or high-dose cytosine arabinoside with or without TBI. While there were significantly less CMV excretion episodes ($P = .04$) and viremia ($P = .01$) in the treatment group, incidences of CMV disease including CMV pneumonia, CMV enteritis, and CMV syndrome were not statistically different. There were also no differences in median times of onset of CMV infection or disease, median number of hospital days, or survival between the two groups. No patients received high-dose acyclovir or other immunoglobulin prophylaxis. Use of CMV HYPERIVIG could not yet be recommended for prophylaxis of primary CMV infection after allogeneic marrow transplant in seronegative patients with seropositive marrow for the ultimate goal of reducing symptomatic CMV disease, especially pneumonia.

Renal Transplantation.   The first indication for CMV HYPERIVIG was approved in 1990 for prophylaxis in seronegative recipients of kidneys from seropositive donors. CMV HYPERIVIG was subsequently shown to be effective for prevention of the considerable morbidity and mortality associated with CMV disease (111). A trial conducted by Conti et al. (112) evaluated CMV HYPERIVIG in renal transplant recipients. Twenty-seven patients received IVIG for 6-week periods or low-dose intravenous Ganciclovir for 3 weeks. While both prophylactic regimens significantly reduced the incidence of invasive CMV infection ($P < .05$), the cost of Ganciclovir was $350 per patient compared to $4000 per patient for IVIG. CMV HYPERIVIG could be used in place of acyclovir for the prevention of primary CMV disease in renal transplant recipients (113). When treatment was started prior to transplantation and continued between 12 and 16 weeks, significant reduction of primary CMV disease was seen, although effectiveness for the prevention of CMV reinfection or reactivation has not yet been established. This study did not take into account the effect IVIG may have had on GvHD and allograft survival.

Finn found CMV HYPERIVIG to have significant benefits in renal transplant patients (114). Multivariant analysis demonstrated that receipt of anti-rejection therapy, a liver transplant, or a donor organ from a CMV-seropositive individual (if the recipient was CMV-seronegative) were major risk factors for the development of CMV disease ($P < .001$), while the difference between Acyclovir and Ganciclovir + IVIG prophylaxis was also significant ($P = .054$). Their conclusions were that CMV transmission or reactivation may best be prevented by long-term antiviral agent administration, and that the primary indicator of CMV morbidity was the need for rehospitalization. Combination therapy that used CMV hyperimmune globulin and Ganciclovir could be used in the most severe forms of the disease. Stratta et al. evaluated four regimens of prophylaxis for CMV in 82 combined pancreas-kidney transplantation (PKT) patients with OKT3 induction during a 4-year period (115). The first 30 patients received standard IVIG at 500 mg/kg for six doses and oral Acyclovir for 3 months. The next 34 recipients received intravenous Ganciclovir (2.5 mg/kg) twice daily for 2 weeks followed by oral Acyclovir for 3 months. In the third group, patients were randomized to five doses over 2 months of either standard IVIG (n = 9) or CMV hyperimmune globulin (CytoGam; n = 9, 100–150 mg/kg) plus 2 weeks of intravenous Ganciclovir followed by 3 months of oral Acyclovir. All four groups were similar with respect to clinical, demographic, and immunological variables, including donor and recipient CMV serologic status and blood transfusions. All patients were monitored in the first 6 months after PKT. Immune globulin prophylaxis appeared to reduce the severity of symptomatic CMV infection. However, the authors could not show any added benefit of either Cytogam or standard IVIG when used in combination with other antiviral agents. They recommended that IVIG preparations be used only in high-risk situations such as primary CMV exposure, not routinely with antilymphocyte therapy.

Lung Transplantation.   Zamora et al. evaluated a CMV HYPERIVIG for the prevention of CMV disease in CMV-seropositive lung transplant recipients (116). Data from a small patient trial suggested that immunoglobulin in combination with Ganciclovir effectively reduced the incidence and delayed the onset of CMV infections in these transplant patients. Not addressed by this study were the optimal dosage and duration of treatment with CMV HYPERIVIG for effective prophylaxis or if it was cost-effective while enhancing allograft survival. These determinations awaited a prospective, random-assignment trial.

A trial by Dunn et al. (117) tested the hypothesis that CMV transmission or reactivation began immediately or soon after solid organ transplantation. Their study compared a short-duration Ganciclovir-based regimen to a more prolonged oral Acyclovir-based prophylaxis (800 mg given orally or 400 mg IV q.i.d. for 12 weeks after transplantation or 6 weeks after any antirejection therapy) versus short-duration GCV (5 mg/kg/12 h IV for 7 days after transplant or after any antirejection therapy) plus IVIG (either Sandoglobulin or the CMV HYPERIVIG) at 100 mg/kg IV administered on days 1, 4, and 7 after transplant or after any antirejection therapy. CMV disease occurred in fewer patients (n = 28, 21.0%) in the Acyclovir group, while significantly more patients (n = 42, 31.6%) in the Ganciclovir + IVIG group developed CMV disease. It was not determined whether or not a higher dose of IVIG, 400 mg/kg, may have yielded differing outcomes, although Andolina et al. (118) also conducted studies using IVIG at 100 mg/kg/day within a protocol for GVHD prophylaxis after a mismatched BMT.

Liver Transplantation. CMV HYPERIVIG was tested for the prevention of CMV disease and its complications in patients receiving liver transplants. The study was a randomized, multicenter, placebo-controlled, double-blind trial; 141 patients completed the study (119). CMV HYPERIVIG or placebo (1% albumin) was given in doses of 150 mg/kg body weight within 72 h of the transplant, then at weeks 2, 4, 6, and 8, and at 100 mg/kg at weeks 12 and 16. Patient follow-up was for 1 year post-transplantation. Immunoglobulin alone was found to reduce the rate of severe CMV-associated disease in patients undergoing orthotopic liver transplantation. No effect of CMV HYPERIVIG on CMV donor-positive, recipient-negative liver transplant recipients was shown, which suggested a need for additional prophylactic strategies. Acyclovir, with or without IVIG, did not prevent primary CMV infection or disease in donor-positive recipient-negative solid organ transplant recipients in studies done by Bailey et al. (120). Moreover, most patients were treated with Ganciclovir despite the use of prophylactic treatment. Reappraisal of the role of CMV prophylaxis by Acyclovir and IVIG was recommended.

Anti–*Pseudomonas aeruginosa* HYPERIVIG

Development of a tetravalent *Pseudomonas* immune globulin (PS HYPERIVIG) was described by Collins and Roby (67). Donors whose plasma contained naturally high levels of antibodies (IgG) to lipopolysaccharide antigens immunotypes 1, 2, 4, and 6 of *P. aeruginosa* were identified using a specific ELISA. PS HYPERIVIG was then prepared from Cohn fraction II as previously described (12). Titers of the product were approximately fivefold higher against immunotypes 1, 2, 4, 5, and 6, but only about twofold higher against immuntypes 3 and 7 than standard IVIG. Until the late 1980s, *P. aeruginosa* was a common lethal pathogen in burn patients. Hunt and Purdue reported on the evaluation of this tetravalent hyperimmune *Pseudomonas* globulin G in 10 burn patients with *Pseudomonas* sepsis and eight with bacteremia (68). This preparation is currently licensed for clinical use in Germany under the name Psomaglobin N (Table 2).

Reformulated Hyperimmune IMIGs

Four products, licensed in the U.S. as intramuscular products, were reformulated as IVIG products. They were currently available only in various areas of Europe. Indicated uses were for prevention and/or treatment of hepatitis B, tetanus, varicella zoster, and alloimmunization of Rh_o-negative mothers by an Rh_o fetus (Table 2).

INVESTIGATIONAL HYPERIVIG

Hyperimmune immunoglobulin preparations described in the following sections were outlined in Table 3 (antibacterial) and Table 4 (antiviral).

Streptococcus pneumoniae

An *S. Pneumoniae* hyperimmune IVIG was developed by Hyland Therapeutics in the early 1980s (121). Normal plasma donors were selected and immunized with 14-valent pneumococcal vaccines (Pneumovax or Pnuimmune). Antibody levels against six or 12 serotypes were measured by a quantitative ELISA (122) and a Farr-type radioimmunoassay (RIA), respectively (49). A geometric mean titer of 3.0 was established as the minimum plasma antibody level required to be suitable for fractionation to a high-titer antipneumococcal IVIG. Hyperimmune globulin (PN HYPERIVIG) was prepared and compared to a variety of standard IVIG preparations. Geometric mean titers (GMT) were three- to fivefold higher in PN IVIG than standard IVIG, and 44-fold higher than the FDA preimmunization plasma standard. Complement-dependent opsonization assays showed that the decreases in colony-forming units (CFU) after 2 h for types 3 and 6A were 78% and 95% for PN HYPERIVIG and 35% and 85% for normal IVIG. Passive immunization of mice with PN HYPERIVIG greatly increased the survival of mice following lethal challenge with pneumococcal types 1, 3, or 8. In control mice injected with human serum albumin (HSA), the LD_{50} values were less than 10 CFU for types 1 and 3 and 6×10^2 for type 8. When the pneumococcal hyperimmune globulin was compared to normal IVIG in the same protection model, increases in LD_{50} values of 1000-, 100-, and 10-fold, respectively, for serotypes 1, 3, and 8 were seen. Survival of female Swiss-Webster mice was studied when 10 mg of either HSA, three normal IVIG peparations (different manufacturers), or PN HYPERIVIG was administered IV 18 h prior to intraperitoneal (IP) bacterial challenge (doses between 10^1 and 10^8 CFU). A second set of protection experiments was performed in which Bicillin (100 units per

Table 3 Investigational Human Antibacterial Intravenous Hyperimmune Globulins

Disease	Sponsor	Status
Pseudomonas aeruginosa (mucoexopolysaccharide)	NABI (HyperGAM+CF)	Phase II
Group B *Streptococcus* (GBS)	NABI (NeoGAM)	Unknown
Pseudomonas aeruginosa/ Klebsiella pneumoniae	SSVI (Nosocuman)	Phase II
Escherichia coli	SSVI	Preclinical
Klebsiella pneumoniae	SSVI (KP-IGIV)	Preclinical
Staphylococcus aureus	NABI (Staph GAM)	Preclinical

Table 4 Investigational Human Antiviral Intravenous Hyperimmune Globulins

Disease	Sponsor	Status
Human immunodeficiency virus	NABI (HIV-IG)	Phase III (U.S.)
	Hemacare Corporation (Immupath)	Phase II
	Verigen (PASSHIV-1)	Phase I
Respiratory syncytial virus	MedImmune/Massachusetts (RespiGam, RSVIG, Respivir)	Awaiting licensure
Hepatitis B virus	NABI (H-BIG IV)	Preclinical
Hepatitis C virus	NABI (H-CIG)	Preclinical

mouse) was given IM 30 min postbacterial challenge. The LD_{50} for PN IVIG alone was 10^5 CFU, 10^4 CFU for HSA + Bicillin, and 7×10^6 CFU for combinations of PN HYPERIVIG and Bicillin. Positive synergy was demonstrated and the same combination yielded the greatest degree of protection in animals. These data strongly suggested that PN HYPERIVIG produced from the plasma of immunized donors would be effective in the treatment of infections due to *Streptococcus pneumoniae*. Phase I and II studies using PN HYPERIGIV in patients were completed. Phase III clinical trials were initiated in 13 Veterans Administration Hospitals but were canceled during the second year.

Staphylococcus epidermidis/Staphyloccus aureus

Hyperimmune IVIG products for treatment of gram-positive infections were under development by UNIVAX prior to a recent merger with NABI (formally North American Biologicals, Inc.). Product development was based on a polysaccharide conjugate vaccine for immunization of donors against *S. aureus* capsular types 5 and 8, which reportedly cause 70–80% of *S. aureus* disease. This vaccine was in Phase II clinical trials and was being used for production of a HYPERIVIG that should be available for clinical studies later in 1996. NABI holds the rights to this vaccine, which was licensed from the NIH and developed by Univax. The current developmental status of the vaccine and/or hyperimmune immunoglobulins is unknown.

Lipid emulsions became a standard component of parenteral nutrition in many nurseries. Recent evidence that lipid emulsions limited immunity against bacterial infections (123,124) were consistent with the recent finding that coagulase-negative staphylococcal bacteremia in neonates was associated with lipid emulsion infusions (125). Fischer studied opsonic antibody to *S. epidermidis* in various IVIG preparations in a lipid-emulsion–induced lethal suckling rat model of neonatal *S. epidermidis* sepsis. Levels of opsonic antibody varied between preparations and different lots of the same preparation (31). IVIG containing ≥90% opsonic activity promoted bacterial clearance from blood and significantly enhanced survival when compared to lots with ≤50% opsonic activity. Further, absorption with IVIG removed in vitro opsonic antibody and in vivo protective activity. Since the level of specific antibody was highly variable among preparations (from a low of 3% to a high of 92%), the authors concluded that standard IVIG may not provide therapy effective in preventing *S. epidermidis* infections and that a HYPERIVIG was desirable (126).

Group B Steptococcus

Studies to date have not firmly established the efficacy of standard IVIG for either treatment or prevention of GBS neonatal bacterial infections. A study by Baker et al., however, suggested that treatment of premature infants weighing between 500 and 1750 g at birth with IVIG reduced the risk of nosocomial infection due to coagulase-negative staphylococci (127). However, even at doses of 900 mg/kg, infants under 1000 g at birth often did not sustain target levels of antibody for 2 weeks. Infections in some infants who received IVIG probably resulted from the failure to achieve optimal protective antibody levels. Well-designed, carefully controlled trials were needed to address the issues of appropriate dosage and the variability of the pathogen-specific antibody activity of various products. These questions wer appropriate for both standard IVIG and HYPERIVIG (39,128,129).

In 1986, Fischer and co-workers reported on their hyperimmune GBS HYPERIVIG, which had been prepared in collaboration with the Sandoz Corporation (130). This hyperimmune was prepared by immunization of plasma donors with a GBS vaccine containing the Ia, Ib, II, and III GBS type-specific polysaccharide antigens (24,131). In parallel studies, it was found that GBS HYPERIVIG increased survival of experimental animals when compared to standard IVIG. Survival of suckling rats was 100% versus ≤20% at identical doses for hyperimmune versus standard IVIG. GBS type-specific opsonic activity was ≥ 90% for GBS HYPERIVIG at a 1280-fold dilution versus a 10-fold dilution in standard IVIG. Fischer et al. also demonstrated that GBS HYPERIVIG protected neonatal rhesus monkeys in a GBS sepsis model (39). Using a limited number of strains, Hill and co-workers showed that both a human IgM monoclonal antibody (HuMAb) and GBS HYPERIVIG (51 µg/ml) gave increased protective (neonatal rat model) and opsonic activities at lower total doses of immunoglobulin than did standard IVIG preparations against type III GBS (38). GBS HYPERIVIG had lower concentrations of type II–specific antibody (15 µg/ml) and less protective activity against type II strains at a 20 mg/kg, but not at a 40 mg/kg, dose than the 500 mg/kg dose of IVIG. The highest concentration of type-specific antibody in the GBS hyperimmune immunoglobulin was directed against the type Ia polysaccharide (150 µg/ml). The HuMAb (20 mg/kg) outperformed both polyclonal preparations. The murine monoclonal IgM was one of the most protective agents available against type II GBS strains (132). However, it was specific for the sialic acid–containing type II capsular antigen and offered no cross-protection against type I or II strains.

Trials were initiated to evaluate these preparations in premature infants and neonates (133). Fischer et al. (130) and Weisman (134) tested the GBS HYPERIVIG preparation in 15 neonates with suspected sepsis using doses of 500, 250, or 100 mg/kg of GBS hyperimmune IVIG. Although IVIG did not significantly increase serum GBS type-specific IgG, GBS HYPERIVIG (500 mg/kg) produced a fourfold rise for >6 weeks, with variable increases seen at lower doses (128). These 15 were compared with five who received 500 mg/kg of standard IVIG. The two groups were similar in gestation, birth weight, and age. Hyperimmune GBS IVIG was also prepared following the immunization of donors with a pentavalent GBS type-specific polysaccharide vaccine (135,136). This preparation contained antibodies with opsonophagocytic titers >1:1000 and ELISA titers >1:20,000, and showed efficacy in GBS-infected rats and monkeys. Serum titers were higher after hyperimmune treatment comparing 500 mg/kg standard IVIG to 500 mg/kg GBS HYPERIVIG ($P < .001$). From this study, the authors concluded that GBS HYPERIVIG appeared safe and resulted in significant GBS type-specific activity. It was suggested that phase II efficacy studies were necessary.

Although the potential target population of individuals infected with GBS was small compared to some, i.e., *Pseudomonas* infections, a GBS HYPERIVIG could make a major impact in a niche market. In addition to neonates diagnosed with GBS infections, any newborn developing a sudden fever could be treated prophylactically, since death was possible within 24 h, and before a diagnostic confirmation of GBS infection could be made.

Hepatitis B and C Virus

NABI is developing an intravenous hyperimmune immunoglobulin for the treatment of hepatitis B virus (HBV HYPERIVIG) (137). Preselected individuals were immunized with hepatitis B vaccine. The resulting high-titer plasma was then processed to a final container and designated hepatitis B immune globulin (H-BIG) (137). The product under an IND entered clinical trials in 1996 to prevent hepatitis B in arthrotopic liver transplants. With an IV formulation, significant drug can be given to the patient to neutralize and reduce viral load and protect the transplants against reinfection.

For several years, manufacturers of human plasma products were required by the U.S. FDA to screen and eliminate donors whose plasma contained detectable levels of antibody to HCV. As a consequence of this screening, individuals may be selected for preparation of high-titer HCV immunoglobulin (virus-negative), which might be useful in individuals such as those suffering from chronic HCV disease of the liver. Taking advantage of this requirement, NABI began development of an HCV HYPERIVIG (H-CIG) (137). Initiation of clinical trials using this preparation was scheduled to begin following approval of the investigational new drug (IND) application by the FDA. A primary target indication for this product was for prophylaxis of either primary or recurrent HCV infection in liver transplant patients.

Klebsiella pneumoniae

In 1986, Cryz et al. produced an experimental *K. pneumoniae* hyperimmune IVIG (KP HYPERIVIG) (75). This preparation was made from the sera of donors immunized with a polyvalent vaccine containing capsular polysaccharide (CPS) from serotypes 2, 3, 10, 21, 30 and 55 antigens (138). Plasma was fractionated using a modified Cohn procedure followed by ion exchange chromatography, and the IgG was concentrated and formulated in a final container at 50 mg/ml in a stabilizing solution. The experimental KP HYPERIVIG and seven standard commercial IVIG preparations were compared for antibody levels to capsular polysaccharides as well as opsonic and protective capacity against *Klebsiella*. All but one of the standard IVIGs reacted immunologically with the various capsular antigens, although titers varied considerably among different products. Antibody titers seen for the KP HYPERIVIG ranged from 32- to 128-fold compared to standard IVIG. Only the hyperimmune globulin was capable of promoting the phagocytosis and killing of six *Klebsiella* test strains. When given prophylactically in mice, standard IVIG gave protection against lethal challenge doses of *Klebsiella* only at doses of 500 mg/kg, whereas the hyperimmune IVIG provided similar protection at doses as low as 5 mg/kg. Standard IVIG was ineffective, while the hyperimmune IVIG was highly protective for therapy of sepsis. Combination antibiotic (Gentamicin, 200 μg IV in 0.2 ml/mouse) immunoglobulin therapy was most effective at reducing mortality.

This vaccine proved to be immunogenic and, in a subsequent study the number of CPS was expanded to 24 to be used in the stimulation of donors in combination with a *Pseudomonas* vaccine described in a later section.

Pseudomonas aeruginosa/Klebsiella pneumoniae Combined Product

NABI, Immuno, the Swiss Serum and Vaccine Institute (SSVI), Scotgen, and others began development of hyperimmune immunoglobulin products for the treatment and/ or prophylaxis of *P. aeruginosa* infection. In addition, the SSVI developed a combined anti–*P. aeruginosa* and anti–*K. pneumoniae* product for treatment of multiple infections.

Approximately 2500 plasma donors were immunized with an octavalent *P. aeruginosa* O-polysaccharide toxin A conjugate vaccine developed at the SSVI (139–141) and found to be safe in healthy adults, cystic fibrosis (CF) patients, and bone marrow transplant recipients (142). These same donors were simultaneously immunized with a *Klebsiella* capsular polysaccharide vaccine (SSVI), which consisted of 24 capsular polysaccharide antigens. Geometric mean antibody concentrations and mean fold antibody rises to the 33 vaccine antigens (including toxin A) were similar in the two groups at 2 months, and the declines in antibody measured at 18 months were also similar (140). Selected donor plasma was pooled, and a hyperimmune intravenous immunoglobulin was produced (PA/KP HYPERIVIG) (143). This hyperimmune IVIG was reported to contain significantly high anti-lipopolysaccharide and anti–toxin A antibody titers, which displayed markedly enhanced opsonic activity and in vivo protective activity compared to standard IVIG. In addition, substantially higher IgG antibody levels to all nine *Pseudomonas* vaccine antigens and to 22 of 24 *Klebsiella* antigens were seen compared to standard IVIG (144). The hyperimmune was more effective in opsonophagocytic assays and neutralized >20 times more toxin A than commercial IVIG. Only the hyperimmune IVIG gave significant protection against *Klebsiella* K2 sepsis and against six of the eight *P. aeruginosa* vaccine serotypes when compared with normal IVIG in a murine burn model of sepsis.

PA/KP HYPERIVIG (Nosocumen, produced by SSVI has now undergone Phase I studies. Results were encouraging, and a definite antibody effect for *Klebsiella* was measured, although higher doses may be required for efficacy in *Pseudomonas* disease. Further, Phase II studies leading to Phase III trials were initiated (145). Nosocumen has a large potential for use in surgery and transplantation and is currently undergoing evaluation in clinical trials for evaluation of efficacy in treatment of infections in the intensive care unit.

Pseudomonas aeruginosa

Lipopolysaccharides (LPS) of virulent smooth strains of *P. aeruginosa* were composed of O-specific polysaccharide antigens which confer immunotype specificity. Also present in LPS were neutral polysaccharide components that expressed antigenic determinants common to many clinical isolates. Hatano et al. demonstrated that antibodies specific to neutral polysaccharides were opsonic for poorly virulent, nonmucoid LPS rough isolates, but offered no protection from challenge with low doses of virulent LPS smooth strains of *P. aeruginosa* at doses of < 103 CFU/mouse (146). On the other hand, antibodies to neutral polysaccharides deposited more complement factor 3 (C3), required for opsonization, onto LPS rough strains than did antibodies to O side chains. Less binding of C3 resulted when isogenic LPS smooth strains were tested. From these data, it appeared that antibodies specific to neutral polysaccharide antigens were not protective against *P. aeruginosa* infection due to inhibition of opsonic killing activity by both O side-chain antigens and the mucoexopolysaccharide antigens of mucoid bacterial forms. Therefore, these antigens were poor candidates as potential components of a *P. aeruginosa* vaccine (146). In contrast, opsonic killing of mucoid *P. aeruginosa* strains, mediated by antibodies specific for MEP (alginate), was shown to be the principal immune effector associated with human (147) and animal (148,149) resistance to chronic lung infection by these organisms. In chronically infected CF patients, nutritional conditions within the microenvironment favored the deflagellation of pseudomonads with resultant conversion to the MEP-secreting mucoid form.

Bacterial colonization of the lungs of CF patients was almost exclusively due to *P. aeruginosa*. Once chronic colonization occurred, the pseudomonads existed primarily in a nonflagellated mucoid form against which therapeutic treatment was mostly unsuccessful. NABI prepared a polyclonal human hyperimmune IVIG from the plasma of donors immunized with a mucoid exopolysaccharide MEP vaccine developed by Pier. This new hyperimmune IVIG was designed for the prevention and treatment of chronic *Pseudomonas* infections in CF patients (147) and is currently undergoing evaluation in Phase II trials in both the U.S. and Europe, using a total of 170 patients (137,150).

In preclinical studies using mice, Collins et al. evaluated a cocktail of five human monoclonal IgM antibodies in burn and pneumonia models with the results suggesting that the monoclonal preparation might be an important adjunct to antimicrobial therapy of life-threatening *P. aeruginosa* infections (151). These studies were extended by Collins et al. using a preparation which included the previously described five human monoclonal IgM antibodies (151) plus a human IgG1 that had exotoxin A–neutralizing activity (31). Studied were 12 noninfected patients and eight patients with either *P. aeruginosa* bacteremia, pneumonia, or both. Patients were evaluated using intravenously administered doses which ranged from 0.3 to 1.2 ml/kg (0.75–3.0 mg/kg IgM protein). After a single infusion of 1.2 ml/kg (3.0 mg/kg IgM protein), serum antibody titers were boosted into the therapeutic range, with serum half-lives ranging from 34 to 99 h. Serum opsonophagocytic activity increased more than 10-fold for all but one antibody. Finally, no patient immunological responses against the MAb preparation were observed. Commercialization of this MAb cocktail was discontinued due to changing priorities within the company.

Escherichia coli

A number of studies have evaluated the potential for the development of hyperimmune IVIGs which contain protective and opsonic antibodies to *E. coli* (152–154). In an initial study, an *E. coli* K1 018 polysaccharide–toxin A conjugate vaccine was developed at the SSVI (155,156). Following the immunization of rabbits, estimates of protective levels of anti-O-specific lipopolysaccharide (LPS) immunoglobulin IgG against bacteremia and death were determined. Passive transfer of immunized rabbit serum was found to confer significant protection from a lethal *E. coli* infection in a neonatal rat model. The overall incidence of bacteremia and mortality was 4% in rat pups receiving undiluted post vaccination serum, while that in control animals was 100% ($P < .001$). Rates of 5% and 72% (bacteremia) and mortality (0% and 72%) were seen for IgG levels greater than 1.0 and less than 1.0 μg/ml, respectively. These results suggested that IgG levels >1.0 μg/ml achieved following administration of a hyperimmune IVIG provided protection against bacteremia and death caused by a homologous *E. coli* K1 infection. As a result, a more complex 12-valent vaccine, which consisted of 12 O-polysaccharide–toxin A conjugates, was designed and formulated. Passive transfer of immune rabbit serum to mice conferred statistically significant ($P < .05$) protection against challenge with nine of the 12 vaccine serotypes. Cryz et al. (156) and Cross et al. (157) produced a hyperimmune IGIV (EC HYPERIVIG) against the K1 O18 strain which gave protection versus lethal challenge in a rat model.

More recently, Cross et al. evaluated a polyvalent *E. coli* vaccine in humans (157). Based on the fact that a limited number of O serogroups account for nearly 70% of bacteremic and meningitic *E. coli* isolates, the vaccine was prepared by formulation of conjugates of O polysaccharides coupled to exotoxin A that represented 12 serogroups of *E. coli* (O1, O2, O4, O6–O8, O12, O15, O16, O18, O25, and O75). Fourfold or greater increases in ELISA antibody levels over baseline were greatest ($>60\%$ of vaccines) for O1, O2, O6–O8, and O15; intermediate ($\sim 50\%$) for O18 and O75; and poorest ($\leq 45\%$) for O4, O12, O16, and O25. Opsonic antibody titers generally paralleled ELISA antibody responses. In addition to the potential use for active immunization, this *E. coli* vaccine would ultimately be combined with existing *Klebsiella* and *Pseudomonas* vaccines in order that a broadly protective, multispecific hyperimmune IVIG(EC/PA/KP HYPERIVIG) might be produced (139–141,144).

Human Immunodeficiency Virus

At least three HIV hyperimmune immunoglobulin preparations (HIV HYPERIVIG) have been evaluated in humans, in animal, and in in vitro studies. Perhaps only one or two are still in development for commercialization. Studies presented here were restricted to HIV HYPERIVIG preparations or high-titer HIV-seropositive plasma.

A 1992 study of passive immunization was done by Osther et al. (Verigen, Inc.) using porcine hyperimmune immunoglobulin (PASSHIV-1) against HIV-1 (158). PASSHIV-1 was used to treat 14 HIV-1 infected individuals for 5–7 days. Two of the 14 patients were retreated for an additional 5 days at 3 months in order to evaluate side effects from retreatment with procine immunoglobulins. Ten patients had no side effects, while three experienced transient urticarial eruptions which responded to antihistamine administration. One patient, who received concomitant standard IVIG, experienced a type 3 hypersensitivity reaction. All patients demonstrated a significant improvement for fatique, weight gain, fever, polyneuropathy, bronchitis candidiasis, diarrhea, and dermatitis. One of five with Kaposi's sarcoma showed improvement. This therapy was well tolerated by HIV-1-infected individuals and appeared to be efficacious in the amelioration of a variety of the clinical symptoms associated with HIV-1 disease.

Key to the efficacy of HIV HYPERIVIG in HIV-positive or AIDS patients may be the requirement that HIV immunoglobulins be delivered to intracellular spaces (site of viral replication) for inhibition of viral replication. An interesting approach to test this hypothesis was done in a recent UCLA study. Both HIVIG and standard IVIG were cationized with hexamethylenediamine to an isoelectric point >9.5 prior to use. Padridge and co-workers then tested cationized forms of IVIG for enhanced absorptive-mediated endocytosis into cells for inhibition of HIV replication (159). This process was found to markedly increase the binding and endocytosis of both HIV HYPERIVIG and IVIG by human peripheral blood lymphocytes (PBL). Levels of 250 μg IgG/ml HIV HYPERIVIG resulted in a 90% inhibition in the amount of p24 released to the medium in HIV-1-infected human PBL.

The efficacy of a HIV HYPERIVIG for prevention of HIV infection in chimpanzees was evaluated by Prince et al. (160). Whereas in previous experiments no protection had been observed when relatively high challenge doses (100 chimpanzee infectious doses) were used (161), the current study showed that HIV HYPERIVIG protected against a challenge dose (10 CID50) 10-fold lower than that used previously (162). Protected animals remained free of HIV infection for up to 1 year as determined by cocultivation and polymerase chain reaction, and did not mount a detectable primary immune response. These results provided an experimental rationale to conduct clinical trials to evaluate prevention of maternal-infant vertical transmission of HIV.

Initial steps for commercial development of HIV HYPERIVIG addressed potential safety issues (163). Methods for the safe fractionation of plasma donated from HIV+ individuals previously developed were utilized (164). Before fractionation, plasma pools were treated with 1% tri-N-butyl phosphate and 1% Tween-80 followed by heating for 4 h at 30 °C for inactivation of HIV and other lipid envelope viruses. The crude IgG (fraction II precipitate) paste was further purified using QAE-50 Sephadex that yielded pure monomeric unfragmented and undenatured human IgG (165). All four IgG subclasses were represented in the preparation, but, interestingly, the HIV HYPERIVIG had a lower percentage of IgG2 and a higher content of IgG1 than standard IVIG. Cummins and collaborators, using these methods, prepared an intravenous solution of 99% pure globulin (HIV HYPERIVIG) from the pooled plasma of selected HIV-1-seropositive, clinically healthy, asymptomatic donors (166). Acceptable donors were those with > 400 CD4+ cells/ml and a high titer of antibodies (>1:128) to HIV-1 p24 protein. Also present in these plasmas were high titers of antibodies to gp41, gp120 (group-specific neutralizing domain), and the gp120 hypervariable region. Donated sera were also required to be HIV Ag, HBsAg, and anti-CMV negative. Over an 18-month period, of 246 asymptomatic HIV-seropositive donors who were screened 39 had an anti-p24 antibody titer >1:128, and all but four had a CD4+ cell count >400/μl. Overall, 14.2% of seropositive donors tested met the selection criteria for inclusion in plasma pools for preparation of HIV HYPERIVIG. Donors were found to maintain stable antibody titers over a period of 6–28 months with a 1.0% decrease in CD4+ cells per month. Validation of these safety methods was assessed by infusion of 1 g/kg administered to chimpanzees and was found to not transmit HIV as measured by several critiera including polymerase chain reaction. The mean half-life for p24 antibody was 15 days.

Anti-HIV antibody activities were measured in virus neutralization assays versus HIV strains MN and III-B, for binding to V3 loop peptides by ELISA, for antibody-dependent cellular cytotoxicity (ADCC), and for their ability to inhibit syncytia formation. Inhibition of syncytia formation occurred at antibody concentrations between 375 and 1800 μg/ml IgG; ADCC activity occurred at 2.5–250 μg/ml, inhibition of cytopathic effects in T cells occurred at 500 μg/ml; and inhibition of in vitro HIV replication occurred at 50–500 μg/mL. Interestingly, these data indicated that HIVIG was less efficient than cationized IgG at inhibition of syncytial formation (159). Assuming a two-compartment distribution, plasma IgG concentrations from a 20 mg/kg dose would provide a HIVIG plasma level of 2085 µg/mL. At an average 15-day $T_{1/2}$ (actual range of 11–19 days) and monthly dosage, IgG levels > 1000 µg/ml could be maintained over time.

NABI has an HIV HYPERIVIG product in development. This product, HIV-IG, was manufactured according to the above described methodology. This preparation is currently undergoing evaluation in Phase III clinical trials for the prevention of HIV vertical transmission in HIV+ pregnant women (137). Other planned studies include evaluation for the prevention of infection in infants at a single non-U.S. site by treating just the neonate for prevention of HIV vertical transmission. An additional study evaluated the HIV HYPERIVIG for treatment of HIV+ children (137).

A randomized study that evaluated the safety and short-term efficacy of serial transfusion of HIV-1-seropositive plasma in 18 patients was conducted by Vittecoq et al. (167). Heat-inactivated, anti-HIV, antibody-rich plasma was compared with seronegative fresh-frozen, antibody-negative plasma given in addition to zidovudine and other conventional prophylactic treatments. A total of seven transfusions at 2-week intervals of immune plasma significantly reduced (2 vs. 8, $P = .06$) the number of opportunistic infections, and antigenemia became undetectable. When transfusions were stopped, positive p24 antigenemia returned at a level higher than that seen prior to treatment and was correlated with a severe clinical deterioration, suggesting a rebound effect. This trial also supported the contention that passive immunotherapy was a promising treatment for AIDS. Also confirmed was the apparent lack of effect of plasma donation upon donors' CD4 count over a 1-year period. In patients with severe immunodeficiency, this study also indicated that special attention should be paid to withdrawal of an effective HIVIG therapy, since virologic relapse may be explosive and poorly tolerated.

Additional impetus for continued development of HIV HYPERIVIG products (Immupath) was based on a study by Levy and co-workers (Hemacare). Their data showed a reduction in the circulating HIV viral burden and potential efficacy in previous small uncontrolled patients studies, which warranted initiation of a larger controlled study of passive hyperimmune therapy in persons with AIDS (168). A total of 220 AIDS subjects were randomized to receive monthly infusions of 500 ml plasma (full dose), 250 ml plasma diluted in 250 ml of 5% human serum albumin (half dose), or 500 ml of 5% human serum albumin (placebo). Positive benefits were seen only in the full-dose group with baseline CD4 cell counts between 50 and 200 cells/mm^3. Reduced mortality was seen with one death in 21 (full dose) versus three deaths in 21 (half dose) and six deaths in 30 (placebo). Also, CD4 counts improved an average of 32.7 cells/mm^3 in the high-dose group, compared to a study by Mofenson et al. that showed that 400 mg/kg standard IVIG every 28 days was only able to slow the decline of CD4+ cells by 13.5 cells/mm^3/month compared to placebo (169). However, the same dose of standard IVIG was found to be effective in reduction of both serious and minor viral and bacterial infections in children with study entry level CD4+ counts of at least 0.20 × 10^3/L (170).

Respiratory Syncytial Virus

Effective prevention of RSV infections had proven elusive, and no effective preventive drugs were currently approved. Studies in animals and humans had shown that the lower respiratory tract can be protected from RSV infection by sufficient circulating RSV-neutralizing antibody levels (171). Early studies using standard IVIG for use in

RSV disease gave unreliable results due to the low and variable levels of their specific anti-RSV antibody contents. However, some decreased severity of RSV disease was seen using standard IVIG in a randomized, controlled trial (RSV-neutralizing antibody titer of 1:950 in 5% solution) over two RSV seasons (172). The nasopharyngeal aspirates of 82 infants less than 12 months of age and hospitalized for acute lower respiratory tract disease were analyzed to determine the distribution of RSV subtypes (173). Subtype A predominated over subtype B, 19 versus 2. While patients with pneumonia had subtype A, both subtypes were found in infants with bronchitis and bronchiolitis. In that study, Tirado et al. concluded that in spite of currently available antiviral therapy for RSV infections (173), and, while it is reasonable to assume that a vaccine for RSV will eventually be licensed (175), new adjunctive therapy was necessary for the treatment of acute cases. In contrast, a study by McIntosh and co-workers showed that, in 444 infants and children, the difference in rates of infection between group A and group B was only 6% (176). Since IVIG at doses up to 750 mg/kg body weight was found to be safe and feasible and to have some beneficial effect in high-risk infants (177), it was thought that an RSV-specific hyperimmune globulin might be useful for both therapy and prophylaxis.

To be clinically *effective*, an RSV HYPERIVIG must contain high titers of the appropriate antibodies. Choice of an appropriate assay for the selection of high-titer plasma donors was therefore critical. Seven different RSV antibody assays were compared in an attempt to identify suitable donors for preparation of plasma pools (178). This plasma contained elevated levels of RSV-neutralizing IgG which would show protection and increased survival in animal models. Of the seven assays, plasma units identified using an RSV microneutralization yielded IgG with the most significant protection in mice against RSV challenge. Three direct ELISAs used purified F protein, G protein, or RSV-infected cell lysate; two competitive ELISAs versus RSV-neutralizing monoclonal antibodies directed to the F2 or F3 epitopes of the F protein; and a plaque reduction neutralization were determined to be unsuitable. Relative to standard IVIG, IVIG prepared from microneutralization-screened plasma was increased fivefold by plaque reduction neutralization assays done with or without complement. It was concluded that the microneutralization assay was the method of choice for identifying plasma donors for preparation of a human hyperimmune globulin with high protective activity against RSV and deserved further evaluation for the prediction of protective antibody concentrations in children.

Estimates of the levels of anti-RSV antibody (RSVIG) for protection were determined in the immunoprophylactic cotton rat model (179). In a recent study, animals were pretreated by intraperitoneal injection of RSVIG with moderate (1:2226) or high (1:15,000) neutralizing antibody titers to RSV (day 0), challenged intranasally with RSV Long at doses ranging from 10^1 to 10^5 plaque-forming units (pfu; day 1) and sacrificed for virus titration (day 5). Moderate titer RSVIG effected complete or near complete nasal protection against low to moderate (10^1–10^3 pfu) RSV challenge doses and a significant reduction in nasal RSV titers at high (10^4–10^5) pfu challenge doses. Pretreatment with high-titer immunoglobulin gave significant or highly significant reductions in nasal RSV titers at challenge doses of 10^4 and 10^5 pfu, respectively. Levels of circulating protective antibodies required have been confirmed in both new animal studies and in human epidemiological studies (180–184). Such levels were variously estimated to be between 1:300 and 1:400 plaque reduction neutralization titers.

An IVIG preparation with a high titer of antibodies against respiratory syncytial virus could offer protection for infants and young children at risk for RSV infection due to cardiac disease or prematurity. Recently, MedImmune has developed and studied an RSV HYPERIVIG in a 3-year multicenter trial to determine safety and efficacy in the prevention of severe RSV disease in children at high risk for severe RSV illness (83,185). Groothius and co-workers (83) studied 249 at-risk infants and young children who had bronchopulmonary dysplasia due to prematurity (n = 102), congenital heart disease (n = 87), or prematurity without complications (n = 60). Patients were randomly placed in high-dose (750 mg/kg, n = 81) or low-dose (150 mg/kg, n = 79) groups or control for no use of immunoglobulin. There were a total of 64 episodes of repiratory syncytial virus infection: 19 in the high-dose group, 16 in the low-dose group, and 29 in the control group. In the high-dose group there were fewer lower RSV tract infections (7, vs. 20 in the control group; $P = .01$), fewer hospitalizations (6, vs. 18 in the control group; $P = .02$), fewer hospital days (43, vs. 128 in the control group; $P = .02$), fewer days in the intensive care unit ($P = .03$), and less use of ribavirin ($P = .05$). In the low-dose group there was a significant reduction only in the number of days in the intensive care unit ($P = .03$). Although a total of six children died—three in the high-dose group, three in the low-dose group, and none in the control group ($P = .15$)—no death was attributed to the use of immunoglobulin or to RSV infection. Further, treated children did not acquire exaggerated RSV illness in the subsequent year. Thus, high-dose RSVIG reduced the incidence and severity of RSV lower respiratory tract infection and was deemed a safe and effective means of RSV prophylaxis in selected high-risk children.

Although the results of this trial were deemed successful (186), the U.S. FDA elected to not license the RSV immunoglobulin in 1994 (187). A repeat of trials comparing two populations of infants stratified by age was conducted during the RSV 1994–1995 season. On December 15, 1995, members of the Blood Products Advisory Committee of the FDA voted to recommend RSV HYPERIVIG (RSV IGIV) for licensure for prevention of RSV disease in children under 24 months with bronchopulmonary dysplasia (chronic lung disease) or a history of premature birth. This product will be marketed in the U.S. under the trade name RespiGam™.

SUMMARY

Treatment of acute and chronic infectious diseases, most of which are nosocomially acquired, continues to be a great medical challenge. Bacteria such as *S. aureus* and *S. epidermidis* are becoming resistant to the last drug to which they are susceptible, vancomycin. Diseases due to other significant bacterial pathogens, i.e., *P. aeruginosa* and *S. pneumoniae*, are more difficult to treat due to the development of antibiotic-resistant strains. Disease due to relatively common viruses such as CMV and RSV remain difficult to treat in the acute phases due to only partial effectiveness of current antiviral therapy. The efficacy of hyperimmune CMV IVIG may be limited to prevention of primary CMV disease in seronegative recipients of seropositive organ transplants. Licensure of RSV IGIV (MedImmune) has been pending completion of post–Phase III clinical trials in order to demonstrate unequivocal benefit to RSV-infected premature and young infants. FDA approval is now expected during 1996.

A large number of hyperimmune globulin products remain under active or pending development. NABI is aggressively pursuing development of a number of products—HIV-IG, H-BIG IV, H-CIG, PSIVIG, and vaccine-stimulated hyperimmunes—for *S. aureus* and *S. epidermidis*. The SSVI is testing a *Pseudomonas-Klebsiella* hyperimmune IVIG (Nosocumen). Eventually, they plan to include E. coli for formation of a three-organism multivalent product. Certain new viruses such as hepatitis D (HDV), E (HEV), and G (HGV) pose relatively unknown risks for infection. Development of a vaccine for HEV is already under way.

Development of hyperimmune immunoglobulin products requires considerable investments of money and time from large commercial companies. During the last 10–15 years, a number of potential products have come, gone, come, and gone again as company priorities and the marketplace change. Efficacious hyperimmune products offer one of the best opportunities for prophylaxis and therapy in combination with antibiotics and antivirals. Only time will decide if these treatments will ultimately become availabel to the clinician.

ACKNOWLEDGMENTS

The authors would like to acknowledge Dr. Christine V. Sapan (NABI) and Dr. Gerry Fischer (Henry M. Jackson Foundation) for their contributions.

REFERENCES

1. Wedgwood RJ, and Riese GR. Touching a cure of an inverterate phrensy by the transfusion of blood. N Engl J Med 1953; 248:902–904.
2. von Behring E, Kitasato S. Uber das zustandekommen der dephtherie-immunitat und der tetanus-immunitat bei theiren. Dtsch Med Wochensch 1890; 16:1113–1114.
3. Hericourt J, Richet C. Sur une microbe pyogene et septique (*Staphylococcus pyosepticus*) et sur la vaccination contre ses effets. C R Acad Sci 1888; 107:690–694.
4. Ehrlich P. Experimentelle untersuchungen uber immunitat: I. Uberabrin. Dtsch Med Wochensch 1891; 17:976–979.
5. Ehrlich P. Experimentelle untersuchungen uber immunitat: II. Uberabrin. Dtsch Med Wochensch 1891; 17:1218–1219.
6. Eibl MM, Wedgwood RJ. Intravenous immunoglobulin: a review. Immunodefic Rev 1989; suppl 1:1–42.
7. Calmette A. Sur la toxicite dusang de cobra capel: L'immunisation artiicielle des animaux contre le venindes serpents et al therapeutique experimentale des morsures venimeuses: au sujet de l'immunisation des animaux contre l'envenimation. C R Soc Biol 1894; 45:204–205.
8. Cenci F. Alcune esperienze di sieroimmunizzazione e sieroterapia nel morbillo. Riv Clin Pediatr 1907; 6:1017–1025.
9. Anicolle C, Conseil E. Pouvoir preventif duserum d'un malade convalescent de rougeole. Bull Mem Soc Med Hopitaux Paris 1918; 42:336–338.
10. Good RA, Lorenz E. Historic aspects of intravenous immunoglobulin therapy. Cancer 1991; 68:1415–1421.
11. Cohn EJ. Blood proteins and their therapeutic value. Science 1945; 101:51–56.

12. Cohn EJ. The history of plasma fractionation. In: Andrus EC et al. eds. Advances in Military Medicine, Vol. 1. Boston: Little, Brown, 1948:364–443.

13. Cohn EJ et al. Preparation and properties of serum and plasma proteins. J Am Chem Soc 1940; 62:3396–3400.

14. Tselius A. A new apparatus for electrophoretic analysis of colloidal mixtures. Trans Faraday Soc 1937; 33:524–531.

15. Tiselius A, Kaat EA. Electrophoresis of immune serum. Science 1938; 87:416–417.

16. Lerman Y et al. Efficacy of different doses of immune serum globulin in the prevention of hepatitis A: a three-year prospective study. Clin Infect Dis 1993; 17(3):411–414.

17. de Man RA et al. Long-term application of human polyclonal hepatitis-B immunoglobulin to prevent hepatic allograft infection. A review of the literature and presentation of five cases. Neth J Med 1993; 43(1–2):74–82.

18. Palmovic D, Crnjakovic-Palmovic J. Prevention of hepatitis B virus (HBV) infection in health-care workers after accidental exposure: a comparison of two prophylactic schedules. Infection 1993; 21(1):42–45.

19. Siber GR et al. Evaluation of bacterial polysaccharide immune globulin for the treatment or prevention of *Haemophilus influenzae* type b and pneumococcal disease. J Infect Dis 1992; 165(suppl 1):S129–133.

20. Singleton RJ et al. Decline of *Haemophilus influenzae* type b disease in a region of high risk: impact of passive and active immunization. Pediatr Infect Dis J 1994; 13(5):362–367.

21. Shuring PA et al. Bacterial polysaccharide immune globulin for prophylaxis of acute otitis media in high-risk children. J Pediatr 1993; 123:801–810.

22. Barandun S et al. Intravenous administration of human gammaglobulin. Vox Sang 1962; 7:157–174.

23. Smith GN et al. Uptake of IgG after intramuscular and subcutaneous injection. Lancet 1972; 2:1208–1212.

24. Fischer GW et al. Intravenous immunoglobulin in the treatment of neonatal sepsis: therapeutic strategies and laboratory studies. Pediatr Infect Dis J 1986; (suppl):S171–S175.

25. Weisman LE et al. Standard versus hyperimmune intravenous immunoglobulin in preventing or treating neonatal bacterial infections. Clin Perinatol 1993; 20(1):211–224.

26. Sullivan KM et al. Immunomodulatory and antimicrobial efficacy of intravenous immunoglobulin in bone marrow transplantation. N Engl J Med 1990; 323:705–712.

27. ASM News. Are We Reentering the Preantibiotic Era? ASM News 1993; 59(12):384.

28. Morbidity Mortality Weekly Reports. Introduction MMWR 1993; 42(14):257.

29. Fischer G. Personal communication.

30. CDC BRIEFS. Antibiotic resistant pneumococci. Curr Issues Prev Health 1993; 4(8):2.

31. Fischer GW. Opsonic antibodies to *Staphyloccus epidermidis*: in vitro and in vivo studies using human intravenous immune globulin. J Infect Dis 1994; 169:324–329.

32. Shapiro R et al. Serum complement and immunoglobulin values in small-for-gestational-age infants J Pediatr. 1981; 99:139–141.

33. Miller ME. Host Defenses in the Human Neonate. New York: Grune and Stratton, 1978.

34. Fleer A et al. Opsonic defense to *Staphylococcus epidermidis* in the premature neonate. J Infect Dis 1985; 152:930–937.

35. Marques MB et al. Functional activity of antibodies to the group B polysaccharide of group B streptococci elicited by a polysaccharide-protein conjugate vaccine. Infect Immun 1994; 62(5):1539–1539.

36. Zangwill KM et al. Group B streptococcal disease in the United States, 1990: report from a multistate active surveillance system. 1992; 41(SS-6):25–32.

37. Gibson RL et al. Group B streptococci (GBS) injure lung endothelium in vitro: GBS invasion and GBS-induced eicosanoid production is greater with microvascular than with pulmonary artery cells. Infect Immun 1995; 63(1):271–279.

38. Hill HR et al. Comparative protective activity of human monoclonal and hyperimmune polyclonal antibody against group B streptococci. J Infect Dis 1991; 163:792–798.

39. Fischer GW et al. Directed immune globulin for the prevention or treatment of neonatal group B streptococcal infections. Clin Immunol Immunopathol 1992; 62(1 Pt 2):S92–S97.

40. Stewardson-Kreiger PB et al. Perinatal immunity to group B streptococcus type Ia. J Infect Dis 1977; 136:649–654.

41. Fischer GW et al. Demonstration of opsonic activity and in vivo protection against group B streptococci type III by *Streptococcus pneumoniae* type 14 antisera. J Exp Med 1978; 148:776–786.

42. Dancis J et al. Placental transfer of proteins in human gestation. Am J Obstet Gynecol 1961; 82:167–171.

43. Ballow M et al. Development of the immune system in very low birth weight (less than 1500 g) premature infants: concentrations of plasma immunoglobulins and patterns of infections. Pediatr Res 1986; 20:899–904.

44. Klesius PH et al. Cellular and humoral response to group B streptococci. J Pediatr 1973; 83:437–443.

45. Baker CJ, Kasper DL. Correlation of maternal antibody deficiency with susceptibility to neonatal group B streptococcal infection. N Engl J Med 1976; 294:753–756.

46. Hemming VG et al. Assessment of group B streptococcal opsonins in human and rabbit serum by neutrophil chemiluminescence. J Clin Invest 1976; 58:1379–1387.

47. Paoletti LC et al. Neonatal mouse protection against infection with multiple group B streptococcal (GBS) serotypes by maternal immunization with a tetravalent GBS polysaccharide-tetanus toxoid conjugate vaccine. Infect Immun 1994; 62(8):3236–3243.

48. Siber GR. Pneumococcal disease: prospects for a new generation of vaccines. Science 1994; 265:1385–1387.

49. Schiffman G et al. J Immunol Methods 1980; 33:133–144.

50. Baltimore RS. New challenges in the development of a conjugate pneumococcal vaccine. JAMA 1992; 268(23):3366–3367.

51. Shapiro ED et al. The protective efficacy of polyvlent pneumococcal polysaccharide vaccine. N Engl J Med 1991; 325:1453–1460.

52. Robbins JB, Schneerson R. Polysaccharide-protein conjugates: a new generation of vaccines. Rev Infect Dis 1990; 161:821–832.

53. Eskola J et al. Epidemiology of invasive pneumococcal infections in children in Finland. JAMA 1992; 268:3323–3327.

54. Dagan R et al. Epidemiology of invasive childhood pneumococcal infections in Israel. JAMA 1992; 268:3328–3332.

55. Baltimore RS, Shapiro ED. In: Evan AS, Brachman PS, eds. Bacterial Infectsion of Humans: Epidemiology and Control. 2nd ed. New York: Plenum Publishing, 1991:525–546.

56. Mufson MA. Pneumococcal infections. JAMA 1981;246:1942–1948.

57. Austrian R. Tracking the identity of Lister's pneumococcal groups T and V (Danish types 45 and 465). Yale J Biol Med 1982; 55:173–178.

58. Artenstein AW, Cross AS. Serious infections caused by *Pseudomonas aeruginosa*. J Intens Care Med 1994; 9(1):34–51.

59. Rogers DE. The changing pattern of life-threatening microbial disease. N Engl J Med 1959; 261:677–683.

60. Finland M, et al. Occurrence of serious bacterial infections since the introduction of antibacterial agents. JAMA 1959; 170:2188–2197.

61. Finland M. Changing patterns of susceptibility of common bacterial pathogens to antimicrobial agents. Ann Intern Med 1972; 76:1009–1036.

62. Schaberg DR et al. Major trends in the microbial etiology of nosocomial infection. Am J Med 1991; 91(suppl 3B):72S–75S.

63. Weinstein RA. Epidemiology and control of nosocomial infections in adult intensive care units. Am J Med 1991; 91(suppl 3B):179S–184S.

64. Rolston KVI, Bodey GP. *Pseudomonas aeruginosa* infection in cancer patients. Cancer Invest 1992; 10(1):43–59.

65. Whitecar JP et al. *Pseudomonas* bacteremia in patients with malignant diseases. Am J Med Sci 1970; 260:216–223.

66. Hatano K et al. Biologic activities of antibodies to the neutral-polysaccharide component of the *Pseudomonas aeruginosa* lipopolysaccharide are blocked by O side chains and mucoid exopolysaccharide (alginate). Infect Immun 1995; 63(1):21–26.

67. Collins MS, Roby RE. Protective activity of an intravenous immune globulin (human) enriched in antibody against lipopolysaccharide antigens of *Pseudomonas aeruginosa*. Am J Med 1984; 76:168–174.

68. Hunt JL, Purdue GF. A clinical trial of IV tetravalent hyperimmune *Pseudomonas* globulin G in burned patients. J Trauma 1988; 28(2):146–151.

69. Bodey GP et al. *Klebsiella* bacteremia. A 10-year review in a cancer institution. Cancer 1989; 64:2368–2376.

70. Carpenter JL. *Klebsiella* pulmonary infections: occurrence at one medical center and review. Rev Infect Dis 1990; 12:672–682.

71. Feldman C et al. *Klebsiella pneumoniae* bacteraemia at an urban general hospital. J Infect 1990; 20:21–31.

72. Held TK et al. Monoclonal antibody against *Klebsiella* capsular polysaccharide reduces severity and prevents hematogenic spread of experimental *Klebsiella pneumoniae* pneumonia. Infect Immun 1992; 60:1771–1778.

73. Lang AB et al. Human monoclonal antibodies specific for capsular polysaccharides of *Klebsiella* recognize clusters of multiple serotypes. J Immunol 1991; 146:3160–3164.

74. Cryz SJ Jr et al. Safety and immunogenicity of *Klebsiella pneumoniae* K1 capsular polysaccharide vaccine in humans. J Infect Dis 1985; 151:665–671.

75. Cryz SJ Jr et al. Activity of intravenous immune globulins against *Klebsiella*. J Lab Clin Med 1986; 108:182–189.

76. Groothuis JR et al. Safety and bioequivalency of three formulations of respiratory synctial virus-enriched immunoglobulin. Antimicrob Agents Chemother 1995; 39(3):668–671.

77. Glezen WP et al. Risk of primary infection and reinfection with respiratory syncytial virus. Am J Dis Child 1988; 140:543.

78. Cunningham CK et al. Rehospitalization for respiratory illness in infants of less than 32 weeks gestation. Pediatrics 1991; 88:527–532.

79. Groothuis JR et al. Respiratory syncytial virus infection in children with bronchopulmonary dysplasia. Am J Dis Child 1988; 140:153–156.

80. King JC Jr et al. Respiratory syncytial virus illnesses in human immunodeficiency virus and non-infected children. Pediatr Infect Dis J 1993; 12(9):733–739.

81. Levin JJ. Treatment and prevention options for respiratory syncytial virus infections. J Pediatr 1994; 124(5 Pt 2):S22–S27.

82. Meyers JD et al. Cytomegalovirus excretion as a predictor of cytomegalovirus disease after marrow transplantation. J Infect Dis 1990; 162:373–380.

83. Groothuis JR et al. Prophylactic administration of respiratory syncytial virus immune globulin to high-risk infants and young children. The Respiratory Syncytial Virus Immune Globulin Study Group. N Engl J Med 1993; 329(21):1524–1530.

84. Cohen J. Bumps on the vaccine road. Science 1994; 265:1371–1373.

85. Gao F et al. Enhancement in the safety of immune globulins prepared from high-risk plasma. Vox Sang 1993; 64(4):204–209.

86. Yap PL et al. Use of intravenous immunoglobulin in acquired immune deficiency syndrome. Cancer 1991; 68(6 suppl):1440–1450.

87. Mofenson LM, Burns DN. Passive immunization to prevent mother-infant transmission of human immunodeficiency virus. Pediatr Infect Dis J 1991; 10(6):456–462.

88. Guglielmo BJ. Immune globulin therapy in allogeneic bone marrow transplant: a critical review. Bone Marrow Transplant 1994; 13(5):499–510.

89. Bowden RA et al. Cytomegalovirus immune globulin and seronegative blood products to prevent primary cytomegalovirus infection after marrow transplantation. N Engl J Med 1986; 314:1006–1010.

90. Miller WJ et al. Prevention of CMV infection following bone marrow transplantation: a randomized trial of blood product screening. Bone Marrow Transplant 1991; 7:227–234.

91. Reichert CM et al. Autopsy pathology in acquired immune deficiency syndrome. Am J Pathol 1983; 112:357–382.

92. Hoover DR et al. Clinical manifestations of AIDS in the era of pneumocystis prophylaxis. N Engl J Med 1993; 329:1022–1026.

93. Gallant JE et al. Zidovudine Epidemiology Study Group. Incidence and natural history of cytomegalovirus disease in patients with advanced human immunodeficiency virus disease treated with zidovudine. J Infect Dis 1992; 166:1223–1227.

94. Zaia JA. Prevention and treatment of cytomegalovirus pneumonia in transplant recipients. Clin Infect Dis 1993; 17(suppl 2):S392–S399.

95. Jacobson MA, Mills J. Serious cytomegalovirus disease in the acquired immuno-deficiency syndrome (AIDS). Ann Intern Med 1988; 108:585–594.

96. Drew WL. Cytomegalovirus infection in patients with AIDS. Clin Infect Dis 1992; 14:608–615.

97. Jacobson MA, O'Donnell JJ. Approaches to the treatment of cytomegalovirus retinitis: Ganciclovir and foscarnet. J AIDS 1991; 4(suppl 1):S11–S15.

98. Siadak MF et al. Reduction in transplant-related complications in patients given intravenous immunoglobulin after allogeneic marrow transplanation. Clin Exp Immunol 1994; 97(suppl 1):53–57.

99. Bass EB et al. Efficacy of immune globulin in preventing complication of bone marrow transplantation: a meta-analysis. Bone Marrow Transplant 1993; 12(3):273–282.

100. Rand KH et al. Pharmacokinetics of intravenous immunoglobulin (Gammagard) in bone marrow transplant patients. J Clin Pharm 1991; 312(12):1151–1154.

101. Whitley RJ. Neonatal herpes simplex virus infections: is there a role for immunoglobulin in disease prevention and therapy? Pediatr Infect Dis J 1994; 13(5):432–438.

102. Barandun S. Die gammaglobulin therapie. Biblio Haematol 1964; 17(suppl):1–134.

103. Barandun S et al. Immunologic deficiency diagnosis, forms and current treatment. In: Bergsma D, Good RA, eds. Immunologic Deficiency Diseases in Man. New York: National Foundation of the March of Dimes, 1968; 40–49.

104. Barandun S, Isliker H. Development of immunoglobulin preparations for intravenous use. Vox Sang 1986; 51:151–160.

105. Barandun S. Replacement therapy in primary immunodeficiencies. In: Morell A, Nydegger UE, eds. Clinical Use of Intravenous Immunoglobulins. London: Academic Press, 1986:63–66.

106. World Health Organization. Appropriate uses of human immunoglobulin in clinical practice: memorandum from an IUIS/WHO meeting. WHO Bull 60:43–47.

107. Weber B et al. Humoral immune response to human cytomegalovirus infection: diagnostic potential of immunoglobulin class and IgG subclass antibody response to human cytomegalovirus early and late antigens. Clin Invest 1993; 71(4):270–276.

108. Winston DJ et al. Intravenous immunoglobulin and CMV-seronegative blood products for prevention of CMV infection and disease in bone marrow transplant recipients. Bone Marrow Transplant 1993; 12(3):283–288.

109. Timar L et al. Immunglobulinok profilaktikus es terapias alkalmazasa csontvelotranszplantalt betegekben. Orvosi Hetilap 1994; 135(8):405–408.

110. Bowden LD et al. Cytomegalovirus (CMV)-specific intravenous immunoglobulin for the prevention of primary CMV infection and disease after marrow transplantation. J Infect Dis 1991; 164:483–487.

111. Syndman DR et al. New developments in cytomegalovirus prevention and management. Am J Kidney Dis 1993; 21(2):217–228.

112. Conti DJ et al. Prophylaxis of primary cytomegalovirus disease in renal transplant recipients. A trial of ganciclovir vs immunoglobulin. Arch Surg 1994; 129(4):443–447.

113. Rondeau E et al. Treatment of cytomegalovirus infections in renal transplants. Nephrologie 1994; 12(4):189–192.

114. Finn WF. CMV-enriched immune globulin produces consistent reliable results in renal transplant patients. Transplantation 1993; 56(2):491.

115. Stratta RJ et al. Viral prophylaxis in combined pancreas-kidney transplant recipients. Transplantation 1993; 57(4):506–512.

116. Zamora MR et al. Use of cytomegalovirus (CMV) hyperimmune globulin for prevention of CMV disease in CMV-seropositive lung transplant recipients. Transplant Proc 1994; 26(5 suppl 1):49–51.

117. Dunn DL et al. A prospective randomized study of Acyclovir versus Ganciclovir plus human immune globulin prophylaxis of cytomegalovirus infection after solid organ transplantation. Transplantation 1994; 57(6):876–884.

118. Andolina M et al. Intravenous immunoglobulins in bone marrow transplantation. Pediatr Med Chirurg 1993; 15(4):347–348.

119. Syndman DR et al. Cytomegalovirus immune globulin prophylaxis in liver transplantation. A randomized, double-blind, placebo-controlled trial. Boston Center for Liver Transplantation CMVIG Study Group. Ann Intern Med 1993; 119(10):984–991.

120. Bailey TC et al. Failure of high-dose oral acyclovir with or without immune globulin to prevent primary cytomegalovirus disease in recipients of solid organ transplants. Am J Med 1993; 95(3):273–278.

121. Landsperger WJ et al. Characterization of pneumococcal hyperimmune intravenous immune globulin prepared from plasma of immunized donors. Abstract 827. Presented at the 24 Interscience Conference on Antimicrobial Agents and Chemotherapy, Washington, D.C., 1984.

122. Landsperger WJ. Unpublished results.

123. Nordenstrom J et al. Decreased chemotactic and random migration of leukocytes during Intralipid infusion. Am J Clin Nutr 1979; 32:2416–2422.

124. Fischer GW et al. Diminished bacterial defenses with Intralipid. Lancet 1980; 2:819–820.

125. Freeman J et al. Association of intravenous lipid emulsion and coagulase-negative staphylococcal bacteremia in neonatal intensive care units. N Engl J Med 1990; 323:301–308.

126. Fischer GW et al. Opsonic antibodies to *Staphylococcus epidermidis*: in vitro and in vivo studies using human intravenous immune globulin. J Infect Dis 1994; 169:324–329.

127. Baker CJ et al. Intravenous immune globulin for the prevention of nosocomial infection in low-birth-weight neonates. N Engl J Med 1992; 327(4):213–219.

128. Weisman LE et al. Standard versus hyperimmune intravenous immunoglobulin in preventing or treating neonatal bacterial infections. Clin Perinatol 1993; 20(1):211–224.

129. Weisman LE et al. Comparison of group B streptococcal hyperimmune globulin and standard intravenously administered immune globulin in neonates. J Pediatr 1993; 122(6):929–937.

130. Fischer GW et al. Enhanced clearance and protection in a group B streptococcal (GBS) sepsis model: standard intravenous immunoglobulin (IVIG) versus human hyperimmune IVIG (GBS-IVIG). Presented at the 26th Interscience Conference on Antimicrobial Agents and Chemotherapy, Washington, D.C., Sept 28–Oct 1, 1986. Abstract.

131. Gloser H et al. Intravenous immunoglobulin with high activity against group B streptococci. Pediatr Infect Dis J 1986; 5(suppl):S176–S179.

132. Shigeoka AO et al. Protective effect of hybridoma type specific antibody against experimental group B streptococcal infection. J Infect Dis 1984; 149:363–372.
133. Fischer GW. Immunoglobulin therapy of neonatal group B streptococcal infections: an overview. Pediatr Infect Dis J 1988; 7(suppl):S13–S16.
134. Weisman LE et al. Group B streptococcal hyperimmune intravenous immunoglobulin in suspected neonatal sepsis. Pediatr Res 1990; 27:278A.
135. Fischer GW et al. Polyvalent group B streptococcal immune globulin for intravenous administration: overview. Rev Infect Dis 1990; 12:S483–S491.
136. Hemming VG et al. Immunoprophylaxis of postnatally acquired group B streptococcal sepsis in neonatal rhesus monkeys. J Infect Dis 1986; 156:655–658.
137. Sapan CV, NABI. Personal communication.
138. Cryz SJ Jr et al. Safety and immunogenicity of a polyvalent *Klebsiella* capsular polysaccharide vaccine in humans. Vaccine 1986; 4:15–20.
139. Cryz SJ Jr et al. Safety and immunogenicity of a *Pseudomonas aeruginosa* O-polysaccharide toxin A conjugate vaccine in humans. J Clin Invest 1987; 80:51–56.
140. Edelman R et al. Phase 1 trial of a 24-valent *Klebsiella* capsular polysaccharide vaccine and an eight-valent *Pseudomonas* O-polysaccharide conjugate vaccine administered simultaneously. Vaccine 1994; 12(14):1288–1294.
141. Cryz SJ Jr et al. Safety and immunogenicity of a polyvalent *Pseudomonas aeruginosa* O-polysaccharide–toxin A vaccine in humans. Antibiot Chemother 1989; 42:177–183.
142. Cryz SJ Jr et al. Active and passive immunization against *Pseudomonas aeruginosa* in high risk patients. Fourth International Symposium on *Pseudomonas*: Biotechnology and Molecular Biology. Vancouver, B.C., 1993:32.
143. Cryz SJ Jr et al. Production and characterization of a human hyperimmune intravenous immunoglobulin against *Pseudomonas aeruginosa* and *Klebsiella pneumoniae* species. J Infect Dis 1991; 163:1055–1061.
144. Granström M et al. Enzyme-linked immunosorbent assay to evaluate the immunogenicity of a polyvalent *Klebsiella* capsular polysaccharide vaccine in humans. J Clin Microbiol 1988; 26:2257–2261.
145. Donta ST et al. (for the Federal Hyperimmune Immunoglobulin Study Group). Immunoprophylaxis of *Klebsiella* and *Pseudomonas* infections. Annual Meeting of the Infectious Diseases Society of America (New Orleans), Chicago, IL, 1993.
146. Hatano K et al. Biologic activities of antibodies to the neutral-polysaccharide component of the *Pseudomonas aeruginosa* lipopolysaccharide are blocked by O side chains and mucoid-exopolysaccharide (alginate). 1995; 63(1):21–26.
147. Pier GB et al. Opsonophagocytic killing antibody to *Pseudomonas aeruginosa* mucoid exopolysaccharide in older, non-colonized cystic fibrosis patients. N Engl J Med 1987; 317:793–798.
148. Pier GB et al. Protection against mucoid *Psuedomonas aeruginosa* in rodent models of endobronchial infection. Science 1990; 249:537–540.
149. Ames P et al. Opsonophagocytic killing activity of rabbit antibodies to *Pseudomonas aeruginosa* mucoid exopolysaccharide. 1985; 49:281–285.
150. Spalding BJ. Using vaccines to develop specific polyclonals. BioTechnology 1993; 11:1214.
151. Collins MS et al. Therapy of established experimental *Pseudomonas aeruginosa* infections with oral ciprofloxacin and five human monoclonal antibodies against lipopolysaccharide antigens. In: Homma JY, Tanimoto H, Holder IA, Høiby N, Döring G, eds. *Pseudomonas aeruginosa* in Human Diseases. Antibiot Chemother 1991; 44:185–195.
152. Bortolussi R, Fischer GW. Opsonic and protective activity of immunoglobulin modified immunoglobulin and serum against neonatal *Escherichia coli* K1 infection. Pediatr Res 1986; 20:175–178.
153. Pluschke G, Achtman M. Antibodies to O antigen of lipopolysaccharide are protective against neonatal infection with *Escherichia coli* K1. Infect Immun 1985; 49:365–370.

154. Kaufman BM et al. Monoclonal antibodies reactive with K1-encapsulated *Escherichia coli* lipopolysaccharide are opsonic and protect mice against lethal challenge. Infect Immun 1986; 52:617–619.

155. Schiff DE et al. Estimation of protective levels of anti-O-specific lipopolysaccharide immunoglobulin G antibody against experimental *Escherichia coli* infection. Infect Immun 1993; 61(3):975–980.

156. Cryz SJ Jr et al. Safety and immunogenicity of *Escherichia coli* O18 O-specific polysaccharide (O-PS)–toxin A and O-PS–cholera toxin conjugate vaccines in humans. J Infect Dis 1991; 163(5):1040–1045.

157. Cross A et al. Safety and immunogenicity of a polyvalent *Escherichia coli* vaccine in human volunteers. J Infect Dis 1994; 170:834–840.

158. Osther K et al. PASSHIV-1 treatment of patients with HIV-1 infection. A preliminary report of a Phase I trial of hyperimmune porcine immunoglobulin to HIV-1. AIDS 1992; 6(12):1457–1464.

159. Pardridge WM et al. Treatment of human immunodeficiency virus–infected lymphocytes with cationized human immunoglobulins. J Infect Dis 1994; 170(3):563–569.

160. Prince AM et al. Prevention of HIV infection by passive immunization with HIV immunoglobulin. AIDS Res Human Retro 1991; 7(12):971–973.

161. Prince AM et al. Failure of a human immunodeficiency virus (HIV) immune globulin to protect chimpanzees against experimental challenge with HIV. Proc Natl Acad Sci USA 1988; 888:6944.

162. Eichberg JW. Experience with thirteen HIV efficacy trials in chimpanzees. Sixth International Conference on AIDS, San Francisco, June 1990.

163. Gao F et al. Enhancement in the safety of immune globulins prepared from high-risk plasma. Vox Sang 1993; 64(4):204–209.

164. Piet MPJ et al. Inactivation of viruses in plasma on treatment with tri(*N*-butyl) phosphate (TNBP) detergent mixtures. Eleventh International Congress on Thrombosis and Haemostasis, Brussels, July 1987.

165. Condie RM. Preparation and intravenous use of undenatured human IgG. In: Alving BM, Finlayson JS, eds. Immunoglobulins: Characteristics and Uses of Intravenous Preparations. Washington, D.C.: U.S. Government Printing Office, 1980:179.

166. Cummins LM et al. Preparation and characterization of an intravenous solution of IgG from human immunodeficiency virus–seropositive donors. Blood 1991; 77(5):111–1117.

167. Vittecoq D et al. Passive immunotherapy in AIDS: a randomized trial of serial human immunodeficiency virus–positive transfusions of plasma rich in p24 antibodies versus transfusions of seronegative plasma. J Infect Dis 1992; 165(2):364–368.

168. Levy J et al. Passive hyperimmune plasma therapy in the treatment of acquired immunodeficiency syndrome: results of a 12-month multicenter double-blind controlled trial. Passive Hyperimmune Therapy Study Group. Blood 1994; 84(7):2130–2135.

169. Mofenson LM et al. Effect of intravenous immunoglobulin (IVIG on CD4+ lymphocyte decline in HIV-infected children in a clinical trial of IVIG infection prophylaxis. National Institute of Child Health and Human Development Intravenous Immunoglobulin Clinical Trial Study Group. J AIDS 1993; 6(10):1103–1113.

170. Mofenson LM et al. Prophylactic intravenous immunoglobulin in HIV-infected children with CD4+ counts of 0.20 × 10(9)/L or more. Effect on viral, opportunistic, and bacterial infections. JAMA 1992; 268(4):483–488.

171. Hemming VG et al. Hyperimmune globulins in prevention and treatment of respiratory syncytial virus infections. Clin Microbiol Rev 1995; 8(1):22–33.

172. Meissner HC et al. Controlled trial to evaluate protection of high-risk infants against respiratory syncytial virus disease by using standard intravenous immune globulin. Antimicrob Agents Chem 1993; 37(8):1655–1658.

173. Tirado R et al. Occurrence of respiratory syncytial virus subtypes in Mexican infants with acute lower respiratory tract disease. Arch Med Res 1995; 26(2):121–126.
174. Hall CB et al. Ribavirin treatment of respiratory syncytial virus infections: a randomized double blind study. N Engl J Med 1983; 308:1443.
175. Tristam DA et al. Immunogenicity and safety of respiratory syncytal virus subunit vaccine in seropositive children 18–36 months old. J Infect Dis 1993; 167:5.
176. McIntosh ED et al. Clinical severity of respiratory syncytial virus group A in Sidney, Australia. Pediatr Infect Dis J 1993; 12(10):815–819.
177. Groothuis JR et al. Use of intravenous gamma globulin to passively immunize high-risk children against respiratory syncytial virus: safety and pharmacokinetics. RSVIG Study Group. Antimicrob Agents Chem 1991; 35(7):1469–1473.
178. Siber GR et al. Protective activity of a human respiratory syncytial virus immune globulin prepared from donors screened by microneutralization assay. J Infect Dis 1992; 165(3):456–463.
179. Sami IR et al. Systemic immunoprophylaxis of nasal respiratory syncytial virus infection in cotton rats. J Infect Dis 1995; 171(2):440–443.
180. Glezen WP et al. Risk of respiratory syncytial virus infection for infants with low income families in relationship to age, sex, ethnic group and maternal antibody level. J Pediatr 1991; 98:708–715.
181. Parrott RH et al. Epidemiology of respiratory syncytial virus infection in Washington, D.C. II. Infection and disease with respect to age, immunologic status, race and sex. Am J Epidemiol 1973; 98:289–300.
182. Prince GA et al. Quantitative aspects of passive immunity to respiratory syncytial virus infection in infant cotton rats. J Virol 1985; 55:517–520.
183. Siber GR et al. Comparison of antibody concentrations and protective activity of respiratory syncytial virus immune globulin and conventional immune globulin. J Infect Dis 1994; 169:1368–1373.
184. Siber GR et al. Protective activity of a human respiratory syncytial virus immune globulin prepared from donors screened by microneutralization assay. J Infect Dis 1992; 165:456–463.
185. Groothuis JR. Role of antibody and use of respiratory syncytial virus (RSV) immune globulin to prevent severe RSV disease in high-risk children. J Pediatr 1994; 124(5 Pt 2):S28–S32.
186. McIntosh K. Respiratory syncytial virus—successful immunoprophylaxis at last. N Engl J Med 1993; 329:1572–1574.
187. Ellenberg SS et al. A trial of RSV immune globulin in infants and young children: the FDA's view. N Engl J Med 1994; 331(3):203–204.

Index

Administration time of IVIG,
methods for reduction, 107–108, 186–187
Adverse effects of IVIG (nonviral),
acute renal failure, 370–371
alopecia, 61
in chronic lymphocytic leukemia, 219
generalized reactions, 58
hematological complications, 60
hypersensitivity and anaphylactic reactions, 58, 183–184
hypothermia, 61
and immunological contaminants, 61
interference with vaccination, 61–62
in low birth weight neonates, 144
management and prevention, 62–63
in multiple myeloma, 219
neurological complications, 59
renal complications, 59–60
in solid organ transplantation, 120
thrombotic complications, 60
Alloimmune thrombocytopenia,
secondary to platelet transfusions, use of IVIG for, 283
use of IVIG in the fetus, 281–282
Alloimmune thrombocytopenia, neonatal,
causes of, 331
frequency of, 331
use of antenatal platelet transfusions for, 331–332
use of IVIG for, 282–283, 332–333
use of maternal platelets for, 262–263, 331
Amyotrophic lateral sclerosis,
use of IVIG in, 447
ANCA-associated vasculitis
mechanism of action of IVIG in, 27–28, 427
use of IVIG in, 425–426
Antibodies in IVIG preparations, 47, 49–51
Anti-factor VIII autoimmune disease,
mechanism of action of IVIG in, 27

Antiphospholipid syndrome (*see also* Recurrent pregnancy loss),
and recurrent pregnancy loss, 439–440
use of anticoagulants for, 440
use of corticosteroids for, 440
use of IVIG in, 440–441
Autoimmune hemolytic anemia,
patient profile for IVIG usage in, 287–288
use of IVIG for, 287–288
Autoimmune neutropenia,
diagnosis of, 285
mechanism of action of IVIG in, 26–27
pathology of, 286
use of IVIG for, 286–287
Autoimmune thrombocytopenia, neonatal,
use of IVIG for, 282–283

Bacterial polysaccharide immunoglobulin (BP16),
prevention of acute otitis media, 470
prevention of *H. influenzae*, 468, 470
Bone marrow transplantation,
and aplastic anemia, 115
hyperimmunoglobulin for CMV infections after, 479–480
and platelet refractoriness, 115
use of IVIG in, 109,113–115, 247, 478–479
and veno-occlusive disease, 115
Bullous pemphigoid,
use of IVIG in, 447
Burn patients,
infections in, 232–236
and local host defenses, 226–227
prophylaxis of infections in,
and GMCSF, 236
and IVIG, 153, 237
and surveillance, 237–238
and patient isolation, 238
and systemic host defenses, 227–232
wound management in, 233–234

Chronic fatigue syndrome,
  adverse effects of IVIG (nonviral) in the
    treatment of, 270–271
  disorders of immunity in, 268–269
  etiology of, 267
  infection and, 268
  rationale for IVIG in, 267
  use of IVIG for, 269–271
Chronic inflammatory demyelinating poly-
    neuropathy (*see also* Guillain-Barré
    syndrome)
  contrasted with Guillain-Barré syndrome,
    349–350, 350–351
  diagnosis of, 349–350
  dosage schedule, 356–357, 358
  immunological mechanisms in, 350–351
  mechanism of IVIG, 357
  and monoclonal protein of undetermined
    significance, 350
  safety of IVIG in, 356–357
  steroid treatment of, 352, 355, 356
  use of IVIG in, 353–356
  use of plasma exchange for, 352–353, 355–
    356
Chronic lymphocytic leukemia,
  adverse effects of IVIG (nonviral) in, 219
  hypogammaglobulinemia in, 206–207
  immune defects in, 206–207, 209
  immunization response in, 208–209
  incidence of, 103–204
  infections in, 204–209
  patient selection for IVIG use in, 219–220
  pharmacoeconomics of IVIG in, 20–21,
    220
  pharmacokinetics of IVIG in, 13–15, 216
  pneumococcal antibody deficiency in, 207
  quality adjusted life years for, 20
  subcutaneous use of IVIG in, 217
  treatment schedule and dose of IVIG in,
    216–217
  use of IVIG in, 20–21, 214–216
Churg-Strauss syndrome,
  use of IVIG in, 427
Coagulase-negative staphylococcal infections,
  use of IVIG for, 145
Components of IVIG preparations, 47, 48
Crohn's disease (*see also* Inflammatory
    bowel diseases),
  characterization of, 451–452
  clinical description, 452–454
  IgM-enriched immunoglobulin for, 457
  immunopathogenesis of, 454–456
  mechanism of action of IVIG in, 456–457
  use of IVIG in, 457–459, 460

Cytomegalovirus (CMV),
  and antiviral agents, 126–127
  and bone marrow transplantation, 478–480
  hyperimmune IVIG for the treatment of,
    244, 245
  infection in solid organ transplantation,
    119–120
  and pneumonia, 113–115
  prevention by ganciclovir, 114
  and renal transplantation, 480
  risk of infection after bone marrow
    transplantation, 113
  standard and hyperimmune IVIG for the
    prevention of, 31, 120–127, 246–248,
    476–477, 478, 479
  standard and hyperimmune IVIG for the
    treatment of, 127–128
  treatment with IVIG and ganciclovir, 115

Dermatomyositis,
  adverse effects of IVIG (nonviral) in the
    treatment of, 405
  clinical features of, 399–400
  histological findings, 401
  immunological findings, 401
  immunosuppressive therapy for, 401–405
  incidence of, 399
  mechanism of action of IVIG in, 30–31,
    404–405
  steroid therapy for, 401
  use of IVIG in, 30–31, 402–404
Diabetes,
  adverse effects of IVIG (nonviral) in, 323
  animal models for, 319
  Coxsackie virus and, 318
  environmental effects and, 318
  genetics of, 317–318
  immunomanipulation in animal models,
    319–320
  immunopathogenesis of, 318–319
  use of IVIG in, 320–324

E. coli infections,
  use of IVIG for, 146
Enteroviruses,
  adverse effects of IVIG (nonviral) in the
    treatment of, 263
  description, 257
  diagnosis of, 259–260
  epidermology of, 257–259
  in vitro activity in IVIG against, 261
  pathogenesis of, 259
  use of intramuscular immunoglobulin to
    treat, 260–261

[Enteroviruses]
use of IVIG for, 248–249, 261–263
Epidermolysis bullosa acquisita,
use of IVIG in, 447
Epstein-Barr virus,
treatment of associated posttransplant lymphoproliferative disorder by standard or hyperimmune IVIG, 129–130
Essential mixed cryoglobulinemia,
use of IVIG in, 427

Factor VIII inhibitors,
use of IVIG for, 447
Felty's syndrome,
use of IVIG in, 410

Graft-versus-host disease,
prevention by IVIG, 114–115, 247
Graves' ophthalmopathy,
use of IVIG in, 447
Group B streptococcal infections,
use of IVIG for, 145–146
Guillain-Barré syndrome (*see also* Chronic inflammatory demyelinating polyneuropathy)
clinical characterization of, 337–338
general care of patients with, 338–339
and high-dose methylprednisolone, 345
mechanism of action of IVIG in, 27, 357
and the Miller-Fisher syndrome, 338, 343
and treatment of the individual patient, 343–345
use of IVIG in, 341–343, 343–345
and cost effectiveness, 343
use of plasma exchange for, 340–341, 341–343, 343–345
and cost effectiveness, 343

Heart transplantation,
use of standard or hyperimmune IVIG in, 121, 125
Hemolytic disease of the fetus and newborn,
use of IVIG for, 288
Henoch-Schonlein purpura,
use of IVIG in, 421, 426–427
Hepatitis A,
use of intramuscular immunoglobulin for the prevention of, 244, 245, 467–478
Hepatitis B virus,
hyperimmunoglobulin for the prophylaxis of, 244, 245, 246, 468, 469, 479, 485
transmission by intramuscular immunoglobulin, 71
transmission by IVIG, 71, 82–83

Hepatitis C virus (*see also* Non-A, non-B hepatitis),
hyperimmunoglobulin for the treatment of, 485
immunoadsorption, 375, 377
compared with IVIG, 375
plasmapheresis, 374–375, 377
compared with IVIG, 374–375, 377
removal in IVIG production, 42, 43
thymectomy, 375–376
compared with other therapies, 376
transmission by IVIG, 69, 75–76, 77–79, 79–81, 184–186, 283–284, 370, 391
Hepatitis G virus,
transmission by IVIG, 81–82
Herpes viruses,
use of IVIG for, 250–251
Herpes simplex virus,
hyperimmunoglobulin for the treatment of, 477
Home therapy of IVIG,
pharmacoeconomics, 21
in primary immunodeficient patients, 187
and subcutaneous administration of IVIG, 110
Host defense in the neonate,
maternal antibodies, 139–141
nonspecific, 136–138
specific, 138–139
Human immunodeficiency virus (HIV),
criteria for use of IVIG in, 164
dosing of IVIG for, 163
hyperimmunoglobulin for the treatment of, 475–476, 488–490
mechanism of action of IVIG for, 160, 162–163
removal in IVIG production, 42, 43, 46
transmission by IVIG, 81
treatment by IVIG in children, 31–32, 159–164, 476
treatment by IVIG in adults, 31–32, 167–173, 476
and treatment of opportunistic infections by IVIG, 172, 173
Hyperimmune immunoglobulins,
advantages over standard IVIG, 470–471
and antibiotic resistance, 471–472
Gram-positive bacteria,
group B streptococcus, 472–473, 484–485
S. aureus, 483
S. epidermidis, 472, 483
S. pneumoniae, 473–474, 482–483

[Hyperimmune immunoglobulins]
Gram-negative bacteria,
E. *coli*, 487–488
K. *pneumoniae*, 475, 485–486
P. *aeruginosa*, 474–475, 479, 481, 486–
487
preparation of, 477–478
properties of, 478

Idiopathic thrombocytopenia purpura,
anti-D IVIG for, 284
corticosteroids and IVIG for, 283
mechanism of action of IVIG in, 26–27,
285
secondary to HIV infection, treatment by
IVIG, 168, 279–280
secondary to pregnancy, treatment by
IVIG, 280–281
and solvent-detergent treated IVIG, 284
Idiopathic thrombocytopenia purpura, acute,
anti-D IVIG for, 277
dose of IVIG in adults for 278
dose of IVIG in children for, 277
use of IVIG in adults for, 278
use of IVIG in children for, 275–277
use of prednisone in children for, 276–277
Idiopathic thrombocytopenia purpura,
chronic,
cost of IVIG in, 21, 277–278
use of IVIG in adults for, 279
use of IVIG in children for, 277–278
IgA-associated nephropathy,
use of IVIG in, 421, 426–427
Immunomodulatory effects of IVIG,
and Fc-dependent interactions, 26–27
and F(ab')$_2$ or V region-dependent interactions, 27–28
and Fc and F(ab')$_2$-dependent interactions,
28–30
long-term effects, 31
reasons for, 24–26
and treatment of HIV disease, 161–162
Immunoglobulin G subclasses,
role in host defense, 193–194
use of IVIG in subclass deficiencies,
194–197
Infections,
and mechanism of action of IVIG, 32
Inflammatory bowel diseases (*see also*
Crohn's disease and ulcerative
colitis)
anti-inflammatory agents for, 459
characterization of, 451–452

[Inflammatory bowel diseases]
clinical description, 452–454
immunomodulating agents for, 459–460
immunopathogenesis of, 454–456
mechanism of action of IVIG in, 456–457
use of IVIG in, 457–459, 460
Intractable childhood epilepsy,
use of IVIG in, 447
Intraperitoneal administration of IVIG, 108
Intrathecal administration of IVIG, 108–109
Intraventricular administration of IVIG, 109
IVIG and autoimmunity, 24

Juvenile rheumatoid arthritis (*see also* Rheumatoid arthritis)
adverse effects of IVIG (nonviral) in, 312
cost of IVIG in, 313
and corticosteroids, 309, 310
definition of, 309
immune alterations in, 309
therapy for, 309
use of IVIG in, 309–313, 410

Kawasaki syndrome,
adverse effects of IVIG (nonviral) in the
treatment of, 300
cardiovascular involvement in, 294
clinical features of, 293–294
epidemiology of, 296
etiology of, 296–297
future direction of IVIG therapy in, 303–
304
immunological features and pathogenesis
of, 297
mechanism of action of IVIG in, 26–27,
28–29, 303, 417, 457
pathology of, 295
pharmacoeconomics of IVIG in, 19–20
therapeutic problems of IVIG in, 302–302
use of IVIG in, 19–20, 28–29
and aspirin, 301
with aspirin versus aspirin alone, 297–
299
and dosage comparisons, 299–300
and product comparisons, 300–301

Lambert-Eaton myasthenic syndrome,
association with small-cell lung carcinoma,
433–434
clinical features and characterization of,
431, 432
diagnosis of, 432, 433
existing treatment for, 434

[Lambert-Eaton myasthenic syndrome]
immunopathology of, 432–433
use of IVIG in, 434–435
Liver transplantation,
prevention of hepatitis B infection by
hyperimmune IVIG, 128
use of acyclovir in, 481
use of ganciclovir in, 481
use of standard or hyperimmune IVIG in,
121, 123–124, 125, 481
Low-birth-weight neonates,
use of IVIG in, 109
Lung transplantation,
hyperimmunoglobulin for CMV infections after, 480–481
use of acyclovir in, 481
use of ganciclovir in, 481
use of standard or hyperimmune IVIG in,
121, 125, 248, 481

Manufacturers of IVIG, 40–41
Measles,
use of intramuscular immunoglobulin for
the prevention of, 244, 245
Meningoencephalitis,
use of IVIG for, 109, 182–183
Multiple myeloma,
adverse effects of IVIG (nonviral) in, 219
hypogammaglobulinemia in, 211–212
immune defects in, 211–212, 213
immunization response in, 213
infections in, 209–213
patient selection for IVIG use in, 219–220
pharmacoeconomics of IVIG in, 21, 220
specific antibody deficiency in, 212
use of IVIG in, 217–219
Multiple sclerosis,
adverse effects of IVIG (nonviral) in the
treatment of, 391
autoimmune nature of, 382
causes of, 382
characterization of, 381–382
clinical trials in, 382
mechanism of action of IVIG in, 29, 385–
391
use of IVIG in, 382–385
and methylprednisolone, 384
Myasthenia gravis,
adverse effects of IVIG (nonviral), in the
treatment of, 369–370, 374
anticholinesterase compounds for, 364–
365, 377, 376–377
assisted ventilation for, 365

[Myasthenia gravis]
association with other autoimmune
diseases, 364
corticosteroids/immunosuppressive drugs
for, 365, 373–374, 375, 376–377
compared with IVIG, 373–374, 375,
376–377
disease course, 363
effect of IVIG on serological markers,
371–372
mechanism of action of IVIG in, 27, 372–
373
mechanism of weakness in, 364
serological changes in, 363–364
symptoms of, 363
use of IVIG in, 364, 365–369, 373–377
cost of, 377
dosage regimen, 367, 369, 376

Non-A, non-B hepatitis, (*see also* Hepatitis
C virus)
transmission by IVIG, 67, 72–75, 76–77
Nonlipid enveloped viruses,
removal in IVIG production, 46
transmission by IVIG, 83

Oral administration of IVIG, 109

Pancreas transplantation,
use of standard or hyperimmune IVIG in,
121, 125
Parvovirus B19,
use of IVIG for, 251
Pharmacokinetics of IVIG,
bone marrow transplantation, 12–14
chronic lymphocytic leukemia, 13–15, 216
pneumococcal antibodies, 14–15
congenital humoral immunodeficiencies,
6–9
and specific antibodies, 7–8
and dosage, 8–9
mathematical model of, 1–5
mechanism of action of IVIG, 30
neonates and infants, 9–12, 147
normal subjects, 4, 5–6
Platelet alloimmunization (*see also* Alloimmune thrombocytopenia)
mechanism of action of IVIG in, 27–28
platelet transfusion guidelines for, 328–329
and platelet alloantigen systems, 327–328
and susceptible patient populations, 328
use of IVIG for, 329–331

Polyarticular juvenile rheumatoid arthritis (*see also* Juvenile rheumatoid arthritis),
    use of IVIG in, 313
Polymyositis,
    adverse effects of IVIG (nonviral) in the treatment of, 405
    clinical features of, 399–400
    histological findings, 401
    immunological findings, 401
    immunosuppressive therapy for, 401–405
    incidence of, 399
    mechanism of action of IVIG in, 404–405
    steroid therapy for, 401
    use of IVIG in, 402–404
Posttransfusion purpura,
    clinical features of, 333–334
    clinical management of, 334
    use of IVIG for, 334
Primary immunodeficiencies,
    characteristics of, 177–178
    classifications of, 175–177
    dose of IVIG for the treatment of, 179–181
    pregnancy and IVIG in, 181–182
    safety of IVIG in, 183–186
    use of IVIG for, 110, 175–188
    use of intramuscular immunoglobulin for, 178–179
Production of IVIG,
    cold ethanol fractionation, 37, 38–42
    and virus removal or inactivation, 42–46
Production of intramuscular immuno-globulins, 38
Psychosis (secondary to SLE),
    use of IVIG for, 447
Pure red cell or white cell aplasia,
    use of IVIG in, 447

Rabies,
    hyperimmunoglobulin for the treatment of, 244, 245, 246, 468, 469
Recurrent pregnancy loss (*see also* Anti-phospholipid syndrome),
    association with antiphospholipid syndrome, 439–440
    association with SLE, 441
    causes of, 442
    and lupus anticoagulant, 440–441
    use of anticoagulants for, 440
    use of corticosteroids for, 440
    use of IVIG in, 440–441, 442

Red blood cell alloimmunization,
    mechanism of action of IVIG in, 27
Renal transplantation,
    use of ganciclovir in, 480
    use of standard or hyperimmune IVIG in, 120–121, 122–123, 125, 247, 480
Respiratory syncytial virus,
    use of standard and hyperimmune IVIG for, 147, 249–250, 475, 490–492
Rheumatoid arthritis (*see also* Juvenile rheumatoid arthritis,
    adverse effects of IVIG (nonviral) in the treatment of, 412
    characteristics of, 409
    mechanism of action of IVIG in, 409, 412–413
    use of IVIG in, 409–412
    use of placenta-eluted gammaglobulin in, 410
$Rh_o(D)$ (anti-D),
    hyperimmunoglobulin for protection against, 468, 479

Selective antibody deficiencies,
    use of IVIG for, 197–198
Stevens-Johnson syndrome,
    use of IVIG in, 28
Subcutaneous administration of IVIG, 110, 186, 217
    home administration and cost, 3
Surgical and trauma patients,
    mechanism of action of IVIG in, 151–152
    use of IVIG for prevention and treatment of infections in, 151–156
Systemic lupus erythematosus,
    association with recurrent pregnancy loss, 441
    etiology of anti-DNA antibodies in, 415–416
    mechanism of action of IVIG in, 27, 28, 416–418
    quality of life and cost of IVIG in, 3
    use of IVIG in, 28, 417, 419–421, 441
Systemic necrotizing vasculitis (*see also* ANCA-associated vasculitis; Henoch-Schonlein purpura; IgA-associated nephropathy; Churg-Strauss syndrome; Wegener's granulomatosis; and essential mixed cryoglobulinemia),

[Systemic necrotizing vasculitis]
  adverse effects of IVIG (nonviral) in the
      treatment of, 428
  characterization of, 425
  mechanism of action of IVIG in, 427
  use of IVIG in, 425

Tetanus,
  hyperimmunoglobulin for the treatment of,
      468, 469, 479
Thrombotic thrombocytopenic purpura,
  use of IVIG in, 447

Ulcerative colitis (*see also* Inflammatory
      bowel diseases),
  antilymphocyte serum for, 457
  characterization of, 451–452
  clinical description, 452–454
  immunopathogenesis of, 454–456
  mechanism of action of IVIG in, 456–457
  use of IVIG in, 457–459, 460

Uveitis,
  use of IVIG in, 447

Vaccinia infection,
  hyperimmunoglobulin for the treatment
      of, 244, 245, 468, 469
Varicella zoster virus,
  hyperimmunoglobulin for the treatment
      of, 244, 245, 468, 469, 470
  prevention by hyperimmune IVIG after
      solid organ transplantation, 128
Viral safety of IVIG (*see also* Hepatitis A,
      hepatitis B virus, hepatitis C virus,
      hepatitis G virus, non-A, non-B
      hepatitis)
  and in vitro infectivity assays, 96
  and multiple viral inactivation steps, 95–
      96
  and PCR testing, 95
  and virus removal or inactivation, 86–95
von Willebrand's disease,
  use of IVIG in, 447